Thieme

Top Score for the Neurosurgery Board Examination

Questions and Answers

Shehzad Safdar Tarar, MBBS
Post Graduate Trainee
Department of Neurosurgery
Punjab Institute of Neurosciences
Lahore, Punjab, Pakistan

Zubair Ahmad Khan, MBBS, FCPS Neurosurgery
Consultant Neurosurgeon
Department of Neurosurgery
Punjab Institute of Neurosciences
Lahore, Punjab, Pakistan

Mubashir Malik, BSc, MBBS, MRCSEd, MS Neurosurgery
Consultant Neurosurgeon
Department of Neurosurgery
Masood Hospital Lahore
Lahore, Punjab, Pakistan.

Syed Asad Ur Rehman Omer, MBBS
Consultant Neurosurgeon
Department of Neurosurgery
Punjab Institute of Neurosciences
Lahore, Punjab, Pakistan.

Memoona Ejaz, MBBS, MRCSEd
Senior Registrar
Department of Neurosurgery
Fauji Foundation Hospital Rawalpindi
Rawalpindi, Punjab, Pakistan

Thieme
New York • Stuttgart • Delhi • Rio de Janeiro

Library of Congress Cataloging-in-Publication Data
is available with the publisher.

Important note: Medicine is an ever-changing science undergoing continual development. Research and clinical experience are continually expanding our knowledge, in particular our knowledge of proper treatment and drug therapy. Insofar as this book mentions any dosage or application, readers may rest assured that the authors, editors, and publishers have made every effort to ensure that such references are in accordance with **the state of knowledge at the time of production of the book**.

Nevertheless, this does not involve, imply, or express any guarantee or responsibility on the part of the publishers in respect to any dosage instructions and forms of applications stated in the book. **Every user is requested to examine carefully** the manufacturers' leaflets accompanying each drug and to check, if necessary, in consultation with a physician or specialist, whether the dosage schedules mentioned therein or the contraindications stated by the manufacturers differ from the statements made in the present book. Such examination is particularly important with drugs that are either rarely used or have been newly released on the market. Every dosage schedule or every form of application used is entirely at the user's own risk and responsibility. The authors and publishers request every user to report to the publishers any discrepancies or inaccuracies noticed. If errors in this work are found after publication, errata will be posted atwww.thieme.com on the product description page.

Some of the product names, patents, and registered designs referred to in this book are in fact registered trademarks or proprietary names even though specific reference to this fact is not always made in the text. Therefore, the appearance of a name without designation as proprietary is not to be construed as a representation by the publisher that it is in the public domain.
Thieme addresses people of all gender identities equally. We encourage our authors to use gender-neutral or gender-equal expressions wherever the context allows.

Thieme Publishers New York
333 Seventh Avenue, 18th Floor
New York, NY 10001, USA
www.thieme.com
+1 800 782 3488, customerservice@thieme.com

Cover design: © Thieme
Cover image source: © Thieme/From Greenberg M, ed. Greenberg's Handbook of Neurosurgery. 10th ed. New York: Thieme; 2023
Typesetting by Thomson Digital, India

Printed in India by Replika Press Pvt. Ltd. 5 4 3 2 1

DOI: 10.1055/b000001027

ISBN: 978-1-68420-661-2

Also available as an e-book:
eISBN (PDF): 978-1-68420-662-9
eISBN (epub): 978-1-68420-663-6

Dedicated to the Punjab Institute of Neurosciences, Lahore, Pakistan.

Contents

Part XIII: Other Tumors and Tumor-Like Conditions

Part XIV: Head Trauma

Preface

Greenberg's Handbook of Neurosurgery is one of the most popular books among neurosurgery residents. It is concise but comprehensive and covers almost all the aspects of neurosurgery including basic concepts as well as advanced operative procedures. Due to its concentrated nature, it is hard to retain all this information well enough to reproduce it in exams efficiently.

This collection of questions is based on chapters as per Greenberg's chapter distribution and will act as a rapid review. We have tried to base the questions according to the exam-oriented high-yield points. It can be added to the list of exam preparation books for any standard neurosurgery examination.

Shehzad Safdar Tarar, MBBS

Zubair Ahmed Khan, MBBS, FCPS Neurosurgery

Mubashir Malik, BSc, MBBS, MRCSEd, MS Neurosurgery

Acknowledgments

We would like to thank our colleagues, Professor Muhammad Anwar Chaudhary, Dr. Rabia Saleem, Dr. Usama Mansoor, Dr. Ahmed Sultan, Dr. Rida Saleem, Dr. Noor ul Ain, Dr. Zayed Qamar, and Dr. Abuzar Rauf from the Punjab Institute of Neurosciences, Lahore, and the team at Thieme Publishers, who have contributed to this project.

Part I

Anatomy and Physiology

I

1 Gross Anatomy, Cranial and Spine

Questions

▸▸ Question 1

According to Brodmann's map of the cytoarchitectonic fields of the human brain, which of the following is Broca's area (motor speech area)?
- A. 41
- B. 42
- C. 43
- D. 44
- E. 45

▸▸ Question 2

According to Brodmann's map of the cytoarchitectonic fields of the human brain, which of the following is Wernicke's area?
- A. 40
- B. 41
- C. 42
- D. 43
- E. 44

▸▸ Question 3

Which of the following Brodmann's area is the precentral gyrus, the primary motor cortex consisting of a large concentration of giant pyramidal cells of Betz?
- A. 4
- B. 6
- C. 8
- D. 10
- E. 12

▸▸ Question 4

The junction of lambdoid, occipitomastoid, and parietomastoid sutures is:
- A. Nasion
- B. Glabella
- C. Stephanion
- D. Asterion
- E. Lambda

▸▸ Question 5

The junction of coronal suture and superior temporal line is also labeled as:
- A. Nasion
- B. Glabella
- C. Stephanion
- D. Asterion
- E. Lambda

▸▸ Question 6

Taylor-Haughton (T-H) lines can be constructed on an angiogram, CT/MRI scout film, or skull X-ray. They can be constructed on the patient in the OR based on visible external landmarks. A line from inferior margin of orbit through the upper margin of the external auditory meatus (EAM) is:
- A. Frankfurt plane
- B. Reid's baseline
- C. Condylar line
- D. Sylvian fissure line
- E. Central sulcal line

▸▸ Question 7

Numerous methods utilize external landmarks to locate the motor strip (pre-central gyrus) or the central sulcus (Rolandic fissure) which separates motor strip anteriorly from primary sensory cortex posteriorly. About how far the motor strip usually lies behind the coronal suture?
- A. 3 cm
- B. 5 cm
- C. 8 cm
- D. 10 cm
- E. Lies anterior to coronal suture

▸▸ Question 8

To access the potential recipient vessels in the angular gyrus for EC/IC bypass surgery, a 4 cm craniotomy should be performed, and it should be centered around:
- A. Reid's line
- B. Condylar line
- C. Chater's point
- D. Mastoid notch
- E. Zygomatic arch

▸▸ Question 9

For non-hydrocephalic ventricles, what is the average length of third ventricles?
- A. 0.6 cm
- B. 1.2 cm
- C. 2.8 cm
- D. 4 cm
- E. 5 cm

▸▸ Question 10

Regarding estimates of spinal levels for spine surgery, at what level is the inferior scapular pole posteriorly?

- A. C6
- B. T2
- C. T4
- D. T6
- E. T10

▸▸ Question 11

Regarding estimates of spinal levels for spine surgery, at what level is the carotid tubercle anteriorly?

- A. C6
- B. T2
- C. T4
- D. T6
- E. T10

▸▸ Question 12

Regarding cranial foramina and their contents, middle meningeal artery and vein pass through which of the following?

- A. Cribriform plate
- B. Optic canal
- C. Foramen rotundum
- D. Foramen ovale
- E. Foramen spinosum

▸▸ Question 13

Which of the following is not a content of porus acusticus?

- A. Facial nerve
- B. Nervus intermedius
- C. Acoustic portion of vestibulocochlear nerve
- D. Superior branch of vestibular nerve
- E. Glossopharyngeal nerve

▸▸ Question 14

What is the average length of frontal horn anterior to foramen of Monro?

- A. 1 cm
- B. 1.5 cm
- C. 2.5 cm
- D. 4 cm
- E. 5 cm

▸▸ Question 15

What is the average length of the fourth ventricle at the level of fastigium?

- A. 0.8 cm
- B. 1.4 cm
- C. 2.2 cm
- D. 2.5 cm
- E. 3 cm

▸▸ Question 16

Regarding the vascular supply of internal capsule, all of the retrolenticular part including optic radiation and ventral part of posterior limb of internal capsule are supplied by which of the following?

- A. Anterior choroidal artery
- B. Lateral striate branches
- C. Direct distal branches of internal carotid artery
- D. Terminal branches of middle meningeal artery
- E. Paramedian artery

▸▸ Question 17

What are the most important structures in maintaining atlantooccipital stability, without which the remaining cruciate ligament and apical dentate ligament are insufficient?

- A. Tectorial membrane and alar ligament
- B. Descending bands of cruciate ligament
- C. Ascending bands of cruciate ligaments
- D. Anterior and posterior atlantal ligaments
- E. Anterior and posterior atlantooccipital membranes

▸▸ Question 18

Flexor muscle tone is a function of which descending motor tracts of spinal cord?

- A. Anterior corticospinal tracts
- B. Lateral corticospinal tracts
- C. Rubrospinal tract
- D. Vestibulospinal tracts
- E. Medullary reticulospinal tracts

▸▸ Question 19

Sensory pain and temperature are the function of which ascending tract?

- A. Fasciculus gracilis
- B. Posterior spinocerebellar tract
- C. Anterior spinocerebellar tract
- D. Anterior spinothalamic tract
- E. Lateral spinothalamic tract

▸▸ Question 20

The receptors for pain and temperature are probably free nerve endings. The 1st order neurons enter the cord at dorsolateral tract (zone of Lissauer) and synapse in substantia gelatinosa that is equivalent to which Rexed lamina?

- A. I
- B. II

- C. III
- D. IV
- E. V

▸▸ Question 21

Brodmann's area 44 in dominant hemisphere (motor speech area) is known as what?
- A. Wernicke's area
- B. Angular gyrus area
- C. Supramarginal area
- D. Broca's area
- E. Frontal eye field area

▸▸ Question 22

What is the significance of Wernicke's area in dominant hemisphere which comprises Brodmann's area 40 and 39?
- A. Motor speech
- B. Voluntary eye movements
- C. Speech and language
- D. Auditory function
- E. Visual function

▸▸ Question 23

The most prominent paired grooves on CT or MRI of brain which is posterior to the widest biparietal diameter in midline is known as what?
- A. Pars opercularis
- B. Pars triangularis
- C. Pars orbitalis
- D. Pars marginalis
- E. Pars terminalis

▸▸ Question 24

The line connecting anterior commissure and posterior commissure (AC–PC line) has following characteristics except?
- A. It is used as baseline for axial MRI of brain
- B. It is used in functional neurosurgery
- C. Orbitomeatal line is 9 degrees steeper than the AC–PC line
- D. AC and PC are white matter tracts that help identify this line
- E. It is also called as Frankfurt's plane

▸▸ Question 25

Homunculus is somatotopic organization of sensory and motor cortex on the brain representing which of the following?
- A. Arm and face are represented on upper medial surface
- B. Foot and leg are represented on convexity of brain
- C. Arm and face are represented by the convexity of brain
- D. Foot and leg are represented on upper medial surface
- E. Both C and D

▸▸ Question 26

Where is the central sulcus located at interhemispheric fissure?
- A. Anterior to pars marginalis
- B. Lateral to pars marginalis
- C. Posterior to pars marginalis
- D. Medial to pars marginalis
- E. Above pars marginalis

▸▸ Question 27

Pterion, which is located two finger breaths above zygomatic arch, is meeting point of what?
- A. Lambdoid, occipitomastoid, and parietomastoid sutures
- B. Coronal suture and superior temporal line
- C. Frontal, temporal, parietal, and sphenoid bones
- D. Frontal, temporal, zygomatic, and sphenoid bones
- E. Coronal suture and sagittal suture

▸▸ Question 28

The point over skull which is used for external and internal carotid bypass craniotomy is called as what?
- A. Keen's point
- B. Taylor Huhgton point
- C. Stephanion
- D. Chater's point
- E. None of the above

▸▸ Question 29

All of the following landmarks do not match the level of spine except?
- A. Scapular spine—T2, T3
- B. Inferior scapular pole—T6
- C. Intercristal line—L4–L5 disk space
- D. Thyroid cartilage—C4, C5
- E. Hyoid bone—C6, C7

▸▸ Question 30

Vertical crest (Bill's bar) separates the internal auditory meatus into which of the following?
- A. Cochlear area anteriorly and vestibular area posteriorly
- B. Facial canal anteriorly and vestibular area posteriorly
- C. Facial canal posteriorly and vestibular area anteriorly
- D. Superior vestibular area, facial canal superiorly and inferior vestibular area, cochlear area inferiorly
- E. Both B and D

▸▸ Question 31

Which is the strongest ligament in the spine which attaches to medial tubercles of C1 and traps dens against C1?
- A. Transverse atlantal ligament (TAL)
- B. Ascending band of cruciate ligament
- C. Alar ligament
- D. Tectorial membrane
- E. Descending band of cruciate ligament

▸▸ Question 32

Fine touch, deep pressure, and proprioception sensations are carried from the body to the brain through which spinal cord tract?
- A. Lateral spinothalamic tract
- B. Posterior spinothalamic tract
- C. Fasciculus gracilis
- D. Fasciculus cuneatus
- E. B, C, and D

Answers

▸▸ Answer 1

Correct answer is D. 44[1]

▸▸ Answer 2

Correct answer is A. 40[1]

▸▸ Answer 3

Correct answer is A. 4[1]

▸▸ Answer 4

Correct answer is D. Asterion[2]

▸▸ Answer 5

Correct answer is C. Stephanion[2]

▸▸ Answer 6

Correct answer is A. Frankfurt plane[2]

▸▸ Answer 7

Correct answer is B. 5 cm[2]

▸▸ Answer 8

Correct answer is C. Chater's point[2]

▸▸ Answer 9

Correct answer is C. 2.8 cm[3]

▸▸ Answer 10

Correct answer is D. T6[4]

▸▸ Answer 11

Correct answer is A. C6[4]

▸▸ Answer 12

Correct answer is E. Foramen spinosum[4]

▸▸ Answer 13

Correct answer is E. Glossopharyngeal nerve[4]

▸▸ Answer 14

Correct answer is C. 2.5 cm[5]

▸▸ Answer 15

Correct answer is B. 1.4 cm[5]

▸▸ Answer 16

Correct answer is A. Anterior choroidal artery[6]

▸▸ Answer 17

Correct answer is A. Tectorial membrane and alar ligament[7]

▸▸ Answer 18

Correct answer is C. Rubrospinal tract[8]

▸▸ Answer 19

Correct answer is E. Lateral spinothalamic tract[9]

▸▸ Answer 20

Correct answer is B. II[9]

▸▸ Answer 21

Correct answer is D. Broca's area[1]

▸▸ Answer 22

Correct answer is C. Speech and language[1]

▸▸ Answer 23

Correct answer is D. Pars marginalis[10]

▸▸ Answer 24

Correct answer is E. It is also called as Frankfurt's plane[11]

▸▸ Answer 25

Correct answer is E. Both C and D[11]

▸▸ Answer 26

Correct answer is A. Anterior to pars marginalis[11]

▸▸ Answer 27

Correct answer is C. Frontal, temporal, parietal, and sphenoid bones[12]

▸▸ Answer 28

Correct answer is D. Chater's point[2]

▸▸ Answer 29

Correct answer is E. Hyoid bone—C6, C7[4]

▸▸ Answer 30

Correct answer is B. Facial canal anteriorly and vestibular area posteriorly[6]

▸▸ Answer 31

Correct answer is A. Transverse atlantal ligament (TAL)[7]

▸▸ Answer 32

Correct answer is E. B, C, and D[9]

References

[1] Greenberg M, ed. Greenberg's Handbook of Neurosurgery. 10th ed. New York: Thieme; 2023:56
[2] Greenberg M, ed. Greenberg's Handbook of Neurosurgery. 10th ed. New York: Thieme; 2023:61
[3] Greenberg M, ed. Greenberg's Handbook of Neurosurgery. 10th ed. New York: Thieme; 2023:62
[4] Greenberg M, ed. Greenberg's Handbook of Neurosurgery. 10th ed. New York: Thieme; 2023:65
[5] Greenberg M, ed. Greenberg's Handbook of Neurosurgery. 10th ed. New York: Thieme; 2023:64
[6] Greenberg M, ed. Greenberg's Handbook of Neurosurgery. 10th ed. New York: Thieme; 2023:66
[7] Greenberg M, ed. Greenberg's Handbook of Neurosurgery. 10th ed. New York: Thieme; 2023:69
[8] Greenberg M, ed. Greenberg's Handbook of Neurosurgery. 10th ed. New York: Thieme; 2023:70
[9] Greenberg M, ed. Greenberg's Handbook of Neurosurgery. 10th ed. New York: Thieme; 2023:71
[10] Greenberg M, ed. Greenberg's Handbook of Neurosurgery. 10th ed. New York: Thieme; 2023:57
[11] Greenberg M, ed. Greenberg's Handbook of Neurosurgery. 10th ed. New York: Thieme; 2023:58
[12] Greenberg M, ed. Greenberg's Handbook of Neurosurgery. 10th ed. New York: Thieme; 2023:60

2 Vascular Anatomy

Questions

▸▸ Question 1

Regarding anatomical segments of intracranial cerebral arteries, the segment of anterior cerebral artery from the branch point of callosomarginal curving around the genu of the corpus callosum to superior surface of corpus callosum 3 cm posterior to the genu is what?

- A. Pre-communicating
- B. Post-communicating
- C. Pre-callosal
- D. Supracallosal
- E. Post-callosal

▸▸ Question 2

Regarding anatomical segments of intracranial cerebral arteries, the segment of middle cerebral artery from bifurcation to emergence from Sylvian fissure is what?

- A. M1
- B. M2
- C. M3
- D. M4
- E. M5

▸▸ Question 3

The segment of posterior cerebral artery that traverses the quadrigeminal plate is what?

- A. P1
- B. P2
- C. P3
- D. P4
- E. P5

▸▸ Question 4

Which of the following is the first anterior branch of external carotid artery?

- A. Superior thyroid
- B. Facial
- C. Superficial temporal
- D. Infra-alveolar
- E. Infraorbital

▸▸ Question 5

Which of the following is the primary feeder for jugular foramen tumors?

- A. Ascending pharyngeal
- B. Lingual
- C. Facial
- D. Occipital
- E. Ophthalmic

▸▸ Question 6

In case of internal cerebral artery occlusion, an important collateral flow is via anastomosis between branches of facial artery and what?

- A. Ascending pharyngeal
- B. Lingual
- C. Facial
- D. Occipital
- E. Ophthalmic

▸▸ Question 7

Petroclival meningiomas are mainly supplied by branches of which segment of internal carotid artery?

- A. Lacerum
- B. Clinoidal
- C. Ophthalmic
- D. Communicating
- E. Cavernous

▸▸ Question 8

Which segment of internal carotid artery begins just proximal to origin of posterior communicating artery?

- A. Lacerum
- B. Clinoidal
- C. Ophthalmic
- D. Communicating
- E. Cavernous

▸▸ Question 9

Postpartum occlusion of inferior hypophysial artery causes pituitary infarcts (Sheehan's necrosis); however, diabetes insipidus is rare because the stalk is spared as it is supplied by what?

- A. Superior hypophysial artery
- B. Anterior choroidal artery
- C. Posterior choroidal artery
- D. Artery of McConnell
- E. Branches from plexal point

▸▸ Question 10

Fetal circulation is present in 15 to 35% of patients where posterior cerebral artery is supplied on one or both sides primarily by the carotid artery instead of via the vertebrobasilar system. The carotid artery provides this supply via what?

- A. Ascending pharyngeal
- B. Anterior communicating

- C. Posterior communicating
- D. Artery of Hubner
- E. Italian artery

▸▸ Question 11

Which of the following is the first branch of subclavian artery?
- A. Basilar artery
- B. Vertebral artery
- C. ICA
- D. ACA
- E. ECA

▸▸ Question 12

V1 prevertebral segment of vertebral artery courses superiorly and posteriorly to usually enter the foramen transversarium of which vertebral body?
- A. C7
- B. C6
- C. C5
- D. C4
- E. C3

▸▸ Question 13

Which of the following is the largest branch of vertebral artery?
- A. Mandibular
- B. Anterior meningeal
- C. Posterior meningeal
- D. Posterior inferior cerebellar
- E. Anterior inferior cerebellar

▸▸ Question 14

Which branch of the peduncular segment P1 of posterior cerebral artery supplies the tectum and cerebral peduncles and also Edinger-Westphal, oculomotor, and trochlear nuclei?
- A. Artery of Percheron
- B. Medial posterior choroidal
- C. Lateral posterior choroidal
- D. Interpeduncular thalamoperforators
- E. Mesencephalic perforating

▸▸ Question 15

Regarding carotid–vertebrobasilar anastomosis, which is the most common of the persistent fetal anastomosis?
- A. Persistent primitive trigeminal artery (PPTA)
- B. Otic
- C. Hypoglossal
- D. Proatlantal intersegmental
- E. Optic

▸▸ Question 16

Vein of Labbe is the inferior anastomotic vein and is prominent on the dominant side while the superficial superior anastomotic vein which is prominent on the non-dominant side is what?
- A. Vein of Percheron
- B. Vein of Trolard
- C. Vein of Labbe
- D. Basal vein of Rosenthal
- E. Vein of Galen

▸▸ Question 17

Which of the following is not a content of cavernous sinus?
- A. Oculomotor nerve (III)
- B. Trochlear nerve (IV)
- C. Ophthalmic division of trigeminal (V1)
- D. Maxillary division of trigeminal (V2)
- E. Mandibular division of trigeminal (V3)

▸▸ Question 18

Triangular space (of Parkinson) is a landmark for surgical entrance to the cavernous sinus. Its superior border is formed by cranial nerves III and IV, and the lower margin is formed by cranial nerve VI and what?
- A. Optic nerve
- B. Ophthalmic division of trigeminal (V1)
- C. Maxillary division of trigeminal (V2)
- D. Mandibular division of trigeminal (V3)
- E. Facial nerve

▸▸ Question 19

Artery of Adamkiewicz also called arteria radicularis anterior magna is the main arterial supply for which levels of the spinal cord?
- A. C3
- B. C6–C8
- C. T4 or T5
- D. T3–T8
- E. T8 to the conus

▸▸ Question 20

Regarding spinal cord vasculature, a normal variant where the anterior spinal artery joins with the paired posterior spinal arteries at the conus medullaris is called as arcade of what?
- A. Parkinson
- B. Willis
- C. Lazorthes
- D. Adamkiewicz
- E. Sulcal

▸▸ Question 21

Recurrent artery of Heubner (AKA medial striate artery) which supplies the head of caudate, putamen, and anterior internal capsule originates most commonly from what?

- A. Pre-communicating segment of anterior cerebral artery (A1)
- B. Post-communicating segment of anterior cerebral artery (A2)
- C. Junction of anterior cerebral artery and anterior communicating artery
- D. From anterior communicating artery
- E. A, B, and C

▸▸ Question 22

All of the following are segments of middle cerebral artery except?

- A. M1—from origin to bifurcation
- B. M2—from bifurcation to emergence from Sylvian fissure
- C. M3, M4—distal branches
- D. M5—terminal branch
- E. M6—cortical branch

▸▸ Question 23

Which of the following are branches of internal carotid artery in the neck?

- A. Ascending pharyngeal, superior thyroid, lingual, facial
- B. Recurrent laryngeal, thyroid, cricoid branches
- C. Mandibular, maxillary, zygomatic branches
- D. Anterior temporal, frontal, orbitofrontal
- E. None of the above

▸▸ Question 24

A patient presented in OPD with MRI of the brain showing petroclival meningioma. Which of the following arteries becomes prominent in this condition?

- A. Anterior choroidal artery
- B. Medial lenticulostriate artery
- C. Posterior cerebral artery
- D. Meningohypophyseal trunk
- E. Anterior clival artery

▸▸ Question 25

In 15 to 30% of the patients the posterior cerebral artery on one or both sides is primarily supplied by the carotids instead of via the vertebrobasilar system. This phenomenon is known as what?

- A. Carotid vertebrobasilar bypass
- B. Persistent primitive circulation
- C. Fetal circulation
- D. Embryonal circulation
- E. Persistent anterior circulation

▸▸ Question 26

Vertebral artery is the first and the largest branch of subclavian artery which has all of the following segments except?

- A. V1 prevertebral
- B. V2 traversing through transverse foramina from C6 to C2
- C. V3 from axis vertebrae to the foramen magnum
- D. V4 pierces the dura and enters the subarachnoid space
- E. V5 vertebral artery of both sides join to form basilar artery

▸▸ Question 27

Posterior inferior cerebellar artery (PICA) is the largest branch of vertebral artery which originates 10 mm distal to the point where vertebral artery becomes intradural. Which of the following segments of PICA must be preserved during surgery?

- A. Anterior medullary
- B. Lateral medullary
- C. Tonsillomedullary
- D. Cortical segments
- E. A, B, and C

▸▸ Question 28

Basilar artery is formed by junction of two vertebral arteries. Which of the following are its branches?

- A. Anterior inferior cerebellar artery (AICA)
- B. Internal auditory (labyrinthine)
- C. Pontine branches
- D. Superior cerebellar artery (SCA)
- E. All of the above

▸▸ Question 29

A patient presents with acute stroke in emergency. On DWI there is infarction on medial side of left frontal lobe of the brain. Which artery is involved in this ischemic stroke?

- A. Anterior cerebral
- B. Middle cerebral
- C. Posterior cerebral
- D. Vertebral arteries
- E. Basilar artery

▸▸ Question 30

All of the following are contents of cavernous sinus except?

- A. Oculomotor and trochlear nerve
- B. V1 and V2 nerves
- C. V3 nerve
- D. Abducens nerve
- E. Carotid artery

▸▸ Question 31

Great cerebral vein of Galen is formed by confluences of which of the following veins?
- A. Vein of Trolard and vein of Labbe
- B. Cortical veins
- C. Precentral cerebellar vein, basal vein of Rosenthal, and internal cerebral vein
- D. Precentral cerebellar vein, internal cerebral vein, and anterior septal vein
- E. Precentral cerebellar vein, basal vein of Rosenthal, and thalamostriate vein

Answers

▸▸ Answer 1

Correct answer is C. Pre-callosal[1]

▸▸ Answer 2

Correct answer is B. M2[2]

▸▸ Answer 3

Correct answer is C. P3[2]

▸▸ Answer 4

Correct answer is A. Superior thyroid[2]

▸▸ Answer 5

Correct answer is A. Ascending pharyngeal[2]

▸▸ Answer 6

Correct answer is E. Ophthalmic[3]

▸▸ Answer 7

Correct answer is E. Cavernous[4]

▸▸ Answer 8

Correct answer is D. Communicating[3]

▸▸ Answer 9

Correct answer is A. Superior hypophysial artery[3]

▸▸ Answer 10

Correct answer is C. Posterior communicating[5]

▸▸ Answer 11

Correct answer is B. Vertebral artery[5]

▸▸ Answer 12

Correct answer is B. C6[6]

▸▸ Answer 13

Correct answer is D. Posterior inferior cerebellar[6]

▸▸ Answer 14

Correct answer is E. Mesencephalic perforating[6]

▸▸ Answer 15

Correct answer is A. Persistent primitive trigeminal artery (PPTA)[7]

▸▸ Answer 16

Correct answer is B. Vein of Trolard[8]

▸▸ Answer 17

Correct answer is E. Mandibular division of trigeminal (V3)
9

▸▸ Answer 18

Correct answer is B. Ophthalmic division of trigeminal (V1)
9

▸▸ Answer 19

Correct answer is E. T8 to the conus[10]

▸▸ Answer 20

Correct answer is C. Lazorthes[11]

▸▸ Answer 21

Correct answer is C. Junction of anterior cerebral artery and anterior communicating artery[1]

▸▸ Answer 22

Correct answer is E. M6—cortical branch[12]

▸▸ Answer 23

Correct answer is E. None of the above[2]

▸▸ Answer 24

Correct answer is D. Meningohypophyseal trunk[4]

▸▸ Answer 25

Correct answer is C. Fetal circulation[5]

▸▸ Answer 26

Correct answer is E. V5 vertebral artery of both sides join to form basilar artery[6]

▸▸ Answer 27

Correct answer is E. A, B, and C[6]

▸▸ Answer 28

Correct answer is E. All of the above[6]

▸▸ Answer 29

Correct answer is A. Anterior cerebral[1]

▸▸ Answer 30

Correct answer is C. V3 nerve[9]

▸▸ Answer 31

Correct answer is C. Precentral cerebellar vein, basal vein of Rosenthal, and internal cerebral vein[8]

References

[1] Greenberg M, ed. Greenberg's Handbook of Neurosurgery. 10th ed. New York: Thieme; 2023:74
[2] Greenberg M, ed. Greenberg's Handbook of Neurosurgery. 10th ed. New York: Thieme; 2023:76
[3] Greenberg M, ed. Greenberg's Handbook of Neurosurgery. 10th ed. New York: Thieme; 2023:78
[4] Greenberg M, ed. Greenberg's Handbook of Neurosurgery. 10th ed. New York: Thieme; 2023:77
[5] Greenberg M, ed. Greenberg's Handbook of Neurosurgery. 10th ed. New York: Thieme; 2023:80
[6] Greenberg M, ed. Greenberg's Handbook of Neurosurgery. 10th ed. New York: Thieme; 2023:81
[7] Greenberg M, ed. Greenberg's Handbook of Neurosurgery. 10th ed. New York: Thieme; 2023:83
[8] Greenberg M, ed. Greenberg's Handbook of Neurosurgery. 10th ed. New York: Thieme; 2023:85
[9] Greenberg M, ed. Greenberg's Handbook of Neurosurgery. 10th ed. New York: Thieme; 2023:86
[10] Greenberg M, ed. Greenberg's Handbook of Neurosurgery. 10th ed. New York: Thieme; 2023:87
[11] Greenberg M, ed. Greenberg's Handbook of Neurosurgery. 10th ed. New York: Thieme; 2023:88
[12] Greenberg M, ed. Greenberg's Handbook of Neurosurgery. 10th ed. New York: Thieme; 2023:75

3 Neurophysiology and Regional Brain Syndromes

Questions

▸▸ Question 1

The blood–brain barrier is present in which of the following areas?

- A. Choroid plexus
- B. Hypophysis
- C. Tuber cinereum
- D. Area postrema
- E. Brain stem

▸▸ Question 2

In head injury, the blood–brain barrier is closed; therefore, there is no protein extravasation and no enhancement on CT or MRI. The cells swell and then shrink. What kind of cerebral edema is this?

- A. Cytotoxic
- B. Vasogenic
- C. Vasospastic
- D. Ischemic
- E. Mixed

▸▸ Question 3

According to classical model of language and speech function, conduction aphasia is caused by a damage to which of the following?

- A. Brodmann's area 39
- B. Brodmann's area 40
- C. Broca's area
- D. Wernicke's area
- E. Arcuate fasciculus

▸▸ Question 4

The afferent limb of the plantar reflex originates in cutaneous receptors restricted to which dermatome?

- A. L1
- B. L4
- C. L5
- D. S1
- E. S2

▸▸ Question 5

In a patient with suspected stroke, the plantar reflex could not be elicited by stimulation of the lateral plantar surface and transverse arch in a single movement, so the examiner pinched the Achilles tendon to elicit the plantar response. What is this maneuver called?

- A. Chaddok
- B. Schaeffer
- C. Oppenheim
- D. Gordon
- E. Bing

▸▸ Question 6

Hoffman's sign is elicited by flicking downward on the nail of the middle or ring finger: a positive (pathologic) response consists of involuntary flexion of the adjacent fingers and/or thumb. It is monosynaptic (synapse in Rexed lamina IX) and indicates a lesion above what?

- A. C3
- B. C5
- C. C8
- D. T1
- E. T3

▸▸ Question 7

Where does the primary coordinating center for bladder function reside within the pons?

- A. Nucleus locus coeruleus
- B. Nucleus V
- C. Area postrema
- D. Lateral medullary nucleus
- E. Medial medullary nucleus

▸▸ Question 8

The detrusor muscle of the bladder contracts and the internal sphincter relaxes under parasympathetic stimulation; the preganglionic cell bodies reside in the intermediolateral gray of which spinal cord segments?

- A. T2–T10
- B. T10–T12
- C. L1–L3
- D. L2–L4
- E. S2–S4

▸▸ Question 9

Regarding bladder physiology, sympathetic cell bodies lie within the intermediolateral gray column of lumbar spinal cord segments T12–L2. Preganglionic axons pass through the sympathetic chain (without synapsing) to the inferior mesenteric ganglion. Detrusor smooth muscle relaxation during bladder filling and storage is carried out by stimulation of which of the following?

- A. Alpha 1
- B. Alpha 2
- C. Beta 1

- D. Beta 2
- E. Beta 3

▸▸ **Question 10**

A patient presented with urinary frequency, urgency, incontinence, and nocturia. Urodynamic findings showed detrusor overactivity (DO) without detrusor sphincter dyssynergia (DSD). What is the level of lesion?

- A. Supraspinal
- B. Suprasacral during spinal shock
- C. Suprasacral after resolution of spinal shock
- D. Infrasacral
- E. Systemic, e.g., diabetes

▸▸ **Question 11**

What is the cut off value of bladder pressure for safe storage?

- A. < 40 cm H_2O
- B. < 60 cm H_2O
- C. < 80 cm H_2O
- D. < 100 cm H_2O
- E. < 120 cm H_2O

▸▸ **Question 12**

Tamsulosin is a prostate alpha1A adrenoreceptor antagonist. What is the initial usual adult daily dose?

- A. 0.1 mg
- B. 0.4 mg
- C. 1 mg
- D. 2 mg
- E. 4 mg

▸▸ **Question 13**

Which of the following is a parietal lobe syndrome with a unilateral asomatognosia, anosognosia, apathy, allocheiria, dressing apraxia, and extinction and inattention to an entire visual field?

- A. Anton Babinski syndrome
- B. Foster Kennedy syndrome
- C. Parinaud's syndrome
- D. Weber syndrome
- E. Gertsmann's syndrome

▸▸ **Question 14**

A patient presented with agraphia without alexia, left–right confusion, digit agnosia and acalculia. This is typical for which syndrome?

- A. Anton Babinski syndrome
- B. Foster Kennedy syndrome
- C. Parinaud's syndrome
- D. Weber syndrome
- E. Gertsmann's syndrome

▸▸ **Question 15**

Which of the following is cranial nerve III palsy with contralateral hemiparesis?

- A. Anton Babinski syndrome
- B. Foster Kennedy syndrome
- C. Parinaud's syndrome
- D. Weber syndrome
- E. Gertsmann's syndrome

▸▸ **Question 16**

Which syndrome is usually associated with olfactory groove or medial third sphenoid wing tumor and presents with the classic triad of ipsilateral anosmia, ipsilateral central scotoma, and contralateral papilledema?

- A. Anton Babinski syndrome
- B. Foster Kennedy syndrome
- C. Parinaud's syndrome
- D. Weber syndrome
- E. Benedikt's syndrome

▸▸ **Question 17**

After resection of a posterior fossa brain tumor, a child presented with speechlessness, ataxia, hypotonia, and irritability along with cranial nerve deficits, neurobehavioral changes, and urinary incontinence. What syndrome is this?

- A. Cerebellar mutism syndrome
- B. Posterior fossa syndrome
- C. Jugular foramen syndrome
- D. Cerebellar syndrome
- E. Fourth ventricle syndrome

▸▸ **Question 18**

Pars vascularis is the larger posterolateral compartment of jugular foramen and it contains which of the following?

- A. Vagus nerve
- B. Glossopharyngeal nerve
- C. Branching Jacobson's nerve
- D. Inferior petrosal sinus
- E. Meningeal branch of the ascending pharyngeal artery

▸▸ **Question 19**

Which of the following is a jugular foramen syndrome with palsies of cranial nerves IX, X, XI, and XII without sympathetic involvement?

- A. Collet-Sicard syndrome
- B. Villaret's syndrome
- C. Tapia syndrome

- D. (Hughlings) Jackson's syndrome
- E. Schmidt's syndrome

▸▸ Question 20

Which of the following is a jugular foramen syndrome with palsies of cranial nerves IX, X, XI, and XII with sympathetic involvement?

- A. Collet-Sicard syndrome
- B. Villaret's syndrome
- C. Tapia syndrome
- D. (Hughlings) Jackson's syndrome
- E. Schmidt's syndrome

▸▸ Question 21

Blood–brain barrier (BBB) which is formed by the tight junctions (zona occludens) between cerebral capillary endothelial cells is absent in following areas of brain except?

- A. Area postrema and posterior eminence of hypothalamus
- B. Pineal gland and choroid plexus
- C. Tuber cinereum and preoptic recess
- D. Anterior pituitary (adenohypophysis)
- E. Posterior pituitary (neurohypophysis)

▸▸ Question 22

A patient presented in OPD with tumor on brain MRI which showed marked perilesional edema. This edema is due to extravasation of protein because of blood–brain barrier disruption. What is this type of edema in this case of brain tumor called?

- A. Cytotoxic edema
- B. Vascular edema
- C. Vasogenic edema
- D. Ischemic edema
- E. Both B and C

▸▸ Question 23

A patient presents in neurosurgical OPD with complaint of fluent speech, and he/she is unable to understand speech of other people. This phenomenon is known as receptive aphasia. In which brain area this patient most likely has a lesion?

- A. Broca's area
- B. Wernicke's area
- C. At arcuate fasciculus
- D. Primary auditory area
- E. Areas of ventral and dorsal stream flow

▸▸ Question 24

Planter reflex also known as Babinski sign is a primitive reflex present in infancy usually up to 10 months. This reflex consists of extension of great toe in response to noxious stimulus applied to the planter aspect of foot. It is not present in adults in which one of the following conditions?

- A. Tumor in left frontal brain region
- B. Cervical spinal cord compression by prolapsed disk
- C. Tumor at L4–L5 spinal cord level
- D. Compression of thoracic spinal cord due to traumatic vertebral fracture
- E. L4–L5 spinal vertebral level disk

▸▸ Question 25

Hoffmann's sign consists of involuntary flexion of adjacent finger and/or thumb on flicking downward on the nail of middle or ring finger. This sign is positive if lesion is found at which cord level?

- A. Above C5
- B. At or above C3
- C. Only at C8
- D. Only at C5 level
- E. Above C8 level

▸▸ Question 26

Primary coordinating center for bladder function resides within nucleus locus coeruleus. This area is supplied by inhibitory signals for voluntary cortical control of micturition from where?

- A. Anteromedial portion of frontal lobe
- B. Genu of corpus callosum
- C. Gyrus rectus
- D. Frontal lobe of brain
- E. Both A and B

▸▸ Question 27

A patient presented in emergency with traumatic large herniated lumbar disk at L4–L5 vertebral level. This lesion can result in which of the following conditions?

- A. Detrusor overactivity (DO) without detrusor sphincter dysnergy (DSD)
- B. DO with DSD
- C. Only detrusor overactivity
- D. Detrusor areflexia with overflow incontinence
- E. None of the above

▸▸ Question 28

Gerstmann's syndrome is because of lesion in the dominant parietal lobe. It consists of which of the following?

- A. Agraphia without alexia
- B. Left–right confusion
- C. Digit agnosia
- D. Acalculia
- E. All of the above

►► **Question 29**

Frontal eye field is located in the posterior frontal lobe and is Brodmann's area 8. Destructive lesion in this area causes which of the following conditions?

- A. Impaired gaze to the contralateral side
- B. Causing gaze toward contralateral side
- C. Patient looks toward the side of lesion
- D. Patient looks away from the side of lesion
- E. Both A and C
- F. Both C and D

►► **Question 30**

Olfactory groove meningioma or medial sphenoid wing meningioma can cause "Foster Kennedy syndrome." All of the following are the features of this syndrome except?

- A. Contralateral optic atrophy
- B. Ipsilateral anosmia
- C. Ipsilateral central scotoma
- D. Contralateral papilledema
- E. All of the above

►► **Question 31**

Speechlessness that develops following cerebellar injury is called as mutism with subsequent dysarthria. It is also known as what?

- A. Cerebellar mutism
- B. Cerebellar mutism syndrome
- C. Posterior fossa syndrome
- D. Cerebellar dysfunction
- E. Both A and B

Answers

►► **Answer 1**

Correct answer is E. Brain stem[1]

►► **Answer 2**

Correct answer is A. Cytotoxic[1]

►► **Answer 3**

Correct answer is E. Arcuate fasciculus[2]

►► **Answer 4**

Correct answer is D. S1[2]

►► **Answer 5**

Correct answer is B. Schaeffer[3]

►► **Answer 6**

Correct answer is C. C8[3]

►► **Answer 7**

Correct answer is A. Nucleus locus coeruleus[3]

►► **Answer 8**

Correct answer is E. S2–S4[4]

►► **Answer 9**

Correct answer is E. Beta 3[4]

►► **Answer 10**

Correct answer is A. Supraspinal[5]

►► **Answer 11**

Correct answer is A. < 40 cm H_2O[6]

►► **Answer 12**

Correct answer is B. 0.4 mg[7]

►► **Answer 13**

Correct answer is A. Anton Babinski syndrome[8]

►► **Answer 14**

Correct answer is E. Gertsmann's syndrome[9]

►► **Answer 15**

Correct answer is D. Weber syndrome[8]

►► **Answer 16**

Correct answer is B. Foster Kennedy syndrome[10]

►► **Answer 17**

Correct answer is B. Posterior fossa syndrome[10]

►► **Answer 18**

Correct answer is A. Vagus nerve[11]

►► **Answer 19**

Correct answer is A. Collet-Sicard syndrome[12]

►► **Answer 20**

Correct answer is B. Villaret's syndrome[13]

▸▸ Answer 21

Correct answer is D. Anterior pituitary (adenohypophysis)[1]

▸▸ Answer 22

Correct answer is C. Vasogenic edema[1]

▸▸ Answer 23

Correct answer is B. Wernicke's area[1]

▸▸ Answer 24

Correct answer is E. L4–L5 spinal vertebral level disk[2]

▸▸ Answer 25

Correct answer is E. Above C8 level[3]

▸▸ Answer 26

Correct answer is E. Both A and B[3]

▸▸ Answer 27

Correct answer is D. Detrusor areflexia with overflow incontinence[5]

▸▸ Answer 28

Correct answer is E. All of the above[9]

▸▸ Answer 29

Correct answer is E. Both A and C[14]

▸▸ Answer 30

Correct answer is A. Contralateral optic atrophy[10]

▸▸ Answer 31

Correct answer is A. Cerebellar mutism[10]

References

[1] Greenberg M, ed. Greenberg's Handbook of Neurosurgery. 10th ed. New York: Thieme; 2023:90
[2] Greenberg M, ed. Greenberg's Handbook of Neurosurgery. 10th ed. New York: Thieme; 2023:91
[3] Greenberg M, ed. Greenberg's Handbook of Neurosurgery. 10th ed. New York: Thieme; 2023:92
[4] Greenberg M, ed. Greenberg's Handbook of Neurosurgery. 10th ed. New York: Thieme; 2023:93
[5] Greenberg M, ed. Greenberg's Handbook of Neurosurgery. 10th ed. New York: Thieme; 2023:94
[6] Greenberg M, ed. Greenberg's Handbook of Neurosurgery. 10th ed. New York: Thieme; 2023:95
[7] Greenberg M, ed. Greenberg's Handbook of Neurosurgery. 10th ed. New York: Thieme; 2023:97
[8] Greenberg M, ed. Greenberg's Handbook of Neurosurgery. 10th ed. New York: Thieme; 2023:101
[9] Greenberg M, ed. Greenberg's Handbook of Neurosurgery. 10th ed. New York: Thieme; 2023:99
[10] Greenberg M, ed. Greenberg's Handbook of Neurosurgery. 10th ed. New York: Thieme; 2023:100
[11] Greenberg M, ed. Greenberg's Handbook of Neurosurgery. 10th ed. New York: Thieme; 2023:102
[12] Greenberg M, ed. Greenberg's Handbook of Neurosurgery. 10th ed. New York: Thieme; 2023:103
[13] Greenberg M, ed. Greenberg's Handbook of Neurosurgery. 10th ed. New York: Thieme; 2023:104
[14] Greenberg M, ed. Greenberg's Handbook of Neurosurgery. 10th ed. New York: Thieme; 2023:98

Part II

General and Neurology

II

4 Neuroanesthesia

Questions

▸▸ **Question 1**

According to the American Society of Anesthesiologists (ASA) grading system to estimate anesthetic risk for various conditions, a patient with severe systemic disease that is a constant threat to life will be assigned which ASA class?

- A. I
- B. II
- C. III
- D. IV
- E. V

▸▸ **Question 2**

Regarding the importance of temperature control in neuroanesthesia, for each 1°C drop in patient's temperature, the cerebral metabolic rate of oxygen ($CMRO_2$) decreases by about what amount?

- A. 1%
- B. 7%
- C. 11%
- D. 15%
- E. 20%

▸▸ **Question 3**

CO_2 is the most potent cerebral vasodilator; hyperventilation reduces $PaCO_2$ (hypocapnea). The goal for safe neurological surgery is generally end tidal CO_2 ($ETCO_2$) of what?

- A. 20–25 mmHg
- B. 25–30 mmHg
- C. 30–35 mmHg
- D. 35–40 mmHg
- E. > 45 mmHg

▸▸ **Question 4**

Regarding drugs used in neuroanesthesia, which of the following is associated with development of tension pneumocephalus?

- A. Nitrous oxide
- B. Propofol
- C. Etomidate
- D. Barbiturates
- E. Ketamine

▸▸ **Question 5**

Most barbiturates are anticonvulsants except which of the following?

- A. Phenobarbital
- B. Pentobarbital
- C. Sodium thiopental
- D. Primidone
- E. Methohexital

▸▸ **Question 6**

Regarding remifentanil, which statement is false?

- A. Reduces intracranial pressure
- B. Reduces cerebral blood volume
- C. Increases $CMRO_2$
- D. Large doses can be neurotoxic to limbic system
- E. Can be used in awake craniotomy

▸▸ **Question 7**

Dexmedetomidine (Precedex®) is used for control of hypertension postoperatively, as well as for its sedating qualities during awake craniotomy either alone or in conjunction with propofol. It is an agonist for which of the following?

- A. Alpha 1 receptors
- B. Alpha 2 receptors
- C. Beta receptors
- D. Beta 2 receptors
- E. Beta 3 receptors

▸▸ **Question 8**

Regarding paralytics for intubation, which of the following is an intermediate-acting, aminosteroid, nondepolarizing muscle relaxant agent approved for rapid sequence intubation?

- A. Succinylcholine
- B. Lidocaine
- C. Rocuronium
- D. Cisatracurium
- E. Etomidate

▸▸ **Question 9**

Which of the following is the ideal modality regarding anesthesia issues related to intraoperative evoked potential (EPs) monitoring?

- A. Total intravenous anesthesia
- B. Intermittent boluses are preferred over continuous infusion
- C. Nitrous/narcotic is the first choice
- D. Monitoring of temperature and blood pressure changes is not mandatory as these do not affect the potentials
- E. Halothane is the ideal inhalational drug

▸▸ Question 10

Malignant hyperthermia is a hypermetabolic state of skeletal muscle due to idiopathic block of calcium re-entry into sarcoplasmic reticulum. Which of the following is the earliest possible sign?

- A. Increased end tidal pCO_2
- B. Bradycardia
- C. Metabolic alkalosis on arterial blood gas analysis
- D. Decreased myoglobin levels
- E. Decreased CPK levels

▸▸ Question 11

Parameters of primary relevance to neurosurgical surgery that can be modulated by anesthesiologist which play a primary role in control of intracranial pressure (ICP) and cerebral metabolic requirements of nutrients include all of the following except?

- A. Blood pressure which affects cerebral perfusion pressure (CPP)
- B. Jugular venous pressure
- C. Arterial CO_2 tension
- D. Body temperature
- E. Elevating hematocrit

▸▸ Question 12

Nitrous oxide (N_2O) is an inhalational anesthetic agent which is 34 times more soluble in blood as compared to nitrogen. When N_2O comes out of blood into the airtight cranial cavity it can produce tension pneumocephalus. Which of the following are steps that can be used to reduce chances of tension pneumocephalus while using N_2O in patients?

- A. Filling the cranial cavity with fluid while doing closure
- B. Doing the operation in more supine position
- C. Turning off N_2O 10 minutes prior to completion of dural closure
- D. All of the above
- E. Aspirating air with needle while doing closure

▸▸ Question 13

Etomidate is an intravenous anesthetic agent which should be avoided in patients with what?

- A. Liver disease
- B. Renal disease
- C. High blood pressure
- D. Respiratory difficulty
- E. All of the above

▸▸ Question 14

Ketamine is usually not used in neurosurgical patients because of its which side effect?

- A. Respiratory depression
- B. Bradycardia
- C. Low blood pressure
- D. Increase in intracranial pressure
- E. All of the above

▸▸ Question 15

Which of the following are disadvantages of using narcotics in neurosurgical patients?

- A. May cause hypotension by histamine release
- B. May cause cerebrovascular vasodilation which can cause increased ICP
- C. Can cause confusion in renal insufficient patient
- D. Can cause confusion in hepatic insufficient patient
- E. All of the above

▸▸ Question 16

Following are the useful characteristics of propofol which make it more suitable for use in neurosurgical patients except?

- A. Reduces cerebral metabolism, cerebral blood flow, and intracranial pressure
- B. It is a cerebral protectant
- C. Short half-life makes it useful for use in awake craniotomy
- D. Produces isoelectric EEG
- E. All of the above

▸▸ Question 17

Which of following is an alpha 2 adrenergic receptor agonist which is used for control of hypertension in postoperative patients and for sedation during awake craniotomy?

- A. Dexmedetomidine (Precede)
- B. Esmolol
- C. Lidocaine
- D. Propofol
- E. None of the above

▸▸ Question 18

Paralytics should not be given until it has been determined that the patient can be ventilated manually unless what?

- A. The patient has cervical spine injury
- B. The patient has brain tumor
- C. Treating the patient with laryngospasm
- D. When treating the patient with botulism
- E. None of the above

▸▸ Question 19

For inhalational anesthetic agent, maximum alveolar concentration (MAC) of drug should ideally be what?

- A. More than 1
- B. Less than 0.5
- C. More than 1.5
- D. Less than 2
- E. Exactly 1

▸▸ Question 20

A patient developed elevated body temperature (> 44 degrees Celsius or 113 degrees Fahrenheit) after giving succinyl choline during induction of anesthesia. It is a malignant hypertension due to idiopathic block of calcium re-entry into the sarcoplasmic reticulum. Which of the following is treatment for this condition?

- A. Eliminating offending agent and hyperventilation
- B. Giving dantrolene sodium with surface and cavity cooling
- C. Giving bicarbonate with IV insulin and glucose
- D. Giving procainamide and diuretics
- E. All of the above

Answers

▸▸ Answer 1

Correct answer is D. IV[1]

▸▸ Answer 2

Correct answer is B. 7%[1]

▸▸ Answer 3

Correct answer is B. 25–30 mmHg[1]

▸▸ Answer 4

Correct answer is A. Nitrous oxide[2]

▸▸ Answer 5

Correct answer is E. Methohexital[3]

▸▸ Answer 6

Correct answer is C. Increases $CMRO_2$[3]

▸▸ Answer 7

Correct answer is B. Alpha 2 receptors[4]

▸▸ Answer 8

Correct answer is C. Rocuronium[4]

▸▸ Answer 9

Correct answer is A. Total intravenous anesthesia[5]

▸▸ Answer 10

Correct answer is A. Increased end tidal pCO_2[5]

▸▸ Answer 11

Correct answer is E. Elevating hematocrit[1]

▸▸ Answer 12

Correct answer is D. All of the above[2]

▸▸ Answer 13

Correct answer is B. Renal disease[3]

▸▸ Answer 14

Correct answer is D. Increase in intracranial pressure[3]

▸▸ Answer 15

Correct answer is E. All of the above[3]

▸▸ Answer 16

Correct answer is D. Produces isoelectric EEG[3]

▸▸ Answer 17

Correct answer is A. Dexmedetomidine (Precede)[4]

▸▸ Answer 18

Correct answer is C. Treating the patient with laryngospasm[4]

▸▸ Answer 19

Correct answer is B. Less than 0.5[5]

▸▸ Answer 20

Correct answer is E. All of the above[5]

References

[1] Greenberg M, ed. Greenberg's Handbook of Neurosurgery. 10th ed. New York: Thieme; 2023:108

[2] Greenberg M, ed. Greenberg's Handbook of Neurosurgery. 10th ed. New York: Thieme; 2023:109

[3] Greenberg M, ed. Greenberg's Handbook of Neurosurgery. 10th ed. New York: Thieme; 2023:110

[4] Greenberg M, ed. Greenberg's Handbook of Neurosurgery. 10th ed. New York: Thieme; 2023:111

[5] Greenberg M, ed. Greenberg's Handbook of Neurosurgery. 10th ed. New York: Thieme; 2023:112

5 Sodium Homeostasis and Osmolality

Questions

▸▸ Question 1

According to the classification of severity of hyponatremia, severe hyponatremia is sodium level (mEq/L) less than what?

- A. 160
- B. 155
- C. 145
- D. 135
- E. 125

▸▸ Question 2

Which of the following is an etiology for hypotonic hyponatremia?

- A. Mannitol therapy
- B. Renal failure
- C. TURP syndrome
- D. Paraproteinemia
- E. Hypertriglyceridemia

▸▸ Question 3

Hyponatremia is acute if duration documented is less than what?

- A. 48 hours
- B. 56 hours
- C. 72 hours
- D. 5 days
- E. 7 days

▸▸ Question 4

The most important differentiating criterion for differentiation between syndrome of inappropriate ADH (SIAD) and cerebral salt wasting (CSW) is what?

- A. Serum sodium level
- B. Urinary sodium level
- C. Glycemic level
- D. Volume status
- E. Potassium level

▸▸ Question 5

Which of the following is not included in the diagnostic criteria for SIAD?

- A. Decreased effective serum osmolality (< 275 mOsm/kg of water)
- B. Urine osmolality > 100 mOsm/kg of water
- C. Clinical euvolemia
- D. Increased thyroid stimulating hormone (TSH) level
- E. No recent diuretic use

▸▸ Question 6

Solute ratio is defined as (Urinary [Na] + Urinary [K])/Plasma [Na]. For a ratio of 1, what is the recommended fluid intake (mL/d) in SIAD?

- A. < 500
- B. 600
- C. 100
- D. 1500
- E. 2000

▸▸ Question 7

During treatment of SIAD, what is the limit of correction that should not be exceeded?

- A. 2–4 mEq/L in 24 hours
- B. 6–8 mEq/L in 24 hours
- C. 8–10 mEq/L in 24 hours
- D. 12–14 mEq/L in 48 hours
- E. 14–15 mEq/L in 48 hours

▸▸ Question 8

During treatment of SIAD, a patient developed insidious flaccid quadriplegia, mental status changes, and cranial nerve abnormalities with a pseudobulbar palsy appearance. What is the most probable diagnosis?

- A. The diagnosis of SIAD was wrong
- B. Central pontine myelinolysis
- C. Weber syndrome
- D. Transverse myelitis
- E. Hydrocephalus

▸▸ Question 9

Which of the following is avoided during treatment of cerebral salt wasting?

- A. Normal saline
- B. 3% saline
- C. Packed red blood cells
- D. Steroids
- E. Furosemide

▸▸ Question 10

Which of the following drugs is effective in treatment of cerebral salt wasting?

- A. Demeclocycline
- B. Conivaptan
- C. Vasopressin receptor antagonists
- D. Lithium
- E. Fludrocortisone acetate

▸▸ Question 11

Within what time frame should the initial half be replaced?

- A. 10–15 minutes
- B. 30 minutes
- C. 1 hour
- D. 2 hours
- E. 24 hours

▸▸ Question 12

For indeterminate cases, polyuria due to diabetes insipidus can be differentiated from psychogenic polydipsia by the water deprivation test. What is the highest urinary osmolality after Pitressin in water deprivation test that is interpreted as normal?

- A. < 5% increase
- B. 10% increase
- C. 20% increase
- D. 45% increase
- E. > 50% increase

▸▸ Question 13

Which of the following is not a diagnostic criterion for diabetes insipidus?

- A. Urine osmolality < 300 mOsm/kg
- B. Inability to concentrate urine to > 300 mOsm/kg in the presence of clinical dehydration
- C. Urine output > 50 mL/kg/24 h
- D. Hyponatremia
- E. Normal adrenal function

▸▸ Question 14

Intravenous fluid management for diabetes insipidus includes base intravenous fluid: D5 1/2 NS + 20 mEqKCl/L at 75–100 mL/h. In addition to that, the urine output above base intravenous rate should be replaced mL for mL with which of the following?

- A. Normal saline
- B. ½ Normal saline
- C. Hypertonic saline
- D. Red cell concentrates
- E. No need for this replacement

▸▸ Question 15

Regarding desmopressin in DDAVP® Nasal Spray 100 µg/mL, about how much each spray delivers?

- A. 1 µg
- B. 10 µg
- C. 30 µg
- D. 50 µg
- E. 100 µg

▸▸ Question 16

A patient is presented to emergency with anorexia, headache, difficulty concentrating, and irritability. On investigations he/she has serum sodium level of 131 mEq/L, serum osmolality of 265 mOsm/kg, and urine osmolality more than 100 mOsm/kg with euvolemia. What is the most probable diagnosis in this patient?

- A. Diabetes insipidus
- B. Cerebral salt wasting
- C. Syndrome of inappropriate antidiuretic hormone secretion (SIADH)
- D. Hyponatremia
- E. Renal failure

▸▸ Question 17

A patient presented with aneurysmal subarachnoid hemorrhage with only symptom of severe headache. After some time he/she developed irritability, difficulty concentrating, and muscle weakness. Her/his plain brain CT showed no new finding. On labs serum osmolality was less than 275 mOsm/kg, urine osmolality was more than 100 mOsm/kg with volume depletion, and urinary sodium more than 20 mEq/L. What is the most probable diagnosis?

- A. Diabetes insipidus
- B. Cerebral salt wasting
- C. SIADH
- D. Hyponatremia
- E. Renal failure

▸▸ Question 18

Which of the following is the cause of syndrome of inappropriate antidiuretic hormone secretion?

- A. CNS infection
- B. Head trauma
- C. Brain tumors
- D. Aneurysmal subarachnoid hemorrhage
- E. All of the above

▸▸ Question 19

A patient presents with hyponatremia in hospital. On lab investigation urine osmolality is less than 500 mOsm/kg. She/he was given normal saline infusion test with 2 liters of normal saline over 24 to 48 hours. What does correction of hyponatremia suggest?

- A. SIADH
- B. CSW
- C. Extracellular fluid volume depletion
- D. DI
- E. None of the above

▸▸ **Question 20**

A patient being treated for hyponatremia suddenly develops flaccid quadriplegia, mental status changes, and some cranial nerve abnormalities. What is the most probable diagnosis in this case?

- A. Osmotic demyelination syndrome
- B. Severe hyponatremia
- C. Severe hypernatremia
- D. Wernicke's encephalopathy
- E. All of the above

▸▸ **Question 21**

A patient presents in emergency with severe hyponatremia with syndrome of inappropriate antidiuretic hormone secretion (SIADH). Which of the following are treatment options for this condition?

- A. Admission in ICU
- B. 3% normal saline at 1 to 2 mL/kg
- C. Furosemide 20 mg
- D. Restriction of water intake
- E. A, B, and C

▸▸ **Question 22**

A patient being treated for hyponatremia with normal saline develops decreased renal cortical blood flow, metabolic acidosis, reduced gastric mucosal perfusion, tachypnea, hypocapnia, and increased risk of vasoconstriction in brain. Which of the following is the cause of these symptoms?

- A. Severe hypernatremia
- B. Fluid overload
- C. Hyperchloremic acidosis
- D. Severe hyponatremia
- E. None of the above

▸▸ **Question 23**

A patient underwent pituitary surgery. After surgery he developed high urine output. Labs showed urine osmolality less than 300 mOsm/kg and urine specific gravity less than 1.003, with normal or high serum osmolality and high serum sodium. What is the most probable diagnosis in this case?

- A. SIADH
- B. Cerebral salt wasting
- C. Diabetes insipidus
- D. Dehydration
- E. Hypernatremia

▸▸ **Question 24**

Treatment of diabetes insipidus consists of which of the following?

- A. Desmopressin 0.1 mg per oral bd
- B. Nasal spray 2.5 μg by nasal insufflation bd
- C. Clofibrate
- D. Chlorpropamide
- E. All of the above

▸▸ **Question 25**

In nonambulatory comatose patient, treatment of diabetes insipidus consists of what?

- A. Admission in ICU with input–output monitoring every 1 hour, urine specific gravity every 4 hours
- B. Measure serum electrolytes with osmolality every 6 hours
- C. Baseline fluid D5 ½ NS plus 20 mEq/L at 75 to 100 mL/h
- D. Arginine vasopressin
- E. All of the above

Answers

▸▸ **Answer 1**

Correct answer is E. 125[1]

▸▸ **Answer 2**

Correct answer is B. Renal failure[2]

▸▸ **Answer 3**

Correct answer is A. 48 hours[2]

▸▸ **Answer 4**

Correct answer is D. Volume status[3]

▸▸ **Answer 5**

Correct answer is D. Increased thyroid stimulating hormone (TSH) level[3]

▸▸ **Answer 6**

Correct answer is B. 600[4]

▸▸ **Answer 7**

Correct answer is C. 8–10 mEq/L in 24 hours[3]

▸▸ **Answer 8**

Correct answer is B. Central pontine myelinolysis[4]

▸▸ **Answer 9**

Correct answer is E. Furosemide[5]

▸▸ **Answer 10**

Correct answer is E. Fludrocortisone acetate[5]

▸▸ Answer 11

Correct answer is E. 24 hours[6]

▸▸ Answer 12

Correct answer is A. < 5% increase[7]

▸▸ Answer 13

Correct answer is D. Hyponatremia[8]

▸▸ Answer 14

Correct answer is B. ½ Normal saline[7]

▸▸ Answer 15

Correct answer is B. 10 µg[9]

▸▸ Answer 16

Correct answer is C. Syndrome of inappropriate antidiuretic hormone secretion (SIADH)[1]

▸▸ Answer 17

Correct answer is B. Cerebral salt wasting[1]

▸▸ Answer 18

Correct answer is E. All of the above[10]

▸▸ Answer 19

Correct answer is C. Extracellular fluid volume depletion[2]

▸▸ Answer 20

Correct answer is A. Osmotic demyelination syndrome[4]

▸▸ Answer 21

Correct answer is E. A, B, and C[11]

▸▸ Answer 22

Correct answer is C. Hyperchloremic acidosis[6]

▸▸ Answer 23

Correct answer is C. Diabetes insipidus[6]

▸▸ Answer 24

Correct answer is E. All of the above[7]

▸▸ Answer 25

Correct answer is E. All of the above[7]

References

[1] Greenberg M, ed. Greenberg's Handbook of Neurosurgery. 10th ed. New York: Thieme; 2023:114
[2] Greenberg M, ed. Greenberg's Handbook of Neurosurgery. 10th ed. New York: Thieme; 2023:117
[3] Greenberg M, ed. Greenberg's Handbook of Neurosurgery. 10th ed. New York: Thieme; 2023:118
[4] Greenberg M, ed. Greenberg's Handbook of Neurosurgery. 10th ed. New York: Thieme; 2023:119
[5] Greenberg M, ed. Greenberg's Handbook of Neurosurgery. 10th ed. New York: Thieme; 2023:123
[6] Greenberg M, ed. Greenberg's Handbook of Neurosurgery. 10th ed. New York: Thieme; 2023:124
[7] Greenberg M, ed. Greenberg's Handbook of Neurosurgery. 10th ed. New York: Thieme; 2023:128
[8] Greenberg M, ed. Greenberg's Handbook of Neurosurgery. 10th ed. New York: Thieme; 2023:126
[9] Greenberg M, ed. Greenberg's Handbook of Neurosurgery. 10th ed. New York: Thieme; 2023:129
[10] Greenberg M, ed. Greenberg's Handbook of Neurosurgery. 10th ed. New York: Thieme; 2023:116
[11] Greenberg M, ed. Greenberg's Handbook of Neurosurgery. 10th ed. New York: Thieme; 2023:121

6 General Neurocritical Care

Questions

▸▸ Question 1

Labetalol is α1 selective and β nonselective blocker. Its effects include ICP reduction or no change, pulse rate decrease or no change, and it does not change cardiac output. What is the dose adjustment for renal failure?

- A. Same dose
- B. < 15%
- C. < 25%
- D. < 50%
- E. Absolutely contraindicated

▸▸ Question 2

Dopamine has α, β, and dopaminergic effects at what dose (μg/kg/min)?

- A. 0.5
- B. 1
- C. 2
- D. > 5
- E. > 10

▸▸ Question 3

Which of the following is a pure alpha sympathomimetic and useful in hypotension associated with tachycardia?

- A. Dopamine
- B. Dobutamine
- C. Phenylephrine
- D. Norepinephrine
- E. Isoproterenol

▸▸ Question 4

What is the mainstay of treatment of rhabdomyolysis?

- A. Antiallergics
- B. Steroids
- C. Mannitol
- D. Sodium carbonate
- E. Expansion of extracellular volume

▸▸ Question 5

Dialysis may be required in patients with rhabdomyolysis in all of the following except?

- A. Oliguric renal failure
- B. Persistent hyperkalemia
- C. Pulmonary edema
- D. Congestive heart failure
- E. Persistent metabolic alkalosis

▸▸ Question 6

Labetalol (Normodyne or Trandate) is an alpha one selective and beta nonselective blocker drug. It is used intravenously as an antihypertensive drug in dosage sequence of 20, 40, 80, 80, and then 80 (total 300 mg) every 10 minutes until the desired blood pressure (BP) is achieved. It is widely used in neurosurgical patients because of which of the following characteristics?

- A. It has no effect on ICP or may reduce ICP
- B. It does not exacerbate coronary ischemia
- C. It does not change cardiac output
- D. It does not affect pulse rate much
- E. All of the above

▸▸ Question 7

Neurogenic shock, which occurs because of paralysis due to spinal cord injury, is caused by which of the following mechanisms?

- A. Dysrhythmias and myocardial infarction
- B. Pooling of blood in the venous capacitance vessels
- C. Because of hemorrhage due to spinal cord injury
- D. Disruption of neuronal signals below the level of injury
- E. All of the above

▸▸ Question 8

Positive inotropic (causing heart to contract with more force) effect of dopamine occurs at what dosage (μg/kg/min)?

- A. 0.5 to 2
- B. 2 to 10
- C. More than 10
- D. 10 to 20
- E. Less than 0.5

▸▸ Question 9

Which of the following drugs is avoided in neurogenic shock due to spinal cord injury?

- A. Dopamine
- B. Dobutamine
- C. Phenylephrine
- D. Norepinephrine
- E. All of the above

▸▸ Question 10

Stress ulcers AKA Cushing's ulcer can occur because of which of the following CNS pathologies?

- A. Brain injury (especially GCS less than 9)
- B. Brain tumor
- C. Intracerebral hemorrhage

- D. CNS infection
- E. All of the above

▸▸ **Question 11**

Acute kidney injury in rhabdomyolysis patient (a syndrome caused by injury to skeletal muscles) is because of which of the following mechanisms?

- A. Excessive ferrihemate which is formed from myoglobin released due to muscle injury at pH < 5.6
- B. Allergic reaction caused due to release of excessive myoglobin at the time of injury
- C. Renal vasoconstriction
- D. Decreased extracellular volume
- E. A, C, and D

▸▸ **Question 12**

Management of patient with rhabdomyolysis involves the following steps except?

- A. Admission in ICU, input–output monitoring, electrolytes correction
- B. Expansion of extracellular fluid volume by giving IV fluid
- C. Use of mannitol and sodium bicarbonate
- D. Minimizing other nephrotoxic agents like nephrotoxic antibiotic or iodinated IV contrast
- E. Surgical removal of the whole muscle causing rhabdomyolysis

▸▸ **Question 13**

Followings are the side effects of using omeprazole (Prilosec) for prolonged period of time except?

- A. Nausea, vomiting, and headache
- B. Vertigo
- C. Diarrhea
- D. Abdominal pain
- E. Rash

▸▸ **Question 14**

Dobutamine acts as vasodilator by acting on beta one receptors and as positive inotrope by acting on beta 2 receptors. Use of dobutamine at doses greater than 20 µg/kg/min can exacerbate what?

- A. Hypertension
- B. Myocardial ischemia
- C. Renal damage
- D. Hyperglycemia
- E. Hepatic failure

▸▸ **Question 15**

Which of the following crystalloids has less tendency to promote cerebral edema?

- A. Normal saline
- B. Ringer lactate
- C. 5% dextrose water
- D. 3% NaCl
- E. None of the above

Answers

▸▸ **Answer 1**

Correct answer is A. Same dose[1]

▸▸ **Answer 2**

Correct answer is E. > 10[2]

▸▸ **Answer 3**

Correct answer is C. Phenylephrine[3]

▸▸ **Answer 4**

Correct answer is E. Expansion of extracellular volume[4]

▸▸ **Answer 5**

Correct answer is E. Persistent metabolic alkalosis[5]

▸▸ **Answer 6**

Correct answer is E. All of the above[1]

▸▸ **Answer 7**

Correct answer is B. Pooling of blood in the venous capacitance vessels[2]

▸▸ **Answer 8**

Correct answer is B. 2 to 10[2]

▸▸ **Answer 9**

Correct answer is C. Phenylephrine[3]

▸▸ **Answer 10**

Correct answer is E. All of the above[3]

▸▸ **Answer 11**

Correct answer is E. A, C, and D[4]

▸▸ **Answer 12**

Correct answer is E. Surgical removal of the whole muscle causing rhabdomyolysis[4]

▸▸ **Answer 13**

Correct answer is B. Vertigo[6]

▸▸ **Answer 14**

Correct answer is B. Myocardial ischemia[2]

▸▸ **Answer 15**

Correct answer is A. Normal saline[2]

References

[1] Greenberg M, ed. Greenberg's Handbook of Neurosurgery. 10th ed. New York: Thieme; 2023:131

[2] Greenberg M, ed. Greenberg's Handbook of Neurosurgery. 10th ed. New York: Thieme; 2023:133

[3] Greenberg M, ed. Greenberg's Handbook of Neurosurgery. 10th ed. New York: Thieme; 2023:134

[4] Greenberg M, ed. Greenberg's Handbook of Neurosurgery. 10th ed. New York: Thieme; 2023:137

[5] Greenberg M, ed. Greenberg's Handbook of Neurosurgery. 10th ed. New York: Thieme; 2023:138

[6] Greenberg M, ed. Greenberg's Handbook of Neurosurgery. 10th ed. New York: Thieme; 2023:136

7 Sedatives, Paralytics, and Analgesics

Questions

▸▸ Question 1

Regarding Richmond agitation–sedation scale, an alert and calm patient will be given a score of what?

- A. 0
- B. 1
- C. 3
- D. 5
- E. 7

▸▸ Question 2

Propofol is a sedative hypnotic and a neuroprotectant. What is the maximum dose (µg/kg/min) for sedation?

- A. 1
- B. 5
- C. 10
- D. 25
- E. 50

▸▸ Question 3

Succinylcholine is an ultra-short muscle relaxant. Its onset is within 1 minute and duration of action is 5 to 10 minutes and spontaneous recovery occurs after long?

- A. 5 minutes
- B. 10 minutes
- C. 20 minutes
- D. 45 minutes
- E. 1 hour

▸▸ Question 4

Regarding analgesic properties of Aspirin, what is the maximum daily dose?

- A. 25 mg
- B. 50 mg
- C. 100 mg
- D. 1 g
- E. 4 g

▸▸ Question 5

For reduction of gastrointestinal side effects of NSAIDs, which of the following is most important?

- A. Taking before meals
- B. Taking with meals
- C. Taking after meals
- D. Antacids
- E. Misoprostol

▸▸ Question 6

A patient is admitted in neurosurgical ICU after sustaining head injury in a road traffic accident. The patient has to be mechanically ventilated but he/she is aggressive, trying to pull and remove tubes and catheters. The on-call doctor has to give sedation to this patient. After 20 minutes of giving sedation the patient is not responding to voice but shows movement or eye opening on physical stimulation. According to Richmond agitation-sedation scale (RASS), what are the agitation and sedation scores, respectively, in this patient?

- A. + 4, −4
- B. + 3, −3
- C. + 4, −3
- D. + 3, −4
- E. + 2, −3

▸▸ Question 7

Thiopental (Pentothal) is a short-acting barbiturate which is used for sedating patients. Following are the side effects of thiopental except?

- A. Dose-related respiratory depression
- B. Myocardial depression
- C. Damage to basal ganglia in brain
- D. Hypotension in hypovolemic patients
- E. Intra-arterial injection can cause necrosis

▸▸ Question 8

Propofol is a sedative hypnotic. It is used for sedation during general anesthesia and acts as neuroprotectant in aneurysm surgery at high doses. If a patient develops hyperkalemia, hepatomegaly, myocardial failure, renal failure, or death after propofol infusion then what is this condition called?

- A. Anaphylaxis reaction due to propofol infusion
- B. Multiorgan failure
- C. Propofol infusion reaction
- D. Propofol infusion syndrome
- E. All of the above

▸▸ Question 9

Following are the characteristics of nonsteroidal anti-inflammatory drugs (NSAIDs) except?

- A. No dependence develops with NSAIDs
- B. NSAIDs do not demonstrate a ceiling effect
- C. Risk of GI upset is common
- D. Most reversibly inhibit platelet function and prolong bleeding time
- E. All of them cause sodium and water retention and carry the risk of NSAID-induced nephrotoxicity

▸▸ Question 10

A patient presented in neurosurgical emergency with severe headache. He is given pain killer after which he develops respiratory depression. Which analgesic overdosage can cause this side effect?
- A. Ketorolac tromethamine (Toradol)
- B. Indomethacin
- C. Tramadol (Ultram)
- D. Naproxen sodium
- E. All of the above

▸▸ Question 11

For percutaneous rhizotomy in which the patient needs to be sedated and awakened repeatedly, which of the following sedative drugs is most suitable?
- A. Methohexital (Brevital)
- B. Thiopental (Pentothal)
- C. Remifentanil (Ultiva)
- D. Propofol
- E. Precede (Dexmedetomidine)

▸▸ Question 12

Precedex (Dexmetomidine), an alpha-2 adrenoceptor agonist, has both sedative and analgesic properties and dramatically reduces the risk of respiratory depression as well. It has to be with caution in the following patients except?
- A. In advanced heart block
- B. In basal bradycardia
- C. Using with other drug that lowers heart rate
- D. Hypovolemic patients
- E. Hypertensive patients

▸▸ Question 13

During intubation of a head injury patient in the emergency department, which of the following muscle relaxants can be used?
- A. Rocuronium (Zemuron)
- B. Cisatracurium (Nimbex)
- C. Succinylcholine (Anectin)
- D. Vecuronium (Norcuron)
- E. All of the above

▸▸ Question 14

Reversal of competitive muscle blockade is achieved by using neostigmine. What is its maximum dosage?
- A. 2.5 mg
- B. 5 mg
- C. 7.5 mg
- D. 10 mg
- E. 15 mg

▸▸ Question 15

For visceral or deafferentation pain, which of the following analgesics is used?
- A. Tricyclic antidepressants
- B. Tryptophan
- C. Carbamazepine
- D. Tegretol
- E. All of the above

Answers

▸▸ Answer 1

Correct answer is A. 0[1]

▸▸ Answer 2

Correct answer is E. 50[2]

▸▸ Answer 3

Correct answer is C. 20 minutes[3]

▸▸ Answer 4

Correct answer is E. 4 g[4]

▸▸ Answer 5

Correct answer is E. Misoprostol[5]

▸▸ Answer 6

Correct answer is D. + 3, −4[1]

▸▸ Answer 7

Correct answer is C. Damage to basal ganglia in brain[2]

▸▸ Answer 8

Correct answer is D. Propofol infusion syndrome[2]

▸▸ Answer 9

Correct answer is B. NSAIDs do not demonstrate a ceiling effect[5]

▸▸ Answer 10

Correct answer is C. Tramadol (Ultram)[6]

▸▸ Answer 11

Correct answer is A. Methohexital (Brevital)[1]

▸▸ Answer 12

Correct answer is E. Hypertensive patients[7]

▸▸ **Answer 13**

Correct answer is C. All of the above[8]

▸▸ **Answer 14**

Correct answer is B. 5 mg[8]

▸▸ **Answer 15**

Correct answer is E. All of the above[5]

References

[1] Greenberg M, ed. Greenberg's Handbook of Neurosurgery. 10th ed. New York: Thieme; 2023:139

[2] Greenberg M, ed. Greenberg's Handbook of Neurosurgery. 10th ed. New York: Thieme; 2023:140

[3] Greenberg M, ed. Greenberg's Handbook of Neurosurgery. 10th ed. New York: Thieme; 2023:142

[4] Greenberg M, ed. Greenberg's Handbook of Neurosurgery. 10th ed. New York: Thieme; 2023:145

[5] Greenberg M, ed. Greenberg's Handbook of Neurosurgery. 10th ed. New York: Thieme; 2023:144

[6] Greenberg M, ed. Greenberg's Handbook of Neurosurgery. 10th ed. New York: Thieme; 2023:147

[7] Greenberg M, ed. Greenberg's Handbook of Neurosurgery. 10th ed. New York: Thieme; 2023:141

[8] Greenberg M, ed. Greenberg's Handbook of Neurosurgery. 10th ed. New York: Thieme; 2023:143

8 Endocrinology

Questions

▸▸ Question 1

What is the mineralocorticoid potency of dexamethasone?
- A. 0
- B. 1 +
- C. 2 +
- D. 3 +
- E. 5 +

▸▸ Question 2

Regarding routine thyroid hormone replacement, what does levothyroxine contain?
- A. T3
- B. T4
- C. TSH
- D. TSH and T3
- E. TSH, T3, and T4

▸▸ Question 3

Posterior pituitary hormones—ADH and oxytocin—are synthesized in supraoptic and paraventricular nuclei of the hypothalamus in?
- A. Neuroendocrine neurons
- B. Neuroendocrine glands
- C. Median eminence of pituitary stalk
- D. Tuber cinereum
- E. Parvocellular system

▸▸ Question 4

Corticotropin also called adrenocorticotrophic hormone (ACTH) is a 39 amino acid trophic hormone synthesized from POMC. It has an active half-life of 10 minutes. It produces a diurnal peak in cortisol. When does the highest peak occur?
- A. Early morning
- B. Noon
- C. Afternoon
- D. 11 p.m.
- E. Midnight

▸▸ Question 5

What is the most powerful physiologic stimulus for ADH release?
- A. Increase in serum osmolality
- B. Hypokalemia
- C. Hyponatremia
- D. Hypoglycemia
- E. Pain

▸▸ Question 6

The posterior pituitary (neurohypophysis AKA pars nervosa) derives from downward evagination of neural crest cells (brain neuroectoderm) while the anterior pituitary (adenohypophysis) develops from an upward evagination of epithelial ectoderm of oropharynx. This upward evagination of ectoderm of oropharynx is known as?
- A. Median eminence
- B. Craniopharyngeal duct
- C. Rathke's pouch
- D. Remnants of Rathke's pouch
- E. Pars intermedius

▸▸ Question 7

The six hormones that are released from anterior pituitary are primarily formed in tuber cinereum nucleus while two hormones (ADH and oxytocin) that are released from posterior pituitary are primarily formed in magnocellular neuroendocrine neurons in the supraoptic and paraventricular nuclei. Where does these three nuclei reside?
- A. Thalamus
- B. Hypothalamus
- C. Basal ganglia
- D. Median eminence
- E. Both A and B

▸▸ Question 8

Growth hormone (GH) is under dual hypothalamic control via the hypophyseal portal system. GH releasing hormone from the arcuate nucleus stimulates synthesis and secretion of GH while GH release is suppressed by which of the following?
- A. Ghrelin, a peptide secreted by GI tract
- B. Somatostatin from the periventricular nucleus
- C. Insulin-like growth factor-1 synthesized by liver
- D. Somatomedin-C
- E. A and B

▸▸ Question 9

Antidiuretic hormone (ADH) AKA arginine vasopressin (AVP) is released from posterior pituitary gland into the systemic circulation. It causes increased reabsorption of water in kidneys and produces concentrated urine. What is the most powerful physiologic stimulus for ADH release?
- A. Reduction of intravascular volume
- B. Activation of thirst center in brain
- C. Increase in serum osmolality
- D. Reduction of water in interstitial spaces
- E. Both A and C

►► **Question 10**

Physiologic replacement therapy (in the absence of stress) for secondary adrenal insufficiency due to deficient corticotrophin (ACTH) release by pituitary is as follows:

- A. Hydrocortisone 10 mg PO a.m. and 20 mg PO p.m.
- B. Hydrocortisone 20 mg PO a.m. and 10 mg PO p.m.
- C. Hydrocortisone 25 mg PO a.m. and 10 mg PO p.m.
- D. Prednisone 5 mg PO every a.m. and 2.5 mg PO every p.m.
- E. Both B and D

►► **Question 11**

A patient presented with fatigue, anorexia, nausea, hypotension, and hypoglycemia in emergency. This patient was previously taking hydrocortisone for a long period for brain edema due to brain tumor, which was stopped abruptly. What is most likely cause of the symptoms in this patient?

- A. Exacerbation of brain edema
- B. Sudden increase in tumor size
- C. Steroid withdrawal
- D. Thyroid deficiency
- E. All of the above

►► **Question 12**

A patient on prolonged steroid use started developing side effects due to prolonged steroid usage. Following are the side effects of steroid except?

- A. Hypertension
- B. Hypokalemic acidosis
- C. Sodium and water retention
- D. Pseudotumor cerebri
- E. Progressive multifocal leukoencephalopathy

►► **Question 13**

A patient on prolonged steroid use develops flu and fever. He developed mental status changes, muscle weakness, and shock. Following are components of treatment of Addisonian crisis except?

- A. Admit the patient in ICU and give fluids for shock and dehydration
- B. Give hydrocortisone sodium (Solu-Cortef) 100 mg IV stat then 50 mg IV every 6 hours
- C. Desoxycorticosterone acetate 5 mg IM BID
- D. Draw serum for cortisol determination
- E. Methylprednisolone 1 g IV stat

►► **Question 14**

A patient with hypothyroidism has to undergo surgery. 0.05 mg levothyroxine is started in this patient. A few days later the patient developed confusion, lethargy, and hypotension. Which of the following is the possible cause of development of these symptoms?

- A. Development of symptoms of hypothyroidism
- B. Development of hyperthyroidism
- C. Adrenal insufficiency
- D. Hypercortisolism
- E. Brain damage

►► **Question 15**

Steroid stress dose on the day of elective surgery is 50 mg cortisone IM followed by 200 mg hydrocortisone IV infused over 24 hours. What is the steroid dose on postoperative day 1?

- A. 100 mg at 8 a.m., 50 mg at 4 p.m.
- B. 50 mg at 8 a.m., 25 mg at 4 p.m.
- C. 50 mg at 8 a.m., 25 mg at 4 p.m., 12.5 mg at 10 p.m.
- D. 50 mg at 8 a.m., 4 p.m., and 10 p.m.
- E. 100 mg at 8 a.m., 50 mg at 4 p.m., 50 mg at 10 p.m.

Answers

►► **Answer 1**

Correct answer is A. 0[1]

►► **Answer 2**

Correct answer is B. T4[2]

►► **Answer 3**

Correct answer is A. Neuroendocrine neurons[3]

►► **Answer 4**

Correct answer is A. Early morning[3]

►► **Answer 5**

Correct answer is A. Increase in serum osmolality[4]

►► **Answer 6**

Correct answer is C. Rathke's pouch[3]

►► **Answer 7**

Correct answer is B. Hypothalamus[3]

►► **Answer 8**

Correct answer is B. Somatostatin from the periventricular nucleus[4]

►► **Answer 9**

Correct answer is C. Increase in serum osmolality[4]

►► **Answer 10**

Correct answer is E. Both B and D[1]

▸▸ **Answer 11**

Correct answer is C. Steroid withdrawal[5]

▸▸ **Answer 12**

Correct answer is B. Hypokalemic acidosis[6]

▸▸ **Answer 13**

Correct answer is E. Methylprednisolone 1 g IV stat[7]

▸▸ **Answer 14**

Correct answer is C. Adrenal insufficiency[2]

▸▸ **Answer 15**

Correct answer is D. 50 mg at 8 a.m., 4 p.m., and 10 p.m.[6]

References

[1] Greenberg M, ed. Greenberg's Handbook of Neurosurgery. 10th ed. New York: Thieme; 2023:154
[2] Greenberg M, ed. Greenberg's Handbook of Neurosurgery. 10th ed. New York: Thieme; 2023:158
[3] Greenberg M, ed. Greenberg's Handbook of Neurosurgery. 10th ed. New York: Thieme; 2023:151
[4] Greenberg M, ed. Greenberg's Handbook of Neurosurgery. 10th ed. New York: Thieme; 2023:153
[5] Greenberg M, ed. Greenberg's Handbook of Neurosurgery. 10th ed. New York: Thieme; 2023:155
[6] Greenberg M, ed. Greenberg's Handbook of Neurosurgery. 10th ed. New York: Thieme; 2023:156
[7] Greenberg M, ed. Greenberg's Handbook of Neurosurgery. 10th ed. New York: Thieme; 2023:157

9 Hematology

Questions

▸▸ Question 1

What is the circulating blood volume (cc/kg) in adults?

- A. 1
- B. 25
- C. 50
- D. 75
- E. 100

▸▸ Question 2

Platelets may be store for up to how long?

- A. 5 days
- B. 10 days
- C. 2 weeks
- D. 3 weeks
- E. 1 month

▸▸ Question 3

Recommended transfusion criteria for cryoprecipitate include all except?

- A. Hemophilia A
- B. Von Willebrand's disease
- C. Documented fibrinogen/factor VIII deficiency
- D. Documented disseminated intravascular coagulation (DIC)
- E. Anemia

▸▸ Question 4

Regarding routine monitoring for rivaroxaban:

- A. PT daily
- B. aPTT daily
- C. INR on alternate days
- D. Bleeding time
- E. No monitoring required

▸▸ Question 5

For reversal of clopidogrel for emergency surgery, platelets may be given. But in cases with continued oozing in the first day or so after discontinuing clopidogrel, which of the following regimen can be started?

- A. Activated factor I
- B. Activated factor V
- C. Activated factor VII
- D. Activated factor XII
- E. Activated factor XIII

▸▸ Question 6

Treatment with which of the following is associated with Coumadin necrosis during the initial days?

- A. Heparin
- B. Warfarin
- C. Massive transfusion
- D. Aspirin
- E. Clopidogrel

▸▸ Question 7

What is a common side effect with chronic use of heparin?

- A. Osteoporosis
- B. Heparin-induced thrombocytopenia
- C. Blindness
- D. Ototoxicity
- E. Hypothyroidism

▸▸ Question 8

For reversal of heparin, what should be given to the patient?

- A. Packed red cell concentrate
- B. Protamine sulphate
- C. Steroids
- D. Vitamin K
- E. Triofiban

▸▸ Question 9

What is the test of choice for diagnosis of pulmonary embolism?

- A. Contrast-enhanced CT of the chest
- B. Postcontrast MRI of the chest
- C. Ultrasound of the chest
- D. Urinary fat globules
- E. Arterial blood gases

▸▸ Question 10

For treatment of pulmonary embolism, heparin is started. For an average 70 kg patient, begin with 5000 to 7500 unit IV bolus, followed by 1000 U/hour drip, and it is titrated by following what?

- A. PT
- B. aPTT
- C. INR
- D. Serum heparin levels
- E. Platelets count

▸▸ Question 11

An adult patient on aspirin comes in neurosurgical emergency with chronic subdural hematoma. He has reduced platelet count as well. Typical dosage of platelets for thrombocytopenic bleeding in adults is 6 to 10 U (where 1 U increases platelet count by 5k to 10k). All of the following are indications of platelet transfusion in a patient except?

- A. Platelet count (PC) less than 10k even if no bleeding
- B. PC less than 20k and bleeding
- C. PC less than 30k and the patient at risk of bleeding; for example, formation of petechiae, continuous bleeding from wound
- D. PC less than 50 and major surgery planned within 12 hours
- E. Patient on aspirin whose surgery can be postponed for 5 days

▸▸ Question 12

A patient on warfarin presented in neurosurgical emergency after road traffic accident. His CT of the brain showed extradural hematoma. On baseline investigations PT, APTT, and INR come out to be deranged. Which of the following are indications of transfusion of fresh frozen plasma (usual dosage of 2 bags equal to 400–600 mL) in a patient?

- A. PT > 18 sec, APTT > 55 sec or INR > 1.6
- B. Previous history of coagulation factor deficiency; for example, factor 2, 5, 7, 10, 11, or 12
- C. Patient taking warfarin and needs emergent surgery
- D. Deficiency of antithrombin 3, protein C, or protein S
- E. All of the above

▸▸ Question 13

All of the following are contraindications to full anticoagulation with heparin except?

- A. Recent severe head injury
- B. Recent craniotomy
- C. Hemorrhagic infarction
- D. Uncontrollable hypertension
- E. Intracranial hypertension due to sinus thrombosis

▸▸ Question 14

Use of warfarin during pregnancy can cause spontaneous abortion and stillbirth. Its use during the first trimester can also cause fetal warfarin syndrome which includes all of the following except?

- A. Scoliosis
- B. Polydactyly
- C. Vertebral column calcifications
- D. Ventriculomegaly
- E. Agenesis of corpus callosum

▸▸ Question 15

A diabetic elderly woman on low-molecular-weight heparin had to undergo an orthopedic procedure at bilateral hip joint. She was given spinal anesthesia for this purpose. After surgery she was given NSAIDs for pain control. The patient developed paralysis of lower limbs after surgery. What can be the possible cause of this?

- A. Damage to bilateral sciatic nerve during surgery
- B. Damage to cord due to wrong-level spinal injunction
- C. Spinal shock due to cord damage during spinal anesthesia
- D. Spinal epidural hematoma
- E. None of the above

▸▸ Question 16

Desmopressin (DDAVP) can be used to increase coagulation activity in the following cases except?

- A. Mild hemophilia A
- B. Von Willebrand's disease type 1
- C. Von Willebrand's disease type 2B
- D. In minor procedures
- E. None of the above

▸▸ Question 17

A patient presents in neurosurgical emergency after road traffic accident with diagnosis of diffuse axonal injury. He has low GCS and is sedated. After some hours he develops diffuse bleeding, petechial hemorrhage, and shock. His lab shows increased PT and APTT and reduced platelets. What is the possible cause of these symptoms in this patient?

- A. Idiopathic thrombocytopenic purpura
- B. Heavy sedation given during intubation
- C. Blood reaction to given medication
- D. Head trauma causing release of thromboplastin into circulation
- E. None of the above

▸▸ Question 18

Q18. Why are neurosurgical patients particularly prone to developing DVTs?

- A. Long operation time of some procedures
- B. Alteration in coagulation status
- C. Use of high doses of steroids
- D. Increased blood viscosity with dehydration and volume loss
- E. All of the above

▸▸ Question 19

An obese patient aged 50 years with brain tumor and bed ridden underwent extensive surgery for a duration 3 hours. What is the estimated risk of calf DVT formation in this patient?

- A. Low risk
- B. Moderately low risk
- C. Moderate risk
- D. Moderately high risk
- E. High risk

▸▸ Question 20

A patient presents with thalassemia major with bilateral weakness in lower limbs from last 3 months. Spinal cord compression is because of enlarged vertebral bodies due to extramedullary hematopoiesis. Following are recommended treatments of this condition except?

- A. Surgical excision with total removal
- B. Surgery followed by radiotherapy
- C. Repeated blood transfusions
- D. Laminectomy and decompression

Answers

▸▸ Answer 1

Correct answer is D. 75[1]

▸▸ Answer 2

Correct answer is A. 5 days[2]

▸▸ Answer 3

Correct answer is E. Anemia[3]

▸▸ Answer 4

Correct answer is E. No monitoring required[4]

▸▸ Answer 5

Correct answer is C. Activated factor VII[5]

▸▸ Answer 6

Correct answer is B. Warfarin[6]

▸▸ Answer 7

Correct answer is A. Osteoporosis[6]

▸▸ Answer 8

Correct answer is B. Protamine sulphate[7]

▸▸ Answer 9

Correct answer is A. Contrast-enhanced CT of the chest[8]

▸▸ Answer 10

Correct answer is B. aPTT[8]

▸▸ Answer 11

Correct answer is E. Patient on aspirin whose surgery can be postponed for 5 days[2]

▸▸ Answer 12

Correct answer is E. All of the above[9]

▸▸ Answer 13

Correct answer is E. Intracranial hypertension due to sinus thrombosis[3]

▸▸ Answer 14

Correct answer is B. Polydactyly[6]

▸▸ Answer 15

Correct answer is D. Spinal epidural hematoma[10]

▸▸ Answer 16

Correct answer is C. Von Willebrand's disease type 2B[11]

▸▸ Answer 17

Correct answer is E. None of the above[12]

▸▸ Answer 18

Correct answer is E. All of the above[12]

▸▸ Answer 19

Correct answer is E. High risk[13]

▸▸ Answer 20

Correct answer is D. Laminectomy and decompression[14]

References

[1] Greenberg M, ed. Greenberg's Handbook of Neurosurgery. 10th ed. New York: Thieme; 2023:160
[2] Greenberg M, ed. Greenberg's Handbook of Neurosurgery. 10th ed. New York: Thieme; 2023:161
[3] Greenberg M, ed. Greenberg's Handbook of Neurosurgery. 10th ed. New York: Thieme; 2023:163
[4] Greenberg M, ed. Greenberg's Handbook of Neurosurgery. 10th ed. New York: Thieme; 2023:166
[5] Greenberg M, ed. Greenberg's Handbook of Neurosurgery. 10th ed. New York: Thieme; 2023:169
[6] Greenberg M, ed. Greenberg's Handbook of Neurosurgery. 10th ed. New York: Thieme; 2023:172
[7] Greenberg M, ed. Greenberg's Handbook of Neurosurgery. 10th ed. New York: Thieme; 2023:174
[8] Greenberg M, ed. Greenberg's Handbook of Neurosurgery. 10th ed. New York: Thieme; 2023:179
[9] Greenberg M, ed. Greenberg's Handbook of Neurosurgery. 10th ed. New York: Thieme; 2023:162

[10] Greenberg M, ed. Greenberg's Handbook of Neurosurgery. 10th ed. New York: Thieme; 2023:173
[11] Greenberg M, ed. Greenberg's Handbook of Neurosurgery. 10th ed. New York: Thieme; 2023:175
[12] Greenberg M, ed. Greenberg's Handbook of Neurosurgery. 10th ed. New York: Thieme; 2023:176
[13] Greenberg M, ed. Greenberg's Handbook of Neurosurgery. 10th ed. New York: Thieme; 2023:177
[14] Greenberg M, ed. Greenberg's Handbook of Neurosurgery. 10th ed. New York: Thieme; 2023:180

10 Neurology for Neurosurgeons

Questions

▸▸ Question 1

Regarding types of migraine, which of the following is a migraine with neurologic symptoms (nausea, vomiting, visual aura) without headache?

- A. Classic migraine
- B. Common migraine
- C. Hemiplegic migraine
- D. Migraine equivalent
- E. Histaminic migraine

▸▸ Question 2

For idiopathic paralysis agitans (IPA), what is the hallmark histological feature?

- A. Lewy bodies
- B. Psammoma bodies
- C. Ki67 index
- D. Stellate microglia
- E. Bence Jones proteins

▸▸ Question 3

Which of the following is classic idiopathic paralysis agitans IPA plus amyotrophic lateral sclerosis (ALS)?

- A. Parkinson-dementia complex of Guam
- B. Riley-Day
- C. Huntington's disease (HD)
- D. Shy-Drager syndrome
- E. Olivopontocerebellar degeneration (OPC)

▸▸ Question 4

Multiple sclerosis is an idiopathic demyelinating disease of the central nervous system producing exacerbating and remitting symptoms that are disseminated in space and time. The McDonald criteria are utilized for the diagnosis. What is the most common finding in CSF analysis?

- A. Raised opening pressure
- B. WBC count > 1000
- C. Proteins > 150
- D. Oligoclonal bands
- E. Mib-I

▸▸ Question 5

Amyotrophic lateral sclerosis is degeneration of anterior horn cells and corticospinal tracts in the cervical spine and medulla. The definitive treatment includes which of the following?

- A. Surgery
- B. Radiotherapy
- C. Antiviral
- D. Antibiotics
- E. None

▸▸ Question 6

Regarding the diagnosis of Guillain-Barre syndrome, which of the following is a universal feature?

- A. Sensory deficit
- B. Areflexia
- C. CSF pleocytosis
- D. Periventricular calcifications
- E. Unilateral facial nerve palsy

▸▸ Question 7

Treatment of Guillain-Barre syndrome includes which of the following?

- A. Steroids
- B. Immunoglobulins
- C. Antivirals
- D. Serial LP drainage
- E. Frontal lobectomy

▸▸ Question 8

For treatment of acute transverse myelitis, which of the following has no role?

- A. Steroids
- B. Plasma exchange
- C. Cyclophosphamide
- D. Surgery
- E. Radiotherapy

▸▸ Question 9

Which of the following is the most common neurologic manifestation of neurosarcoidosis?

- A. Diabetes insipidus
- B. Intracranial hypotension
- C. Foix-Alajouanine syndrome
- D. Radiculopathy
- E. Sudden-onset blindness

▸▸ Question 10

Regarding treatment of neurosarcoidosis, which of the following has no role?

- A. Steroids
- B. Surgery

- C. Radiotherapy
- D. Methotrexate
- E. Antivirals

▸▸ Question 11

A patient presents in OPD with history of headache with nausea, vomiting, and photophobia. The patient also complains of pungent smell before start of headache. Along with headache the patient also has occasional neurologic deficit that resolves spontaneously within 24 hours. What kind of headache this patient has?

- A. Common migraine
- B. Classic migraine
- C. Complicated migraine
- D. Migraine equivalent
- E. Cluster headache

▸▸ Question 12

Patients with parkinsonism can be treated with surgery. Previously stereotactic thalamotomy used to be done for parkinsonism which relieves tremor more than bradykinesia. Which nucleus of thalamus is targeted during this procedure?

- A. Anterolateral
- B. Posterolateral
- C. Ventrolateral
- D. Medial geniculate nucleus
- E. Lateral geniculate nucleus

▸▸ Question 13

Multiple sclerosis is an idiopathic demyelinating disease of the CNS, disseminated in time and space, with classic clinical findings of optic neuritis, paresthesias, and bladder symptoms. Which of the following is the most common pattern of multiple sclerosis at onset?

- A. Relapsing remitting
- B. Secondary progressive
- C. Primary progressive
- D. Progressive relapsing
- E. None of the above

▸▸ Question 14

A patient presents in OPD with slowly progressive weakness and atrophy in hands. With time the patient developed spasticity in lower extremities. The patient also developed dysarthria and dysphagia along with tongue atrophy. EMG showed fibrillation potentials in tongue and slightly elevated protein in CSF. What is the most likely diagnosis in this patient?

- A. Cervical spondylotic myelopathy
- B. Motor neuron disease
- C. Amyotrophic lateral sclerosis
- D. Primary lateral sclerosis
- E. Progressive muscular and spinal atrophy

▸▸ Question 15

A patient presents in emergency with weakness in lower extremities that is symmetrical in both limbs and occurred some days after sore throat. The patient gives history of slight weakness in upper limbs as well with no sensory symptoms in upper or lower limbs. CSF examination shows elevated protein. What is the most likely diagnosis in this patient?

- A. Motor neuron disease
- B. Myasthenia gravis
- C. Guillain-Barre syndrome
- D. Myelitis
- E. Parkinson disease

▸▸ Question 16

A patient presented with backache in the midthoracic region that progressed in 24 hours to muscles weakness in lower extremities. With time it involved sensory system and sphincter disturbance as well. He was diagnosed with acute transverse myelitis. What are treatment options in this patient?

- A. Steroids
- B. Plasma exchange
- C. Immune suppression
- D. Surgical decompression
- E. All of the above

▸▸ Question 17

A patient presents in neurosurgical OPD with multiple cranial nerve palsies. Progressively he developed hydrocephalus and diabetes insipidus. CSF showed increased pressure with elevated protein and mild eosinophilia. Chest X-ray showed lymph node enlargement. What is the most likely disease in this patient?

- A. Hodgkin's disease
- B. CNS lymphoma
- C. Sarcoidosis
- D. Pseudotumor cerebri
- E. None of the above

▸▸ Question 18

Parkinsonism is because of degeneration of substantia nigra which results in reduced levels of what?

- A. Acetylcholine
- B. Dopamine
- C. GABA
- D. Serotonin
- E. Glutamic acid

▸▸ Question 19

Following are the sensory findings in multiple sclerosis except?

- A. Loss of proprioception

- B. Paresthesias of extremities
- C. Lhermitte's sign
- D. Trigeminal neuralgia
- E. Perianal anesthesia

▸▸ **Question 20**

What are the treatment options for Guillain-Barre syndrome?

- A. Immunoglobulins and plasmapheresis
- B. Steroids
- C. Cyclophosphamide
- D. Methotrexate
- E. All of the above

Answers

▸▸ **Answer 1**

Correct answer is D. Migraine equivalent[1]

▸▸ **Answer 2**

Correct answer is A. Lewy bodies[2]

▸▸ **Answer 3**

Correct answer is A. Parkinson-dementia complex of Guam[3]

▸▸ **Answer 4**

Correct answer is D. Oligoclonal bands[4]

▸▸ **Answer 5**

Correct answer is E. None[5]

▸▸ **Answer 6**

Correct answer is B. Areflexia[6]

▸▸ **Answer 7**

Correct answer is B. Immunoglobulins[7]

▸▸ **Answer 8**

Correct answer is E. Radiotherapy[8]

▸▸ **Answer 9**

Correct answer is A. Diabetes insipidus[9]

▸▸ **Answer 10**

Correct answer is E. Antivirals[10]

▸▸ **Answer 11**

Correct answer is B. Classic migraine[1]

▸▸ **Answer 12**

Correct answer is C. Ventrolateral[3]

▸▸ **Answer 13**

Correct answer is A. Relapsing remitting[4]

▸▸ **Answer 14**

Correct answer is C. Amyotrophic lateral sclerosis[11]

▸▸ **Answer 15**

Correct answer is C. Guillain-Barre syndrome[6]

▸▸ **Answer 16**

Correct answer is E. All of the above[8]

▸▸ **Answer 17**

Correct answer is C. Sarcoidosis[9]

▸▸ **Answer 18**

Correct answer is B. Dopamine[12]

▸▸ **Answer 19**

Correct answer is E. Perianal anesthesia[13]

▸▸ **Answer 20**

Correct answer is A. Immunoglobulins and plasmapheresis[7]

References

[1] Greenberg M, ed. Greenberg's Handbook of Neurosurgery. 10th ed. New York: Thieme; 2023:183
[2] Greenberg M, ed. Greenberg's Handbook of Neurosurgery. 10th ed. New York: Thieme; 2023:185
[3] Greenberg M, ed. Greenberg's Handbook of Neurosurgery. 10th ed. New York: Thieme; 2023:186
[4] Greenberg M, ed. Greenberg's Handbook of Neurosurgery. 10th ed. New York: Thieme; 2023:187
[5] Greenberg M, ed. Greenberg's Handbook of Neurosurgery. 10th ed. New York: Thieme; 2023:192
[6] Greenberg M, ed. Greenberg's Handbook of Neurosurgery. 10th ed. New York: Thieme; 2023:193
[7] Greenberg M, ed. Greenberg's Handbook of Neurosurgery. 10th ed. New York: Thieme; 2023:195
[8] Greenberg M, ed. Greenberg's Handbook of Neurosurgery. 10th ed. New York: Thieme; 2023:197

[9] Greenberg M, ed. Greenberg's Handbook of Neurosurgery. 10th ed. New York: Thieme; 2023:198
[10] Greenberg M, ed. Greenberg's Handbook of Neurosurgery. 10th ed. New York: Thieme; 2023:200
[11] Greenberg M, ed. Greenberg's Handbook of Neurosurgery. 10th ed. New York: Thieme; 2023:191
[12] Greenberg M, ed. Greenberg's Handbook of Neurosurgery. 10th ed. New York: Thieme; 2023:184
[13] Greenberg M, ed. Greenberg's Handbook of Neurosurgery. 10th ed. New York: Thieme; 2023:188

11 Neurovascular Disorders and Neurotoxicology

Questions

▸▸ Question 1

Other than addressing the underlying etiology, the treatment of posterior reversible encephalopathy syndrome (PRES) includes tight control of what?

- A. Glycemic levels
- B. Hemoglobin
- C. Hematocrit
- D. Blood pressure
- E. Input–output balance

▸▸ Question 2

In crossed cerebellar diaschisis, the cerebellar cortex contralateral to a cerebral hemispheric lesion suffers from what?

- A. Autoimmune destruction
- B. Hypometabolism
- C. Increased temperature
- D. Direct pressure effects
- E. Hypermyelination

▸▸ Question 3

Which of the following has the least role in the diagnosis of giant cell arteritis?

- A. Temporal artery biopsy
- B. CT angiography of temporal artery
- C. ESR
- D. CRP
- E. CBC showing mild normochromic anemia

▸▸ Question 4

Polymyalgia rheumatica (PMR) has an increased frequency of HLA-DR4 and systemic monocyte activation. 15% of patients with PMR eventually develop which of the following?

- A. Fibromuscular dysplasia
- B. Guillain-Barre syndrome
- C. Transverse myelitis
- D. Amyotrophic lateral sclerosis
- E. Giant cell arteritis

▸▸ Question 5

Periarteritis nodosa is a group of necrotizing vasculitides including classic periarteritis nodosa (PAN) and systemic necrotizing vasculitis. The treatment involves which of the following?

- A. Steroids
- B. Acetaminophen
- C. Cyclophosphamide
- D. Maintaining high urine output
- E. Avoiding latex

▸▸ Question 6

Relapsing ocular lesions and recurrent oral and genital ulcers, with occasional skin lesions, thrombophlebitis, arthritis, and headache is what?

- A. Polyarteritis nodosa
- B. Granulomatosis with polyangiitis
- C. Behcet syndrome
- D. Wegener granulomatosis
- E. Gustatory migraine

▸▸ Question 7

The gold standard test for the diagnosis of fibromuscular dysplasia is the angiogram, which shows multiple, irregularly spaced, concentric narrowings with normal or dilated intervening segments "string of pearls" in which type?

- A. I
- B. II
- C. III
- D. IV
- E. V

▸▸ Question 8

On day 5 of alcohol withdrawal, the patient presented with profound disorientation, agitation, tremor, insomnia, hallucinations, tachycardia, hypertension, diaphoresis, and fever. What is the most probable diagnosis?

- A. Delirium tremens
- B. Wernicke-Korsakoff syndrome
- C. Malignant hyperthermia
- D. Parkinsonism
- E. Acute dementia

▸▸ Question 9

Wernicke's encephalopathy is common in alcoholics. It has classical triad of encephalopathy, ophthalmoplegia, and ataxia. It is caused by deficiency of what?

- A. Iron
- B. Zinc
- C. Manganese
- D. Thiamine
- E. Thyroid stimulating hormone

▸▸ Question 10

A test dose of intravenous naloxone 0.2 mg avoids sudden complete reversal of all opioid effects. But reversal with naloxone may precipitate narcotic withdrawal symptoms in opioid-dependent patients who may require treatment with what?

- A. Vitamin B12

- B. Vitamin B6
- C. Octreotide
- D. Dopamine
- E. Clonidine

▸▸ Question 11

A patient presents in neurosurgical emergency with complaints of headache, seizures, and focal neurological deficit. CT and MRI of the brain were done which showed widespread vasogenic edema predominantly in parietal and occipital regions. This patient was diagnosed with posterior reversible encephalopathy syndrome (PRES) (also known as reversible posterior encephalopathy syndrome). Which of the following conditions are associated with this syndrome?

- A. Malignant hypertension
- B. Infection, sepsis, and shock
- C. Autoimmune disease like lupus, scleroderma, or polyarteritis nodosa
- D. Cancer chemotherapy
- E. All of the above

▸▸ Question 12

A patient presents in neurosurgical OPD with complaint of unilateral temporal headache from 1 year which progressed to jaw claudication and now decreased vision on the side of headache from last some days. On palpation, there is tenderness over temporal muscle on the side of headache. Biopsy of the frontal branch of superior temporal artery showed inflammatory infiltrates. What is the most likely treatment option of this condition?

- A. Immunomodulators
- B. High dose steroids
- C. Interleukin 1 inhibitors like anakinra or rilonacept
- D. Cyclophosphamide and methotrexate
- E. All of the above

▸▸ Question 13

A 70-year-old woman presents in neurosurgical OPD with complaints of fever, anorexia, weight loss, morning ache, and stiffness in the cervical region, shoulder, and pelvic girdle from last 2 months. On labs her ESR is more than 40 mm/h. She responded well to steroids. What is the most likely diagnosis in this patient?

- A. ANCA-associated vasculitis
- B. Atherosclerotic occlusive disease
- C. Wegener's granulomatosis
- D. Behcet's disease
- E. Polymyalgia rheumatica (PMR)

▸▸ Question 14

Granulomatosis with polyangiitis (GPA) formerly known as Wegener's granulomatosis is an ANCA-associated vasculitis which is treated with steroids, immune modulators, and antibodies. Which of the following are the most likely presenting symptoms of this condition?

- A. Isolated kidney involvement
- B. Joint stiffness, granulomas in kidneys, and respiratory involvement
- C. Multiple vessel disease with inflammatory infiltrates
- D. Cranial nerve involvement, peripheral neuropathies, and multiple joint pain
- E. Cough, hemoptysis, kidney involvement, cranial nerves involvement, and diabetes insipidus

▸▸ Question 15

A patient presents with relapsing ocular lesions, recurrent oral and genital ulcers, cerebellar ataxia, seizures, and pseudotumor cerebri. He is diagnosed with Behcet's disease. What is the most likely treatment in this condition?

- A. Steroids
- B. Cytotoxic agents
- C. Thalidomide
- D. Antiepileptics if seizures occur
- E. All of the above

▸▸ Question 16

Fibromuscular dysplasia (FMD) is a vasculopathy primarily affecting branches of aorta, renal artery, or internal carotid arteries with increased chances of stenosis, aneurysm formation, or dissection. The gold standard for the diagnosis of FMD is angiogram. What is the most common angiographic pattern seen in FMD?

- A. String of pearls appearance
- B. Focal tubular necrosis
- C. Atypical FMD with diverticular formation
- D. Type 4
- E. None of the above

▸▸ Question 17

Cerebral autosomal dominant arteriopathy with subcortical infarcts and leukoencephalopathy (CADASIL) is a type of vasculopathy with subcortical infarcts, progressive dementia, depression, and migraine. What is the treatment for this condition?

- A. Aspirin
- B. NSAID
- C. Steroids
- D. Warfarin
- E. Cyclophosphamide

▸▸ Question 18

Pan-cerebellar degeneration is a paraneoplastic syndrome which presents with vertigo, gait disturbance, ataxia, dysarthria, diplopia, and nystagmus. What is the most common primary which can cause this?

- A. Ovarian cancer
- B. Breast cancer
- C. Lung cancer
- D. Hodgkin's lymphoma
- E. All of the above

▸▸ Question 19

A chronic alcohol abuser decides to quit alcohol but begins to suffer from tremulousness, insomnia, autonomic hyperactivity, myalgias, and confusion. What is the mainstay of treatment of alcohol withdrawal syndrome?

- A. Benzodiazepines like chlordiazepoxide, lorazepam, diazepam
- B. Beta blockers like atenolol
- C. Phenobarbital
- D. Thiamine
- E. All of the above

▸▸ Question 20

A patient presents with gait ataxia, oculomotor abnormalities, vomiting, and fever. MRI of brain shows high signal intensities on T2WI and flair around the thalamus, floor of the 4th ventricle, and periaqueductal area. This patient is diagnosed with Wernicke's encephalopathy. What is the mainstay of treatment for this condition?

- A. IV glucose 100 mg for 5 days
- B. Steroids in high dosage
- C. Thiamine 100 mg IV or IM for 5 days
- D. Immune modulator drugs like cyclophosphamide
- E. Ventriculoperitoneal shunt placement

Answers

▸▸ Answer 1

Correct answer is D. Blood pressure[1]

▸▸ Answer 2

Correct answer is B. Hypometabolism[2]

▸▸ Answer 3

Correct answer is B. CT angiography of temporal artery[3]

▸▸ Answer 4

Correct answer is E. Giant cell arteritis[4]

▸▸ Answer 5

Correct answer is C. Cyclophosphamide[5]

▸▸ Answer 6

Correct answer is C. Behcet syndrome[5]

▸▸ Answer 7

Correct answer is A. I[6]

▸▸ Answer 8

Correct answer is A. Delirium tremens[7]

▸▸ Answer 9

Correct answer is D. Thiamine[7]

▸▸ Answer 10

Correct answer is E. Clonidine[8]

▸▸ Answer 11

Correct answer is E. All of the above[1]

▸▸ Answer 12

Correct answer is B. High dose steroids[4]

▸▸ Answer 13

Correct answer is E. Polymyalgia rheumatica (PMR)[4]

▸▸ Answer 14

Correct answer is E. Cough, hemoptysis, kidney involvement, cranial nerves involvement, and diabetes insipidus[9]

▸▸ Answer 15

Correct answer is E. All of the above[5]

▸▸ Answer 16

Correct answer is A. String of pearls appearance[6]

▸▸ Answer 17

Correct answer is D. Warfarin[10]

▸▸ Answer 18

Correct answer is E. All of the above[11]

▸▸ Answer 19

Correct answer is A. Benzodiazepines like chlordiazepoxide, lorazepam, diazepam[12]

▸▸ Answer 20

Correct answer is C. Thiamine 100 mg IV or IM for 5 days[8]

References

[1] Greenberg M, ed. Greenberg's Handbook of Neurosurgery. 10th ed. New York: Thieme; 2023:202
[2] Greenberg M, ed. Greenberg's Handbook of Neurosurgery. 10th ed. New York: Thieme; 2023:203
[3] Greenberg M, ed. Greenberg's Handbook of Neurosurgery. 10th ed. New York: Thieme; 2023:205
[4] Greenberg M, ed. Greenberg's Handbook of Neurosurgery. 10th ed. New York: Thieme; 2023:206
[5] Greenberg M, ed. Greenberg's Handbook of Neurosurgery. 10th ed. New York: Thieme; 2023:208
[6] Greenberg M, ed. Greenberg's Handbook of Neurosurgery. 10th ed. New York: Thieme; 2023:210
[7] Greenberg M, ed. Greenberg's Handbook of Neurosurgery. 10th ed. New York: Thieme; 2023:214
[8] Greenberg M, ed. Greenberg's Handbook of Neurosurgery. 10th ed. New York: Thieme; 2023:215
[9] Greenberg M, ed. Greenberg's Handbook of Neurosurgery. 10th ed. New York: Thieme; 2023:207
[10] Greenberg M, ed. Greenberg's Handbook of Neurosurgery. 10th ed. New York: Thieme; 2023:211
[11] Greenberg M, ed. Greenberg's Handbook of Neurosurgery. 10th ed. New York: Thieme; 2023:212
[12] Greenberg M, ed. Greenberg's Handbook of Neurosurgery. 10th ed. New York: Thieme; 2023:213

Part III

Imaging and Diagnostics

III

12 Plain Radiology and Contrast Agents

Questions

▸▸ **Question 1**

Which of the following marks the anterior limit of spinal canal?

- A. Anterior marginal line
- B. Middle marginal line
- C. Posterior marginal line
- D. Posterior spinal line
- E. Spinolaminar line

▸▸ **Question 2**

What is the average normal anterior dentate interval in adult male?

- A. < 3 mm
- B. 7 mm
- C. 9 mm
- D. 11 mm
- E. 15 mm

▸▸ **Question 3**

On cervical spine anteroposterior X-ray, a fracture-dislocation or ligament disruption may be diagnosed if the interspinous distance (measured from center of spinous processes) relative to that at both adjacent levels is what?

- A. 0.25 times
- B. 0.5 times
- C. Equal
- D. > 1.5 times
- E. Not related

▸▸ **Question 4**

In C2 vertebra, how many primary ossification centers are there at birth?

- A. 1
- B. 2
- C. 3
- D. 4
- E. 5

▸▸ **Question 5**

Butterfly vertebra is an uncommon congenital anomaly thought to arise from failure of fusion of the lateral halves of the vertebral bodies due to persistent notochord tissue on AP X-rays or coronal CT scan reconstructions. On lateral views, what may it mimic?

- A. Locked facets
- B. Burst fracture
- C. Compression fracture
- D. Fracture dislocation
- E. Teardrop fracture

▸▸ **Question 6**

For basilar invagination, what is the line drawn across foramen magnum (basion to opisthion)?

- A. McRae's line
- B. Chamberlain's line
- C. McGregor's baseline
- D. Wackenheim's clivus-canal line
- E. Fischgold's digastric line

▸▸ **Question 7**

For basilar invagination, posterior hard palate to posterior margin of foramen magnum-opisthion is what?

- A. McRae's line
- B. Chamberlain's line
- C. McGregor's baseline
- D. Wackenheim's clivus-canal line
- E. Fischgold's digastric line

▸▸ **Question 8**

What is the primary approved contrast agent for intrathecal use?

- A. Iohexol
- B. Iopromide
- C. Ioversol
- D. Iodixanol
- E. Ultravist

▸▸ **Question 9**

What is the U.S. Nuclear Regulatory Commission (NRC) recommended maximal annual occupational dose limits for radiation (rem/y) for whole body?

- A. 5
- B. 10
- C. 15
- D. 20
- E. 50

▸▸ **Question 10**

For minimizing the occupational radiation exposure, ALARA ("As Low As Reasonably Achievable") involves making every reasonable effort to keep radiation dose as far below the limits as possible and it is believed that lead aprons and shields may or may not work, but distance always works. What distance (ft) the American Association of Neurological Surgeons (AANS) has recommended to be kept?

- A. 1
- B. 2
- C. 3
- D. 5
- E. 10

▸▸ **Question 11**

On lateral c spine X-ray, there are four contour lines which normally form smooth gentle curve. Which of these four lines forms the anterior margin of spinal canal?

- A. Anterior marginal line along the anterior cortical surface
- B. Posterior marginal line along the posterior cortical surface
- C. Spinolaminar line
- D. Posterior spinous line
- E. None of above

▸▸ **Question 12**

According to the rule of Spence, the transverse atlantal ligament (TAL) is probably disrupted if the sum total overhang of both C1 lateral masses over C2 is more than or equal to what?

- A. 3 cm
- B. 5 cm
- C. 7 cm
- D. 9 cm
- E. 11 cm

▸▸ **Question 13**

Posterior atlantodental interval, which is the distance from the back of odontoid to the anterior aspect of posterior C1 arch, forms the spinal canal diameter at this level. Stenosis of cervical spinal canal is present if the canal diameter is less than what?

- A. 10 mm
- B. 11 mm
- C. 12 mm
- D. 13 mm
- E. 15 mm

▸▸ **Question 14**

Which of the following statements is true?

- A. On oblique X-ray view of lumbar sacral spine, discontinuation in the neck of scotty dog shows defect of spinous process
- B. AP X-ray view of lumbar sacral spine: nonvisualization of owl's eyes shows pedicle erosion which is due to lytic tumor
- C. Butterfly vertebra is due to failure of fusion of two halves of posterior vertebral arches
- D. In axis vertebrae, the anterior synchondroses normally fuse between 6 and 9 years of age
- E. All of the above statements are correct

▸▸ **Question 15**

The depth and length of the sella turcica on lateral view of normal skull X-ray are 8.1 and 10.6 mm, respectively. How does pituitary adenoma changes the dimensions of sella turcica?

- A. It tends to enlarge the sella
- B. It erodes posterior clinoids and does not enlarge sella
- C. It balloons the sella symmetrically
- D. It does not enlarge sella but causes enlargement of sphenoid sinus
- E. None of the above

▸▸ **Question 16**

Basilar invagination/basilar impression (BI) is upward displacement of odontoid process through foramen magnum into the posterior fossa. Which of the following is best statement regarding BI?

- A. Basilar impression implies abnormal softening of skull base bones with atlantooccipital fusion
- B. Basilar invagination means normal skull base bones
- C. Platybasia is abnormal basal angle at skull base with > 145 degrees angle
- D. Type 1 BI means BI with Chiari malformation
- E. Type 2 BI denotes BI without Chiari malformation

▸▸ **Question 17**

McRae's line is drawn from basion to opisthion and it is used in measurements in basilar invagination (BI). What is the relationship of odontoid tip with this line for excluding the diagnosis of BI?

- A. No part of odontoid tip should be above this line
- B. Dens should not be more than 3 mm above this line
- C. Dens should not be more than 4.5 mm above this line
- D. Odontoid tip should be 3 mm below this line
- E. None of the above

▸▸ **Question 18**

Which of the following conditions are associated with basilar invagination (BI)?

- A. Congenital conditions like Down syndrome, Klippel-Feil syndrome, Chiari malformation, or syringomyelia
- B. Acquired conditions like rheumatoid arthritis
- C. Post-traumatic
- D. Conditions with softening of bone like Paget's disease, osteogenesis imperfecta, osteomalacia, rickets, or hyperparathyroidism
- E. All of the above

▸▸ **Question 19**

What medication can be used in a patient going to use intravenous contrast agent with previous history of mild reaction with iodinated contrast medium for prevention of reaction again?

- A. Prednisone 50 mg po
- B. Solumedrol 25 mg IV

- C. Diphenhydramine 50 mg IM
- D. Hydrocortisone 100 mg IV
- E. All of the above

Answers

▸▸ **Answer 1**

Correct answer is C. Posterior marginal line[1]

▸▸ **Answer 2**

Correct answer is A. < 3 mm[2]

▸▸ **Answer 3**

Correct answer is D. > 1.5 times[3]

▸▸ **Answer 4**

Correct answer is D. 4[4]

▸▸ **Answer 5**

Correct answer is C. Compression fracture[5]

▸▸ **Answer 6**

Correct answer is A. McRae's line[6]

▸▸ **Answer 7**

Correct answer is B. Chamberlain's line[6]

▸▸ **Answer 8**

Correct answer is A. Iohexol[7]

▸▸ **Answer 9**

Correct answer is A. 5[8]

▸▸ **Answer 10**

Correct answer is E. 10[8]

▸▸ **Answer 11**

Correct answer is B. Posterior marginal line along the posterior cortical surface[1]

▸▸ **Answer 12**

Correct answer is C. 7 cm[2]

▸▸ **Answer 13**

Correct answer is C. 12 mm[3]

▸▸ **Answer 14**

Correct answer is B. AP X-ray view of lumbar sacral spine: nonvisualization of owl's eyes shows pedicle erosion which is due to lytic tumor[4]

▸▸ **Answer 15**

Correct answer is A. It tends to enlarge the sella[5]

▸▸ **Answer 16**

Correct answer is C. Platybasia is abnormal basal angle at skull base with > 145 degrees angle[6]

▸▸ **Answer 17**

Correct answer is A. No part of odontoid tip should be above this line[6]

▸▸ **Answer 18**

Correct answer is E. All of the above[9]

▸▸ **Answer 19**

Correct answer is E. All of the above[10]

References

[1] Greenberg M, ed. Greenberg's Handbook of Neurosurgery. 10th ed. New York: Thieme; 2023:222
[2] Greenberg M, ed. Greenberg's Handbook of Neurosurgery. 10th ed. New York: Thieme; 2023:223
[3] Greenberg M, ed. Greenberg's Handbook of Neurosurgery. 10th ed. New York: Thieme; 2023:224
[4] Greenberg M, ed. Greenberg's Handbook of Neurosurgery. 10th ed. New York: Thieme; 2023:226
[5] Greenberg M, ed. Greenberg's Handbook of Neurosurgery. 10th ed. New York: Thieme; 2023:227
[6] Greenberg M, ed. Greenberg's Handbook of Neurosurgery. 10th ed. New York: Thieme; 2023:228
[7] Greenberg M, ed. Greenberg's Handbook of Neurosurgery. 10th ed. New York: Thieme; 2023:230
[8] Greenberg M, ed. Greenberg's Handbook of Neurosurgery. 10th ed. New York: Thieme; 2023:235
[9] Greenberg M, ed. Greenberg's Handbook of Neurosurgery. 10th ed. New York: Thieme; 2023:229
[10] Greenberg M, ed. Greenberg's Handbook of Neurosurgery. 10th ed. New York: Thieme; 2023:232

13 Imaging and Angiography

Questions

▸▸ Question 1

Originally, axial CT scan slices were taken parallel to the orbitomeatal line which connects the lateral canthus of the eye to the midpoint of the external auditory meatus. Current volumetric CT scanners tend to create axial slices parallel to what?
- A. McRae's line
- B. Chamberlain's line
- C. AC-PC line
- D. McGregor's baseline
- E. Wackenheim's clivus-canal line

▸▸ Question 2

A noncontrast CT scan is usually employed in emergency situations for diagnosis and screening. However, diffusion-weighted (DWI) MRI is preferred in which of the following?
- A. Acute stroke
- B. Subarachnoid hemorrhage
- C. Intraparenchymal hemorrhage
- D. Acute subdural hemorrhage
- E. Pneumocephalus

▸▸ Question 3

For CT perfusion to assess cerebral blood volume and flow, which of the following tests is used?
- A. Acetazolamide challenge test
- B. Dexamethasone challenge test
- C. Insulin tolerance test
- D. Oral glucose tolerance test
- E. Water deprivation

▸▸ Question 4

In fluid-attenuated inversion recovery (FLAIR), the gray/white intensity pattern is reversed from T1WI and it resembles a T2WI except the CSF which is more what?
- A. Bright
- B. Hyperintense
- C. Same density
- D. Dark
- E. White

▸▸ Question 5

Regarding gradient echo MRI, which of the following appears white?
- A. Bone
- B. Calcium
- C. Heavy metals
- D. Intraparenchymal blood
- E. CSF

▸▸ Question 6

Which of the following is the most sensitive study for ischemia of the brain?
- A. DWI MRI
- B. Fluid-attenuated inversion recovery (FLAIR)
- C. Perfusion-weighted (PWI) MRI
- D. CT of brain with intrathecal contrast
- E. EEG

▸▸ Question 7

Regarding peaks on magnetic resonance spectroscopy (MRS), which of the following is the marker of membrane synthesis?
- A. Lipid
- B. Acetate
- C. Creatinine
- D. Choline
- E. N-acetyl aspartate

▸▸ Question 8

Which of the following is the most useful to permit planning surgical approaches that minimize disruption of critical white matter tracts during brain surgery for deep lesions?
- A. DWI MRI
- B. Fluid-attenuated inversion recovery (FLAIR)
- C. PWI MRI
- D. Diffusion tensor imaging (DTI) MRI
- E. Proton magnetic resonance spectroscopy (MRS)

▸▸ Question 9

Usual convention for color coding tracts on diffusion tensor imaging (DTI). Superior longitudinal fasciculus is colored what?
- A. Red
- B. Blue
- C. Green
- D. White
- E. Black

▸▸ Question 10

Three-phase bone scan uses technetium 99m-HDP and has three phases: flow phase, blood pooling, and bone imaging. Osteomyelitis causes increased uptake in which phase?

- A. 1st phase
- B. 2nd phase
- C. 3rd phase
- D. All three phases
- E. No intake

▸▸ Question 11

Attenuation of the X-ray beam on a CT scan is quantified in Hounsfield units. What are the Hounsfield units for air and dense bone, respectively?

- A. + 1000, −1000
- B. −1000, + 1000
- C. −100, + 100
- D. + 5, −5
- E. 0, + 1000

▸▸ Question 12

CT perfusion (CTP) uses iodinated contrast (40 mL IV at 5 mL/sec) in which scans are repeated through region of interest at small intervals. Acetazolamide challenge is given (1000 mg IV) and scans are repeated at intervals again. Which of the following parameters can be calculated by this method?

- A. Cerebral blood volume
- B. Cerebral blood flow
- C. Mean transit time
- D. Time to peak
- E. All of the above

▸▸ Question 13

The radiation dose to a fetus from head or cervical spine CT is small and can be reduced by lead shielding. The risk from fetal exposure to X-rays is highest during which time of pregnancy?

- A. The first 2 weeks of gestation
- B. Between 8 and 16 weeks of gestation
- C. In the first 3 months of gestation
- D. In the 4th and 5th months of gestation
- E. Both A and B

▸▸ Question 14

Following statements are correct regarding T1WI MRI except?

- A. Fat including bone marrow, blood > 48 hours old, and melanin appears bright
- B. CSF and bone appear dark
- C. Anatomic image which somewhat resembles CT
- D. Most pathology is high signal
- E. White matter has higher signal than gray matter

▸▸ Question 15

Which of the following statements are true regarding T2WI MRI images?

- A. Most pathology shows up as high signal including surrounding edema
- B. Brain edema, water, and fat appear bright
- C. Bone appears dark
- D. Clues to recognize are CSF is white, long TR and TE
- E. Fluid-attenuated inversion recovery (FLAIR) resembles T2WI except that CSF is nulled out (appears dark)
- F. All of the above

▸▸ Question 16

Following statements are correct except?

- A. GRASS (gradient recalled acquisition in a steady state) MRI images are useful for visualizing myelographic cervical spine image, bony spurs, and small old cerebral blood
- B. STIR (short tau inversion recovery) is a fat suppression image which is good to visualize bone edema, periventricular lesion, or intraorbital fat
- C. FIESTA (fast imaging employing steady state acquisition) is useful to visualize pathology at cerebellopontine angle
- D. CISS (constructive interference in steady state) is useful for imaging cranial nerves, CSF leaks, and aqueductal stenosis
- E. Gradient echo images also known as T2 GRE images are useful for seeing brainstem lesions

▸▸ Question 17

MRI with pituitary protocol is used to visualize pituitary gland with detailed imaging. It has all of the following components except?

- A. MRI is done without contrast
- B. Thin coronal cuts are taken through sella, cavernous sinus, and optic chiasma
- C. Dynamic images at intervals are taken to differentiate adenoma from pituitary as pituitary enhances before adenoma
- D. Microadenomas can be visualized using this method
- E. It is done by using MRI with and without contrast

▸▸ Question 18

All of the following are common contraindications to MRI except?

- A. Cardiac pacemakers, defibrillators, implanted neurostimulators, cochlear implants, and infusion pumps
- B. Nonferromagnetic aneurysm clips
- C. Ferromagnetic aneurysm clips
- D. Metallic implants or foreign bodies with iron in it
- E. Placement of vascular stents, coil, filter within past 6 weeks

▸▸ Question 19

Intraparenchymal areas of bright signal on DWI that are not bright on apparent diffusion coefficient (ADC) map are abnormal and represent regions of restricted diffusion. It is useful in the diagnosis of which of the following pathologies in brain?

- A. Ischemic brain tissue
- B. Cerebral abscess
- C. Active MS plaques
- D. Some tumors like epidermoids, lymphoma, or some meningiomas
- E. All of the above

▸▸ Question 20

All of the following are true regarding magnetic resonance spectroscopy (MRS) except?

- A. Lactate is a marker of hypoxia and indicates ischemia, infection, or demyelinating disease
- B. N-acetyl aspartate (NAA) is decreased in brain tumor, MS, brain abscess, and brain injury
- C. Choline is increased in brain neoplasms
- D. Abscess causes decreased succinate and acetate peaks
- E. Tumor causes increased lactate, lipid, choline, and decreased NAA

▸▸ Question 21

Diffusion tensor imaging also known as diffusion tensor tractography is an MRI technique that demonstrates white matter tracts in brain. Surgical trajectory is kept parallel to the long axis of white matter tract to avoid its damage. What are the fibers that connect regions within the same hemisphere?

- A. Optic radiations
- B. Uncinate fasciculus
- C. Arcuate fasciculus
- D. Cingulum
- E. All of the above

▸▸ Question 22

All of the following are the contraindications to myelography except?

- A. Anticoagulation
- B. Allergy to iodinated contrast
- C. Obese patient
- D. Infection at desired puncture site
- E. Extensive midline lumbar spinal fusion

▸▸ Question 23

Technetium-99 is a radioisotope that may be attached to various substrates for use in bone scan. Bone scan can be used to aid in the diagnosis of which of the following?

- A. Bone infections
- B. Bony tumor
- C. Craniosynostosis
- D. Fracture
- E. All of the above

Answers

▸▸ Answer 1

Correct answer is C. AC-PC line[1]

▸▸ Answer 2

Correct answer is A. Acute stroke[1]

▸▸ Answer 3

Correct answer is A. Acetazolamide challenge test[2]

▸▸ Answer 4

Correct answer is D. Dark[3]

▸▸ Answer 5

Correct answer is E. CSF[4]

▸▸ Answer 6

Correct answer is C. Perfusion-weighted (PWI) MRI[5]

▸▸ Answer 7

Correct answer is D. Choline[5]

▸▸ Answer 8

Correct answer is D. Diffusion tensor imaging (DTI) MRI[6]

▸▸ Answer 9

Correct answer is C. Green[7]

▸▸ Answer 10

Correct answer is D. All three phases[8]

▸▸ Answer 11

Correct answer is B. −1000, + 1000[1]

▸▸ Answer 12

Correct answer is E. All of the above[2]

▸▸ Answer 13

Correct answer is E. Both A and B[2]

▸▸ Answer 14

Correct answer is D. Most pathology is high signal[2]

▸▸ Answer 15

Correct answer is F. All of the above[3]

▸▸ Answer 16

Correct answer is E. Gradient echo images also known as T2 GRE images are useful for seeing brainstem lesions[4]

▸▸ Answer 17

Correct answer is A. MRI is done without contrast[4]

▸▸ Answer 18

Correct answer is B. Nonferromagnetic aneurysm clips[9]

▸▸ Answer 19

Correct answer is E. All of the above[10]

▸▸ Answer 20

Correct answer is D. Abscess causes decreased succinate and acetate peaks[5]

▸▸ Answer 21

Correct answer is E. All of the above[6]

▸▸ Answer 22

Correct answer is C. Obese patient[8]

▸▸ Answer 23

Correct answer is E. All of the above[8]

References

[1] Greenberg M, ed. Greenberg's Handbook of Neurosurgery. 10th ed. New York: Thieme; 2023:238
[2] Greenberg M, ed. Greenberg's Handbook of Neurosurgery. 10th ed. New York: Thieme; 2023:239
[3] Greenberg M, ed. Greenberg's Handbook of Neurosurgery. 10th ed. New York: Thieme; 2023:240
[4] Greenberg M, ed. Greenberg's Handbook of Neurosurgery. 10th ed. New York: Thieme; 2023:241
[5] Greenberg M, ed. Greenberg's Handbook of Neurosurgery. 10th ed. New York: Thieme; 2023:244
[6] Greenberg M, ed. Greenberg's Handbook of Neurosurgery. 10th ed. New York: Thieme; 2023:245
[7] Greenberg M, ed. Greenberg's Handbook of Neurosurgery. 10th ed. New York: Thieme; 2023:246
[8] Greenberg M, ed. Greenberg's Handbook of Neurosurgery. 10th ed. New York: Thieme; 2023:247
[9] Greenberg M, ed. Greenberg's Handbook of Neurosurgery. 10th ed. New York: Thieme; 2023:242
[10] Greenberg M, ed. Greenberg's Handbook of Neurosurgery. 10th ed. New York: Thieme; 2023:243

14 Electrodiagnostics

Questions

▸▸ **Question 1**

Bilateral periodic lateralizing epileptiform discharges (PLEDs) on EEG is diagnostic of which of the following?

- A. Creutzfeldt-Jakob disease
- B. Anoxic encephalopathy
- C. Brain death
- D. Herpes simplex encephalitis
- E. Bacterial meningitis

▸▸ **Question 2**

Regarding common EEG rhythms, a frequency of > 13 Hz is what?

- A. Alpha
- B. Beta
- C. Theta
- D. Delta
- E. Epsilon

▸▸ **Question 3**

Regarding brainstem auditory evoked responses (BAER), vestibular schwannoma may be suggested by which of the following?

- A. I peak latency
- B. I-III peak latency
- C. V peak latency
- D. N9-N18 peak latency
- E. P100 absolute latency

▸▸ **Question 4**

Regarding cervical electromyography (EMG), there are no good muscles to reliably test which of the following?

- A. C4
- B. C5
- C. C6
- D. C7
- E. C8

▸▸ **Question 5**

Reduction of sensory nerve action potential (SNAP) with no paraspinal muscle fibrillations suggests which of the following?

- A. Monoradiculopathy
- B. Plexopathy
- C. Traumatic herniated lumbar disk
- D. Transverse myelitis
- E. Motor neuron disease

▸▸ **Question 6**

The primary use of electroencephalogram (EEG) is the diagnosis and management of seizure disorder. Following statements regarding differential diagnosis on the basis of EEG pattern are correct except?

- A. Herpes simplex encephalitis causes periodic lateralizing epileptiform discharges on EEG
- B. Subacute sclerosing panencephalitis causes periodic high voltage with 4 to 15 seconds separation
- C. Creutzfeldt-Jakob disease causes bilateral sharp waves 1.5 to 2 per second
- D. Cannot differentiate between hydranencephaly and severe hydrocephalus
- E. Used as a clinical confirmation test in the determination of brain death

▸▸ **Question 7**

Somatosensory evoked potential (SSEP) and brain stem auditory evoked potential (BAER) are used by neurosurgeons for intraoperative monitoring purposes. What should cause the surgeon to assess all variables (retractors, instruments, blood pressure) and do surgery more carefully?

- A. A 10% increased latency of a major evoked potential peak
- B. A drop in amplitude of more than or equal to 50%
- C. Complete loss of waveform
- D. Increase in 50% latency
- E. A, B, and C

▸▸ **Question 8**

Impulses during somatosensory evoked potential monitoring during spine surgery are carried through which tract of spinal cord?

- A. Spinothalamic tract
- B. Ipsilateral posterior column
- C. Dorsolateral fasciculus
- D. Both B and C
- E. Spinocerebellar tract

▸▸ **Question 9**

Transcranial motor evoked potentials (TCMEPs) are generated by stimulation of motor cortex of brain or descending axons in spinal cord using EMG recordings of motor potentials from representative muscle groups. What is the contraindication of using TCMEP?

- A. History of epilepsy or seizures
- B. Past surgical skull defects
- C. Metal in head or neck
- D. Implanted electronic devices
- E. All of the above

▸▸ Question 10

Following statements regarding checklist for changes in SSEP or TCMEPs during spine surgery are correct except?
- A. Technical defect in recording such as connections or electrodes position
- B. Pause the surgery and eliminate possible distractions
- C. Stagnara wake up test is not useful in this situation
- D. Metabolic considerations such as anemia, mean arterial pressure, change in pH, body temperature
- E. Patient positions, retractors, instruments

▸▸ Question 11

Nerve conduction study (NCS) (nerve conduction velocity) is performed by applying electrical stimulation through surface electrodes at specified location, and electrical stimulation is recorded at receiving electrodes. Which of the following components of a nerve can be studied using NCS?
- A. Nerve conduction velocity
- B. Amplitude of nerve
- C. Latency
- D. Duration of motor and sensory nerves
- E. All of the above

▸▸ Question 12

All of the following are the components of electromyographic study except?
- A. Sensory nerve action potential (SNAP)
- B. F-wave
- C. B-wave
- D. H-reflex
- E. Polyphasic potentials

▸▸ Question 13

An EMG examination has three phases: insertional activity, spontaneous activity, and volitional activity. Which of the following are potentials or discharges that are observed in nerve disorders?
- A. Fibrillation potentials that are observed in lower motor neuron death or denervation
- B. Complex repetitive discharges that are seen in neuropathic or myopathic disorders
- C. Fasciculation potentials that are seen in motor neuron disease
- D. Motor unit action potential analysis in which change in amplitude or duration of nerve action potential shows disorder of LMN or myopathic disorder
- E. All of the above

▸▸ Question 14

What are the EMG criteria for radiculopathy?
- A. Fibrillation potential or positive sharp waves in at least two muscles innervated by a single nerve root in question, with single peripheral nerve
- B. Fibrillation potential or positive sharp waves in at least two muscles innervated by a single nerve root in question but by two different peripheral nerves
- C. Fibrillation potential or positive sharp waves in two muscles innervated by two nerve roots with two different peripheral nerves
- D. Fibrillation potential in muscles irrespective of nerve root in question
- E. None of above

▸▸ Question 15

On healing radiculopathy, which potential return first on EMG?
- A. Sensory potential
- B. Motor potential
- C. Fibrillation potential
- D. Fasciculation potential
- E. Positive sharp waves

Answers

▸▸ Answer 1

Correct answer is D. Herpes simplex encephalitis[1]

▸▸ Answer 2

Correct answer is B. Beta[1]

▸▸ Answer 3

Correct answer is B. I-III peak latency[2]

▸▸ Answer 4

Correct answer is A. C4[3]

▸▸ Answer 5

Correct answer is B. Plexopathy[4]

▸▸ Answer 6

Correct answer is D. Cannot differentiate between hydranencephaly and severe hydrocephalus[1]

▸▸ Answer 7

Correct answer is E. A, B, and C[5]

▸▸ Answer 8

Correct answer is D. Both B and C[2]

▸▸ **Answer 9**

Correct answer is E. All of the above[6]

▸▸ **Answer 10**

Correct answer is C. Stagnara wake up test is not useful in this situation[5]

▸▸ **Answer 11**

Correct answer is E. All of the above[5]

▸▸ **Answer 12**

Correct answer is C. B-wave[7]

▸▸ **Answer 13**

Correct answer is E. All of the above[7]

▸▸ **Answer 14**

Correct answer is B. Fibrillation potential or positive sharp waves in at least two muscles innervated by a single nerve root in question but by two different peripheral nerves[3]

▸▸ **Answer 15**

Correct answer is B. Motor potential[4]

References

[1] Greenberg M, ed. Greenberg's Handbook of Neurosurgery. 10th ed. New York: Thieme; 2023:249
[2] Greenberg M, ed. Greenberg's Handbook of Neurosurgery. 10th ed. New York: Thieme; 2023:252
[3] Greenberg M, ed. Greenberg's Handbook of Neurosurgery. 10th ed. New York: Thieme; 2023:256
[4] Greenberg M, ed. Greenberg's Handbook of Neurosurgery. 10th ed. New York: Thieme; 2023:257
[5] Greenberg M, ed. Greenberg's Handbook of Neurosurgery. 10th ed. New York: Thieme; 2023:254
[6] Greenberg M, ed. Greenberg's Handbook of Neurosurgery. 10th ed. New York: Thieme; 2023:253
[7] Greenberg M, ed. Greenberg's Handbook of Neurosurgery. 10th ed. New York: Thieme; 2023:255

Part IV

Developmental Anomalies

IV

15 Primary Intracranial Anomalies

Questions

▸▸ **Question 1**

What is the Galassi type of a small, biconvex arachnoid cyst located in anterior temporal tip causing no mass effect and communicating with subarachnoid space on water-soluble contrast CT cisternogram (WS-CTC)?

- A. 0
- B. I
- C. II
- D. III
- E. IV

▸▸ **Question 2**

"Bobble-head doll syndrome" is repetitive anteroposterior head movements usually associated with expansile lesions in the region of the third ventricle. What is the recommended treatment for suprasellar arachnoid cysts?

- A. Endoscopic third ventriculostomy
- B. Ventriculoperitoneal shunt
- C. Bilateral external ventricular drains
- D. Neuroendoscopic ventriculocystocisternostomy
- E. Biopsy followed by radiotherapy

▸▸ **Question 3**

Excluding suprasellar cysts, what is the definitive treatment for intracranial arachnoid cysts?

- A. Needle aspiration
- B. Burr hole evacuation
- C. Craniotomy, excising cyst wall and fenestrating it into basal cisterns
- D. Endoscopic cyst fenestration through a burr hole
- E. Shunting of cyst into peritoneum or into vascular system

▸▸ **Question 4**

Which one is true about hypothalamic hamartoma (HH)?

- A. HH is the least common cause of precocious puberty
- B. Pedunculated and sessile are the two subtypes
- C. Stereotactic radiosurgery used for large sessile type or for near-total resection
- D. Precocious puberty failing to respond to medicine is not an indication of surgery
- E. Endoscopic app used for lesion > 1.5 cm in diameter

▸▸ **Question 5**

Which one is false about agenesis of corpus callosum?

- A. It may present as an incidental finding
- B. Patient presents with hydrocephalus and seizures
- C. Failure of comissuration occurs at > 3 weeks of conception
- D. There is separation of lateral ventricles
- E. There may be absence of anterior or posterior CC

▸▸ **Question 6**

Craniofacial dysmorphic syndromes are due to mutations in which gene?

- A. FGFR
- B. p53
- C. Chromosome 19
- D. WNT signaling pathway
- E. EFGR

▸▸ **Question 7**

Bilateral arachnoid cyst may occur in which of the following?

- A. Hunter syndrome
- B. Hurler syndrome
- C. Neurofibromatosis type 2
- D. Neurofibromatosis type 1
- E. von Hippel lindau syndrome

▸▸ **Question 8**

Which of the following is the most common craniosynostosis (CSO) affecting a single suture producing a palpable keel-like sagittal ridge and dolichocephaly (elongated skull with high forehead/frontal bossing)?

- A. Sagittal CSO
- B. Coronal CSO
- C. Metopic CSO
- D. Lambdoid CSO
- E. Multiple synostoses

▸▸ **Question 9**

Which is true about plagiocephaly?

- A. Premature ossification of lambdoid and sagittal suture
- B. It is always bilateral
- C. Positional plagiocephaly is associated with anterior displacement of ear
- D. Posterior plagiocephaly is associated with anterior displacement of ear
- E. Children can be managed conservatively for up to 1 year

▸▸ **Question 10**

Which of the following is the only group of encephaloceles which does not produce a visible soft tissue mass and may present as CSF leak or recurrent meningitis?

- A. Occipital
- B. Cranial vault
- C. Frontoethmoidal
- D. Basal
- E. Posterior fossa

▸▸ Question 11

Mastoid process and air cells form at what age?

- A. 2 years and 5 years
- B. 2 years and 6 years
- C. 3 years and 6 years
- D. 2 years and 7 years
- E. 1 year

▸▸ Question 12

In which of the following vermis is intact?

- A. Dandy–Walker malformation (DWM) and Dandy–Walker variant (DWV)
- B. Black pouch cyst
- C. Retrocerebellar arachnoid cyst and cisterna magna
- D. Joubert's syndrome
- E. All of the above

▸▸ Question 13

What is the rate of occurrence of hydrocephalus in DWM?

- A. 2 to 4%
- B. 75 to 95%
- C. 50 to 70%
- D. 10%
- E. 30 to 40%

▸▸ Question 14

A mother brought her 2 months old child with pointed shaped head. What is this type of craniosynostosis?

- A. Sagittal CSO
- B. Coronal CSO
- C. Metopic CSO
- D. Lambdoid CSO
- E. Multiple synostoses

▸▸ Question 15

Hypoplasia of the optic nerves and optic chiasm is seen in which of the following?

- A. Hurler syndrome
- B. de Morsier syndrome
- C. Hypothalamic hamartomas
- D. DWV
- E. BPC

▸▸ Question 16

Arachnoid cyst is a congenital fluid containing abnormality of the arachnoid membrane which is most common in the middle fossa, CPA, suprasellar region, and posterior fossa. According to the classification scheme of Galassi et al for middle fossa cysts all of the following are true except?

- A. Type 1 is a small biconvex cyst located at temporal tip
- B. Type 2 involves proximal and intermediate segments of the middle fossa
- C. Type 3 involves the entire sylvian fissure
- D. Type 4 involves agenesis of the temporal horn
- E. None of the above

▸▸ Question 17

What are the different treatment options of arachnoid cyst?

- A. Drainage by needle aspiration or burr hole evacuation
- B. Craniotomy with excision of cyst wall and fenestrating it into basal cisterns
- C. Shunting of cyst into peritoneum
- D. Endoscopic cyst fenestration through burr hole
- E. All of the above

▸▸ Question 18

Anterior fontanelle (the largest fontanelle, diamond shaped, 4 × 2.5 cm in size) and posterior fontanelle (small, irregular in shape) normally close, respectively, by what age?

- A. 2 years and 3 to 4 months
- B. 2.5 years and 2 to 3 months
- C. 2 years and 1 to 2 months
- D. 2.5 years and 4 to 5 months
- E. None of the above

▸▸ Question 19

Diploe appears in skull bone by the age of 2 years and reach maximum (when diploic veins form) by what age?

- A. 25 years
- B. 30 years
- C. 35 years
- D. 40 years
- E. None of the above

▸▸ Question 20

Craniosynostosis is premature ossification of a cranial suture. The diagnosis of craniosynostosis is aided by all of the following except?

- A. On palpation by palpating bony prominence or gentle firm pressure with thumbs fail to cause relative movement of bones
- B. Plain skull X-ray will show lack of normal lucency or beaten copper calvaria

- C. Plain CT of brain demonstrates thickening or ridging at synostosis
- D. Technetium bone scan should be used in questionable cases
- E. MRI demonstrates thickening of bone and ridging

▸▸ Question 21

The most common craniosynostosis (CSO) affecting a single suture which produces a palpable ridge and reduced biparietal diameter is known as dolichocephaly or scaphocephaly. CSO of which suture causes this abnormality?

- A. Sagittal suture
- B. Coronal suture
- C. Lambdoid suture
- D. Both coronal and sagittal sutures
- E. None of the above

▸▸ Question 22

Coronal synostosis can accompany with Crouzon's syndrome or Apert's syndrome with unilateral coronal synostosis producing anterior plagiocephaly. Which of the following are the signs in case of unilateral coronal synostosis?

- A. Forehead on the affected side flattened or concaved with compensatory prominence of contralateral forehead
- B. Harlequin eye sign on the affected side (supraorbital margin is higher than the normal side)
- C. Orbit rotates out on the affected side producing amblyopia
- D. Deviation of nose toward the normal side (the root of the nose tends to rotate toward the deformity)
- E. All of the above

▸▸ Question 23

It is important to distinguish lazy lambdoid (positional flattening) from posterior plagiocephaly. What are the distinguishing features between the two?

- A. Posterior plagiocephaly produces a trapezoid-shaped deformity, while the other produces a parallelogram
- B. The ipsilateral ear is displaced posteriorly in posterior plagiocephaly, while it is displaced anteriorly in the other one
- C. There is contralateral frontal bossing in posterior plagiocephaly, while it is ipsilateral frontal bossing in postural plagiocephaly
- D. Postural plagiocephaly is associated with decreased mobility, abnormal posture, or intentional positioning
- E. All of the above

▸▸ Question 24

Encephalocele (cranium bifidum) is a defect in the fusion of the cranial bone through which either meninges and CSF herniate (meningocele) or meninges and cerebral tissue protrude (encephalocele). What is the most common type of encephalocele?

- A. Occipital
- B. Cranial vault
- C. Frontoethmoidal
- D. Basal
- E. Posterior fossa

▸▸ Question 25

Dandy Walker malformation is a congenital defect with classic triad of absence or hypoplasia of cerebellar vermis, cystic dilatation of the 4th ventricle, and enlarged posterior fossa. All of the following are included in the differential diagnosis except?

- A. Cerebellar hamartomal cyst
- B. Persistent Blake's pouch
- C. Epidermoid cyst
- D. Retrocerebellar arachnoid cyst
- E. Joubert's syndrome

Answers

▸▸ Answer 1

Correct answer is B. I[1]

▸▸ Answer 2

Correct answer is D. Neuroendoscopic ventriculocystocisternostomy[2]

▸▸ Answer 3

Correct answer is E. Shunting of cyst into peritoneum or into vascular system[3]

▸▸ Answer 4

Correct answer is B. Pedunculated and sessile are the two subtypes[4]

▸▸ Answer 5

Correct answer is C. Failure of comissuration occurs at < 3 weeks of gestation[5]

▸▸ Answer 6

Correct answer is A. FGFR[6]

▸▸ Answer 7

Correct answer is B. Hurler syndrome[7]

▸▸ Answer 8

Correct answer is A. Sagittal CSO[8]

▸▸ Answer 9

Correct answer is C. Positional plagiocephaly is associated with anterior displacement of ear[9]

▸▸ Answer 10

Correct answer is D. Basal[6]

▸▸ Answer 11

Correct answer is B. 2 years and 6 years[3]

▸▸ Answer 12

Correct answer is C. Retrocerebellar arachnoid cyst and cisterna magna[10]

▸▸ Answer 13

Correct answer is B. 75 to 95%[11]

▸▸ Answer 14

Correct answer is C. Metopic CSO[12]

▸▸ Answer 15

Correct answer is B. de Morsier syndrome[13]

▸▸ Answer 16

Correct answer is D. Type 4 involves agenesis of the temporal horn[1]

▸▸ Answer 17

Correct answer is E. All of the above[3]

▸▸ Answer 18

Correct answer is B. 2.5 years and 2 to 3 months[3]

▸▸ Answer 19

Correct answer is C. 35 years[3]

▸▸ Answer 20

Correct answer is E. MRI demonstrates thickening of bone and ridging[8]

▸▸ Answer 21

Correct answer is A. Sagittal suture[8]

▸▸ Answer 22

Correct answer is E. All of the above[9]

▸▸ Answer 23

Correct answer is E. All of the above[9]

▸▸ Answer 24

Correct answer is A. Occipital[6]

▸▸ Answer 25

Correct answer is A. Cerebellar hamartomal cyst[10]

References

[1] Greenberg M, ed. Greenberg's Handbook of Neurosurgery. 10th ed. New York: Thieme; 2023:261
[2] Greenberg M, ed. Greenberg's Handbook of Neurosurgery. 10th ed. New York: Thieme; 2023:263
[3] Greenberg M, ed. Greenberg's Handbook of Neurosurgery. 10th ed. New York: Thieme; 2023:264
[4] Greenberg M, ed. Greenberg's Handbook of Neurosurgery. 10th ed. New York: Thieme; 2023:277
[5] Greenberg M, ed. Greenberg's Handbook of Neurosurgery. 10th ed. New York: Thieme; 2023:274
[6] Greenberg M, ed. Greenberg's Handbook of Neurosurgery. 10th ed. New York: Thieme; 2023:269
[7] Greenberg M, ed. Greenberg's Handbook of Neurosurgery. 10th ed. New York: Thieme; 2023:260
[8] Greenberg M, ed. Greenberg's Handbook of Neurosurgery. 10th ed. New York: Thieme; 2023:265
[9] Greenberg M, ed. Greenberg's Handbook of Neurosurgery. 10th ed. New York: Thieme; 2023:266
[10] Greenberg M, ed. Greenberg's Handbook of Neurosurgery. 10th ed. New York: Thieme; 2023:271
[11] Greenberg M, ed. Greenberg's Handbook of Neurosurgery. 10th ed. New York: Thieme; 2023:270
[12] Greenberg M, ed. Greenberg's Handbook of Neurosurgery. 10th ed. New York: Thieme; 2023:267
[13] Greenberg M, ed. Greenberg's Handbook of Neurosurgery. 10th ed. New York: Thieme; 2023:276

16 Primary Spinal Developmental Anomalies

Questions

▸▸ **Question 1**

Surgical closure of myelomeningocele should be done within what time?

- A. 24 hours
- B. 48 hours
- C. 56 hours
- D. 3 days
- E. 7 days

▸▸ **Question 2**

What is the most common complicating condition associated with myelomeningocele?

- A. Neural injury
- B. Aseptic meningitis
- C. Hydrocephalus
- D. CSF leak
- E. Bladder injury

▸▸ **Question 3**

Myelomeningocele most commonly involves which region of spine?

- A. Thoracic
- B. Lumbosacral
- C. Thoracolumbar
- D. Lumbar
- E. Sacral

▸▸ **Question 4**

If a myelomeningocele patient has increasing scoliosis, increasing spasticity, worsening gait, or deteriorating urodynamics, what should be the first workup for?

- A. Syrinx
- B. Brain stem compression
- C. Dermal sinus
- D. Lipoma
- E. Shunt malfunction

▸▸ **Question 5**

It is difficult to differentiate a tethered cord from congenitally low-lying conus. In congenitally low-lying conus, the filum diameter is generally normal, and the conus should not be below which level?

- A. L3
- B. L4
- C. L5
- D. S1
- E. S2

▸▸ **Question 6**

A patient with SCM type 1 is has which of the following?

- A. Two hemicords in one dural sac
- B. Two hemicords in separate dural sac
- C. Anterior sacral meningocele
- D. Open myelomeningocele
- E. Thoracic dermal sinus tract

▸▸ **Question 7**

Which of the following is true about spinal neuroenteric cyst?

- A. Anterior to the spinal cord and extradural
- B. Posterior to the cord and extradural
- C. Anterior to the cord and intradural
- D. Anterior and posterior to the cord
- E. Intradural and intramedullary

▸▸ **Question 8**

Which of the following is the clinical triad of Klippel-Feil syndrome?

- A. Low anterior hairline, bervicollis, and limitation of movement
- B. Low posterior hairline, bervicollis, and limitation of movement
- C. Low posterior hairline, bervicollis, and normal range of movement
- D. Low posterior hairline, bervicollis, and fusion of two vertebrae
- E. Torticollis, bervicollis, and fusion of two vertebrae

▸▸ **Question 9**

What is the most common presenting sign and symptom in tethered cord?

- A. Hypertrichosis
- B. Posterior spina bifida
- C. Gait difficulty
- D. Subcutaneous lipoma
- E. Sensory deficit

▸▸ **Question 10**

What is the congenital anomaly in lumbosacral nerve root type 3?

- A. Conjoined nerve root with common dural sheath
- B. Two nerve roots exit through one foramen

- C. Adjacent nerve roots are connected by anastomosis
- D. Two nerve roots exit through separate foramen
- E. None of the above

▸▸ Question 11

Spinal arachnoid cysts are almost always dorsal and most common in thoracic spine. Following statements regarding arachnoid cysts are correct except?

- A. Etiologies can be congenital, post-traumatic, or post-infectious
- B. Symptoms of myelopathy are strong indication of surgery
- C. Pain is a strong indication of surgery
- D. It can be treated with percutaneous procedures like needle aspiration or needle fenestration
- E. Open procedures for its treatment are surgical resection, cyst fenestration, or shunting

▸▸ Question 12

Myelomeningocele (MM) is a spinal defect called spina bifida aperta or spina bifida cystica in which there is congenital defect in vertebral arches, with cystic dilatation of meninges and structural or functional abnormality of spinal cord. Its incidence can be lowered down by using prenatal folate. What percentage of MM patients develop hydrocephalus?

- A. 45 to 65%
- B. 65 to 85%
- C. 35 to 45%
- D. 85 to 90%
- E. 25 to 35%

▸▸ Question 13

Surgical closure of meningomyelocele defect should be done within 36 hours after birth. Following are steps of management of myelomeningocele before surgical closure of the defect except?

- A. If the lesion is ruptured, antibiotics are started and the defect is covered with Telfa soaked in N/S or R/L
- B. Lowest level of neurological function is identified for correlation after surgical repair
- C. Orbitofrontal circumference is taken and head US is also done to rule out hydrocephalus
- D. No need for orthopedic consultation for kyphotic or scoliotic deformities
- E. The patient is started on regular urinary catheterization and urological consultation is taken

▸▸ Question 14

Lipomyeloschisis is dorsal spinal dysraphism with lipoma which includes dural lipoma, lipomyelomeningocele, or fibrolipoma of filum terminale. What is lipomyelomeningocele?

- A. A visible defect on back with protrusion of fat and meninges
- B. A lipoma on back with protrusion of meninges and neural tissue
- C. A tuft of hair on skin with a subcutaneous lipoma that passes through the defect in lumbosacral fascia, vertebral neural arch, and dura
- D. A subcutaneous lipoma that does not merges with low-lying tethered cord
- E. Lipoma and meninges with protruding neural tissue separately visible on skin surface

▸▸ Question 15

All of the following statements are true regarding lipomyeloschisis except?

- A. It consists of removing abnormal fatty tissue
- B. Untethering of cord is done during surgery
- C. Surgery is essentially performed before 2 months of age
- D. Plain lumbosacral spine X-ray will show spinal bifida in most cases
- E. Most common presentations are back mass and bladder problems

▸▸ Question 16

What is the suggested treatment of filum terminale lipoma?

- A. Prophylactic division of fatty filum terminale without symptoms
- B. Removal of only fat with no division of filum terminale
- C. Division of fatty filum terminale if symptomatic
- D. Fatty filum sectioning for asymptomatic lesion if surgery is being performed for some other reason
- E. Both C and D

▸▸ Question 17

Following statements about spinal dermal sinus are correct except?

- A. Failure to separate neural ectoderm from dermal ectoderm at the time of closure results in myelomeningoceledefect
- B. It is recommended that surgical excision should only be done if symptomatic causing neurologic or infection symptoms
- C. There can be epidermoid cyst or dermoid cyst along the path of sinus
- D. These are potential pathways for intradural infection with chances of meningitis
- E. If present at birth, ultrasound is the best means to evaluate for spina bifida or mass inside the canal

▸▸ Question 18

Congenital fusion of two or more cervical vertebrae is a defect that results from failure of normal segmentation of cervical somites between 3 and 8 weeks of gestation. This condition presents with classic clinical triad of low posterior hairline, shortened neck, and limitation of neck movements. What is this condition is called?

- A. Fused cervical deformity
- B. Cervical myelopathy with fused vertebrae
- C. Klippel-Feil syndrome
- D. Platybasia
- E. Basilar invagination

▸▸ Question 19

Which of the following is true regarding tethered cord syndrome?

- A. It is low-lying conus medullaris with thickened filum terminale and intradural lipoma
- B. The most common presenting symptom of tethered cord syndrome in adults is pain
- C. Filum terminale is distinguished from nerve root by the presence of characteristic squiggly vessel on the surface and whiter appearance under microscope
- D. Diagnosis must be made clinically in patients with myelomeningocele as all of these patients will have tethering radiographically
- E. All of the above

▸▸ Question 20

All of the following are true regarding split cord malformation (SCM) except?

- A. Type 1 SCM is two hemicords each with central canal and surrounding pia in a separate dural tube
- B. Type 1 is also called diastematomyelia
- C. There is no rule of untethering of cord in these patients
- D. Type 2 is two hemicords within a single tube
- E. Type 2 is also called diplomyelia

Answers

▸▸ Answer 1

Correct answer is A. 24 hours[1]

▸▸ Answer 2

Correct answer is C. Hydrocephalus[2]

▸▸ Answer 3

Correct answer is B. Lumbosacral[2]

▸▸ Answer 4

Correct answer is E. Shunt malfunction[3]

▸▸ Answer 5

Correct answer is A. L3[4]

▸▸ Answer 6

Correct answer is B. Two hemicords in separate dural sac[4]

▸▸ Answer 7

Correct answer is A. Anterior to the spinal cord and extradural[5]

▸▸ Answer 8

Correct answer is B. Low posterior hairline, bervicollis, and limitation of movement[6]

▸▸ Answer 9

Correct answer is B. Posterior spina bifida[6]

▸▸ Answer 10

Correct answer is C. Adjacent nerve roots are connected by anastomosis[7]

▸▸ Answer 11

Correct answer is C. Pain is a strong indication of surgery[5]

▸▸ Answer 12

Correct answer is B. 65 to 85%[2]

▸▸ Answer 13

Correct answer is D. No need for orthopedic consultation for kyphotic or scoliotic deformities[1]

▸▸ Answer 14

Correct answer is C. A tuft of hair on skin with a subcutaneous lipoma that passes through the defect in lumbosacral fascia, vertebral neural arch, and dura[8]

▸▸ Answer 15

Correct answer is C. Surgery is essentially performed before 2 months of age[9]

▸▸ Answer 16

Correct answer is E. Both C and D[10]

▸▸ Answer 17

Correct answer is B. It is recommended that surgical excision should only be done if symptomatic causing neurologic or infection symptoms[11]

▸▸ Answer 18

Correct answer is C. Klippel-Feil syndrome[12]

▸▸ **Answer 19**

Correct answer is E. All of the above[6]

▸▸ **Answer 20**

Correct answer is C. There is no rule of untethering of cord in these patients[4]

References

[1] Greenberg M, ed. Greenberg's Handbook of Neurosurgery. 10th ed. New York: Thieme; 2023:282

[2] Greenberg M, ed. Greenberg's Handbook of Neurosurgery. 10th ed. New York: Thieme; 2023:281

[3] Greenberg M, ed. Greenberg's Handbook of Neurosurgery. 10th ed. New York: Thieme; 2023:283

[4] Greenberg M, ed. Greenberg's Handbook of Neurosurgery. 10th ed. New York: Thieme; 2023:292

[5] Greenberg M, ed. Greenberg's Handbook of Neurosurgery. 10th ed. New York: Thieme; 2023:280

[6] Greenberg M, ed. Greenberg's Handbook of Neurosurgery. 10th ed. New York: Thieme; 2023:290

[7] Greenberg M, ed. Greenberg's Handbook of Neurosurgery. 10th ed. New York: Thieme; 2023:293

[8] Greenberg M, ed. Greenberg's Handbook of Neurosurgery. 10th ed. New York: Thieme; 2023:284

[9] Greenberg M, ed. Greenberg's Handbook of Neurosurgery. 10th ed. New York: Thieme; 2023:285

[10] Greenberg M, ed. Greenberg's Handbook of Neurosurgery. 10th ed. New York: Thieme; 2023:286

[11] Greenberg M, ed. Greenberg's Handbook of Neurosurgery. 10th ed. New York: Thieme; 2023:287

[12] Greenberg M, ed. Greenberg's Handbook of Neurosurgery. 10th ed. New York: Thieme; 2023:288

17 Primary Craniospinal Anomalies

Questions

▸▸ Question 1

A 40-year-old female patient presents in neurosurgical OPD with complaints of occipital headache which is exacerbated by coughing. On examination, she has numbness in right upper limb and downbeat nystagmus is found to be positive. MRI of brain shows cerebellar tonsillar herniation 7 mm below foramen with stasis of CSF flow at foramen magnum level and cervical syringomyelia. What is this condition called?

- A. Type 1 Chiari malformation
- B. Type 2 Chiari malformation
- C. Arnold Chiari malformation
- D. Chiari type 1.5 malformation
- E. Cerebellar tonsillar herniation syndrome

▸▸ Question 2

Chiari pseudotumor cerebri syndrome is a condition in which CSF obstruction due to Chiari leads to elevated ICP without hydrocephalus. Following are the features of this condition except?

- A. CSF shunting is an initial therapy
- B. Posterior fossa decompression is done for patients with papilledema and Chiari
- C. Papilledema is uncommon in this condition
- D. LP is relatively contraindicated
- E. None of the above

▸▸ Question 3

A female with obesity presents with visual field constriction and only abducens nerve palsy. On examination, there is papilledema without hydrocephalus. Following are true statements regarding pseudotumor cerebri except?

- A. For patients with severe pseudotumor cerebri VP shunt or ONSF is the treatment of choice
- B. On LP if opening pressure is more than 25 cm of CSF, consider pseudotumor cerebri
- C. If findings are not suggestive of pseudotumor, then posterior fossa decompression is done
- D. For deterioration of vision, shunt is the only treatment
- E. None of the above

▸▸ Question 4

A neonate presents in neurosurgical emergency with sudden respiratory arrest. He/she had previous history of swallowing difficulties with poor feeding, cyanosis during feeding, and nasal regurgitation. There is also history of previous apneic spells and stridor. MRI of brain showed low caudally displaced cervicomedullary junction, small posterior fossa, and tectal beaking. What is the most likely diagnosis?

- A. Chiari malformation type 1
- B. Chiari malformation type 3
- C. Arnold–Chiari malformation
- D. Chiari type 1.5
- E. Chiari malformation type 4

▸▸ Question 5

What are the features of Chiari type 1.5?

- A. Dislocation of cerebellum below foramen magnum
- B. Cerebellar hypoplasia without cerebellar herniation and small posterior fossa
- C. Cerebellar tonsils herniated ventrally with brain stem compression
- D. Entire cervicomedullary junction situated below foramen magnum
- E. Syringohydromyelia without hindbrain herniation

▸▸ Question 6

What is the most frequently performed procedure for Chiari malformation which decompresses brain stem and reestablish normal flow of CSF at cervicomedullary junction?

- A. c1, c2, and c3 laminectomy
- B. Suboccipital craniectomy without dural patch grafting
- C. Suboccipital craniectomy with dural patch grafting but with no upper cervical laminectomy
- D. Suboccipital craniectomy with dural patch grafting and upper cervical laminectomy
- E. Suboccipital craniectomy only

▸▸ Question 7

All of the following are postneurulation defects except?

- A. Microcephaly
- B. Anencephaly
- C. Holoprosencephaly
- D. Lissencephaly
- E. Porencephaly

▸▸ Question 8

Which of the following is a postneurulation defect that is considered migration abnormality?

- A. Lissencephaly (maldevelopment of cerebral contusion)
- B. Heteropia (abnormal foci of gray matter)
- C. Schizencephaly (a cleft that communicates with ventricle)
- D. Cortical dysplasia (a cleft that does not communicate with ventricles)
- E. All of the above

▸▸ **Question 9**

Following are tests can differentiate hydranencephaly (absence or near-total absence of cerebrum) from maximal hydrocephalus except?

- A. EEG
- B. Occipitofrontal circumference measurement
- C. CT, MRI, or ultrasound
- D. Transillumination of skull
- E. CT brain angiography

▸▸ **Question 10**

Microcephaly is defined as head circumference more than 2 standard deviations below the mean for sex and gestational age. It is a postneurulation defect. What are the possible causes of this condition?

- A. Infection during pregnancy (rubella, toxoplasmosis, zika virus, cytomegalovirus)
- B. Severe malnutrition
- C. Maternal exposure to certain drugs such as cocaine or alcohol during pregnancy
- D. Interruption of blood supply to brain during pregnancy
- E. All of the above

▸▸ **Question 11**

All of the following are risk factors for macrocrania except?

- A. Lack of prenatal folic acid
- B. Maternal cold exposure from cold water
- C. Use of valproic acid
- D. Obesity
- E. Maternal cocaine abuse

Answers

▸▸ **Answer 1**

Correct answer is A. Type 1 Chiari malformation[1]

▸▸ **Answer 2**

Correct answer is C. Papilledema is uncommon in this condition[2]

▸▸ **Answer 3**

Correct answer is D. For deterioration of vision, shunt is the only treatment[2]

▸▸ **Answer 4**

Correct answer is C. Arnold–Chiari malformation[3]

▸▸ **Answer 5**

Correct answer is D. Entire cervicomedullary junction situated below foramen magnum[4]

▸▸ **Answer 6**

Correct answer is D. Suboccipital craniectomy with dural patch grafting and upper cervical laminectomy[5]

▸▸ **Answer 7**

Correct answer is B. Anencephaly[6]

▸▸ **Answer 8**

Correct answer is E. All of the above[7]

▸▸ **Answer 9**

Correct answer is B. Occipitofrontal circumference measurement[8]

▸▸ **Answer 10**

Correct answer is E. All of the above[9]

▸▸ **Answer 11**

Correct answer is B. Maternal cold exposure from cold water[9]

References

[1] Greenberg M, ed. Greenberg's Handbook of Neurosurgery. 10th ed. New York: Thieme; 2023:295
[2] Greenberg M, ed. Greenberg's Handbook of Neurosurgery. 10th ed. New York: Thieme; 2023:301
[3] Greenberg M, ed. Greenberg's Handbook of Neurosurgery. 10th ed. New York: Thieme; 2023:303
[4] Greenberg M, ed. Greenberg's Handbook of Neurosurgery. 10th ed. New York: Thieme; 2023:305
[5] Greenberg M, ed. Greenberg's Handbook of Neurosurgery. 10th ed. New York: Thieme; 2023:306
[6] Greenberg M, ed. Greenberg's Handbook of Neurosurgery. 10th ed. New York: Thieme; 2023:308
[7] Greenberg M, ed. Greenberg's Handbook of Neurosurgery. 10th ed. New York: Thieme; 2023:309
[8] Greenberg M, ed. Greenberg's Handbook of Neurosurgery. 10th ed. New York: Thieme; 2023:310
[9] Greenberg M, ed. Greenberg's Handbook of Neurosurgery. 10th ed. New York: Thieme; 2023:312

Part V

Coma and Brain Death

V

18 Coma and Coma Scales

Questions

▸▸ Question 1

A 30-year-old male with traumatic head injury is admitted in ICU with a GCS of E1VTM3. The decorticate posturing is attributed to what?

- A. Disinhibition of vestibulospinal tract
- B. Disinhibition of pontine reticular formation
- C. Disinhibition by removal of corticospinal pathways above the midbrain
- D. Disinhibition of medullary reticular formation
- E. Transection at inter-collicular level

▸▸ Question 2

A patient admitted in ICU for monitoring developed an abnormal breathing pattern: the breathing gradually crescendos in amplitude and then trails off, followed by an expiratory pause, and then the pattern repeats. Cheyne-Stokes breathing indicates dysfunction of which of the following?

- A. High medulla
- B. Lower medulla
- C. Pons
- D. Bilateral cerebral hemispheres
- E. Basilar artery occlusion

▸▸ Question 3

Which of the following is usually a pre-terminal breathing pattern?

- A. Cheyne-Stokes
- B. Cluster
- C. Ataxic
- D. Apneustic
- E. Apneic

▸▸ Question 4

On examination of a middle-aged female patient on assisted ventilation in ICU, bilateral pin point pupils were noted. This finding is due to what?

- A. Unopposed sympathetic input
- B. Loss of sympathetic input
- C. Loss of parasympathetic output
- D. Medullary lesion
- E. Midbrain lesion

▸▸ Question 5

Which of the following may be a manisfestation of a lesion in medial longitudinal fasciculus?

- A. Ocular blobbing
- B. Ping pong gaze
- C. Windshield wiper eye
- D. Internuclear ophthalmoplegia
- E. Wrong way gaze

▸▸ Question 6

While testing oculovestibular reflex, contralateral eye fails to adduct. This finding may be labeled as what?

- A. Ocular blobbing
- B. Ping pong gaze
- C. Windshield wiper eye
- D. Internuclear ophthalmoplegia
- E. Wrong way gaze

▸▸ Question 7

A patient develops subfalcine herniation where cingulate gyrus herniates under the falx. Which of the following vessels is at risk of occlusion?

- A. ICA
- B. ACA
- C. MCA
- D. PCA
- E. PICA

▸▸ Question 8

A patient with mass effect on CT scan deteriorated after lumbar puncture was done. Which of the following herniation syndrome is most likely in this case?

- A. Central
- B. Uncal
- C. Subfalcine
- D. Upward cerebellar
- E. Tonsillar

▸▸ Question 9

A comatosed patient in ICU had high urinary output. Diabetes insipidus may result from which herniation syndrome?

- A. Central
- B. Uncal
- C. Subfalcine
- D. Upward cerebellar
- E. Tonsillar

▸▸ Question 10

A patient diagnosed with left temporoparietal brain tumor was brought to emergency department. His examination revealed regular and shallow respiration at 30 breaths/min; pupils were midposition (3–5 mm) and fixed; Doll's eyes reflex was unelicitable; bilateral Babinski was positive with occasional lower extremity flexion to pain. These findings are consistent with which stage of tentorial herniation?

- A. Diencephalic
- B. Midbrain
- C. Midbrain–upper pontine
- D. Lower pons–upper medullary
- E. Medullary

▸▸ Question 11

A patient with traumatic brain injury had sustained a hematoma in the lateral middle fossa. His examination revealed sustained hyperpnea breathing, with both pupils in mid position (5–6 mm) and fixed; oculomotor was impaired and there was bilateral decerebrate rigidity. These finding favor which stage of uncal herniation?

- A. Diencephalic
- B. Midbrain
- C. Midbrain–upper pontine
- D. Lower pons–upper medullary
- E. Medullary

▸▸ Question 12

A middle-aged male presented to ER after roadside accident. His brain CT revealed left temporal hematoma and motor examination revealed ipsilateral hemiplegia. Which of the following is a false localizing sign?

- A. Kernohan's phenomenon
- B. Internuclear ophthalmoplegia
- C. Ocular blobbing
- D. Ataxic respiration
- E. Doll's eye reflex

▸▸ Question 13

Anoxemic anoxia in hypoxic shock severely affects which of the following?

- A. Caudate nucleus
- B. Putamen
- C. Globus pallidus
- D. Incisura
- E. Tentorium

▸▸ Question 14

A 3-year-old boy was brought to ER by her mother after fall from stairs. On examination, he opened his eyes to pain, was inconsolable, and had a decorticate posture. What is his GCS score?

- A. 4
- B. 5
- C. 6
- D. 7
- E. 8

▸▸ Question 15

Oculocephalic reflex is contraindicated in which of the following?

- A. Ventilated patient
- B. Cervical spine injury
- C. Pyrexia
- D. Severe head injury
- E. Post craniotomy

▸▸ Question 16

Coma is the severest impairment of arousal and is defined as inability to obey commands, speak, or open the eyes to pain. What GCS score is generally accepted as operational definition of coma?

- A. Less than 9
- B. Less than 8
- C. Less than 6
- D. Less than 7
- E. Less than 5

▸▸ Question 17

A patient presents to neurosurgical emergency after road traffic accident. The on-call resident decides to intubate after assessing that GCS score is less than 9. The patient opens his eyes to pain, has incomprehensible verbal response, and has flexion (decorticate) posturing. What is the GCS score in this patient?

- A. 8
- B. 7
- C. 6
- D. 5
- E. 4

▸▸ Question 18

A 3-year-old child presented in neurosurgical emergency after road traffic accident. This child opens his/her eyes to pain, is inconsistently consolable, is moaning, and localizes to pain. What is the GCS score in this patient?

- A. 12
- B. 11
- C. 10
- D. 9
- E. 8

▸▸ Question 19

Decorticate posturing (abnormal flexion in upper extremities and extension in lower extremities) has slightly better prognosis than decerebrate posturing (abnormal extension in both upper and lower extremities). What pathways are removed or damaged in decorticate posturing and decerebrate posturing, respectively?

- A. Vestibulospinal tract and corticospinal tract
- B. Corticospinal tract and pontine reticular formation
- C. Corticospinal tract and vestibulospinal tract
- D. Corticospinal tract and vestibulospinal tract + pontine reticular formation
- E. Corticospinal tract and vestibulobulbar tract

▸▸ Question 20

Structural causes of coma include vascular obstruction (like bilateral carotid or thalamo-perforators supplying both medial thalamic areas), any abscess, hemorrhagic contusion or hematoma, brain tumor, and herniation. What amount of midline shift causes stuporous stage of unconsciousness?

- A. 8 to 13 mm
- B. 6 to 8.5 mm
- C. 4 to 6 mm
- D. 3 to 4 mm
- E. None of the above

▸▸ Question 21

A comatose patient is brought to emergency for unknown reason. Following are the steps in emergency management of this patient except?

- A. Establishment of airway, stabilization of BP, 25 mL of dextrose 50% given IV, and attachment of oxygen with saturation monitoring
- B. Blood is obtained for electrolytes and toxicology screen
- C. Emergency medicines such as solocurtef, Avil, adrenaline, fluid, naloxone, flumazenil, or thiamine are given if there is suspicion of anaphylactic shock narcotic overdose or benzodiazepine overdose, or Wernicke's suspected, respectively
- D. No need of core neuro examination in this patient to avoid wasting time
- E. If signs of raised ICP noted, measures to lower ICP started and STAT CT brain plain is obtained

▸▸ Question 22

Following statements regarding pupil examination in a comatose patient are correct except?

- A. Equal and reactive pupils indicate toxic or metabolic cause with few exceptions such as glutethimide toxicity, anoxic encephalopathy, anticholinergics or narcotics overdose
- B. Anisocoria is produced by afferent pupillary defect
- C. Most common causes of anisocoria are herniation syndrome and Horner syndrome
- D. Bilateral fixed and dilated pupil (7–10 mm) is seen in subtotal damage to medulla or immediate post anoxia or hypothermia
- E. Bilateral fixed and mid position pupil (4–6 mm) are due to more extensive midbrain lesion

▸▸ Question 23

A breathing pattern that gradually crescendos in amplitude and then trails off followed by an expiratory pause and then the pattern repeats is most commonly seen in diencephalic lesion or bilateral cerebral hemisphere dysfunction. What is this pattern of breathing called?

- A. Cheyne-Stokes breathing
- B. Hyperventilation
- C. Cluster breathing
- D. Apneustic breathing
- E. Ataxic breathing

▸▸ Question 24

All of the following are causes of bilateral conjugate deviation of eyes except?

- A. Frontal lobe lesion
- B. Pontine lesion
- C. Lesion in medial longitudinal fasciculus
- D. Medial thalamic hemorrhage
- E. Midbrain pretectal lesions

▸▸ Question 25

Which of the following statements is true regarding herniation syndrome?

- A. Central and uncal herniations are types of supratentorial herniation
- B. Upward cerebellar herniation is seen in posterior fossa mass, and it is exacerbated by ventriculostomy
- C. Tonsillar herniation can be due to supra- or infratentorial masses, elevated ICP from cerebral edema, or obstruction to CSF flow at foramen magnum, and it is exacerbated by LP
- D. Temporal lobe or middle lobe mass lesion produces uncal herniation
- E. All of the above

Answers

▸▸ Answer 1

Correct answer is C. Disinhibition by removal of corticospinal pathways above the midbrain[1]

▸▸ Answer 2

Correct answer is D. Bilateral cerebral hemispheres[2]

▸▸ Answer 3

Correct answer is C. Ataxic[2]

▸▸ Answer 4

Correct answer is B. Loss of sympathetic input[3]

▸▸ **Answer 5**

Correct answer is D. Internuclear ophthalmoplegia[4]

▸▸ **Answer 6**

Correct answer is D. Internuclear ophthalmoplegia[4]

▸▸ **Answer 7**

Correct answer is D. PCA[5]

▸▸ **Answer 8**

Correct answer is E. Tonsillar[6]

▸▸ **Answer 9**

Correct answer is A. Central[6]

▸▸ **Answer 10**

Correct answer is D. Lower pons–upper medullary[7]

▸▸ **Answer 11**

Correct answer is C. Midbrain–upper pontine[8]

▸▸ **Answer 12**

Correct answer is A. Kernohan's phenomenon[8]

▸▸ **Answer 13**

Correct answer is C. Globus pallidus[9]

▸▸ **Answer 14**

Correct answer is D. 7[10]

▸▸ **Answer 15**

Correct answer is B. Cervical spine injury[4]

▸▸ **Answer 16**

Correct answer is B. Less than 8[10]

▸▸ **Answer 17**

Correct answer is B. 7[10]

▸▸ **Answer 18**

Correct answer is C. 10[10]

▸▸ **Answer 19**

Correct answer is D. Corticospinal tract and vestibulospinal tract + pontine reticular formation[1]

▸▸ **Answer 20**

Correct answer is B. 6 to 8.5 mm[11]

▸▸ **Answer 21**

Correct answer is D. No need of core neuro examination in this patient to avoid wasting time[11]

▸▸ **Answer 22**

Correct answer is B. Anisocoria is produced by afferent pupillary defect[3]

▸▸ **Answer 23**

Correct answer is A. Cheyne-Stokes breathing[3]

▸▸ **Answer 24**

Correct answer is C. Lesion in medial longitudinal fasciculus[2]

▸▸ **Answer 25**

Correct answer is E. All of the above[5]

References

[1] Greenberg M, ed. Greenberg's Handbook of Neurosurgery. 10th ed. New York: Thieme; 2023:319
[2] Greenberg M, ed. Greenberg's Handbook of Neurosurgery. 10th ed. New York: Thieme; 2023:322
[3] Greenberg M, ed. Greenberg's Handbook of Neurosurgery. 10th ed. New York: Thieme; 2023:321
[4] Greenberg M, ed. Greenberg's Handbook of Neurosurgery. 10th ed. New York: Thieme; 2023:323
[5] Greenberg M, ed. Greenberg's Handbook of Neurosurgery. 10th ed. New York: Thieme; 2023:324
[6] Greenberg M, ed. Greenberg's Handbook of Neurosurgery. 10th ed. New York: Thieme; 2023:325
[7] Greenberg M, ed. Greenberg's Handbook of Neurosurgery. 10th ed. New York: Thieme; 2023:326
[8] Greenberg M, ed. Greenberg's Handbook of Neurosurgery. 10th ed. New York: Thieme; 2023:327
[9] Greenberg M, ed. Greenberg's Handbook of Neurosurgery. 10th ed. New York: Thieme; 2023:328
[10] Greenberg M, ed. Greenberg's Handbook of Neurosurgery. 10th ed. New York: Thieme; 2023:318
[11] Greenberg M, ed. Greenberg's Handbook of Neurosurgery. 10th ed. New York: Thieme; 2023:320

19 Brain Death and Organ Donation

Questions

▸▸ Question 1

Absence of brain stem reflexes is considered as brain death. Which of the following is a brain stem reflex that should be absent to declare a patient brain dead?

- A. Corneal reflex
- B. Oculovestibular reflex
- C. Oculocephalic reflex
- D. Oropharyngeal reflex
- E. All of the above

▸▸ Question 2

Apnea test is used as a confirmatory test for brain death. A patient is confirmed to be brain dead if he/she does not breathe for at least 2 minutes when $PaCO_2$ is kept above what?

- A. 80 mmHg
- B. 70 mmHg
- C. 60 mmHg
- D. 20 mmHg above baseline
- E. Both C and D

▸▸ Question 3

A patient cannot be declared as brain dead in the absence of brain stem reflexes if which of following criteria is met?

- A. Core body temperature less than 36 degrees Celsius
- B. Blood alcohol content more than 0.08%
- C. Neuromuscular blocking agents given to the patient
- D. Systolic blood pressure more than 100 mmHg
- E. A, B, and C

▸▸ Question 4

Following are ancillary confirmatory tests for brain death except?

- A. Cerebral angiography
- B. EEG
- C. Cerebral radionuclide angiogram (CRAG)
- D. ECG
- E. None of the above

▸▸ Question 5

Cerebral radionuclide angiogram (CRAG) is an ancillary confirmatory test for brain death. In which of the following setting is this test useful?

- A. When complicating conditions are present such as hypotension, hypothermia, drug intoxication, or metabolic abnormalities
- B. In patients with severe facial trauma where evaluation of ocular findings is difficult
- C. In patients with severe COPD or CHF where apnea test may not be valid
- D. To shorten the observation period
- E. All of the above

▸▸ Question 6

Hollow skull phenomenon where there is lack of blood uptake in the ACA and MCA distributions is seen in which test?

- A. CT angiography of brain
- B. MR angiography of brain
- C. CRAG
- D. Transcranial Doppler
- E. All of the above

▸▸ Question 7

There can be movement of body parts after brain death which is due to spinal cord discharges as it undergoes cell death. Following features of these movements differentiate them from normal movements except?

- A. These movements are repetitive
- B. Decerebrate posturing
- C. These movements are stereotypical
- D. These do not change with changing stimuli
- E. Finger tremors

▸▸ Question 8

What is the most reliable means of diagnosis of brain death in term newborns, infants, and children?

- A. Clinical diagnosis
- B. Ancillary tests
- C. Single apnea test
- D. EEG
- E. All of the above

▸▸ Question 9

Following are the physiologic aberrations that occur in a brain-dead patient which need to be corrected in order to preserve body organs for transplantation except?

- A. Hypotension
- B. Diabetes insipidus
- C. Hypothermia
- D. Electrolytes imbalance
- E. None of the above

▸▸ Question 10

Which of the following are requirements of organ donation?

- A. Ventilator-dependent patient
- B. Family agreed to withdraw support
- C. Medical team suspects that the patient would go into asystole in less than 60 minutes after stopping the support
- D. The transplant team cannot participate in end-of-life care or declaration of death
- E. All of the above

Answers

▸▸ Answer 1

Correct answer is E. All of the above[1]

▸▸ Answer 2

Correct answer is E. Both C and D[1]

▸▸ Answer 3

Correct answer is E. A, B, and C[2]

▸▸ Answer 4

Correct answer is D. ECG[3]

▸▸ Answer 5

Correct answer is E. All of the above[3]

▸▸ Answer 6

Correct answer is C. CRAG[4]

▸▸ Answer 7

Correct answer is B. Decerebrate posturing[5]

▸▸ Answer 8

Correct answer is A. Clinical diagnosis[5]

▸▸ Answer 9

Correct answer is D. Electrolytes imbalance[6]

▸▸ Answer 10

Correct answer is E. All of the above[7]

References

[1] Greenberg M, ed. Greenberg's Handbook of Neurosurgery. 10th ed. New York: Thieme; 2023:331
[2] Greenberg M, ed. Greenberg's Handbook of Neurosurgery. 10th ed. New York: Thieme; 2023:332
[3] Greenberg M, ed. Greenberg's Handbook of Neurosurgery. 10th ed. New York: Thieme; 2023:333
[4] Greenberg M, ed. Greenberg's Handbook of Neurosurgery. 10th ed. New York: Thieme; 2023:334
[5] Greenberg M, ed. Greenberg's Handbook of Neurosurgery. 10th ed. New York: Thieme; 2023:335
[6] Greenberg M, ed. Greenberg's Handbook of Neurosurgery. 10th ed. New York: Thieme; 2023:336
[7] Greenberg M, ed. Greenberg's Handbook of Neurosurgery. 10th ed. New York: Thieme; 2023:337

Part VI

Infection

VI

20 Bacterial Infections of the Parenchyma and Meninges and Complex Infections

Questions

▸▸ Question 1

A comatose middle-aged male was brought to emergency after roadside accident. After 3 days, he still showed no improvement in consciousness level and was observed to have cerebrospinal fluid (CSF) rhinorrhea. His vaccination status was not known. According to the CDC recommendation, which vaccination should be given in this case to prevent post-traumatic meningitis?

- A. Tetanus toxoid
- B. MMR
- C. IPV
- D. Pneumococcal
- E. Recommence EPI schedule

▸▸ Question 2

What is the most common cause of Waterhouse–Friderichsen syndrome?

- A. *Neisseria meningitidis*
- B. *Cryptococcus neoformans*
- C. WFS prions
- D. Herpes simplex
- E. Varicella zoster

▸▸ Question 3

What is the most common etiology for aseptic meningitis?

- A. Carcinomatous meningitis
- B. Viral meningitis
- C. Fungal meningitis
- D. TB meningitis
- E. Intraoperative rupture of cyst leading to spilling of contents

▸▸ Question 4

Surgical excision for cerebral abscess should be attempted when the abscess is in which histological phase?

- A. Early cerebritis
- B. Late cerebritis
- C. Delayed cerebritis
- D. Early capsule
- E. Late capsule

▸▸ Question 5

Histopathology of a tissue obtained from brain abscess shows neovascularity, necrotic center, and reticular network surrounds (less well-developed alongside-facing ventricles). What will be the histological grade in this case?

- A. Early cerebritis
- B. Late cerebritis
- C. Early capsule
- D. Late capsule
- E. Inconclusive

▸▸ Question 6

For medical treatment of meningitis and cerebral abscess, the dose of vancomycin to achieve trough of 15 to 20 mg/dL is what?

- A. 5 mg/kg TDS
- B. 10 mg/kg TDS
- C. 15 mg/kg BD-TDS
- D. 30 mg/kg BD-TDS
- E. 100 mg/kg OD

▸▸ Question 7

What is the most common pathogen to cause cerebral abscess in AIDS patient?

- A. MRSA
- B. MSSA
- C. *Streptococcus pyogenes*
- D. *Toxoplasma gondii*
- E. *Cryptococcus neoformans*

▸▸ Question 8

According to modified Vellore grading system (mVG) for hydrocephalus in tuberculous meningitis, patient with GCS score 9–14 (altered sensorium but easily arousable) ± dense neurologic deficit is which grade?

- A. Grade 0
- B. Grade I
- C. Grade II
- D. Grade III
- E. Grade IV

▸▸ Question 9

Lyme disease (LD) is a complex multisystem disease caused by various species of what?

- A. Cryptococcus
- B. Yeasts
- C. *Borrelia spirochetes*
- D. Nocardia
- E. *Pneumocystis carinii*

▸▸ **Question 10**

Which of the following is the most common cause of bilateral Bell's palsy?

- A. Toxoplasmosis
- B. Lyme's disease
- C. PCNSL
- D. Cysticercosis
- E. Nocardiosis

▸▸ **Question 11**

A 21-year-old female presents to OPD with tuberculous meningitis. She is started on ATT and is given rifampicin, INH, pyrazinamide, and ethambutol for initial 2 months. For how long will INH and rifampicin be continued in the next phase?

- A. 9 to 12 months
- B. 7 to 10 months
- C. 4 to 6 months
- D. 12 to 18 months

▸▸ **Question 12**

To which of the following drugs should a mycobacteria strain be resistant to, to be labeled as MDR TB?

- A. Isoniazid and rifampin
- B. Isoniazid and pyrazinamide
- C. Rifampicin and ethambutol
- D. Isoniazid and ethambutol
- E. Rifampicin and pyrazinamide

▸▸ **Question 13**

A 17-year-old boy is started on ATT for MDR TB. How long should the treatment be continued according to the WHO guidelines?

- A. 9 to 12 months
- B. 12 to 18 months
- C. 18 to 24 months
- D. 20 to 24 months
- E. 18 to 36 months

▸▸ **Question 14**

A 25-year-old boy presents with new-onset seizures and weight loss along with fever. He undergoes MRI of brain which reveals a ring enhancing frontal lesion with perilesional edema. There is low signal on DWI in the center of the lesion. What is the type of lesion?

- A. Caseating granuloma
- B. Noncaseating granuloma
- C. Liquefactive necrosis
- D. Healed tuberculoma
- E. Calcified lesion

▸▸ **Question 15**

A patient presented with meningitis 6 days after a neurosurgical procedure. Usual organisms in this patient could be staphylococci coagulase negative, *S. aureus*, Enterobacteriaceae, pseudomonas, or pneumococci. What are the empiric antibiotics in this patient?

- A. Vancomycin 15 mg/kg every 8 to 12 hours + cefepime 2 g IV every 8 hours
- B. Aztreonam 2 g IV every 6 to 8 hours + ciprofloxacin 400 mg IV every 8 hours
- C. Intrathecal antibiotics like vancomycin, gentamycin, amikacin, colistin
- D. Liposomal amphotericin B 3–4 mg/kg IV daily + flucytosine 25 mg/kg PO QID for 2 weeks
- E. A, B, and C

▸▸ **Question 16**

Post-traumatic meningitis is mostly caused by organism Gram-positive cocci (*Staphylococcus haemolyticus*, *S. warneri*, *S. cohnii*, *S. epidermis*, and *Streptococcus pneumoniae*) and Gram-negative bacilli (*E. coli*, *Klebsiella pneumonia*, *Acinetobacter anitratus*). Following are suggested recommendations of pneumococcal vaccination for patients with CSF leak except?

- A. Children 6 to 18 years of age who have not received pneumococcal conjugate vaccine (PCV 13) before should receive a single dose of PCV 13
- B. Children 2 to 18 years of age should receive a dose of pneumococcal polysaccharide vaccine (PPSV23) at least 8 weeks after any dose of PCV 13
- C. For adults with unknown vaccination status or with no pervious vaccination, one dose of PCV 13 should be given
- D. One dose of PPSV23 at least 8 weeks after giving PCV 13
- E. Patients above 65 years of age do not need more dose of PPSV23

▸▸ **Question 17**

Following statements are true regarding chemical meningitis except?

- A. Chemical meningitis cannot occur spontaneously
- B. It can occur after intrathecal administration of certain drugs such as methotrexate or contrast agents
- C. CSF WBC is found no more than 7,500/µL in most patients
- D. CSF glucose should not be less than 10 mg/dL
- E. Treatment is removal of the offending agent, systemic steroid, and serial lumbar punctures

▸▸ **Question 18**

Cerebral abscess is most likely to be formed in patients with pulmonary abscess or AV fistula, congenital cyanotic heart disease, immunocompromised host, chronic sinusitis, or after

dental procedures. What is the most common pathogen in general for cerebral abscess?
- A. *Streptococcus*
- B. *Staphylococcus aureus*
- C. Enterobacteriaceae
- D. *Actinomyces*
- E. *Staphylococcus epidermidis*

▸▸ Question 19

Which of the following is true regarding histologic staging of cerebral abscess?
- A. Early cerebritis stage (1–3 days) is early infection and inflammation with poor demarcation from surrounding brain and no resistance to aspirating needle
- B. Late cerebritis (4–9 days) is formation of reticular matrix and developing necrotic center with intermediate resistance to aspirating needle
- C. Early capsule (10–13 days) is formation of neovascularity, necrotic center, and reticular network with no resistance to aspirating needle
- D. Late capsule (> 14 days) is formation of collagen capsule and necrotic center with no resistance to intermediate resistance to aspirating needle
- E. Abscess leaves a glial scar after healing

▸▸ Question 20

Cerebral abscess shows which of the following characteristics on MRI of brain?
- A. On diffusion-weighted MRI, it is bright on DWI and dark on ADC
- B. MR spectroscopy shows peaks of lactate and acetate
- C. Cerebritis stage is hypointense on T1 and hyperintense on T2
- D. Capsular stage is shown as hypointense center with bright capsule on T1 and hyperintense center with dark capsule on T2
- E. All of the above are true

▸▸ Question 21

Medical management for cerebral abscess is indicated for patients in early cerebritis stage and size of abscess less than 3 cm with vancomycin, meropenem given IV for 6 to 8 weeks. Following are indications for surgical management of these lesions except?
- A. Significant mass effect exerted by lesion
- B. Lesion far from ventricle
- C. Traumatic abscess with foreign material
- D. Fungal abscess
- E. Multiloculated abscess

▸▸ Question 22

What is the mainstay of surgical treatment of cerebral abscess along with IV antibiotics?
- A. Needle aspiration
- B. Surgical excision
- C. External drainage
- D. Instillation of antibiotics
- E. All of the above

▸▸ Question 23

A patient presents in neurosurgical OPD with history of fever, headache, and signs of meningismus and hemiparesis. MRI shows crescentic extracerebral lesion with high signal on T2 MRI. What is the most likely diagnosis?
- A. Brain abscess
- B. Chronic subdural hematoma with meningitis
- C. Subdural empyema
- D. EDH with meningitis
- E. None of the above

▸▸ Question 24

Following statements are true except?
- A. Toxoplasmosis in brain usually shows more than five lesions in brain while primary CNS lymphoma (PCNSL) shows multiple lesions in brain but less than five in number
- B. Toxoplasmosis lesions show ring enhancement while PCNSL shows homogenous enhancement and PML shows no enhancement
- C. Lesion in toxoplasmosis is in basal ganglia and gray–white junction; in PCNSL it is subependymal while limited to white matter in PML
- D. All three lesions (toxoplasmosis, PCNSL, and PML) produce mass effect
- E. PML is high signal on T2 and low signal on T1 MRI

Answers

▸▸ Answer 1

Correct answer is D. Pneumococcal[1]

▸▸ Answer 2

Correct answer is A. Neisseria meningitidis[2]

▸▸ Answer 3

Correct answer is B. Viral meningitis[3]

▸▸ Answer 4

Correct answer is E. Late capsule[4]

▸▸ Answer 5

Correct answer is C. Early capsule[4]

▸▸ Answer 6

Correct answer is C. 15 mg/kg BD-TDS[5]

▸▸ Answer 7

Correct answer is D. ***Toxoplasma gondii***[4]

▸▸ Answer 8

Correct answer is D. Grade III[6]

▸▸ Answer 9

Correct answer is C. ***Borrelia spirochetes***[7]

▸▸ Answer 10

Correct answer is B. Lyme's disease[7]

▸▸ Answer 11

Correct answer is B. 7 to 10 months[8]

▸▸ Answer 12

Correct answer is A. Isoniazid and rifampin[8]

▸▸ Answer 13

Correct answer is C. 18 to 24 months[8]

▸▸ Answer 14

Correct answer is A. Caseating granuloma[9]

▸▸ Answer 15

Correct answer is A. Vancomycin 15 mg/kg every 8 to 12 hours + cefepime 2 g IV every 8 hours[1]

▸▸ Answer 16

Correct answer is E. Patients above 65 years of age do not need more dose of PPSV23[1]

▸▸ Answer 17

Correct answer is A. Chemical meningitis cannot occur spontaneously[3]

▸▸ Answer 18

Correct answer is A. ***Streptococcus***[10]

▸▸ Answer 19

Correct answer is E. Abscess leaves a glial scar after healing[4]

▸▸ Answer 20

Correct answer is E. All of the above are true[11]

▸▸ Answer 21

Correct answer is B. Lesion far from ventricle[12]

▸▸ Answer 22

Correct answer is A. Needle aspiration[13]

▸▸ Answer 23

Correct answer is C. Subdural empyema[14]

▸▸ Answer 24

Correct answer is D. All three lesions (toxoplasmosis, PCNSL, and PML) produce mass effect[15]

References

[1] Greenberg M, ed. Greenberg's Handbook of Neurosurgery. 10th ed. New York: Thieme; 2023:341
[2] Greenberg M, ed. Greenberg's Handbook of Neurosurgery. 10th ed. New York: Thieme; 2023:340
[3] Greenberg M, ed. Greenberg's Handbook of Neurosurgery. 10th ed. New York: Thieme; 2023:342
[4] Greenberg M, ed. Greenberg's Handbook of Neurosurgery. 10th ed. New York: Thieme; 2023:345
[5] Greenberg M, ed. Greenberg's Handbook of Neurosurgery. 10th ed. New York: Thieme; 2023:348
[6] Greenberg M, ed. Greenberg's Handbook of Neurosurgery. 10th ed. New York: Thieme; 2023:362
[7] Greenberg M, ed. Greenberg's Handbook of Neurosurgery. 10th ed. New York: Thieme; 2023:364
[8] Greenberg M, ed. Greenberg's Handbook of Neurosurgery. 10th ed. New York: Thieme; 2023:358
[9] Greenberg M, ed. Greenberg's Handbook of Neurosurgery. 10th ed. New York: Thieme; 2023:359
[10] Greenberg M, ed. Greenberg's Handbook of Neurosurgery. 10th ed. New York: Thieme; 2023:343
[11] Greenberg M, ed. Greenberg's Handbook of Neurosurgery. 10th ed. New York: Thieme; 2023:346
[12] Greenberg M, ed. Greenberg's Handbook of Neurosurgery. 10th ed. New York: Thieme; 2023:347
[13] Greenberg M, ed. Greenberg's Handbook of Neurosurgery. 10th ed. New York: Thieme; 2023:349
[14] Greenberg M, ed. Greenberg's Handbook of Neurosurgery. 10th ed. New York: Thieme; 2023:350
[15] Greenberg M, ed. Greenberg's Handbook of Neurosurgery. 10th ed. New York: Thieme; 2023:355

21 Skull, Spine, and Postsurgical Infections

Questions

▸▸ Question 1

The most common organism involved in VP or VA shunt infection is *Staphylococcus epidermidis*. Following statements regarding shunt infection is true except?

- A. Over 50% of *Staphylococcus* infections occur within 2 weeks post shunt
- B. Children with shunt infection have an increased mortality rate
- C. Risk of seizure post shunt infection increases in children
- D. In MMC patient, waiting for shunt insertion until the child is 2 weeks old significantly lowers the infection rate
- E. In MMC patient, ventriculitis after shunting have no effect on IQ of the patient

▸▸ Question 2

An 8-month-old child presented in neurosurgical emergency with fever, nausea, vomiting, and lethargy 10 days after placement of ventricular shunt. The patient had CSF analysis which showed WBC count to be > 20,000, protein elevated, glucose normal, and CSF culture negative. The patient is not shunt dependent with Candida spp. infection. What is most appropriate treatment in this patient?

- A. Completely remove the contaminated shunt
- B. Completely remove the shunt, place EVD, and start antifungal therapy
- C. Completely remove the shunt and start antifungal therapy
- D. No need to remove the shunt and start antifungal therapy
- E. Place a fresh shunt immediately and continue antifungal therapy

▸▸ Question 3

In most instances of shunt infection, the shunt is either externalized or completely removed with placement of EVD. Treatment of shunt infection with antibiotics without shunt removal is acceptable in all of the following patients except?

- A. In terminally ill patient
- B. In patient with poor anesthetic risk
- C. In patients with slit ventricles
- D. In patients with septicemia
- E. None of the above

▸▸ Question 4

After removal of shunt hardware in case of shunt infection with shunt dependency, placement of EVD can serve which of the following functions?

- A. Easy monitoring of CSF flow
- B. Control of ICP
- C. Repeated sampling of CSF for signs of resolution of infection
- D. Administration of intrathecal antibiotics
- E. All of the above

▸▸ Question 5

A patient with EVD placed develops signs and symptoms of CSF infection. On CSF analysis, WBC count is more than 1,000/µL, CSF to blood glucose ratio is < 0.2 but negative Gram stain and culture. What is this called?

- A. Contamination
- B. Ventriculostomy colonization
- C. Possible ventriculostomy-related infection
- D. Probable ventriculostomy-related infection
- E. Definitive meningitis

▸▸ Question 6

Intraventricular or intrathecal administration of antibiotics may be required if systemic treatment is ineffective or for resistant organism. Following are the antimicrobials that can be used intrathecally except?

- A. Vancomycin
- B. Aminoglycosides like gentamicin, amikacin, tobramycin
- C. Cefepime
- D. Daptomycin
- E. Colistimethate sodium

▸▸ Question 7

A patient presented with severe backache which is exacerbated by any movement, fever, and point tenderness 3 weeks after laminectomy and diskectomy. On MRI of lumbosacral spine with contrast, there is contrast enhancement in vertebral bone marrow, disk space, and posterior annulus fibrosus. What is the most likely diagnosis in this case?

- A. Epidural abscess
- B. Recurrent/residual disk herniation
- C. Vertebral bone marrow infection
- D. Postoperative diskitis
- E. Postoperative arachnoiditis

▸▸ Question 8

What is a Pott puffy tumor?

- A. Vertebral osteomyelitis with edema and swelling
- B. Spine infection with spread into spinal canal
- C. Skull infection without edema and swelling
- D. Skull infection with surrounding edema and swelling
- E. Skull infection with smoke-like pattern on X-ray around the tumor

▸▸ Question 9

A patient with history of IV drug abuse presented with severe backache at midthoracic region which started spontaneously. He has point tenderness on examination and elevated ESR and CRP levels. On MRI, there is hypointense epidural mass on T1 and hyperintense epidural mass on T2 which enhances with contrast. Diagnosis of epidural abscess is confirmed with needle-guided aspiration. What is the most common pathogen in this case?

- A. *Streptococcus epidermidis*
- B. *Staphylococcus aureus*
- C. *Pseudomonas aeruginosa*
- D. *E. coli*
- E. Brucellosis

▸▸ Question 10

A patient with diabetes mellitis presents with chronic backache in neurosurgical OPD. MRI findings showed T1 low signal in vertebral bodies and intervertebral disk while increased intensity in vertebral bodies and intervertebral disk on T2. CT-guided needle biopsy confirmed Pott's disease or tuberculous vertebral osteomyelitis. What is the most commonly involved structure in this scenario?

- A. Posterior elements of vertebrae
- B. Intervertebral disk
- C. Vertebral body
- D. Both vertebral body and intervertebral disk
- E. Vertebral body and pedicles

Answers

▸▸ Answer 1

Correct answer is E. In MMC patient, ventriculitis after shunting have no effect on IQ of the patient[1]

▸▸ Answer 2

Correct answer is C. Completely remove the shunt and start antifungal therapy[2]

▸▸ Answer 3

Correct answer is D. In patients with septicemia[2]

▸▸ Answer 4

Correct answer is E. All of the above[2]

▸▸ Answer 5

Correct answer is C. Possible ventriculostomy-related infection[3]

▸▸ Answer 6

Correct answer is C. Cefepime[4]

▸▸ Answer 7

Correct answer is D. Postoperative diskitis[5]

▸▸ Answer 8

Correct answer is D. Skull infection with surrounding edema and swelling[6]

▸▸ Answer 9

Correct answer is B. *Staphylococcus aureus*[7]

▸▸ Answer 10

Correct answer is C. Vertebral body[8]

References

[1] Greenberg M, ed. Greenberg's Handbook of Neurosurgery. 10th ed. New York: Thieme; 2023:371
[2] Greenberg M, ed. Greenberg's Handbook of Neurosurgery. 10th ed. New York: Thieme; 2023:373
[3] Greenberg M, ed. Greenberg's Handbook of Neurosurgery. 10th ed. New York: Thieme; 2023:375
[4] Greenberg M, ed. Greenberg's Handbook of Neurosurgery. 10th ed. New York: Thieme; 2023: 377
[5] Greenberg M, ed. Greenberg's Handbook of Neurosurgery. 10th ed. New York: Thieme; 2023: 378
[6] Greenberg M, ed. Greenberg's Handbook of Neurosurgery. 10th ed. New York: Thieme; 2023:380
[7] Greenberg M, ed. Greenberg's Handbook of Neurosurgery. 10th ed. New York: Thieme; 2023:381
[8] Greenberg M, ed. Greenberg's Handbook of Neurosurgery. 10th ed. New York: Thieme; 2023:387

22 Other Nonbacterial Infections

Questions

▸▸ Question 1

What is the treatment of choice for Creutzfeldt-Jakob disease?

- A. Penicillin
- B. Cephalosporins
- C. Carbapenems
- D. Antifungals
- E. No known treatment

▸▸ Question 2

Herpes simplex encephalitis has a predilection for what?

- A. Temporal lobe
- B. Parietal lobe
- C. Occipital lobe
- D. Medulla oblongata
- E. Peripheral nerves

▸▸ Question 3

What is the drug of choice for treatment of herpes simplex encephalitis?

- A. Acyclovir
- B. Oseltamivir
- C. Zanamivir
- D. Adefovir
- E. Interferons

▸▸ Question 4

Which of the following is the most common parasitic infection involving CNS?

- A. Cysticercosis
- B. Schistosomiasis
- C. Amoebiasis
- D. Trypanosomiasis
- E. Malaria

▸▸ Question 5

What is the treatment for hydatid cyst of brain?

- A. Antibiotics
- B. Femicyclovir
- C. Prednisolone
- D. Needle aspiration
- E. Surgical excision

▸▸ Question 6

Which of the following is the only amoeba to cause CNS infection in human beings?

- A. *Amoeba histolytica*
- B. *Amoeba proteus*
- C. *Dictyostelium*
- D. *Naegleria fowleri*
- E. *Entamoeba dysentrii*

▸▸ Question 7

The 2009 CDC guidelines for CNS cryptococcal infection in HIV-infected individuals recommend which antifungal agent?

- A. Amphotericin B plus fluconazole
- B. Amphotericin B plus ketoconazole
- C. Amphotericin B plus lucovorin
- D. Clotrimazole plus fluconazole
- E. Amphotericin B plus clotrimazole

▸▸ Question 8

An 8-year-old boy presents in neurosurgical emergency with complaints of irritability, altered mentation, malaise, and seizure. CSF analysis showed leukocytosis, and raised RBC and protein. MRI of brain showed edema in bilateral temporal lobe with transsylvian sign. EEG showed periodic lateralizing epileptiform discharges (PLEDs). Acyclovir is started in this patient to treat the suspected pathology. Which part of the brain is most affected by this pathology?

- A. Temporal lobe
- B. Orbitofrontal lobes
- C. Limbic system
- D. Parietal lobe
- E. A, B, and C

▸▸ Question 9

A patient presents in neurosurgical OPD with complaint of dementia which progressively increased over time. Later the patient develops pyramidal tract findings (limb weakness, stiffness, and pathologic reflexes) and myoclonus. MRI of brain shows hyperintensities in the striatum and in multiple cortical regions. EEG showed bilateral sharp waves. This disease has no known treatment with median survival of only 5 months. What is the most likely diagnosis in this patient?

- A. Neurocysticercosis
- B. Creutzfeldt-Jakob disease
- C. Multifocal varicella-zoster leukoencephalitis
- D. Herpes simplex encephalitis
- E. Progressive multifocal leukoencephalopathy

▸▸ **Question 10**

A patient with history of fits presents with multiple ring enhancing lesions within the brain. Blood test shows eosinophilia. Diagnosis of neurocysticercosis (*Taenia solium* or tapeworm) was made. Which of the following is the location of cyst within brain?

- A. Meningeal
- B. Parenchymal
- C. Ventricular
- D. Mixed
- E. All of the above

▸▸ **Question 11**

All of the following are true regarding treatment of neurocysticercosis except?

- A. Praziquantel and albendazole are given
- B. Antiepileptics may be needed for seizures
- C. Steroids are not given because it decreases immunity
- D. Surgical resection of lesion is done when appropriate
- E. CSF diversionary procedure is done when needed

▸▸ **Question 12**

Echinococcus is a condition which is caused by encysted larvae of the dog tapeworm Echinococcus granulosa and is also called as hydatid disease (cyst). On CT of the brain, it presents as single cyst confined to brain white matter. All of the following are included in Dowling technique for cyst removal except?

- A. The head is positioned so that the cyst points straight up toward ceiling
- B. Low power bipolar cautery is used to avoid cyst rupture
- C. Open the dura close to the dome of the cyst as it may be adherent to the dura
- D. Keep the surface of the cyst moist
- E. The cyst is removed without rupturing it

▸▸ **Question 13**

Following are fungal CNS infection of brain except?

- A. Cryptococcosis
- B. Candidiasis
- C. Aspergillosis
- D. Echinococcosis
- E. Coccidiomycosis

▸▸ **Question 14**

Cryptococcal CNS infection is the most common fungal infection diagnosed in living patients. Which of the following is true regarding cryptococcal CNS infection?

- A. Cryptococcoma almost exclusively occurs in AIDS patients
- B. Cryptococcal meningitis can occur without AIDS and usually occurs with raised ICP
- C. CSF opening pressure is usually more than 20 cm of water
- D. Recommended medical treatment is amphotericin B deoxycholate plus fluconazole
- E. All of the above

▸▸ **Question 15**

Amebic infection of CNS is caused by Naegleria fowleri which can cause diffuse encephalitis with hemorrhagic necrosis and purulent meningitis involving the brain and spinal cord. What is the drug of choice for medical treatment of this condition?

- A. Albendazole
- B. Praziquantel
- C. Amphotericin B
- D. Miconazole
- E. Fluconazole

▸▸ **Question 16**

Following are parasitic infections of CNS except?

- A. Cysticercosis
- B. Toxoplasmosis
- C. Echinococcus
- D. Mucormycosis
- E. Schistosomiasis

▸▸ **Question 17**

Which of the following is the fully operative operating room sterilization procedure for Creutzfeldt-Jakob disease?

- A. Immersion in 1N NaOH for 1 hour at room temperature
- B. Steam autoclaving at 121 degrees Celsius for 15 to 30 minutes
- C. Steam autoclaving at 132 degrees Celsius for 15 to 30 minutes
- D. Immersion in sodium hypochlorite for 1 hour
- E. All of the above

Answers

▸▸ **Answer 1**

Correct answer is E. No known treatment[1]

▸▸ **Answer 2**

Correct answer is A. Temporal lobe[2]

▸▸ **Answer 3**

Correct answer is A. Acyclovir[2]

▸▸ **Answer 4**

Correct answer is A. Cysticercosis[1]

▸▸ **Answer 5**

Correct answer is E. Surgical excision[3]

▸▸ Answer 6

Correct answer is D. ***Naegleria fowleri***[4]

▸▸ Answer 7

Correct answer is A. Amphotericin B plus fluconazole[4]

▸▸ Answer 8

Correct answer is E. A, B, and C[2]

▸▸ Answer 9

Correct answer is B. Creutzfeldt-Jakob disease[5]

▸▸ Answer 10

Correct answer is E. All of the above[1]

▸▸ Answer 11

Correct answer is C. Steroids are not given because it decreases immunity[6]

▸▸ Answer 12

Correct answer is C. Open the dura close to the dome of the cyst as it may be adherent to the dura[3]

▸▸ Answer 13

Correct answer is D. Echinococcosis[7]

▸▸ Answer 14

Correct answer is E. All of the above[7]

▸▸ Answer 15

Correct answer is C. Amphotericin B[4]

▸▸ Answer 16

Correct answer is D. Mucormycosis[1]

▸▸ Answer 17

Correct answer is A. Immersion in 1N NaOH for 1 hour at room temperature[8]

References

[1] Greenberg M, ed. Greenberg's Handbook of Neurosurgery. 10th ed. New York: Thieme; 2023:404
[2] Greenberg M, ed. Greenberg's Handbook of Neurosurgery. 10th ed. New York: Thieme; 2023:397
[3] Greenberg M, ed. Greenberg's Handbook of Neurosurgery. 10th ed. New York: Thieme; 2023:408
[4] Greenberg M, ed. Greenberg's Handbook of Neurosurgery. 10th ed. New York: Thieme; 2023:410
[5] Greenberg M, ed. Greenberg's Handbook of Neurosurgery. 10th ed. New York: Thieme; 2023:399
[6] Greenberg M, ed. Greenberg's Handbook of Neurosurgery. 10th ed. New York: Thieme; 2023:407
[7] Greenberg M, ed. Greenberg's Handbook of Neurosurgery. 10th ed. New York: Thieme; 2023:409
[8] Greenberg M, ed. Greenberg's Handbook of Neurosurgery. 10th ed. New York: Thieme; 2023:402

Part VII

Hydrocephalus and Cerebrospinal Fluid (CSF)

VII

23 Cerebrospinal Fluid

Questions

▸▸ **Question 1**

Cerebrospinal fluid (CSF) surrounds the brain and spinal cord and circulates within the subarachnoid space. Following statements regarding CSF is true except?

- A. Formation rate is 0.3 to 0.35 mL/min in adults and total volume is 150 mL
- B. Absorption of CSF is in arachnoid villi, choroid plexuses, and glymphatics
- C. In normal adults, lymphocytes are 0 to 5/mm^3 while there are no RBCs or polymorphonuclear cells
- D. Produced only in the choroid plexus in the ventricles
- E. Normal glucose in CSF is 60 mg/dL while protein is 35 mg/dL

▸▸ **Question 2**

What is the most accurate confirmatory test for fluid to be CSF?

- A. Halo sign
- B. Beta 2 transferrin
- C. Reservoir sign
- D. Quantitative glucose within fluid
- E. CT cisternography

▸▸ **Question 3**

A patient presents with signs of meningitis. On CSF examination, there is increased opening pressure with turbid appearance of fluid, increased protein, decreased glucose, and few 1000 WBCs (mostly PMNs). What is the most likely diagnosis in this patient?

- A. Viral meningitis
- B. TB meningitis
- C. Fungal meningitis
- D. Acute purulent meningitis
- E. Multiple sclerosis

▸▸ **Question 4**

Which of the following is the cause of nontraumatic CSF fistula?

- A. Empty sella syndrome
- B. Increased ICP or hydrocephalus
- C. Infection of paranasal sinuses
- D. A persistent remnant of craniopharyngeal canal
- E. All of the above

▸▸ **Question 5**

A child presents with complaint of recurrent meningitis without any identifiable cause. A diagnosis of spontaneous posterior fossa fistula is made. Which of the following is a possible site of egress of CSF in this patient?

- A. Facial canal which can fistulize into the middle ear
- B. Petromastoid canal: along the path of arterial supply to the mucosa of mastoid air cells
- C. Hyrtl's fissure also known as tympanomeningeal fissure which links posterior fossa to hypotympanum
- D. Anomaly of labyrinthine in Mundini dysplasia
- E. All of the above

▸▸ **Question 6**

Pneumococcal meningitis is the most common pathogen in CSF fistula meningitis. Meningitis most commonly occurs in which type of CSF fistula?

- A. Fistula following a neurosurgical procedure
- B. Posttraumatic fistula
- C. Spontaneous fistula
- D. Fistula due to basal skull fracture
- E. All of the above

▸▸ **Question 7**

What is investigation of choice to determine the site of CSF fistula?

- A. CT of brain with and without contrast
- B. Water-soluble, contrast CT cisternography
- C. MRI with and without contrast
- D. MRI only without contrast
- E. Radionuclide cisternography

▸▸ **Question 8**

Following statements are true regarding treatment of CSF fistula except?

- A. Prophylactic antibiotics are recommended while there is no rule of pneumococcal vaccine
- B. Conservative treatment includes bed rest, acetazolamide, avoidance from straining, and modest fluid restriction
- C. Serial LPs or continuous lumbar drainage with head of bed elevation
- D. Waiting for 2 weeks before surgical treatment for posttraumatic fistula that does not settle with conservative therapy
- E. Spontaneous leaks usually requires surgery

▸▸ **Question 9**

A patient has spontaneous intracranial hypotension (SIH) with low CSF pressure and orthostatic hypotension in the absence of antecedent trauma or dural puncture. Following are characteristics finding on imaging except?

- A. Sagging brain
- B. Pachy-meningeal enhancement

- C. Engorged veins
- D. Pituitary hyperemia
- E. Subdural space absence

▸▸ **Question 10**

In SIH, there is usually a spontaneous CSF leak which can occur due to spinal diverticula, underlying weakness of meninges as in some connective tissue disorder such as Ehlers and Marfan syndrome and CSF leak because of dural injury due to degenerative disk, osteophyte, or bony spurs. What is the study of choice for diagnosing and localizing intermittent leaks?

- A. CT myelogram with iodinated contrast
- B. MRI with intrathecal gadolinium
- C. Radioisotope cisternography
- D. Spinal MRI
- E. CT of brain

Answers

▸▸ **Answer 1**

Correct answer is D. Produced only in the choroid plexus in the ventricles[1]

▸▸ **Answer 2**

Correct answer is B. Beta 2 transferrin[2]

▸▸ **Answer 3**

Correct answer is D. Acute purulent meningitis[3]

▸▸ **Answer 4**

Correct answer is E. All of the above[4]

▸▸ **Answer 5**

Correct answer is E. All of the above[4]

▸▸ **Answer 6**

Correct answer is C. Spontaneous fistula[4]

▸▸ **Answer 7**

Correct answer is B. Water-soluble, contrast CT cisternography[5]

▸▸ **Answer 8**

Correct answer is A. Prophylactic antibiotics are recommended while there is no rule of pneumococcal vaccine[6]

▸▸ **Answer 9**

Correct answer is E. Subdural space absence[7]

▸▸ **Answer 10**

Correct answer is A. CT myelogram with iodinated contrast[7]

References

[1] Greenberg M, ed. Greenberg's Handbook of Neurosurgery. 10th ed. New York: Thieme; 2023:414
[2] Greenberg M, ed. Greenberg's Handbook of Neurosurgery. 10th ed. New York: Thieme; 2023:415
[3] Greenberg M, ed. Greenberg's Handbook of Neurosurgery. 10th ed. New York: Thieme; 2023:417
[4] Greenberg M, ed. Greenberg's Handbook of Neurosurgery. 10th ed. New York: Thieme; 2023:418
[5] Greenberg M, ed. Greenberg's Handbook of Neurosurgery. 10th ed. New York: Thieme; 2023:419
[6] Greenberg M, ed. Greenberg's Handbook of Neurosurgery. 10th ed. New York: Thieme; 2023:420
[7] Greenberg M, ed. Greenberg's Handbook of Neurosurgery. 10th ed. New York: Thieme; 2023:423

24 Hydrocephalus: General Aspects

Questions

▸▸ Question 1

Hydrocephalus (HCP) is abnormal accumulation of CSF within ventricles of brain. What is the most common cause of communicating hydrocephalus in pediatric population?
- A. Chiari type 2 malformation with MMC
- B. Chiari type 1 malformation without MMC
- C. Periaqueductal stenosis
- D. Infection
- E. Post hemorrhagic

▸▸ Question 2

A 2-month-old child presents with irritability, N/V, and poor head control. On examination, he/she has bulging fontanelle, engorged scalp veins, setting sun sign, and positive Macewan's sign. MRI of brain showed periaqueductal gliosis in this patient. Following are the causes of congenital hydrocephalus in pediatric population except?
- A. Chiari type 2 with MMC
- B. Chiari type 1 without MMC
- C. Secondary aqueductal gliosis
- D. Dandy Walker malformation
- E. Colloid cyst blocking CSF flow at aqueduct

▸▸ Question 3

Occipital frontal circumference is used to monitor head growth and to assess possible pathological process causing change in head measurement from normal. Active hydrocephalus, subdural hematoma, or subdural effusion is signified by which of the following?
- A. Progressive upward deviation from the normal curve
- B. Continued head growth of more than 1.25 cm/wk
- C. OFC measuring 2 standard deviations above normal
- D. Head circumference out of proportion to body length or weight
- E. All of the above

▸▸ Question 4

Pregeniculate blindness is because of lesion anterior to the lateral geniculate body while postgeniculate blindness is because of lesion posterior to the lateral geniculate body. Following are the causes of blindness from hydrocephalus except?
- A. Occlusion of posterior cerebral arteries (caused by downward transtentorial herniation)
- B. Diffuse hypoxic injury to occipital lobes caused by hypotension
- C. Chronic papilledema causing injury to optic nerve at optic disk
- D. Dilatation of third ventricle with compression of optic chiasma
- E. Compression of PCA caused by upward herniation of cerebellum

▸▸ Question 5

Following are the specific radiologic criteria for the diagnosis of hydrocephalus except?
- A. Evans ratio (FH/BPD) more than 0.3 shows hydrocephalus
- B. Size of both temporal horns > 2 mm shows HCP
- C. Slit third ventricle
- D. Periventricular low density on plain CT of brain and hyperintensity on MRI of brain
- E. Ballooning of lateral and frontal ventricles

▸▸ Question 6

Following are features indicative of chronic hydrocephalus except?
- A. Beaten copper cranium
- B. Third ventricle herniating into sella
- C. Erosion of sella turcica
- D. The temporal horns are markedly prominent
- E. Atrophy and upward bowing of corpus callosum

▸▸ Question 7

Pseudohydrocephalus refers to conditions that may mimic hydrocephalus but are not due to inadequate CSF absorption. Which of the following can be called as pseudohydrocephalus?
- A. Hydrocephalus ex vacuo due to cerebral atrophy
- B. Developmental anomalies like agenesis of corpus callosum, septo-optic dysplasia, or hydranencephaly
- C. Otic hydrocephalus
- D. External hydrocephalus
- E. All of the above

▸▸ Question 8

A 4-month-old child presents with macrocrania and frontal bossing. Plain CT of brain showed enlarged subarachnoid spaces over the cortical sulci of frontal poles. Basal cisterns and anterior hemispheric fissure are also seen to be enlarged. A diagnosis of external hydrocephalus or benign external hydrocephalus is made. What is the most appropriate treatment for this condition?
- A. Usually resolves spontaneously before 2 years of age
- B. Parents may need to periodically reposition the head while the child is sleeping
- C. Shunt may be needed for cosmetic reasons in severe macrocrania
- D. Parents are reinsured that this is not cortical atrophy
- E. All of the above are correct

▸▸ Question 9

A disconnected ventriculoperitoneal shunt may continue to function through an endothelialized subcutaneous tract. Which of the following statements is true regarding repair or removing of a VP shunt?

- A. Indications for shunt repair are marginally functioning shunt with signs and symptoms of increased ICP
- B. Most of the patients with spina bifida or aqueductal stenosis are not shunt dependent
- C. If a shunt is nonfunctioning and the patient is not shunt dependent then the shunt should be removed regardless of shunt infection or not
- D. A patient with nonfunctioning shunt with no symptoms does not need to be followed up
- E. All of the above are correct

▸▸ Question 10

A patient above 60 years of age presents with gait disturbance (wide based, short shuffling steps like glued to the ground), dementia with slowing of thoughts (bradyphrenia), and urinary incontinence with urgency. On examination, there is no papilledema, hyperreflexia, or lateralizing signs. LP was done which showed normal pressure. MRI showed ventricular enlargement without any blockage. Following are features that correlate with favorable response to shunt in this condition except?

- A. Periventricular low density on plain CT of brain and high intensity on T2WI MRI
- B. Compression of convexity sulci
- C. Rounding of the frontal horns
- D. Dilated subarachnoid spaces in high convexity
- E. Upward bowing and thinning of corpus collosum

▸▸ Question 11

Which of the following is a component of iNPH Radscale?

- A. Evans ratio increased
- B. Tight high convexity
- C. Sylvian fissure enlargement
- D. Decrease of callosal angle
- E. All of the above are true

▸▸ Question 12

Which of the following is true regarding treatment of normal pressure hydrocephalus?

- A. Positive response on tap test increase the likelihood of responding to shunting
- B. VP shunt is the procedure of choice with use of medium pressure valve
- C. ETV has been advocated by some authors
- D. Most likely symptom to improve with shunting is incontinence then gait disturbance and then dementia
- E. All of the above

Answers

▸▸ Answer 1

Correct answer is D. Infection[1]

▸▸ Answer 2

Correct answer is E. Colloid cyst blocking CSF flow at aqueduct[1]

▸▸ Answer 3

Correct answer is E. All of the above[2]

▸▸ Answer 4

Correct answer is B. Diffuse hypoxic injury to occipital lobes caused by hypotension[3]

▸▸ Answer 5

Correct answer is C. Slit third ventricle[4]

▸▸ Answer 6

Correct answer is D. The temporal horns are markedly prominent[5]

▸▸ Answer 7

Correct answer is E. All of the above[5]

▸▸ Answer 8

Correct answer is E. All of the above are correct[6]

▸▸ Answer 9

Correct answer is A. Indications for shunt repair are marginally functioning shunt with signs and symptoms of increased ICP[7]

▸▸ Answer 10

Correct answer is D. Dilated subarachnoid spaces in high convexity[8]

▸▸ Answer 11

Correct answer is E. All of the above are true[9]

▸▸ Answer 12

Correct answer is E. All of the above[10]

References

[1] Greenberg M, ed. Greenberg's Handbook of Neurosurgery. 10th ed. New York: Thieme; 2023:426
[2] Greenberg M, ed. Greenberg's Handbook of Neurosurgery. 10th ed. New York: Thieme; 2023:428
[3] Greenberg M, ed. Greenberg's Handbook of Neurosurgery. 10th ed. New York: Thieme; 2023:429
[4] Greenberg M, ed. Greenberg's Handbook of Neurosurgery. 10th ed. New York: Thieme; 2023:432
[5] Greenberg M, ed. Greenberg's Handbook of Neurosurgery. 10th ed. New York: Thieme; 2023:433
[6] Greenberg M, ed. Greenberg's Handbook of Neurosurgery. 10th ed. New York: Thieme; 2023:434
[7] Greenberg M, ed. Greenberg's Handbook of Neurosurgery. 10th ed. New York: Thieme; 2023:436
[8] Greenberg M, ed. Greenberg's Handbook of Neurosurgery. 10th ed. New York: Thieme; 2023:441
[9] Greenberg M, ed. Greenberg's Handbook of Neurosurgery. 10th ed. New York: Thieme; 2023:443
[10] Greenberg M, ed. Greenberg's Handbook of Neurosurgery. 10th ed. New York: Thieme; 2023:447

25 Treatment of Hydrocephalus

Questions

▸▸ Question 1

Diuretic therapy may be tried in premature infants with bloody CSF as long as there is no evidence of active hydrocephalus, and satisfactory control is reported in about half of the infants. What is the initial dose of acetazolamide in mg/kg/d in divided doses?

- A. 1
- B. 5
- C. 10
- D. 25
- E. 50

▸▸ Question 2

A 4-year-old child was admitted with hydrocephalus and tectal glioma. He had no previous surgery. What is the ETV success score?

- A. 10
- B. 20
- C. 30
- D. 60
- E. 80

▸▸ Question 3

What is the most common cause of shunt malfunction?

- A. Proximal end blockade
- B. Distal end blockade
- C. Shunt fracture
- D. Silicone allergy
- E. *Streptococcus viridians* infection

▸▸ Question 4

Upward gaze palsy or setting sun sign is associated with which of the following?

- A. Parinaud's syndrome
- B. Pulfrich syndrome
- C. Anton's syndrome
- D. Ridoch's phenomenon
- E. Weber syndrome

▸▸ Question 5

Contrast medium commonly used for X-ray shuntogram is what?

- A. Gadolinium
- B. Iohexol
- C. 99m-technetium pertechnetate
- D. Gadopentate dimeglumine
- E. Ferric ammonium citrate

▸▸ Question 6

What is the shunt malfunction rate in percentage during the first year of placement in the pediatric population?

- A. 1
- B. 3
- C. 7
- D. 17
- E. 49

▸▸ Question 7

What is the treatment of choice for short-term symptoms of intracranial hypotension due to over-shunting of a VP shunt?

- A. Antibiotics
- B. Steroids
- C. Antisiphon device
- D. Shunt removal
- E. Y connector shunt

▸▸ Question 8

What do the three dots visible on the shunt valve on X-ray represent?

- A. Very low pressure
- B. Low pressure
- C. Medium pressure
- D. High pressure
- E. Very high pressure

▸▸ Question 9

Diuretic therapy is used in premature infants for bloody CSF with no evidence of active hydrocephalus as an adjunct to definitive treatment or as a temporizing measure. Satisfactory control of hydrocephalus can also be achieved in children less than 1 year of age with stable vital signs, normal renal function, and no symptoms of elevated ICP (apnea, lethargy, vomiting) using diuretic therapy. Following are true regarding diuretic therapy except?

- A. Acetazolamide is started at 25 mg/kg/d with simultaneous start of furosemide at 1 mg/kg/d
- B. To counteract acidosis, tricitrate is used at a dose of 4 mL/kg/d
- C. There is no need to measure electrolytes along with diuretic therapy
- D. Weekly ultrasound or CT of brain is performed and ventricular shunt is inserted if ventriculomegaly occurs
- E. This therapy is used for 6 months and then dosage is tapered over 2 to 4 weeks

▸▸ Question 10

Surgical methods to control hydrocephalus include third ventriculostomy, various shunting methods, eliminating the obstruction like tumor, and choroid plexectomy. What is the goal of surgery in such patients?

- A. Normal sized ventricles
- B. Opened basal cisterns
- C. Optimum neurologic function and good cosmetic result
- D. Opened subarachnoid spaces
- E. Both A and B

▸▸ Question 11

Endoscopic third ventriculostomy is an endoscopic method of dealing with hydrocephalus. Which of the following is an indication of endoscopic third ventriculostomy?

- A. It is used in patients with obstructive hydrocephalus
- B. In managing shunt infection as a means to remove all hardware without subjecting the patient to increased ICP
- C. It is also proposed as an option for patients who developed subdural hematomas after shunting in which the shunt is removed before ETV is performed
- D. It is also indicated for slit ventricle syndrome
- E. All of the above are indications of ETV

▸▸ Question 12

During ETV complications can occur such as injury to basilar artery, PCom, or PCA, injury to pituitary stalk and hypothalamus, or transient 3rd and 6th nerve palsies. ETV has low success rate in infants because of which of the following?

- A. There are higher chances of complications to occur
- B. It is difficult to do ventriculostomy in infants
- C. Mortality in infants in high after ETV
- D. They may not have a normally developed subarachnoid space
- E. All of the above

▸▸ Question 13

ETV success score is used to predict the likelihood of success of ETV. Scores less than 40% correlate with very low chance of success while scores more than 80% show better chance of success compared to shunting. A child 3 years of age with tectal tumor and no history of previous shunt has ETV success score of what?

- A. 60%
- B. 70%
- C. 80%
- D. 90%
- E. 50%

▸▸ Question 14

There are various types of shunts including ventriculoperitoneal shunt (VP), ventriculoatrial shunt (VA), Torkildsen shunt (shunts ventricles to CSF space), ventriculopleural shunt, and lumboperitoneal shunt. VP shunt is the most commonly used shunt in modern era. What are indications of VA shunt instead of VP shunt in a patient?

- A. Extensive abdominal surgery
- B. Peritonitis
- C. Morbid obesity
- D. In patients who have had NEC
- E. All of the above

▸▸ Question 15

What is the most common complication of a shunt?

- A. Obstruction
- B. Disconnection at a junction or breakage at any point
- C. Infection
- D. Seizures
- E. Extraneural metastasis of certain tumors

▸▸ Question 16

A child underwent VP shunting with reprogrammable shunt, the pressure setting on which can be seen using an X-ray perpendicular to the shunt valve. This boy after some time presents with N/V, headache, lethargy, and ataxia. On physical examination, this child has bulging fontanelles and upward gaze palsy. What is the appropriate method for evaluation of shunt malfunction?

- A. Shunt series (plain X-rays to visualize the entire shunt)
- B. Using ultrasound in patient with open fontanelles
- C. Plain CT of brain
- D. MRI of brain
- E. All of the above

▸▸ Question 17

What are possible complications of over-shunting of VP shunt?

- A. Dilated ventricles
- B. Intracranial hypertension
- C. Subdural hematomas
- D. Wide opened sylvian aqueduct
- E. All of the above

▸▸ Question 18

A patient after VP shunting presents after 1 year with intermittent headaches, nausea, vomiting, irritability, and impaired mentation. Plain CT of brain showed totally collapsed ventricles. What is the procedure of choice in this patient?

- A. Expectant management
- B. Upgradation to a higher-pressure valve
- C. Upgradation to low-pressure valve
- D. Removal of shunt and reinserting again
- E. Antisiphon devices have no role in these patients

Answers

▸▸ Answer 1

Correct answer is D. 25[1]

▸▸ Answer 2

Correct answer is E. 80[2]

▸▸ Answer 3

Correct answer is A. Proximal end blockade[3]

▸▸ Answer 4

Correct answer is A. Parinaud's syndrome[4]

▸▸ Answer 5

Correct answer is B. Iohexol[5]

▸▸ Answer 6

Correct answer is D. 17[5]

▸▸ Answer 7

Correct answer is C. Antisiphon device[6]

▸▸ Answer 8

Correct answer is D. High pressure[7]

▸▸ Answer 9

Correct answer is C. There is no need to measure electrolytes along with diuretic therapy[8]

▸▸ Answer 10

Correct answer is C. Optimum neurologic function and good cosmetic result[1]

▸▸ Answer 11

Correct answer is E. All of the above are indications of ETV[8]

▸▸ Answer 12

Correct answer is D. They may not have a normally developed subarachnoid space[8]

▸▸ Answer 13

Correct answer is C. 80%[2]

▸▸ Answer 14

Correct answer is E. All of the above[2]

▸▸ Answer 15

Correct answer is A. Obstruction[3]

▸▸ Answer 16

Correct answer is A. Shunt series (plain X-rays to visualize the entire shunt)[4]

▸▸ Answer 17

Correct answer is C. Subdural hematomas[9]

▸▸ Answer 18

Correct answer is B. Upgradation to a higher-pressure valve[10]

References

[1] Greenberg M, ed. Greenberg's Handbook of Neurosurgery. 10th ed. New York: Thieme; 2023:452
[2] Greenberg M, ed. Greenberg's Handbook of Neurosurgery. 10th ed. New York: Thieme; 2023:454
[3] Greenberg M, ed. Greenberg's Handbook of Neurosurgery. 10th ed. New York: Thieme; 2023:455
[4] Greenberg M, ed. Greenberg's Handbook of Neurosurgery. 10th ed. New York: Thieme; 2023:459
[5] Greenberg M, ed. Greenberg's Handbook of Neurosurgery. 10th ed. New York: Thieme; 2023:460
[6] Greenberg M, ed. Greenberg's Handbook of Neurosurgery. 10th ed. New York: Thieme; 2023:462
[7] Greenberg M, ed. Greenberg's Handbook of Neurosurgery. 10th ed. New York: Thieme; 2023:467
[8] Greenberg M, ed. Greenberg's Handbook of Neurosurgery. 10th ed. New York: Thieme; 2023:453
[9] Greenberg M, ed. Greenberg's Handbook of Neurosurgery. 10th ed. New York: Thieme; 2023:461
[10] Greenberg M, ed. Greenberg's Handbook of Neurosurgery. 10th ed. New York: Thieme; 2023:464

Part VIII

Seizures

VIII

26 Seizures: Classification and Syndromes

Questions

▸▸ Question 1

A patient was brought to the OPD with history of seizures. His mother showed you a video recording of seizure episode where you noticed fairly symmetric, bilateral, synchronous, semirhythmic jerking of the upper and lower extremities, with elbow flexion and knee extension. What are these?

- A. Partial seizures
- B. Tonic seizures
- C. Clonic seizures
- D. Atonic seizures
- E. Astatic seizures

▸▸ Question 2

A patient presented to you with history of seizures. On further inquiry you find that there is no history of aura, motor involvement, and postictal confusion. His EEG revealed spike and wave at exactly 3/sec. These features are most consistent which of the following?

- A. Uncal seizures
- B. Mesial temporal seizures
- C. Absence seizures
- D. Partial seizures
- E. Grand mal seizures

▸▸ Question 3

What is the most common cause of intractable temporal lobe epilepsy?

- A. Absence seizures
- B. Uncal epilepsy
- C. Mesial temporal sclerosis
- D. Superior temporal gyrus syndrome
- E. Temporal lobe hemorrhagic contusion

▸▸ Question 4

A patient with recently diagnosed epilepsy presented to the OPD for follow-up. During the review of the radiology, the clinician notices hippocampal atrophy on MRI. What is the most likely diagnosis?

- A. West syndrome
- B. Lennox Gustate syndrome
- C. Mesial temporal lobe epilepsy
- D. Juvenile myoclonic epilepsy
- E. Uncinate seizures

▸▸ Question 5

A patient with known case of temporal lobe epilepsy presents with kakosmia. This subtype of seizures is classified as?

- A. Uncinate seizures
- B. Complex seizures
- C. Focal seizures
- D. Sensory seizures

▸▸ Question 6

Factors that lower the seizure threshold (make it easier to provoke a seizure) include sleep deprivation, hyperventilation, photic stimulation, infection, metabolic disturbances, and head trauma. Todd's paralysis is a phenomenon that occurs after seizure activity. Which of the following is true regarding Todd's paralysis?

- A. Partial or total paralysis usually occurs in areas involved in a partial seizure
- B. It occurs more commonly in nonstructural lesion
- C. The paralysis usually resolves over days to weeks
- D. Postictal aphasia or hemianopia are not included in this
- E. All of the above are true

▸▸ Question 7

A patient presents in neurosurgical emergency with complaint of first occurrence of focal seizure with retained consciousness (simple partial seizure). As a rule of thumb, what is the cause of such seizure?

- A. Metabolic cause
- B. Insult to brain within previous 2 weeks
- C. Structural lesion within brain
- D. Febrile seizure
- E. None of the above

▸▸ Question 8

Tonic–clonic seizure is a type of motor seizure which is a generalized seizure that evolves from tonic to clonic motor activity. A patient presenting with other type of motor seizure in which there is shock-like body jerks (one or more in succession) with generalized EEG discharges is said to have which type of seizure?

- A. Clonic
- B. Tonic
- C. Myoclonic tonic clonic
- D. Myoclonic
- E. Myoclonic-tonic

▸▸ Question 9

A patient with known family history of seizure is presented with complex partial seizure that begins with arrest and stare, and oroalimentary and complex automatism signs with posturing of arm. This seizure activity lasts for 1 to 2 minutes and there is preictal olfactory aura for few seconds as well. He is suspected to have mesial temporal lobe epilepsy or mesial

temporal sclerosis. Which of the following will help in the diagnosis in this case?
- A. MRI of brain showing hippocampal atrophy and signal alteration with ipsilateral dilatation of temporal horn of lateral ventricle
- B. Unilateral or bilateral independent anterior temporal EEG spikes with maximal amplitude in basal electrodes
- C. PET scan showing hypometabolism in temporal lobe
- D. Neuropsychological testing showing memory dysfunction specific to involved temporal lobe
- E. All of the above

▸▸ Question 10

A patient with strong family history of epilepsy presents with history of myoclonic jerks on waking up in morning. EEG shows poly spike discharges and MRI shows no structural lesion. The patient is suspected to have a generalized epilepsy syndrome with generalized tonic clonic and absence types in addition to the type mentioned above. What is this syndrome called?
- A. West syndrome
- B. Lennox–Gastaut syndrome
- C. Juvenile myoclonic epilepsy
- D. Temporal lobe syndrome
- E. Juvenile tonic clonic epilepsy

▸▸ Question 11

Which of the following is true regarding West syndrome?
- A. It is a seizure disorder that typically begins in first year of life
- B. It consists of recurrent gross fixation and occasionally extension of trunks and limbs
- C. It is usually associated with mental retardation with EEG showing interictal hypsarrhythmia or modified hypsarrhythmia
- D. Seizures usually respond dramatically to ACTH or corticosteroids
- E. All of the above

▸▸ Question 12

Hippocampus is composed of Ammon's horn and dentate gyrus. The dorsal hippocampus subserves aspects of spatial memory, verbal memory, and learning conceptual information. Hippocampal sclerosis can cause which of the following?
- A. Total memory impairment
- B. Loss of all functions of basal ganglia
- C. Olfactory loss
- D. Intractable temporal lobe epilepsy
- E. All of the above

▸▸ Question 13

Following are motor seizures except?
- A. Tonic
- B. Gelastic seizures
- C. Clonic
- D. Atonic
- E. Epileptic spasms

▸▸ Question 14

Symptomatic seizure also known as secondary seizure results from structural abnormality within the brain. Which of the following is included in this type of seizure?
- A. Cavernous malformation
- B. Stroke
- C. Brian tumor
- D. Mesial temporal sclerosis
- E. All of the above

▸▸ Question 15

Mortality in patients with epilepsy is 2 to 4 times that of general population. Which of the following deaths are directly related to seizure?
- A. Status epilepticus
- B. Accidents during seizure activity
- C. Suicides
- D. Sudden unexplained death in epilepsy
- E. All of the above

Answers

▸▸ Answer 1

Correct answer is C. Clonic seizures[1]

▸▸ Answer 2

Correct answer is C. Absence seizures[1]

▸▸ Answer 3

Correct answer is C. Mesial temporal sclerosis[1]

▸▸ Answer 4

Correct answer is C. Mesial temporal lobe epilepsy[1]

▸▸ Answer 5

Correct answer is A. Uncinate seizures[2]

▸▸ Answer 6

Correct answer is A. Partial or total paralysis usually occurs in areas involved in a partial seizure[3]

▸▸ Answer 7

Correct answer is C. Structural lesion within brain[4]

▸▸ Answer 8

Correct answer is D. Myoclonic[1]

▸▸ Answer 9

Correct answer is E. PET scan showing hypometabolism in temporal lobe[2]

▸▸ Answer 10

Correct answer is C. Juvenile myoclonic epilepsy[5]

▸▸ Answer 11

Correct answer is E. All of the above[5]

▸▸ Answer 12

Correct answer is D. Intractable temporal lobe epilepsy[2]

▸▸ Answer 13

Correct answer is B. Gelastic seizures[4]

▸▸ Answer 14

Correct answer is E. All of the above[3]

▸▸ Answer 15

Correct answer is A. Status epilepticus[3]

References

[1] Greenberg M, ed. Greenberg's Handbook of Neurosurgery. 10th ed. New York: Thieme; 2023:482
[2] Greenberg M, ed. Greenberg's Handbook of Neurosurgery. 10th ed. New York: Thieme; 2023:483
[3] Greenberg M, ed. Greenberg's Handbook of Neurosurgery. 10th ed. New York: Thieme; 2023:480
[4] Greenberg M, ed. Greenberg's Handbook of Neurosurgery. 10th ed. New York: Thieme; 2023:481
[5] Greenberg M, ed. Greenberg's Handbook of Neurosurgery. 10th ed. New York: Thieme; 2023:484

27 Antiseizure Medication (ASM)

Questions

▸▸ Question 1

A patient is on antiepileptic drugs (AED) for 2 years. On follow-up, his liver function tests were deranged. AED should be discontinued based on derangement of which parameter?

- A. Fatty liver on USG
- B. Acute decrease in ALT
- C. Decrease in ALT/AST ratio
- D. GGT levels twice the normal
- E. Hyperalbuminemia

▸▸ Question 2

What is the dose adjustment of phenytoin in renal failure?

- A. Continue same dosage
- B. Two-thirds of the previous dosage
- C. Half the previous dose
- D. Double the previous dose
- E. Only give on SOS basis

▸▸ Question 3

What is the parenteral loading dose of phenytoin for adults?

- A. 16 mg/kg
- B. 18 mg/kg
- C. 20 mg/kg
- D. 22 mg/kg
- E. 25 mg/kg

▸▸ Question 4

What is the most common electrolyte imbalance associated with carbamazepine?

- A. Hypernatremia
- B. Hyponatremia
- C. Hypochloremia
- D. Hyperchloremia
- E. Hypermagnesia

▸▸ Question 5

Carbamazepine should be discontinued when CBC shows a WBC count of what?

- A. < 10,000
- B. < 7000
- C. < 6000
- D. < 5000
- E. < 4000

▸▸ Question 6

Oxcarbazepine was prescribed to a patient for epilepsy. Which blood tests should be employed to monitor the side effects?

- A. CBC
- B. RFTs
- C. Electrolytes
- D. Urinalysis
- E. No blood tests required

▸▸ Question 7

What is the maximum recommended adult dose of valproic acid?

- A. 20 mg/kg/d
- B. 30 mg/kg/d
- C. 40 mg/kg/d
- D. 50 mg/kg/d
- E. 60 mg/kg/d

▸▸ Question 8

What is the therapeutic level of valproic acid?

- A. 5 to 10 µg/mL
- B. 10 to 20 µg/mL
- C. 20 to 30 µg/mL
- D. 30 to 40 µg/mL
- E. 50 to 100 µg/mL

▸▸ Question 9

What is the loading dose of phenobarbital in adults?

- A. 10 mg/kg
- B. 12 mg/kg
- C. 15 mg/kg
- D. 18 mg/kg
- E. 20 mg/kg

▸▸ Question 10

What is the recommended daily dose of ethosuximide in adults?

- A. 500 to 1,500 mg/d
- B. 500 to 1,000 mg/d
- C. 250 to 500 mg/d
- C. 100 to 200 mg/d
- D. 100 to 300 mg/d

▸▸ Question 11

What is the initial dose of levetiracetam in adults?

- A. 500 mg oral twice daily
- B. 400 mg oral twice daily
- C. 300 mg oral twice daily
- D. 250 mg oral twice daily
- E. 100 mg thrice daily

▸▸ Question 12

What is the maximum daily dose of levetiracetam for adults?

- A. 1,000 mg
- B. 1,500 mg
- C. 2,000 mg
- D. 3,000 mg
- E. 1 g

▸▸ Question 13

When given for epilepsy, what is the usual target dosage of gabapentin?

- A.100 mg/d
- B. 1,000 mg/d
- C. 500 to 1,000 mg/d
- D. 800 to 1,800 mg/d
- E. 5 g/d

▸▸ Question 14

The anticonvulsant effect of lamotrigine is due to presynaptic inhibition of release of what?

- A. Calcium
- B. Potassium
- C. Albumin
- D. Glutamate
- E. Serotonin

▸▸ Question 15

The maximum effect of topiramate for seizures control is observed at what dose?

- A. 100 mg/d
- B. 200 mg/d
- C. 400 mg/d
- D. > 600 mg/d
- E. 1 g/d

▸▸ Question 16

Fetal hydantoin syndrome is associated with which of the following?

- A. Valproic acid
- B. Levetiracetam
- C. Lamotrigine
- D. Phenytoin
- E. Benzodiazepines

▸▸ Question 17

Ethosuximide is drug of choice for what?

- A. Absence seizures
- B. GTC seizures
- C. Myoclonic seizures
- D. Tonic seizures
- E. Atonic seizures

▸▸ Question 18

Aside from some specific agents for some particular seizure types, there is generally no significant difference in efficacy of antiseizure medication. Hence, choices are made on the basis of tolerability, adverse effects, effects on comorbidities, drug-drug interactions, or availability of dosing form. What is the goal of antiseizure medication?

- A. Seizure control which is seizure-free time for at least 3 years for an epileptic patient and no or minimum chances of seizure in future
- B. Seizure control which is reduction of seizure frequency and severity to very low
- C. Seizure control which is reduction of seizure frequency and severity so that the patient can live normal life without epilepsy-related limitations
- D. Seizure control which is reduction of seizure frequency and severity so that the patient can live normal life without epilepsy-related limitations with minimal or no drug toxicity
- E. None of above

▸▸ Question 19

In person with focal onset seizure with or without retained awareness and with or without secondary generalization, the indicated antiseizure medications (ASM) are carbamazepine, phenytoin, phenobarbital, and primidone. Which of the following is the drug indicated in absence seizure?

- A. Ethosuximide
- B. Valproic acid
- C. Clonazepam
- D. Methsuximide
- E. All of the above

▸▸ Question 20

Valproic acid, lamotrigine, levetiracetam, and zonisamide are considered as broad spectrum ASM. A patient presenting with low platelet counts in neurosurgical OPD with primary generalized tonic clonic seizures is to be started with ASM. Which ASM is indicated in this patient as first-line medication?

- A. Valproic acid
- B. Phenytoin

- C. Levetiracetam
- D. Phenobarbital
- E. Lamotrigine

▸▸ Question 21

Following statements regarding antiseizure medication are true except?

- A. A given medication dose is increased until seizures are controlled or side effects become intolerable
- B. Monotherapy is tried with different drugs before resorting to two drugs together as 80% of epileptics can be controlled with monotherapy
- C. When more than two ASMs are needed, it is considered that the patient is having nonepileptic seizure
- D. An ASM is discontinued if GGT levels exceed normal levels
- E. When first evaluating a patient on multiple drugs, the most sedating ones are withdrawn first

▸▸ Question 22

Oral loading dose of phenytoin is 300 mg every 4 hours until 17 mg/kg is given while IV loading dose is 18 mg/kg slow IV. Maintenance dose in adults is 200 to 500 mg/d and 4 to 7 mg /kg/d in children. It is diluted only in normal saline and given at slow rate of 20 mg/min or maximum up to 40 mg/min because of risk of which following side effect?

- A. Hypotension
- B. Arrythmias
- C. Laryngeal spasm
- D. Acute kidney failure
- E. Both A and B

▸▸ Question 23

Carbamazepine is indicated for focal onset seizures, generalized tonic clonic seizures with or without secondary generalization, and trigeminal neuralgia. Dosage range in adults is 600 to 2,000 mg/d, while in children it is 20 to 30 kg/mg/d but it is started at low dosage and increased slowly like 200 mg per oral every day for 1st week, then 200 mg twice a day for next week, then 200 mg thrice a day for next week, and so on. Which test is necessary before starting carbamazepine therapy?

- A. CBC
- B. Platelet count
- C. Serum iron
- D. Liver enzymes
- E. A, B, and C

▸▸ Question 24

What is the most effective ASM for generalized genetic epilepsies with generalized tonic clonic seizures, which is also effective for all focal onset seizures, and generalized onset seizures including absence seizure and myoclonic seizures? (Adult dosage range of this drug is 600 to 3,000 mg/d, while in children it is 15 to 60 mg/kg/d, while it is contraindicated in pregnancy or in patients below 2 years of age.)

- A. Levetiracetam
- B. Valproate
- C. Phenytoin
- D. Phenobarbital
- E. Lamotrigine

▸▸ Question 25

Levetiracetam is used as an adjunctive therapy for partial onset seizures with secondary generalization in patients 4 years of age and older. It is also used in myoclonic seizure (juvenile myoclonic epilepsy) and generalized tonic clonic seizures. It can cause somnolence, fatigue, dizziness, asthenia, or infection as side effect. What is the maximum safe recommended dose of this medication per day?

- A. 2,000 mg
- B. 2,500 mg
- C. 3,000 mg
- D. 3,500 mg
- E. 4,000 mg

▸▸ Question 26

After cessation of ASM, which of the following factors are found to affect the likelihood of relapse after seizure-free interval of 2 years?

- A. Seizure type: more relapse in patients with generalized seizures as compared to partial seizures
- B. More the number of seizures before control is attained, the more the chance of relapse
- C. Use of multiple ASM is related with more chance of relapse
- D. EEG class 4 has worst prognosis for relapse
- E. All of the above

▸▸ Question 27

For most women of child-bearing potential, monotherapy with the lowest dose of carbamazepine is indicated. What is the second indicated drug in such patients if therapy with carbamazepine is ineffective?

- A. Levetiracetam
- B. Valproic acid
- C. Phenytoin
- D. Lamotrigine
- E. Phenobarbital

Answers

▸▸ Answer 1

Correct answer is D. GGT levels twice the normal[1]

▸▸ Answer 2

Correct answer is A. Continue same dosage[2]

▸▸ Answer 3

Correct answer is B. 18 mg/kg[3]

▸▸ Answer 4

Correct answer is B. Hyponatremia[4]

▸▸ Answer 5

Correct answer is E. < 4000[3]

▸▸ Answer 6

Correct answer is E. No blood tests required[4]

▸▸ Answer 7

Correct answer is E. 60 mg/kg/d[5]

▸▸ Answer 8

Correct answer is E. 50 to 100 µg/mL[5]

▸▸ Answer 9

Correct answer is E. 20 mg/kg[6]

▸▸ Answer 10

Correct answer is A. 500 to 1,500 mg/d[7]

▸▸ Answer 11

Correct answer is A. 500 mg oral twice daily[8]

▸▸ Answer 12

Correct answer is D. 3,000 mg[8]

▸▸ Answer 13

Correct answer is D. 800 to 1,800 mg/d[9]

▸▸ Answer 14

Correct answer is D. Glutamate[9]

▸▸ Answer 15

Correct answer is D. > 600 mg/d[10]

▸▸ Answer 16

Correct answer is D. Phenytoin[11]

▸▸ Answer 17

Correct answer is A. Absence seizures[12]

▸▸ Answer 18

Correct answer is D. Seizure control which is reduction of seizure frequency and severity so that the patient can live normal life without epilepsy-related limitations with minimal or no drug toxicity[13]

▸▸ Answer 19

Correct answer is E. All of the above[12]

▸▸ Answer 20

Correct answer is A. Valproic acid[13]

▸▸ Answer 21

Correct answer is D. An ASM is discontinued if GGT levels exceed normal levels[1]

▸▸ Answer 22

Correct answer is E. Both A and B[3]

▸▸ Answer 23

Correct answer is E. A, B, and C[3]

▸▸ Answer 24

Correct answer is B. Valproate[5]

▸▸ Answer 25

Correct answer is C. 3,000 mg[8]

▸▸ Answer 26

Correct answer is E. All of the above[14]

▸▸ Answer 27

Correct answer is B. Valproic acid[15]

References

[1] Greenberg M, ed. Greenberg's Handbook of Neurosurgery. 10th ed. New York: Thieme; 2023:487
[2] Greenberg M, ed. Greenberg's Handbook of Neurosurgery. 10th ed. New York: Thieme; 2023:488
[3] Greenberg M, ed. Greenberg's Handbook of Neurosurgery. 10th ed. New York: Thieme; 2023:490
[4] Greenberg M, ed. Greenberg's Handbook of Neurosurgery. 10th ed. New York: Thieme; 2023:491
[5] Greenberg M, ed. Greenberg's Handbook of Neurosurgery. 10th ed. New York: Thieme; 2023:492
[6] Greenberg M, ed. Greenberg's Handbook of Neurosurgery. 10th ed. New York: Thieme; 2023:493

[7] Greenberg M, ed. Greenberg's Handbook of Neurosurgery. 10th ed. New York: Thieme; 2023:494
[8] Greenberg M, ed. Greenberg's Handbook of Neurosurgery. 10th ed. New York: Thieme; 2023:495
[9] Greenberg M, ed. Greenberg's Handbook of Neurosurgery. 10th ed. New York: Thieme; 2023:497
[10] Greenberg M, ed. Greenberg's Handbook of Neurosurgery. 10th ed. New York: Thieme; 2023:498
[11] Greenberg M, ed. Greenberg's Handbook of Neurosurgery. 10th ed. New York: Thieme; 2023:501
[12] Greenberg M, ed. Greenberg's Handbook of Neurosurgery. 10th ed. New York: Thieme; 2023:486
[13] Greenberg M, ed. Greenberg's Handbook of Neurosurgery. 10th ed. New York: Thieme; 2023:485
[14] Greenberg M, ed. Greenberg's Handbook of Neurosurgery. 10th ed. New York: Thieme; 2023:499
[15] Greenberg M, ed. Greenberg's Handbook of Neurosurgery. 10th ed. New York: Thieme; 2023:292

28 Special Seizure Consideration

Questions

▸▸ **Question 1**

What is the most common cause of first type seizures in pediatric age group?

- A. Febrile
- B. Hydrocephalus
- C. Electrolyte imbalance
- D. Vascular event
- E. Idiopathic

▸▸ **Question 2**

Prophylactic antiepileptic drugs reduce the incidence of late post-traumatic epilepsy by how much?

- A. One-fourth
- B. One-third
- C. Half
- D. No effect
- E. Increase the incidence by drug resistance

▸▸ **Question 3**

What is the most common cause of nonepileptic seizures?

- A. Psychogenic
- B. Basilar migraine
- C. Cardiac arrhythmias
- D. Cyclic vomiting syndrome
- E. Dyskinesias

▸▸ **Question 4**

According to the definition of status epilepticus, seizure lasting more than how many minutes warrants management according to status epilepticus protocol?

- A. 1
- B. 3
- C. 5
- D. 30
- E. 60

▸▸ **Question 5**

What is the most common cause of status epilepticus?

- A. Low levels of antiepileptic drugs
- B. Metabolic
- C. Hypoxia
- D. Tumor
- E. Cerebrovascular event

▸▸ **Question 6**

What is the first-line treatment for status epilepticus?

- A. Benzodiazepine
- B. Fosphenytoin
- C. Phenytoin
- D. Valproic acid
- E. Phenobarbital

▸▸ **Question 7**

What is the drug of choice for myoclonic status epilepticus?

- A. Benzodiazepine
- B. Fosphenytoin
- C. Phenytoin
- D. Valproic acid
- E. Phenobarbital

▸▸ **Question 8**

Antiseizure medication can be tapered off in which of the following cases after 7 days?

- A. Penetrating brain injury
- B. Development of late PTS
- C. Prior seizures history
- D. Patient undergoing craniotomy
- E. Linear skull fracture

▸▸ **Question 9**

The etiologies of first-time seizure include neurologic insult (stroke, head trauma, CNS infection, birth asphyxia), underlying CNS abnormality (congenital, degenerative, CNS tumor, hydrocephalus, AVM), acute systemic metabolic disturbance (electrolyte disorders, alcohol withdrawal, cocaine toxicity, opioids, phenothiazine antiemetics), and idiopathic. Which of the following neurologic insult is the most common cause of first-onset seizure in pediatric population?

- A. CNS infection
- B. Birth asphyxia
- C. Febrile seizures
- D. Idiopathic
- E. Head trauma

▸▸ **Question 10**

An adult person comes in neurosurgical OPD with history of new-onset seizure in the absence of obvious cause like alcohol withdrawal. His/her MRI with and without contrast and systemic workup come out to be negative. How this adult should be followed up?

- A. No need for further follow-up in absence of seizure

- B. Follow-up after 6 months with repeat MRI which if found negative then no need for further follow-up
- C. Further follow-up if seizure occurs again
- D. Further follow-up after 6 months with repeat MRI, then at 1 year with repeat MRI, and possibly at 2 years to rule out tumor in brain
- E. Start antiepileptic medication and follow-up after 6 months

▸▸ Question 11

Post-traumatic seizures (PTS) can occur in patients after head injury. These can adversely affect the patient as it may elevate ICP, may adversely affect blood pressure or oxygen delivery, and may worsen other injuries. Hence, antiseizure medication (levetiracetam, phenytoin, carbamazepine) should be started within 24 hours in patients meeting high-risk criteria for PTS. These high-risk criteria include the following except?

- A. ASD hematoma, EDH, ICH, or open depressed skull fracture with parenchymal injury
- B. No history of significant alcohol abuse
- C. Seizures within the first 24 hours after injury
- D. Penetrating head injury
- E. GCS less than 10 or cortical contusion

▸▸ Question 12

Antiseizure medications (ASMs) are given for 1 week and then tapered as it prevents from early-onset post-traumatic seizure (within 7 days of injury). However, ASMs are continued for 6 to 12 months in patients after head injury in which of the following conditions?

- A. Penetrating head injury
- B. Development of late PTS (a seizure lasting more than 7 days following head injury)
- C. Prior seizure history
- D. Patients undergoing craniotomy
- E. All of the above

▸▸ Question 13

Alcohol withdrawal seizure can occur within 7 to 30 hours of cessation or reduction of alcohol intake in habituated drinkers. These seizures are treated with diazepam or lorazepam if they continue for 3 to 4 minutes or phenytoin. What is the loading dose (mg/kg) of phenytoin for such patients?

- A. 16
- B. 18
- C. 20
- D. 22
- E. 24

▸▸ Question 14

Differentials of nonepileptic seizures include psychologic disorders (anxiety, dissociative, psychonic, impulse control, attention deficit), cardiovascular disorders (syncope, cardiac arrythmias, TIAs), migraine syndrome, movement disorders (tremors, dyskinesias, tic), parasomnias with sleep-related disorders, and others like malingering or cognitive disorders. Following are features associated with nonepileptic seizure disorder except?

- A. Manifestations altered by distraction
- B. Intermittent arrhythmic and out-of-phase convulsive activity
- C. Nonfluctuating intensity and severity during seizure
- D. Bilateral motor activity with preserved consciousness
- E. Absence of stereotypy

▸▸ Question 15

A febrile seizure is said to be a seizure in infants or children associated with fever with no defined cause and unaccompanied by acute neurologic illness. Which statement is most appropriate regarding management of these seizures?

- A. There are recommendations for prescribing antiseizure medication in these cases
- B. Phenobarbital can be used with no effect on kid's IQ
- C. Valproate has no serious risks in the kids younger than 2 years
- D. Recurrence of febrile seizures in children can be reduced using diazepam 0.33 mg/kg per oral every 8 hours during a febrile episode and continuing until 24 hours after the fever subsides
- E. None of the above

▸▸ Question 16

Status epilepticus is a continuous seizure activity or more than equal to two sequential seizures without full recovery of consciousness between seizures for more than 30 minutes. The goal of treatment in such patients is rapid termination of clinical and electrical seizure activity as continuation of seizure activity for more than 30 minutes can cause permanent neurologic deficit. What is the most common cause of status epilepticus?

- A. Low level of prescribed ASM in a patient with a seizure disorder
- B. Remote symptomatic cause
- C. Stroke
- D. Metabolic disturbance
- E. Hypoxia

▸▸ Question 17

Treatment of status epilepticus is divided into four phases with phase 1 comprising from 0 to 5 minutes, phase 2 from 5 to 20 minutes, phase 3 from 20 to 40 minutes, and phase 4 from 40 to 60 minutes. First 0 to 5 minutes phase is called as stabilization phase. Following are the components of this phase except?

- A. ABC, that is, assessment and correction of airway, breathing, circulation with adequate oxygenation and arterial blood gases (ABG) monitoring
- B. 50 mL of dextrose 50 is given by IV push before giving 100 mg thiamine IV
- C. Baseline investigation is sent for with start of IV fluid and neurologic examination
- D. Initial additional measures include EEG monitoring if possible, head CT without contrast, correction of any suspected electrolyte imbalance, and CNS sampling for suspected CNS infection with start of antibiotics
- E. General medication for unknown suspected poisoning cases includes naloxone 0.4 mg IV for narcotics, bicarbonate to counter acidosis, and for neonates less than 2 years, pyridoxine 100 mg IV push is given

►► Question 18

During the second phase of status epilepticus treatment, which last from 5 to 20 minutes, benzodiazepine is the drug of choice with IM midazolam or IV lorazepam or IV diazepam in dosage of 10 mg (for adult) or 0.1 mg/kg/dose or 0.15 to 0.2 mg/kg/dose given, respectively, once. If all the above meds are unavailable or contraindicated, then IV phenobarbital (15 mg/kg/dose) or rectal diazepam (0.2 to 0.5 mg/kg) or intranasal midazolam or buccal midazolam can be given. What is the component of the second therapy phase which lasts from 20 to 40 minutes?

- A. IV phosphenytoin
- B. IV valproic acid 40 mg/kg/dose up to max 3,000 mg/dose
- C. IV levetiracetam 60 mg/kg/dose up to max 4,500 mg/dose
- D. IV phenobarbital 15 mg/kg/dose
- E. All of the above

Answers

►► Answer 1

Correct answer is A. Febrile[1]

►► Answer 2

Correct answer is D. No effect[2]

►► Answer 3

Correct answer is A. Psychogenic[3]

►► Answer 4

Correct answer is C. 5[4]

►► Answer 5

Correct answer is A. Low levels of antiepileptic drugs[4]

►► Answer 6

Correct answer is A. Benzodiazepine[5]

►► Answer 7

Correct answer is D. Valproic acid[6]

►► Answer 8

Correct answer is E. Linear skull fracture[7]

►► Answer 9

Correct answer is C. Febrile seizures[1]

►► Answer 10

Correct answer is D. Further follow-up after 6 months with repeat MRI, then at 1 year with repeat MRI, and possibly at 2 years to rule out tumor in brain[2]

►► Answer 11

Correct answer is B. No history of significant alcohol abuse[7]

►► Answer 12

Correct answer is E. All of the above[8]

►► Answer 13

Correct answer is B. 18[8]

►► Answer 14

Correct answer is C. Nonfluctuating intensity and severity during seizure[9]

►► Answer 15

Correct answer is D. Recurrence of febrile seizures in children can be reduced using diazepam 0.33 mg/kg per oral every 8 hours during a febrile episode and continuing until 24 hours after the fever subsides[4]

►► Answer 16

Correct answer is A. Low level of prescribed ASM in a patient with a seizure disorder[4]

►► Answer 17

Correct answer is B. 50 mL of dextrose 50 is given by IV push before giving 100 mg thiamine IV[10]

►► Answer 18

Correct answer is E. All of the above[6]

References

[1] Greenberg M, ed. Greenberg's Handbook of Neurosurgery. 10th ed. New York: Thieme; 2023:509
[2] Greenberg M, ed. Greenberg's Handbook of Neurosurgery. 10th ed. New York: Thieme; 2023:504
[3] Greenberg M, ed. Greenberg's Handbook of Neurosurgery. 10th ed. New York: Thieme; 2023:507
[4] Greenberg M, ed. Greenberg's Handbook of Neurosurgery. 10th ed. New York: Thieme; 2023:510
[5] Greenberg M, ed. Greenberg's Handbook of Neurosurgery. 10th ed. New York: Thieme; 2023:513
[6] Greenberg M, ed. Greenberg's Handbook of Neurosurgery. 10th ed. New York: Thieme; 2023:514
[7] Greenberg M, ed. Greenberg's Handbook of Neurosurgery. 10th ed. New York: Thieme; 2023:505
[8] Greenberg M, ed. Greenberg's Handbook of Neurosurgery. 10th ed. New York: Thieme; 2023:506
[9] Greenberg M, ed. Greenberg's Handbook of Neurosurgery. 10th ed. New York: Thieme; 2023:508
[10] Greenberg M, ed. Greenberg's Handbook of Neurosurgery. 10th ed. New York: Thieme; 2023:512

Part IX

Pain

IX

29 Pain

Questions

▸▸ Question 1

A 35-year-old young woman presents with left-sided facial pain without any numbness. She had several episodes in the last few months, and her pain triggers after eating, talking, and touching her cheek. MRI shows a vessel compressing cranial nerve V. Which vessel is most commonly involved?

- A. Superior cerebral artery
- B. AICA
- C. PICA
- D. PCA

▸▸ Question 2

A 25-year-old young male presented with painful vesicular eruption. It was in dermatomal distribution on one side of thorax. What is the effective treatment for the pain of acute attack?

- A. Epidural
- B. Intercostal block
- C. Antiviral
- D. Both A and B

▸▸ Question 3

A 60-year-old female with history of breast cancer, with metastasis to bone and pain in right arm, reports 3 weeks of worsening of pain (burning in right hand—brachial plexus neuropathy). She was prescribed tricyclic antidepressant, use of which is limited by which of the following?

- A. Anticholinergic effect
- B. Central effects
- C. Limited pain relief
- D. All of the above

▸▸ Question 4

Ramsay Hunt syndrome is characterized by which of the following triads?

- A. Contralateral facial paralysis, ear pain, and vesicle on face, ear, or in the ear
- B. Recurrent oral ulcers, genital ulcers, and iridocyclitis
- C. Sixth cranial n. palsy, persistent ear discharge, deep-seated retro-orbital pain
- D. Ipsilateral facial paralysis, ear pain, and vesicle on face, ear, or in the ear

▸▸ Question 5

Which of the following is correct regarding primary otalgia?

- A. More common in children
- B. Mostly unilateral
- C. Cold, air, and water most common triggers
- D. 75% associated with aural symptoms (hearing loss, tinnitus, and vertigo)
- E. All of the above

▸▸ Question 6

A European solider presented to the emergency department after 24 hours of being shot, with classical triad of burning pain, autonomic dysfunction, and trophic change (complex regional pain syndrome) on his upper extremity. Which of the following statements is true?

- A. Medical therapy is sufficient
- B. Sympathetic block may not help
- C. Guanethidine commonly used intravenous injection
- D. No role of tricyclic antidepressants
- E. All of the above

▸▸ Question 7

There are three major types of pain, namely, nociceptive pain (somatic and visceral), deafferentation pain, and sympathetically maintained pain. Pain which is caused by lesion or compression of peripheral or central nervous system manifesting as sensory signs and symptoms is called as neuropathic pain. Following are peripheral neuropathic pain syndromes except?

- A. Acute and chronic inflammatory demyelinating polyneuropathy
- B. Entrapment neuropathies
- C. Cervical spondylotic myelopathy
- D. Post herpetic neuralgia
- E. Painful diabetic neuropathy

▸▸ Question 8

Which of the following statements regarding medical treatment of neuropathic pain is true?

- A. Traditional treatment includes narcotic analgesic and tricyclic antidepressants (amitriptyline 75 mg daily)
- B. Gabapentin is effective for post herpetic neuralgia, painful diabetic neuropathy, trigeminal neuralgia, postoperative state, spinal cord injury, cancer, MS, and migraine
- C. Lidocaine patch is applied for 12 hours/d over the most painful area
- D. Tramadol is a centrally acting analgesic which is effective for these patients
- E. All of the above

▸▸ Question 9

Possible pathways for facial pain include trigeminal nerve, facial nerve, and cranial nerve eight. Which of the following is a cause of cephalic neuralgia?

- A. Tic convulsif: otalgia and deep prosopalgia
- B. Diabetic neuritis of oculomotor nerve
- C. Nerve injury to superior or inferior alveolar nerves
- D. Sinusitis of frontal, maxillary, sphenoidal, or ethmoidal sinus
- E. All of the above

▸▸ Question 10

Primary otalgia is unilateral in most cases, and it is mostly triggered by cold air or water. It is associated with aural symptoms like hearing loss, vertigo, and tinnitus. Following is true regarding the management of primary otalgia except?

- A. An initial trial with medications used in trigeminal neuralgias like carbamazepine, phenytoin, and baclofen is the first line of defense
- B. Suboccipital exploration of the 7th cranial nerve or lower cranial nerve with MVD has no role in these cases
- C. Ultimate treatment is sectioning of nervus intermedius, the 9th and upper two fibers of 10th nerve, and a geniculate ganglionectomy
- D. Pain relief with nerve block of pharyngeal tonsils suggests glossopharyngeal neuralgia
- E. CT or MRI should be done in any case where no cause is found

▸▸ Question 11

A woman 50 years of age presented with unilateral pain in forehead with tenderness on one side of forehead. The pain is temporarily relieved with nerve block in the region of orbital roof. This condition responds to gabapentin, pregabalin, or topical capsaicin. What is the most likely diagnosis in this case?

- A. Trigeminal neuralgia
- B. Migraine
- C. Supraorbital neuralgia
- D. Hemi crania continua
- E. Trochleitis

▸▸ Question 12

Herpes varicella zoster virus is responsible for painful vesicular cutaneous eruptions mostly in the area of thorax or in distribution of trigeminal neuralgia. If pain from this condition persists for more than 1 month, then this condition is called post herpetic neuralgia. The recommended medical treatment for this condition includes which of the following?

- A. Acyclovir 800 mg every 4 hours for 7 days
- B. Tricyclic antidepressants
- C. Gabapentin
- D. Lidocaine patch
- E. All of the above

▸▸ Question 13

For post herpetic neuralgia, gabapentin is started at a dose of 300 mg once a day for first day, 300 mg twice a day on second day, and 300 mg thrice a day on third day. Which side effect of gabapentin makes a surgeon to start it at night with slow increments of doses?

- A. Ataxia and fatigue
- B. Drowsiness
- C. Peripheral edema and confusion
- D. Depression
- E. All of the above

▸▸ Question 14

Capsaicin patches or lidocaine patches are helpful in post herpetic neuralgia patients. Intrathecal steroid with methylprednisolone plus 3% lidocaine once every week for 4 weeks has shown good to excellent pain relief for up to 2 years. What is the surgical treatment that is uniformly successful in treating post herpetic neuralgias?

- A. Nerve block
- B. Neurectomies
- C. Cordotomy
- D. Rhizotomy
- E. None of the above

▸▸ Question 15

Complex regional pain syndrome also known as causalgia is a disproportionate pain syndrome which can cause burning pain, autonomic dysfunction, or trophic changes. Which of the following is true regarding the cause of this syndrome?

- A. These are high velocity missile injuries (also known as CRPS type 2)
- B. Sympathetic dystrophy or causalgia minor is caused by nonpenetrating injury and is called as CRPS type 1
- C. It can occur in postoperative patients following carpal tunnel surgery or surgery on lumbar or cervical spine
- D. It can occur because of direct injury to nerve or because of injury to surrounding soft tissue
- E. All of the above

▸▸ Question 16

CRPS mostly affects limbs with hand and foot involvement. Examination (in such patients is difficult because of tenderness) may show vasodilatation, vasoconstriction, or trophic changes. Following are recommended treatment options in these patients except?

- A. Gabapentin
- B. Tricyclic antidepressants
- C. Sympathetic block
- D. Surgical sympathectomy
- E. Spinal cord stimulation

Answers

▸▸ Answer 1

Correct answer is A. Superior cerebral artery[1]

▸▸ Answer 2

Correct answer is D. Both A and B[2]

▸▸ Answer 3

Correct answer is D. All of the above[1]

▸▸ Answer 4

Correct answer is D. Ipsilateral facial paralysis, ear pain, and vesicle on face, ear, or in the ear[1]

▸▸ Answer 5

Correct answer is E. All of the above[3]

▸▸ Answer 6

Correct answer is C. Guanethidine commonly used intravenous injection[4]

▸▸ Answer 7

Correct answer is C. Cervical spondylotic myelopathy[5]

▸▸ Answer 8

Correct answer is E. All of the above[1]

▸▸ Answer 9

Correct answer is A. Tic convulsif: otalgia and deep prosopalgia[1]

▸▸ Answer 10

Correct answer is B. Suboccipital exploration of the 7th cranial nerve or lower cranial nerve with MVD has no role in these cases[3]

▸▸ Answer 11

Correct answer is C. Supraorbital neuralgia[3]

▸▸ Answer 12

Correct answer is E. All of the above[6]

▸▸ Answer 13

Correct answer is B. Drowsiness[7]

▸▸ Answer 14

Correct answer is E. None of the above[8]

▸▸ Answer 15

Correct answer is E. All of the above[8]

▸▸ Answer 16

Correct answer is A. Gabapentin[4]

References

[1] Greenberg M, ed. Greenberg's Handbook of Neurosurgery. 10th ed. New York: Thieme; 2023:519
[2] Greenberg M, ed. Greenberg's Handbook of Neurosurgery. 10th ed. New York: Thieme; 2023:523
[3] Greenberg M, ed. Greenberg's Handbook of Neurosurgery. 10th ed. New York: Thieme; 2023:521
[4] Greenberg M, ed. Greenberg's Handbook of Neurosurgery. 10th ed. New York: Thieme; 2023:527
[5] Greenberg M, ed. Greenberg's Handbook of Neurosurgery. 10th ed. New York: Thieme; 2023:518
[6] Greenberg M, ed. Greenberg's Handbook of Neurosurgery. 10th ed. New York: Thieme; 2023:522
[7] Greenberg M, ed. Greenberg's Handbook of Neurosurgery. 10th ed. New York: Thieme; 2023:524
[8] Greenberg M, ed. Greenberg's Handbook of Neurosurgery. 10th ed. New York: Thieme; 2023:525

Part X

Peripheral Nerves

X

30 Peripheral Nerves

Questions

▸▸ Question 1

A 16-year-old boy presented to the OPD for follow-up after 2 months of brachial plexus injury. Initially, his reflexes were absent. Which maneuver will help you to further support your finding?

- A. Jendrassick maneuver
- B. Hamlick maneuver
- C. tENS
- D. Stimulation

▸▸ Question 2

A 35-year-old female is suffering from wrist drop after getting IM injection from a quack. Her tone is decreased and reflexes are absent. What kind of lesion is this?

- A. Upper motor neuron
- B. Mixed
- C. Myopathic
- D. Lower motor neuron

▸▸ Question 3

There are three innervations of thumb. Pick up the correct sequence.

- A. Median nerve: opposition; ulnar nerve: adduction; and radial nerve: extension
- B. Median nerve: extension; ulnar nerve: abduction; and radial nerve: extension
- C. Median nerve: flexion; ulnar nerve: abduction; and radial nerve: extension
- D. None of the above

▸▸ Question 4

A patient suffered from foot drop after peroneal nerve injury during car accident. Which of the following statements is true regarding nerve injury?

- A. After 24 months of denervation, most muscle cannot recover useful function even with reinnervation
- B. The longer the distance from the injury site to the function unit to be innervated, the earlier the surgical intervention should be considered
- C. There is some degree of continuity in > 60% of nerve injury
- D. All of the above

▸▸ Question 5

A 30-year-old weight lifter presented to the OPD with severe back ache which started right after his workout. Since then his right foot is numb, and he cannot move his lower limb without pain. MRI spine shows disk prolapse at L5–S1. Which is best way to test L5 clinically?

- A. Extensor hallucis longus
- B. Plantar flexion of big toe
- C. Tibialis anterior and extensor digitorum
- D. None of the above

▸▸ Question 6

A young patient came to electrophysiology department for NCS/EMG for carpel tunnel syndrome. Despite complete absence of a median nerve evoked compound muscle action potential from the thenar eminence, the patient had significant preservation of function and minimal muscle atrophy. Activation of the ulnar nerve at both the wrist and elbow generated easily obtainable compound muscle action potentials from the thenar eminence with initial negative onset. This observed preservation of function and electrophysiologic responses are best explained by the presence of what?

- A. Martin Gruber anastomosis
- B. Medial and radial nerve anastomosis
- C. Radial and anterior interosseous nerve anastomosis
- D. Richie–Cannieu anastomosis

▸▸ Question 7

A young male was referred to the OPD 6 weeks after a fall from the roof. Immediately after the fall he was not able to extend his wrist and unable to extend his fingers, along with weakness of brachioradialis muscle. The most likely radial nerve injury is where?

- A. Axillary area
- B. Spiral groove
- C. At wrist
- D. Forearm

▸▸ Question 8

The peripheral nervous system consists of nerve fibers and axons that connect the central nervous system with motor and sensory, somatic, and visceral end organs. Following are included in peripheral nervous system except?

- A. Cranial nerves one and two
- B. Cranial nerves three to twelve
- C. Spinal nerves
- D. Nerves of extremities
- E. Cervical, brachial, and lumbosacral plexus

▸▸ Question 9

Medical Research Council scale (MRC scale) is used for muscle strength grading. A patient presented to neurosurgical

OPD with reduced power of right upper limb. The patient can move the limb actively with gravity eliminated. What is MRC grade of this patient?

- A. 1
- B. 2
- C. 3
- D. 4
- E. 5

►► Question 10

Muscle stretch reflex grading scale is used for deep tendon reflex. It typically ranges from 0 to 4 +. Which of the following statements is true regarding these reflexes?

- A. 2 + is normal while 3 + is less brisk than normal
- B. 0.5 + means reflex is elicitable only with reinforcement
- C. In the lower extremities, reinforcement consists of having patients clench their teeth
- D. In the upper extremities, reinforcement consists of hooking tip of fingers of right hand into left hand and pulling (Jendrassik maneuver)
- E. 5 + means hyperreflexic with clonus

►► Question 11

Possible etiologies of upper motor neuron (UMN) paralysis are stroke, spinal cord injury, and cervical spondylotic myelopathy while of lower motor neuron (LMN) paralysis are herniated intervertebral disk, nerve entrapment syndrome, polio, and progressive muscular atrophy. Which of the following statements is incorrect regarding difference between UMN paralysis and LMN paralysis?

- A. Muscle tone in UMN paralysis is initially flaccid then later spastic with clasping resistance while in LMN paralysis it is flaccid
- B. Tendon reflexes are hyperactive in UMN paralysis while these are absent in LMN paralysis
- C. Pathologic reflexes like Babinski and Hoffman are present in UMN paralysis while these are absent in LMN paralysis
- D. Atrophy does not occur in UMN paralysis while it does occur in LMN paralysis
- E. Spontaneous spasms may occur in UMN paralysis while in LMN paralysis fibrillations and fasciculations occur

►► Question 12

Fasciculations are coarse muscle contractions that are visible to the naked eye while fibrillations are not visible and require EMG to detect. Fasciculations most often occur in diseases involving anterior horn cells which includes which of the following?

- A. Amyotrophic lateral sclerosis
- B. Spinal muscular atrophy
- C. Polio
- D. Syringomyelia
- E. All of the above

►► Question 13

What is the common root value of deltoid muscle (abducts arm from 30 to 90), biceps brachii (flex forearm and supinate forearm), and brachialis (flex forearm)?

- A. C4, c5
- B. C6, c7
- C. C5, c6
- D. C5, c6, c7
- E. C4, c5, c6

►► Question 14

C7, C8, and T1 roots collectively supply which muscle in upper extremities?

- A. Flexor pollicis longus (flex distal phalanx of thumb)
- B. Flexor digitorum profundus 1 and 2 (radial part) (flex distal phalanx of digits 2 and 3, also flexes wrist)
- C. Palmaris longus (wrist flexion)
- D. Flexor digitorum superficialis (flexion of middle phalanx of digits 2 to 5, flexes wrist)
- E. All of the above

►► Question 15

Flexion and extension of thumb occurs in the plane of palm while adduction and abduction occur in plane at right angle to the palm and opposition is bringing the thumb across the hand to the little finger. All of the following statements regarding innervation of thumb muscles is correct except?

- A. Median nerve innervates abductor pollicis brevis which causes abduction
- B. Ulnar nerve supplies adductor pollicis which causes adduction of thumb
- C. Radial nerve supplies extensor pollicis brevis and longus which cause extension of thumb
- D. Radial nerve also supplies opponens brevis which causes opposition
- E. Median nerve also supplies flexor pollicis brevis which causes flexion

►► Question 16

Which muscle is supplied by only L5 and S1 nerve roots?

- A. Extensor digitorum longus which causes extension of toes 2 to 5 and foot dorsiflexion
- B. Extensor hallucis longus which causes great toe extension and foot dorsiflexion
- C. Extensor digitorum brevis which causes extension of great toe and toes 2 to 5
- D. Peroneus longus and brevis which cause planter flexion of pronated foot and eversion
- E. All of the above

▸▸ Question 17

A nerve action potential (NAP) is produced if a normal healthy nerve fiber is stimulated with an electrical stimulus that has an amplitude and duration which exceed nerve fiber threshold. Presence of NAP (regardless of amplitude and latency) distal to lesion in continuity in the first few months after injury usually indicates that operative intervention will not be needed. What is the recommended timing to obtain NAP recording?

- A. 2–4 months for relatively focal contusions
- B. 4–5 months for stretch injuries such as brachial plexus
- C. Any time for partial injuries, entrapments, compressive lesions, and tumors
- D. Acutely to identify an area of nerve block
- E. All of the above are true

Answers

▸▸ Answer 1

Correct answer is A. Jendrassick maneuver[1]

▸▸ Answer 2

Correct answer is D. Lower motor neuron[1]

▸▸ Answer 3

Correct answer is A. Median nerve: opposition; ulnar nerve: adduction; and radial nerve: extension[2]

▸▸ Answer 4

Correct answer is D. All of the above[3]

▸▸ Answer 5

Correct answer is A. Extensor hallucis longus[4]

▸▸ Answer 6

Correct answer is D. Richie–Cannieu anastomosis[5]

▸▸ Answer 7

Correct answer is B. Spiral groove[6]

▸▸ Answer 8

Correct answer is A. Cranial nerves one and two[7]

▸▸ Answer 9

Correct answer is B. 2[7]

▸▸ Answer 10

Correct answer is B. 0.5 + means reflex is elicitable only with reinforcement[1]

▸▸ Answer 11

Correct answer is D. Atrophy does not occur in UMN paralysis while it does occur in LMN paralysis[1]

▸▸ Answer 12

Correct answer is E. All of the above[1]

▸▸ Answer 13

Correct answer is C. C5, c6[8]

▸▸ Answer 14

Correct answer is E. All of the above[8]

▸▸ Answer 15

Correct answer is D. Radial nerve also supplies opponens brevis which causes opposition[2]

▸▸ Answer 16

Correct answer is E. All of the above[4]

▸▸ Answer 17

Correct answer is E. All of the above are true[3]

References

[1] Greenberg M, ed. Greenberg's Handbook of Neurosurgery. 10th ed. New York: Thieme; 2023:531
[2] Greenberg M, ed. Greenberg's Handbook of Neurosurgery. 10th ed. New York: Thieme; 2023:533
[3] Greenberg M, ed. Greenberg's Handbook of Neurosurgery. 10th ed. New York: Thieme; 2023:535
[4] Greenberg M, ed. Greenberg's Handbook of Neurosurgery. 10th ed. New York: Thieme; 2023:534
[5] Greenberg M, ed. Greenberg's Handbook of Neurosurgery. 10th ed. New York: Thieme; 2023:540
[6] Greenberg M, ed. Greenberg's Handbook of Neurosurgery. 10th ed. New York: Thieme; 2023:537
[7] Greenberg M, ed. Greenberg's Handbook of Neurosurgery. 10th ed. New York: Thieme; 2023:530
[8] Greenberg M, ed. Greenberg's Handbook of Neurosurgery. 10th ed. New York: Thieme; 2023:532

31 Entrapment Neuropathy

Questions

▸▸ Question 1

Pick the false statement about entrapment neuropathy.

- A. It can be either an external force or a force by nearby structure
- B. One or repetitive insult
- C. Most common symptom is pain which frequently occurs at rest and is more severe at night
- D. Never consider the possibility of systemic disease
- E. None of the above

▸▸ Question 2

A young female presented with pain in occiput with trigger point at the back of head. Any pressure on that reproduces the pain which radiates up along the vertex. She was diagnosed with occipital nerve entrapment. Treatment options for this patient are the following except?

- A. Idiopathic cases are self-limiting
- B. Temporary relief with occipital nerve block
- C. TENS provide no relief
- D. Collar for 2 weeks may help
- E. C and D

▸▸ Question 3

A coal mine worker presented with weak grip in his dominant hand His hands get fatigued easily now with poorly localized paresthesia in index finger and thumb. What are the salient features to differentiate pronator teres syndrome from carpal tunnel syndrome (CTS)?

- A. Pain in palm rule out CTS
- B. Nocturnal exacerbation
- C. More common than CTS
- D. Involvement of ulnar nerve

▸▸ Question 4

A young female with moderate obesity often visits OPD with tingling in the hand, on palmar side of thumb, index finger, middle finger, and radial half of ring finger. Now all of sudden it has become severe. Acute carpel tunnel syndrome is uncommon and is associated with which of the following?

- A. Exertion or trauma
- B. Median artery thrombosis
- C. Hematoma in transverse carpal ligament (TCL)
- D. All of the above

▸▸ Question 5

A young female complains about tingling on palmer side of hand involving the thumb, index, middle, and half of ring finger, which wakes her up at night with painful numbness. Her grip gradually became weak. How much increase in carpel tunnel pressure produces sensory and motor dysfunction?

- A. 40 mmHg
- B. Less than 20
- C. 30
- D. 20–30

▸▸ Question 6

Regarding carpel tunnel syndrome, which statement is false?

- A. Most common entrapment neuropathy
- B. Females are 4 times more affected
- C. Pain at palmer area is characteristic of pronator teres syndrome
- D. Neutral position splint relieves only 20% of patients
- E. Steroid injection may improve symptoms in 75% of patients

▸▸ Question 7

In carpel tunnel syndrome, surgical intervention is recommended for which of the following?

- A. Constant numbness
- B. Symptoms lasting > 1 year
- C. Sensory loss
- D. Thenar atrophy
- E. All of the above

▸▸ Question 8

A 32-year-old male presented to the OPD with discomfort in little finger and medial half of ring finger, with slight hand weakness of 4 + power and mild muscle atrophy. What is the grade of ulnar nerve injury classification of this patient?

- A. Grade 1
- B. Grade 2
- C. Grade 3
- D. Grade 4

▸▸ Question 9

Which one is a wrong statement about ulnar nerve?

- A. Elbow is most vulnerable for entrapment
- B. Tardy ulnar palsy is due to delayed onset following bony injury at the elbow
- C. NCS shows 4 m/sec faster than median nerve
- D. Early symptoms of ulnar nerve entrapment may be purely motor

▸▸ Question 10

A manual labor worker with frequent use of pneumatic drill presented to the OPD with Froment's sign and claw hand de-

formity with no sensory loss at dorsum of hand. Most probably injury to which of the following has caused the lesion?
- A. Cubital tunnel
- B. Osborne ligament
- C. Guyon's canal
- D. Struther's arcade

▸▸ Question 11

How can radial nerve injury be distinguished from posterior cord injury?
- A. Involvement of all forearm extensor
- B. Patchy sensory loss in the distribution of radial nerve
- C. Sparing of deltoid and latissimus dorsi muscles
- D. Purely motor involvement

▸▸ Question 12

Injury to radial nerve proximal to radial groove of humerus will involve which of the following?
- A. Wrist extensors only
- B. Finger extensors only
- C. Triceps only
- D. Triceps, wrist, and finger extensors

▸▸ Question 13

A young male was hit by a car while he was riding a bike. He is unable to dorsiflex his ankle and shows weakness of lateral hamstring. Which nerve will be involved in this case?
- A. Common peroneal nerve
- B. Posterior tibial nerve
- C. Deep peroneal nerve
- D. Superficial peroneal nerve

▸▸ Question 14

A male presented to the OPD with complains of spontaneous rubbing or massaging of upper lateral aspect of thigh, along with burning dysesthesia and hyperpathia. How can meralgia paresthetica be differentiated from femoral neuropathy?
- A. Sensory changes on upper lateral aspect
- B. Purely sensory involvement
- C. No motor weakness
- D. None of the above

▸▸ Question 15

A patient presented with complaint of pain that is more severe at night, frequently at rest, often with retrograde radiation, causing more proximal lesion to be suspected. The patient also has tenderness at the site of pain. He is suspected to have entrapment neuropathy. What are most common associations with entrapment neuropathy?
- A. Diabetes mellitus and hypothyroidism
- B. Acromegaly and amyloidosis
- C. Carcinomatosis and polymyalgia rheumatica
- D. Rheumatoid arthritis
- E. All of the above

▸▸ Question 16

What is the mechanism of injury in case of entrapment neuropathy?
- A. Chronic compression can cause axonolysis and Wallerian degeneration
- B. Acute compression can compromise axoplasmic flow, which can reduce membrane excitability
- C. There can be ischemia due to vascular supply compromise
- D. Venous stasis can produce ischemia which can lead to edema outside the axonal sheath, which can further exacerbate ischemia
- E. All of the above

▸▸ Question 17

A patient after trauma to back of the head presents with headache mostly in back and myofascial spasm. Diagnosis of occipital nerve entrapment was made which occurs due to entrapment of the great occipital nerve, which is a sensory branch of C2. All of the following are surgical options for treatment of occipital neuralgia except?
- A. Decompression of C2 nerve root if compressed between c1 and c2
- B. Occipital neurectomy
- C. Occipital nerve block with local anesthetic and steroids
- D. Occipital nerve stimulators
- E. Ganglionectomy

▸▸ Question 18

The median nerve is supplied by nerve roots C5 through T1 and it arises from medial and lateral cords of brachial plexus. In the cubital fossa, it passes just behind the lacertus fibrosus (bicipital aponeurosis) and enters the upper forearm between the two heads of pronator teres and supplies this muscle. Following statements regarding median nerve are correct except?
- A. Anterior interosseous nerve is purely motor branch of median nerve that supplies all but two muscles of finger and wrist flexion
- B. Near the wrist, it lies medial to the tendon of flexor carpi radialis and passes under transverse carpal ligament which also contains the tendons of FDP and FDS deep to the median nerve
- C. The second motor branch of the median nerve arises deep to the TCL and supplies LOAF muscles in the hand
- D. Palmaris cutaneous branch of the median nerve passes under the TCL and provides sensory innervation to the base of thenar eminence
- E. In the case of main trunk injury of the median nerve, a benediction hand is made when trying to make a fist (due to weakness of flexor digitorum 1 and 2)

▸▸ **Question 19**

A patient presents in neurosurgical emergency with complaint of difficulty in grasping small objects between the thumb and the index finger with no sensory loss. Pinch sign is positive. EMG assesses pronator quadratus and flexor pollicis longus. What is the diagnosis in this patient?

- A. Anterior interosseus neuropathy
- B. Pronator teres syndrome
- C. Carpal tunnel syndrome
- D. Injury to the main trunk of median nerve
- E. None of the above

▸▸ **Question 20**

A bulky female of 45 years of age presents in the OPD with complaints of pain in the palmer aspect of radial three and half fingers, dorsal side of these same fingers distal to PIP, and radial half of palm. The patient gets awakened at night by painful numbness in the hands. There is also hand weakness especially grip. Phalen's test (wrist flexion to 90 degrees angle reproduces the pain) is positive. What is the diagnosis in this patient?

- A. Cervical radiculopathy
- B. Pronator teres syndrome
- C. Carpal tunnel syndrome
- D. Reflex sympathetic atrophy
- E. De Quervain's syndrome

▸▸ **Question 21**

In case of carpal tunnel syndrome patient, EMG shows sensory latencies of 3.7 to 4 and 4.1 to 5 in mild and moderate CTS, respectively, while motor latencies are 4.4 to 6.9 and 7 to 9.9 in mild and moderate CTS. Laboratory workup for these patients include all of the following except?

- A. Thyroid hormone levels
- B. CBC
- C. There is no role of serum electrolytes in CTS patients
- D. HbA1c and glucose
- E. Vitamin B12, folate, and MMA

▸▸ **Question 22**

Which statement is true regarding treatment of carpal tunnel syndrome?

- A. NSAIDs, pyridoxine, and diuretics have strong evidence of good efficacy with no obvious benefits of neutral position splint for 2 to 4 weeks or steroid injection of 10 to 25 mg hydrocortisone into carpal tunnel
- B. Surgery is recommended for symptoms less than 1 year duration with no sensory or motor symptoms
- C. Recurrent motor branch which innervates muscles of the thenar eminence is also called as million dollar nerve because its injury can lead to loss of thumb function and a possible malpractice lawsuit
- D. Kaplan's cardinal line runs from the base of the thumb web space to the hook of hamate which has no link with anastomosis between superficial and deep palmer arches
- E. Incision extends from the proximal wrist flexion crease up to Kaplan's cardinal line between digits 3 and 4

▸▸ **Question 23**

Ulnar nerve has components of c7, c8, and T1. It is second most common entrapment neuropathy after CTS. Potential sites of its compression are above the elbow by arcade of Struthers, at the elbow in retroepicondylar groove (ulnar groove), cubital tunnel, at the point of exit from flexor carpi ulnaris, and in the wrist at Guyon's canal. What are the motor findings in ulnar entrapment neuropathy?

- A. Wasting of interossei may occur
- B. Wartenberg's sign: patients may complaint that the little finger does not make it in when they reach into their pocket due to abducted little finger because of the weakness of the third palmer interosseous muscle
- C. Froment's prehensile thumb sign: grasping a piece of paper between the thumb and the extended index finger results in extension of the proximal phalanx of the thumb and flexion of the distal phalanx
- D. Claw deformity of hand: benediction sign when trying to open the fist from closed position, which is fingers 4 and 5 are hyperextended at MCP joints and flexed at the interphalangeal joint
- E. All of the above

▸▸ **Question 24**

Electrodiagnostic criteria for ulnar neuropathy at the elbow are absolute motor nerve conduction velocity (NCV) less than 50 m/sec from below the elbow (BE) to above the elbow (AE), drop of NCV to more than 10 m/sec when comparing BE to the wrist segment to the AE to BE segment and decrease in compound myogenic action potential (CMAP) by more than 20% from BE to AE. Which of the following statements is true regarding Stewart classification system for severity of ulnar nerve injury?

- A. Grade 1 is mild which shows sensory symptoms, with or without motor symptoms, with or without sensory loss, with no muscle atrophy or weakness
- B. Grade 2 is moderate which shows sensory symptoms, with detectable sensory loss, with mild atrophy and 4 or 4 + muscle strength
- C. Grade 3 is severe which shows usually constant sensory symptoms, with detectable sensory loss, with moderate to marked atrophy and 4 or less muscle strength
- D. All of the above
- E. None of the above

Answers

▸▸ Answer 1

Correct answer is D. Never consider the possibility of systemic disease[1]

▸▸ Answer 2

Correct answer is E. C and D[2]

▸▸ Answer 3

Correct answer is A. Pain in palm rule out CTS[3]

▸▸ Answer 4

Correct answer is D. All of the above[4]

▸▸ Answer 5

Correct answer is A. 40 mmHg[5]

▸▸ Answer 6

Correct answer is D. Neutral position splint relieves only 20% of patients[6]

▸▸ Answer 7

Correct answer is E. All of the above[6]

▸▸ Answer 8

Correct answer is B. Grade 2[7]

▸▸ Answer 9

Correct answer is C. NCS shows 4 m/sec faster than median nerve[7]

▸▸ Answer 10

Correct answer is C. Guyon's canal[8]

▸▸ Answer 11

Correct answer is C. Sparing of deltoid and latissimus dorsi muscles[9]

▸▸ Answer 12

Correct answer is D. Triceps, wrist, and finger extensors[9]

▸▸ Answer 13

Correct answer is A. Common peroneal nerve[10]

▸▸ Answer 14

Correct answer is A. Sensory changes on upper lateral aspect[11]

▸▸ Answer 15

Correct answer is E. All of the above[1]

▸▸ Answer 16

Correct answer is E. All of the above[1]

▸▸ Answer 17

Correct answer is C. Occipital nerve block with local anesthetic and steroids[2]

▸▸ Answer 18

Correct answer is D. Palmaris cutaneous branch of the median nerve passes under the TCL and provides sensory innervation to the base of thenar eminence[12]

▸▸ Answer 19

Correct answer is A. Anterior interosseus neuropathy[13]

▸▸ Answer 20

Correct answer is C. Carpal tunnel syndrome[5]

▸▸ Answer 21

Correct answer is C. There is no role of serum electrolytes in CTS patients[14]

▸▸ Answer 22

Correct answer is C. Recurrent motor branch which innervates muscles of the thenar eminence is also called as million dollar nerve because its injury can lead to loss of thumb function and a possible malpractice lawsuit[6]

▸▸ Answer 23

Correct answer is E. All of the above[15]

▸▸ Answer 24

Correct answer is D. All of the above[7]

References

[1] Greenberg M, ed. Greenberg's Handbook of Neurosurgery. 10th ed. New York: Thieme; 2023:541
[2] Greenberg M, ed. Greenberg's Handbook of Neurosurgery. 10th ed. New York: Thieme; 2023:542
[3] Greenberg M, ed. Greenberg's Handbook of Neurosurgery. 10th ed. New York: Thieme; 2023:544
[4] Greenberg M, ed. Greenberg's Handbook of Neurosurgery. 10th ed. New York: Thieme; 2023:547
[5] Greenberg M, ed. Greenberg's Handbook of Neurosurgery. 10th ed. New York: Thieme; 2023:546

[6] Greenberg M, ed. Greenberg's Handbook of Neurosurgery. 10th ed. New York: Thieme; 2023:550
[7] Greenberg M, ed. Greenberg's Handbook of Neurosurgery. 10th ed. New York: Thieme; 2023:555
[8] Greenberg M, ed. Greenberg's Handbook of Neurosurgery. 10th ed. New York: Thieme; 2023:558
[9] Greenberg M, ed. Greenberg's Handbook of Neurosurgery. 10th ed. New York: Thieme; 2023:559
[10] Greenberg M, ed. Greenberg's Handbook of Neurosurgery. 10th ed. New York: Thieme; 2023:563
[11] Greenberg M, ed. Greenberg's Handbook of Neurosurgery. 10th ed. New York: Thieme; 2023:561
[12] Greenberg M, ed. Greenberg's Handbook of Neurosurgery. 10th ed. New York: Thieme; 2023:543
[13] Greenberg M, ed. Greenberg's Handbook of Neurosurgery. 10th ed. New York: Thieme; 2023:545
[14] Greenberg M, ed. Greenberg's Handbook of Neurosurgery. 10th ed. New York: Thieme; 2023:549
[15] Greenberg M, ed. Greenberg's Handbook of Neurosurgery. 10th ed. New York: Thieme; 2023:554

32 Nonentrapment Peripheral Neuropathies

Questions

▸▸ Question 1

What is the most common cause for peripheral neuropathy?
- A. Diabetes
- B. Arteritis
- C. Monoclonal gammopathy
- D. Acute idiopathic polyneuritis
- E. Sjogren syndrome

▸▸ Question 2

In critical illness polyneuropathy (CIP), CPK levels are normal or mildly elevated while EMG shows what?
- A. Decrease in amplitudes of compound muscle action potentials
- B. Increase in amplitudes of compound muscle action potentials
- C. Amplitudes of compound muscle action potentials remain unchanged
- D. Two spikes per second
- E. Nonlocalizing changes

▸▸ Question 3

Idiopathic brachial plexitis usually starts to show some improvement by when?
- A. 3rd day
- B. 2nd week
- C. 4th week
- D. 2nd month
- E. 3rd month

▸▸ Question 4

EMG changes can be appreciated in neuralgic amyotrophy of the upper extremity after how long?
- A. 24 hours
- B. 48 hours
- C. 72 hours
- D. 2 weeks
- E. 3 weeks

▸▸ Question 5

A diabetic patient presents with abrupt onset of asymmetric pain in back, hip, buttocks, thigh, and leg usually deep aching/burning with superimposed lancinating paroxysms, severe at night. Progressive weakness in proximal and distal muscles was preceded by weight loss. Patellar reflexes are absent. Sensory loss is minimal. EMG findings consistent with demyelination are invariably accompanied by axonal degeneration, with involvement of paraspinals and no evidence of myopathy. These findings are consistent with what?
- A. Guillain Barre syndrome
- B. Bruns-Garland syndrome
- C. Ramsay Hunt syndrome
- D. Tolosa Hunt syndrome
- E. Brachial plexitis

▸▸ Question 6

Which of the following is not associated with drug-induced neuropathy?
- A. Metronidazole
- B. Ciprofloxacin
- C. Phenytoin
- D. Thallium
- E. Cisplatin

▸▸ Question 7

What is the most common cause of femoral neuropathy?
- A. Diabetes
- B. Nerve entrapment
- C. Intra-abdominal tumor
- D. Femoral artery catheterization
- E. Retroperitoneal hematoma

▸▸ Question 8

Peripheral nerves regeneration rate in mm/d is about how much?
- A. 1
- B. 2
- C. 3
- D. 5
- E. 10

▸▸ Question 9

According to the Sunderland system for classification of peripheral nerve injury what is neurotmesis?
- A. First degree
- B. Second degree
- C. Third degree
- D. Fourth degree
- E. Fifth degree

▸▸ Question 10

In which of the following complete interruption of axons and myelin sheaths takes place and Wallerian degeneration occurs whereas supporting structures including endoneurium remain intact?

- A. Neuropraxia
- B. Axonotmesis
- C. Neurotmesis
- D. Axonolysis
- E. First degree injury of Sunderland system

▸▸ Question 11

Lesions of peripheral nerves can produce somatic findings (combination of weakness, sensory disturbance, and reflex changes) and/or autonomic disturbances. Etiologies of nonentrapment peripheral neuropathies include which of the following?

- A. Diabetes
- B. Alcoholism
- C. Guillain-Barre syndrome
- D. Vasculitis/arteritis
- E. All of the above

▸▸ Question 12

A patient admitted in ICU developed critical illness neuropathy (CIP) also known as neuropathy of critical illness or ICU neuropathy. For evaluation of the patient, blood work with fasting electrolytes, Hgb-A1C, CBC, ESR, CRP, vitamin B12, methylmalonic acid, serum protein electrophoresis with serum immunofixation, and electrodiagnostics (EMG/NCV) are done to rule out the cause of neuropathy. Following are the diagnostic criteria of CIP except?

- A. Presence of sepsis, multiorgan failure, septic inflammatory response syndrome, or respiratory failure
- B. Difficulty weaning from ventilator or extremity weakness
- C. EMG showing increased amplitudes of compound muscle action potentials
- D. Widespread muscle denervation potentials
- E. Normal or only mild increase in serum CPK levels

▸▸ Question 13

A male patient 30 years of age develops acute onset of intense pain in right upper extremity some days after a viral illness. Weakness of the same limb developed acutely after 2 weeks of pain onset. Arm movements exacerbated the pain. EMG/NCV showed the portion of brachial plexus involved. What is the most probable diagnosis in this patient?

- A. Parsonage Turner syndrome
- B. Immune-mediated brachial plexus neuropathy
- C. Neuralgic amyotrophy of the upper extremity
- D. Brachial plexitis
- E. All of the above

▸▸ Question 14

A patient presents to neurosurgical OPD with history of sudden onset of pain in lower extremity with weakness of quadriceps femoris muscle, SLR positive. EMG/NCV was done which showed patchy denervation involving at least two segmental levels with sparing of the paraspinal muscles. What is the most likely diagnosis in this case?

- A. L4 and L5 acute rupture of intervertebral disk
- B. Lumbosacral plexus neuropathy
- C. Rupture of AVM at L4 and L5 level
- D. Sudden compression of lumbosacral plexus
- E. None of the above

▸▸ Question 15

About 50% of patients with diabetes mellitus develop neuropathic symptoms or show slowing of nerve conduction velocities on electrodiagnostic studies. What is the most appropriate treatment of diabetic amyotrophy?

- A. Mexiletine started at 150 mg every 8 hours
- B. Gabapentin 1800 to 3600 mg every day
- C. Pregabalin up to a maximum of 100 mg TID
- D. Amitriptyline and fluphenazine
- E. All of the above

▸▸ Question 16

Drugs that are most notorious for peripheral neuropathy include all of the following except?

- A. Thalidomide
- B. Macrolides
- C. Phenytoin
- D. Amitriptyline
- E. Metronidazole

▸▸ Question 17

AIDS patients can develop vague numbness, tingling, and sometimes painful feet. There may be reduction of light touch and vibratory sense. What is this condition called?

- A. Distal symmetric polyneuropathy
- B. Mononeuropathy multiplex
- C. Meralgia paresthetica
- D. Lumbar polyradiculopathy
- E. All of the above

▸▸ Question 18

Following are most common nerves that can be involved in perioperative neuropathy except?

- A. Ulnar nerve
- B. Brachial plexus
- C. Median nerve
- D. Radial nerve
- E. Common peroneal nerve

▸▸ Question 19

Which of the following statements is incorrect regarding the Sunderland system of peripheral nerve injury classification?

- A. First degree is physiologic transection with local conduction block with usually complete recovery in 2 to 3 weeks and is also called neuropraxia
- B. Second degree is complete interruption of axons and myelin sheath, with supporting structures including endoneurium intact with recovery at 1 mm/d and is also called axonotmesis
- C. Third degree is endoneurium disrupted with intact epineurium and perineurium and is also called axonotmesis
- D. Fourth degree is interruption of all neural and supporting elements with only epineurium intact and is also called neurotmesis
- E. Fifth degree is complete transection with loss of continuity

►► Question 20

Brachial plexus injuries include Erb's palsy (Duchene) from c5, c6, and may be c7 injury, Klumke's paralysis from c8, T1, and may be c7, or birth brachial plexus injuries which involves arm hanging at side, internally rotated, extended at elbow, and flexed at wrist (Bellhop's tip position), and claw deformity with weakness and wasting of small arm muscles. What are indications of neurosurgical intervention in gun shot wound to the brachial plexus?

- A. Complete loss in distribution of at least one element evident by no improvement clinically or in EMG for 2 to 5 months
- B. Incomplete loss with failure to control pain medically
- C. Pseudoaneurysm, fistula, or clot involving plexus
- D. True causalgia requiring sympathectomy
- E. All of the above

Answers

►► Answer 1

Correct answer is A. Diabetes[1]

►► Answer 2

Correct answer is A. Decrease in amplitudes of compound muscle action potentials[2]

►► Answer 3

Correct answer is C. 4th week[3]

►► Answer 4

Correct answer is E. 3 weeks[4]

►► Answer 5

Correct answer is B. Bruns-Garland syndrome[5]

►► Answer 6

Correct answer is B. Ciprofloxacin[6]

►► Answer 7

Correct answer is A. Diabetes[7]

►► Answer 8

Correct answer is A. 1[8]

►► Answer 9

Correct answer is E. Fifth degree[9]

►► Answer 10

Correct answer is B. Axonotmesis[9]

►► Answer 11

Correct answer is E. All of the above[10]

►► Answer 12

Correct answer is C. EMG showing increased amplitudes of compound muscle action potentials[2]

►► Answer 13

Correct answer is E. All of the above[3]

►► Answer 14

Correct answer is B. Lumbosacral plexus neuropathy[4]

►► Answer 15

Correct answer is E. All of the above[5]

►► Answer 16

Correct answer is B. Macrolides[6]

►► Answer 17

Correct answer is A. Distal symmetric polyneuropathy[7]

►► Answer 18

Correct answer is D. Radial nerve[11]

►► Answer 19

Correct answer is D. Fourth degree is interruption of all neural and supporting elements with only epineurium intact and is also called neurotmesis[9]

►► Answer 20

Correct answer is E. All of the above[12]

References

[1] Greenberg M, ed. Greenberg's Handbook of Neurosurgery. 10th ed. New York: Thieme; 2023:562
[2] Greenberg M, ed. Greenberg's Handbook of Neurosurgery. 10th ed. New York: Thieme; 2023:569
[3] Greenberg M, ed. Greenberg's Handbook of Neurosurgery. 10th ed. New York: Thieme; 2023:570
[4] Greenberg M, ed. Greenberg's Handbook of Neurosurgery. 10th ed. New York: Thieme; 2023:571
[5] Greenberg M, ed. Greenberg's Handbook of Neurosurgery. 10th ed. New York: Thieme; 2023:572
[6] Greenberg M, ed. Greenberg's Handbook of Neurosurgery. 10th ed. New York: Thieme; 2023:573
[7] Greenberg M, ed. Greenberg's Handbook of Neurosurgery. 10th ed. New York: Thieme; 2023:574
[8] Greenberg M, ed. Greenberg's Handbook of Neurosurgery. 10th ed. New York: Thieme; 2023:577
[9] Greenberg M, ed. Greenberg's Handbook of Neurosurgery. 10th ed. New York: Thieme; 2023:578
[10] Greenberg M, ed. Greenberg's Handbook of Neurosurgery. 10th ed. New York: Thieme; 2023:568
[11] Greenberg M, ed. Greenberg's Handbook of Neurosurgery. 10th ed. New York: Thieme; 2023:575
[12] Greenberg M, ed. Greenberg's Handbook of Neurosurgery. 10th ed. New York: Thieme; 2023:580

Part XI

Neuro-Ophthalmology and Neurotology

XI

33 Neuro-Ophthalmology

Questions

▸▸ Question 1

A lesion in diencephalon will present with which nystagmus type?
- A. See-saw
- B. Convergence
- C. Retractorius
- D. Downbeat
- E. Upbeat

▸▸ Question 2

Brun's nystagmus is associated with lesion in which of the following?
- A. Medial longitudinal fasciculus
- B. Lateral longitudinal fasciculus
- C. Pontomedullary junction
- D. Midbrain tegmentum
- E. Medulla

▸▸ Question 3

Low degree of papilledema with elevation of nasal margin, 360-degree disk swelling (circumferential halo) but no obscuration of major vessels on fundoscopy characterize which modified Frisen grade papilledema?
- A. Grade I
- B. Grade II
- C. Grade III
- D. Grade IV
- E. Grade V

▸▸ Question 4

Homonymous superior quadrantanopsia in the contralateral visual field ("pie in the sky" deficit) is caused by lesion of which of the following?
- A. Optic tract
- B. Optic chiasma
- C. Meyer's loop
- D. Optic radiation
- E. Occipital cortex

▸▸ Question 5

Aneurysm of which of the following most commonly presents with third nerve palsy?
- A. A comm
- B. P comm
- C. ACA
- D. MCA trifurcation
- E. DACA

▸▸ Question 6

Which of the following is not a part of complete Horner syndrome?
- A. Miosis
- B. Ptosis
- C. Enophthalmos
- D. Hyperemia of internal ear
- E. Anhidrosis of half of face

▸▸ Question 7

What is the most common cause of bilateral internuclear ophthalmoplegia in young adults?
- A. Ocular tuberculosis
- B. Herpes zoster
- C. Congenital
- D. Multiple sclerosis
- E. Horner syndrome

▸▸ Question 8

Which of the following is not a cause of pupil-sparing oculomotor palsy?
- A. Uncal herniation
- B. Diabetic neuropathy
- C. Atherosclerosis
- D. Giant cell arteritis
- E. Myasthenia gravis

▸▸ Question 9

Which of the following nerves is not involved in superior orbital fissure syndrome?
- A. III
- B. IV
- C. V1
- D. V2
- E. VI

▸▸ Question 10

Mastoiditis with involvement of petrous apex presenting with classic triad of abducens palsy, retro-orbital pain, and draining ear is which of the following?
- A. Raeder's neuralgia
- B. Tolosa Hunt syndrome
- C. Gradenigo's syndrome
- D. Orbital apex syndrome
- E. Inferior orbital fissure syndrome

▸▸ Question 11

Nystagmus is involuntary rhythmic oscillations of the eyes, usually conjugate, most common form of which is jerk nystagmus in which the direction of the nystagmus is defined by the direction of the fast component. A patient with structural lesion in the posterior fossa at the cervicomedullary junction including Chiari malformation type 1, basilar impression, basilar impression, or syringobulbia has which type of nystagmus?

- A. Upbeat nystagmus
- B. Vestibular nystagmus
- C. Downbeat nystagmus
- D. See-saw nystagmus
- E. Convergence nystagmus

▸▸ Question 12

Papilledema also known as choked optic is optic disk swelling caused by increased intracranial pressure (ICP). Elevated ICP is transmitted through the subarachnoid space of the optic nerve sheath to the region of the optic disk which causes axoplasmic stasis and papilledema. How long it typically takes to develop papilledema after development of a sustained rise in ICP?

- A. 6 to 24 hours
- B. > 6 hours
- C. 12 to 24 hours
- D. 24 to 48 hours
- E. 48 to 72 hours

▸▸ Question 13

Papilledema can cause posterior globe flattening or elevation of the optic nerve head and dilatation of the optic nerve sheath (optic nerve sheath hydrops) which can be demonstrated on MRI or CT brain. Following statements regarding modified Frisen scale for papilledema on fundoscopic examination are correct except?

- A. Grade 0 is normal optic disk with minimal swelling of nasal margin, nerve fiber layer is clear, vessels are not obscured, and cup is also not obscured
- B. Grade 1 is minimal papilledema with 230-degree C-shaped swelling of nasal superior and inferior borders with normal temporal margin, and cup, if present, is maintained
- C. Grade 2 is low degree of papilledema with elevation of nasal margin, 360-degree disk swelling, and obscuration of major vessel starting from margins of disk
- D. Grade 3 is moderate degree of papilledema with elevation of entire disk, 360-degree disk swelling, obscuration of greater than or equal to 1 segment of major blood vessel at disk margin, and cup may be obscured
- E. Grade 4 is marked degree of papilledema with nerve fiber layer opaque, 360-degree disk swelling. Vessels obscured at disk margin, not completely obscured at disk surface

▸▸ Question 14

Which of the following is not an etiology of unilateral papilledema?

- A. Compressive lesions like intraorbital meningiomas, optic nerve sheath schwannoma, or optic nerve glioma
- B. Local inflammatory disorders
- C. Foster Kennedy syndrome
- D. Demyelinating disease such as multiple sclerosis
- E. Elevated ICP due to frontal lobe glioma

▸▸ Question 15

The normal eye can detect stimuli as far as 60 degrees superiorly, 70 degrees inferiorly, 60 degrees nasally, and 100 degrees temporally. Confrontational method is a bed side test to detect any gross peripheral field defect while Humphrey visual field, octopus perimeters, and Goldmann perimetry are more accurate in detecting visual field defect. Which of the following statements is incorrect?

- A. Optic nerve and knee of Wilbrand injury on one side will cause junctional scotoma of ipsilateral eye (monocular blindness) while superior temporal quadrantanopsia of the same side eye
- B. Injury to optic chiasma causes bitemporal hemianopia
- C. Injury to right optic nerve or optic radiation causes left homonymous hemianopia with macular splitting of the left visual field
- D. Injury to right Meyer's loop causes homonymous left superior quadrantanopsia with macular sparing of left visual field
- E. Partial lesion of right optic radiation or visual cortex causes left homonymous hemianopsia with macular sparing of left visual field

▸▸ Question 16

Macular splitting can occur both in lesions anterior and posterior to lateral geniculate body (LGB) while macular sparing tends to occur in lesions posterior to LGB. Homonymous hemianopsia with macular sparing usually occurs with the lesion of the optic radiation or infarcts of the primary visual cortex. What is the reason for macular sparing in lesions posterior to LGB?

- A. Input from macula is spread over large portion of optic radiation or primary visual cortex
- B. In some cases the occipital pole receives dual blood supply
- C. Occipital pole receives anomalous blood supply from the MCA
- D. Macula is resistant to lesion in this area
- E. A, B, and C

▸▸ Question 17

A patient presents with ipsilateral central scotoma and contralateral superior temporal quadrantanopsia. This condition is also called as anterior chiasmal syndrome. This injury occurs due to which of the following?

- A. Lesion causing this deficit is close to anterior chiasma
- B. Ipsilateral optic nerve injury
- C. Damage to decussating knee of Wilbrand fibers
- D. All of the above
- E. Damage to only optic nerve close to chiasma

▸▸ Question 18

Pupillodilator muscle fibers are sympathetically innervated and are arranged radially in iris while pupilloconstrictor muscles are parasympathetically innervated and are arranged as sphincter in the iris. Which statement is incorrect regarding the path of sympathetic fibers for pupilodilator muscles?

- A. First-order neuron arises in the anteromedial hypothalamus and descends uncrossed in the lateral tegmentum of the midbrain, pons, medulla, and the cervical spinal cord
- B. Second-order neurons arise from intermediolateral cell column of the spinal cord from C8 to T1 (ciliospinal center of Budge-Waller) which are preganglionic fibers. These exit at T1 and ascend in sympathetic chain
- C. Third-order neurons arise from superior cervical ganglion also known as postganglionic and ascend with common carotid artery
- D. Postganglionic fibers follow ICA through carotid canal, carotid sinus where they follow the 6th nerve and accompany V1 into orbit, then these enter ciliary ganglion and supply pupilodilator muscle
- E. Some fibers travel with ophthalmic artery to supply lacrimal gland and Muller's muscle

▸▸ Question 19

Pupillary light reflex involves cranial nerves 2, 3, neurons in Edinger-Westphal nucleus, and pretectal nuclear complex. Which of the following is true regarding pupillary light reflex?

- A. Cranial nerve 2 acts as afferent pathway
- B. Cranial nerve 2 fibers of light reflex lead to pretectal nuclear complex of superior colliculus without synapsing in the lateral geniculate body
- C. Edinger-Westphal nucleus is a parasympathetic motor nuclei
- D. Efferent is carried by the 3rd nerve
- E. All of the above

▸▸ Question 20

Light near dissociation is pupillary constriction of convergence but absence of light response. This condition can occur with syphilis, Parinaud's syndrome, oculomotor neuropathy, or Adie's pupil. What is this condition called?

- A. Argyll Robertson pupil
- B. Marcus Gunn pupil
- C. Swinging flashlight pupil
- D. Anisocoria
- E. None of the above

Answers

▸▸ Answer 1

Correct answer is A. See-saw[1]

▸▸ Answer 2

Correct answer is C. Pontomedullary junction[1]

▸▸ Answer 3

Correct answer is B. Grade II[2]

▸▸ Answer 4

Correct answer is C. Meyer's loop[3]

▸▸ Answer 5

Correct answer is B. P comm[4]

▸▸ Answer 6

Correct answer is D. Hyperemia of internal ear[5]

▸▸ Answer 7

Correct answer is D. Multiple sclerosis[6]

▸▸ Answer 8

Correct answer is A. Uncal herniation[7]

▸▸ Answer 9

Correct answer is D. V2[8]

▸▸ Answer 10

Correct answer is C. Gradenigo's syndrome[9]

▸▸ Answer 11

Correct answer is C. Downbeat nystagmus[1]

▸▸ Answer 12

Correct answer is D. 24 to 48 hours[1]

▸▸ Answer 13

Correct answer is C. Grade 2 is low degree of papilledema with elevation of nasal margin, 360-degree disk swelling, and obscuration of major vessel starting from margins of disk[2]

▸▸ Answer 14

Correct answer is E. Elevated ICP due to frontal lobe glioma[10]

▸▸ Answer 15

Correct answer is A. Optic nerve and knee of Wilbrand injury on one side will cause junctional scotoma of ipsilateral

eye (monocular blindness) while superior temporal quadrantanopsia of the same side eye[3]

▸▸ Answer 16

Correct answer is E. A, B, and C[11]

▸▸ Answer 17

Correct answer is D. All of the above[3]

▸▸ Answer 18

Correct answer is A. First-order neuron arises in the anteromedial hypothalamus and descends uncrossed in the lateral tegmentum of the midbrain, pons, medulla, and the cervical spinal cord[3]

▸▸ Answer 19

Correct answer is E. All of the above[3]

▸▸ Answer 20

Correct answer is A. Argyll Robertson pupil[12]

References

[1] Greenberg M, ed. Greenberg's Handbook of Neurosurgery. 10th ed. New York: Thieme; 2023:586
[2] Greenberg M, ed. Greenberg's Handbook of Neurosurgery. 10th ed. New York: Thieme; 2023:587
[3] Greenberg M, ed. Greenberg's Handbook of Neurosurgery. 10th ed. New York: Thieme; 2023:590
[4] Greenberg M, ed. Greenberg's Handbook of Neurosurgery. 10th ed. New York: Thieme; 2023:592
[5] Greenberg M, ed. Greenberg's Handbook of Neurosurgery. 10th ed. New York: Thieme; 2023:594
[6] Greenberg M, ed. Greenberg's Handbook of Neurosurgery. 10th ed. New York: Thieme; 2023:596
[7] Greenberg M, ed. Greenberg's Handbook of Neurosurgery. 10th ed. New York: Thieme; 2023:597
[8] Greenberg M, ed. Greenberg's Handbook of Neurosurgery. 10th ed. New York: Thieme; 2023:599
[9] Greenberg M, ed. Greenberg's Handbook of Neurosurgery. 10th ed. New York: Thieme; 2023:601
[10] Greenberg M, ed. Greenberg's Handbook of Neurosurgery. 10th ed. New York: Thieme; 2023:588
[11] Greenberg M, ed. Greenberg's Handbook of Neurosurgery. 10th ed. New York: Thieme; 2023:589
[12] Greenberg M, ed. Greenberg's Handbook of Neurosurgery. 10th ed. New York: Thieme; 2023:591

34 Neurotology

Questions

▸▸ **Question 1**

For treatment of Meniere's disease, which procedure should be avoided?
- A. Middle ear perfusion with gentamicin
- B. Bilateral selective vestibular neurectomy
- C. Salt restriction
- D. Vestibular suppressants (e.g., Valium, meclizine)
- E. Endolymphatic shunting

▸▸ **Question 2**

Which of the following diagnostic studies shows normal latencies in Meniere's disease?
- A. ENG with bithermal caloric stimulation
- B. Audiogram
- C. BAER
- D. CT/MRI
- E. VDRL

▸▸ **Question 3**

What is the most common cause of Bell's palsy?
- A. Diabetes
- B. Herpes zoster infection
- C. Trauma/basal skull fracture
- D. Tumor
- E. Idiopathic

▸▸ **Question 4**

For Bell's palsy, if there is complete paralysis of facial nerve at onset, what proportion of patients will have an incomplete recovery despite management?
- A. 30%
- B. 50%
- C. 80%
- D. 90%
- E. 95%

▸▸ **Question 5**

A 70-year-old male presented in OPD with complaints of decreased hearing in right ear. On examination, he is having positive Rinne test (bilaterally AC > BC) and Weber is lateralizing to left ear. What type of hearing loss he is having?
- A. Conductive hearing loss in right ear
- B. Sensorineural hearing loss in right ear
- C. Combined conductive + SNHL
- D. Combined sensorineural hearing loss
- E. Both A and B

▸▸ **Question 6**

Regarding Bell's palsy if treatment is administered, which of the following is the most widely accepted for improvement?
- A. Tarsorrhaphy
- B. Direct brow lift
- C. Transposition of the temporalis muscle
- D. Corticosteroids
- E. Eye ointment and tear drops

▸▸ **Question 7**

Which of the following is a characteristic of grade IV Bell's palsy?
- A. Eye closure is incomplete
- B. Forehead motion is slight to moderate
- C. A slightly weak mouth movement is noted with maximal effort
- D. Asymmetry is noted at rest
- E. Both A and B

▸▸ **Question 8**

Which of the following is not a typical feature of Ménière's disease?
- A. Insidious and progressive hearing loss
- B. Tinnitus
- C. Vertigo
- D. Otolithic crisis of Tumarkin
- E. Fluctuating deafness

▸▸ **Question 9**

Which of the following is recommended regarding steroid treatment in patients with Bell's palsy?
- A. Corticosteroids treatment in Bell's palsy is only recommended within the first 24 hours after symptom onset
- B. Prednisolone 25 mg per oral, twice daily for 10 days
- C. Antiviral treatment should be given as monotherapy prior to steroid treatment
- D. Antiviral combined with prednisolone
- E. Steroid therapy is given along with ceftriaxone

▸▸ **Question 10**

A patient suffers injury to facial nerve during surgery for CP angle space occupying lesion (SOL). Primary repair is done. What is the expected failure rate in these cases?
- A. 13%
- B. 23%
- C. 33%
- D. 43%
- E. 53%

▸▸ Question 11

A patient presents with vertigo (sensation of movement usually spinning) in neurosurgical OPD. Following should be kept in mind as differentials for this disease except?

- A. Inner ear dysfunction which can be caused by labyrinthitis, Meneire's disease, trauma, drugs like aminoglycosides, syphilis, or vertebrobasilar insufficiency
- B. Vestibular nerve dysfunction which can include vestibular neuronitis, vestibular nerve compression by meningioma or schwannoma
- C. Brain stem dysfunction because of vertebrobasilar insufficiency, basilar artery migraine, or multiple sclerosis
- D. Dysfunction of dorsal proprioceptors as in osteoarthritis
- E. Vascular compression of vestibular nerve which can cause disabling positional vertigo

▸▸ Question 12

Complete loss of vestibular function from one side is thought to produce transient vertigo due to mismatch of vestibular input from the two ears. Unilateral selective vestibular neurectomy (SVN) may convert the fluctuating or partial loss to a complete cessation of input and facilitate compensation. What surgical approach is adopted for SVN in case of Meniere's disease?

- A. Retrosigmoid approach
- B. Retrolabyrinthine approach
- C. Middle fossa approach
- D. Translabyrinthine approach
- E. All of the above

▸▸ Question 13

Three surgical approaches for selective vestibular neurectomy (SVN) are retrolabyrinthine approach (which is anterior to sigmoid sinus and requires mastoidectomy with skeletonization of the semicircular canals and endolymphatic sac), retrosigmoid approach (posterior fossa suboccipital approach which is posterior to sigmoid sinus), and middle fossa approach (which is middle fossa extradural approach). Which approach is more suitable for complete section of vestibular nerve when other approaches fail?

- A. Retrolabyrinthine
- B. Retrosigmoid
- C. Translabyrinthine
- D. Middle fossa
- E. None of the above

▸▸ Question 14

A neurosurgeon is going to do selective vestibular neurectomy (SVN). He/she should have following points in mind to have safe surgery and achieve surgical goals except?

- A. The vestibular nerve is the superior half of eighth nerve and is slightly more gray in color than the cochlear nerve (due to less myelin)
- B. Facial nerve is whiter than the eighth nerve complex, lies anterior and superior to eighth nerve complex. EMG monitoring is also recommended while direct stimulation during surgery can also confirm facial nerve identification
- C. Any artery present on eighth nerve bundle may be sacrificed
- D. If no cleavage plane is identified between vestibular and cochlear division then superior half of nerve bundle is divided
- E. The ELC lies midway between posterior edge of external auditory meatus and the sigmoid sinus

▸▸ Question 15

A patient presents in OPD with attacks of violent vertigo, nausea, vomiting, diaphoresis, and tinnitus with progressive hearing loss which is fluctuating and low frequency. These attacks last for 5 to 30 minutes. What is most probable diagnosis in this case?

- A. Meniere's disease which is due to increased endolymphatic pressure
- B. Benign positional vertigo
- C. Vestibular neuronitis
- D. Vertebrobasilar insufficiency
- E. Disabling positional vertigo

▸▸ Question 16

Diagnostic studies for Meniere's disease are electronystagmography with bithermal caloric stimulation abnormal and audiogram with low frequency hearing loss. Its medical management include reduced intake of salt, diuretics including acetazolamide, vestibular suppressants like diazepam, meclizine HCL, and vasodilators. What is the surgical treatment of Meniere's disease for serviceable hearing loss?

- A. Endolymphatic shunting procedure to mastoid cavity or subarachnoid space
- B. Direct application of corticosteroids to inner ear
- C. Nonselective vestibular ablation like surgical labyrinthectomy, middle ear perfusion with gentamicin
- D. Selective vestibular neurectomy
- E. Both A and D

▸▸ Question 17

Vestibular nerve section results in relief of vertigo in 90%, unchanged in 5%, and worse in 5%, while 9% incidence of facial paralysis in which 3% is permanent paralysis. On other hand selective vestibular nerve section results in improved hearing in 10%, unchanged in 28%, and worse in 48% while deafness in 14%. In postoperative failure, if ENG shows any vestibular nerve function on operated side then what is the next management step?

- A. Treatment only with medication
- B. Radiofrequency is done
- C. Chemotherapy is given
- D. Reoperation is considered
- E. All of the above

▸▸ Question 18

Which of the following statements regarding path of facial nerve is incorrect?

- A. The seventh nerve exits the brain stem at the pontomedullary junction and enters the supero-anterior portion of internal auditory canal to enter the geniculate ganglion
- B. The first branch from geniculate ganglion is greater superficial petrosal nerve which passes to the pterygopalatine ganglion, innervates nasal mucosa, palatine mucosa, and lacrimal gland of eye
- C. The second branch is branch to stapedius muscle, and lesions proximal to this produce hyperacusis
- D. Third is chordae tympani which joins the facial nerve bringing sensations from posterior one-third of tongue, and along chordae tympani are fibers to submandibular and sublingual glands
- E. Facial nerve exits skull through stylomastoid foramen where it enters parotid gland and splits into five terminal branches

▸▸ Question 19

What is the recommended management option for Bell's palsy?

- A. General supportive measure
- B. Eye protection and steroid prednisolone 25 mg per oral BID for 10 days
- C. Acyclovir
- D. Surgical decompression
- E. All of the above

Answers

▸▸ Answer 1

Correct answer is B. Bilateral selective vestibular neurectomy[1]

▸▸ Answer 2

Correct answer is C. BAER[2]

▸▸ Answer 3

Correct answer is E. Idiopathic[3]

▸▸ Answer 4

Correct answer is B. 50%[4]

▸▸ Answer 5

Correct answer is B. Sensorineural hearing loss in right ear[5]

▸▸ Answer 6

Correct answer is D. Corticosteroids[4]

▸▸ Answer 7

Correct answer is E. Both A and B[3]

▸▸ Answer 8

Correct answer is A. Insidious and progressive hearing loss[2]

▸▸ Answer 9

Correct answer is B. Prednisolone 25 mg per oral, twice daily for 10 days[4]

▸▸ Answer 10

Correct answer is C. 33%[4]

▸▸ Answer 11

Correct answer is D. Dysfunction of dorsal proprioceptors as in osteoarthritis[6]

▸▸ Answer 12

Correct answer is B. Retrolabyrinthine approach[1]

▸▸ Answer 13

Correct answer is D. Middle fossa[7]

▸▸ Answer 14

Correct answer is C. Any artery present on eighth nerve bundle may be sacrificed[7]

▸▸ Answer 15

Correct answer is A. Meniere's disease which is due to increased endolymphatic pressure[7]

▸▸ Answer 16

Correct answer is E. Both A and D[1]

▸▸ Answer 17

Correct answer is D. Reoperation is considered[8]

▸▸ Answer 18

Correct answer is D. Third is chordae tympani which joins the facial nerve bringing sensations from posterior one-third of tongue, and along chordae tympani are fibers to submandibular and sublingual glands[8]

▸▸ Answer 19

Correct answer is B. Eye protection and steroid prednisolone 25 mg per oral BID for 10 days[4]

References

[1] Greenberg M, ed. Greenberg's Handbook of Neurosurgery. 10th ed. New York: Thieme; 2023:606
[2] Greenberg M, ed. Greenberg's Handbook of Neurosurgery. 10th ed. New York: Thieme; 2023:605
[3] Greenberg M, ed. Greenberg's Handbook of Neurosurgery. 10th ed. New York: Thieme; 2023:608
[4] Greenberg M, ed. Greenberg's Handbook of Neurosurgery. 10th ed. New York: Thieme; 2023:609
[5] Greenberg M, ed. Greenberg's Handbook of Neurosurgery. 10th ed. New York: Thieme; 2023:612
[6] Greenberg M, ed. Greenberg's Handbook of Neurosurgery. 10th ed. New York: Thieme; 2023:603
[7] Greenberg M, ed. Greenberg's Handbook of Neurosurgery. 10th ed. New York: Thieme; 2023:604
[8] Greenberg M, ed. Greenberg's Handbook of Neurosurgery. 10th ed. New York: Thieme; 2023:607

Part XII

Tumors of the Nervous and Related Systems

XII

35 Tumor Classification and General Information

Questions

▸▸ Question 1

In WHO classification of CNS tumors 2021, what does suffix NOS (not otherwise specified) indicate?

- A. Nonconcordance between histological and molecular types
- B. Noncanonical results
- C. New emerging tumor type
- D. Molecular testing not done or uncertain

▸▸ Question 2

Which of the following is no more a subtype of adult type diffuse gliomas?

- A. Astrocytoma IDH mutant, grade 2
- B. Astrocytoma IDH wildtype, grade 2
- C. Astrocytoma IDH mutant, grade 3
- D. Astrocytoma IDH mutant, grade 4

▸▸ Question 3

According to WHO 2021 classification, which lineage of pituitary tumors secretes GH > PRL and a subunit?

- A. Mammosomatotroph pitNET
- B. Mature plurihormonal PIT1 lineage pitNET
- C. Immature PIT1 lineage pit NET
- D. Acidophil stem cell pitNET
- E. Mixed somatotroph–lactotroph PitNET

▸▸ Question 4

During the first 6 months of life, infratentorial tumors comprise what percentage of all intracranial tumors?

- A. 15%
- B. 27%
- C. 53%
- D. 74%
- E. 60%

▸▸ Question 5

A 45-year-old male presented with abulia, dementia, personality changes, apraxia, hemiparesis, and dysphasia. These suggest lesion localized in which area?

- A. Left frontal
- B. Right temporal
- C. Parietal
- D. Occipital
- E. Posterior fossa

▸▸ Question 6

A 40-year-old female presented with auditory and olfactory hallucinations, déja vu, memory impairment, and right superior quadrantanopsia. These suggest lesion localized in which area?

- A. Right frontal
- B. Left temporal
- C. Parietal
- D. Occipital
- E. Posterior fossa

▸▸ Question 7

What is the most common supratentorial tumor in children as well as in adults?

- A. Astrocytoma
- B. Medulloblastoma
- C. Craniopharyngioma
- D. Teratoma
- E. Choroid plexus papilloma

▸▸ Question 8

What is the most common brain tumor in neonates?

- A. Astrocytoma
- B. Medulloblastoma
- C. Craniopharyngioma
- D. Teratoma
- E. Choroid plexus papilloma

▸▸ Question 9

A middle-aged patient presented with first-time seizures. CT of brain showed brain tumor. Dexamethasone 10 mg was given intravenously. What will be the usual adult maintenance dose?

- A. 10 mg postoperatively 12 hourly
- B. 6 mg postoperatively 6 hourly
- C. 4 mg postoperatively 6 hourly
- D. 2 mg postoperatively 8 hourly
- E. Repeat 10 mg as needed

▸▸ Question 10

An old patient undergoes excision of glioblastoma multiforme. What is the alkylating agent used in chemotherapy?

- A. Carmustine
- B. Lomustine
- C. Temozolamine
- D. Vincristine
- E. Procarbazine

▸▸ Question 11

During histochemical analysis of a tumor specimen, which agent is used to stain myelin?

- A. Ziehl Neelsen
- B. Gram stain
- C. Reticulin stain
- D. Luxol fast blue
- E. Periodic acid Schiff

▸▸ Question 12

A patient presented with headache, seizures, and monoplegia. What is the tumor marker for meningioma?

- A. Glial fibrillary acidic protein
- B. Epithelial membrane antigen
- C. S-100
- D. Chromogranin A
- E. Synaptophysin

▸▸ Question 13

Ki-67 is expressed in all phases of cell cycle except?

- A. G0
- B. G1
- C. G2
- D. S1
- E. S2

▸▸ Question 14

Any metastatic small-cell tumors to the brain staining positive for neuroendocrine stains are almost all due to primaries in which of the following?

- A. Liver
- B. Bone
- C. Pancreas
- D. Lungs
- E. Prostate

▸▸ Question 15

The common pediatric brain tumors are gliomas and glioneural tumors (cerebellum, brain stem, and optic nerve) (which accounts for 45% of primary CNS tumors in pediatrics), embryonal tumors (12.3% of pediatric CNS tumors, 67% of which are medulloblastoma), pituitary tumors (6.2%), nerve sheath tumors (4.2%), and craniopharyngioma (3.8%). What are the most common supratentorial tumors in children as well as in adults?

- A. Astrocytomas
- B. Meningiomas
- C. Choroid plexus papilloma
- D. Ependymomas
- E. Craniopharyngiomas

▸▸ Question 16

A patient presents in neurosurgical OPD with complaints of auditory and olfactory hallucinations, déjà vu, memory impairment, and contralateral superior quadrantanopsia. What is the most likely part of brain involved by brain tumor in this patient?

- A. Frontal lobe
- B. Parietal lobe
- C. Temporal lobe
- D. Occipital lobe
- E. Posterior fossa

▸▸ Question 17

Tumor headache is classically described as headache which is worse in morning, often exacerbated by coughing, straining, bending forward, and associated with nausea and vomiting with temporarily relieved by vomiting. Following are etiologies of tumor headache except?

- A. Increased ICP which may be due to tumor mass effect, hydrocephalus, mass effect from associated edema, or mass effect from associated hemorrhage
- B. Invasion or compression of brain sensitive structures like dura, vessels, periosteum, and cranial nerves with sensory functions
- C. Difficulty vision which may be because of diplopia due to direct compression of third, fourth, or fifth cranial nerves, abducens palsy from increased ICP
- D. Extreme hypotension resulting from increased ICP
- E. Psychogenic due to stress from loss of functional capacity

▸▸ Question 18

A pediatric patient presents in OPD with complaints of headache, nausea, vomiting, papilledema, vertigo, diplopia, ataxia of extremities, dysmetria, and intention tremors. What is the most likely location of this tumor within brain of this patient?

- A. Lesion of cerebellar vermis
- B. Lesion of cerebellar hemisphere
- C. Brain stem lesion
- D. Supratentorial lesion
- E. Lesion in cerebellopontine angle

▸▸ Question 19

A patient presents with posterior fossa tumor and the surgeon decides to place a VP shunt in this patient and operate after 2 weeks. Which of the following is a theoretical risk of using this approach?

- A. Placing shunt is a lifelong commitment whereas not all patients with hydrocephalus from posterior fossa tumor requires shunting
- B. Seeding of peritoneum with malignant tumor cells is possible, for example, with medulloblastoma
- C. Shunt infection can occur prior to surgery

- D. Definitive treatment is delayed and there are chances of upward transtentorial herniation
- E. All of the above

▸▸ **Question 20**

An adult patient presents to you with MRI of brain showing multiple brain lesions, and round ring enhancing between gray and white matter with history of weight loss. Steroids are started in this patient with a dosage of 10 mg IV loading dose and 6 mg every 6 hours postoperatively or IV (pediatric loading dose is 0.5 to 1 mg/kg IV then 0.25 to 0.5 mg/kg/d divided every 6 hours). What is the most likely diagnosis in this patient?

- A. Cerebral abscesses
- B. Cerebral metastasis
- C. Multiple gliomas
- D. Neurofibromatosis type 1
- E. None of the above

▸▸ **Question 21**

A patient with brain tumor with no previous history of seizure has to undergo craniotomy for excision of tumor. Prophylactic antiseizure medication (ASM) was started in this patient before surgery. Post surgery, the patient is stable with no distressing event. How long should ASM be continued in this patient?

- A. For 2 years
- B. Taper off ASM starting 2 weeks postoperatively
- C. Taper off ASM starting 1 week postoperatively
- D. Continue for 2 months
- E. There is no need to give postoperative ASM in this patient

▸▸ **Question 22**

Procarbazine, CCNU (lomustine), and vincristine combination therapy is used as either an adjunct (following radiotherapy) or concomitant (simultaneously with radiotherapy) therapy in a number of tumors. What factors make these chemotherapeutic agents efficient instead of presence of blood–brain barrier?

- A. Some CNS tumors may partially disrupt BBB
- B. Lipophilic agents, for example, nitrosoureas, may cross BBB more easily
- C. Selective intraarterial, for example, intracarotid or intervertebral, injection produces higher local concentration which increases penetration
- D. The BBB may be iatrogenically disrupted, for example, by giving mannitol or may be bypassed by intrathecal administration
- E. All of the above

▸▸ **Question 23**

A patient underwent craniotomy for brain tumor. CT of brain without contrast was done after 6 to 12 hours of surgery to assess for acute complications like intraparenchymal hematoma, subdural or epidural hematoma, or for hydrocephalus or pneumocephalus. When should MRI with and without contrast be done in this patient?

- A. It should be delayed at least up to 30 days
- B. It should be done within 2 to 3 days
- C. It should be done after 6 months
- D. It should be done only if symptoms appear
- E. Both A and B

▸▸ **Question 24**

Stains for organisms include tissue gram stains for bacteria, periodic acid-Schiff stain for fungi, Ziehl-Neelsen stain for acid fast bacilli like tuberculosis, and special stains like Luxol fast blue stains for demyelinating lesions which stain myelin sheath. Which statement is incorrect regarding immunohistochemical stain response of different tumors?

- A. Oligodendroglioma stains positive for glial fibrillary acidic protein (GFAP)
- B. Ependymoma, choroid plexus, chordoma, and oligodendroglioma stains positive for S-100
- C. Chordoma, craniopharyngioma, carcinoma, and PitNET stain positive for both CAM 5.2 (cytokeratins) and EMA epithelial membrane protein
- D. Meningioma stains positive for EMA
- E. All of the above statements are correct

Answers

▸▸ **Answer 1**

Correct answer is D. Molecular testing not done or uncertain[1]

▸▸ **Answer 2**

Correct answer is B. Astrocytoma IDH wildtype, grade 2[1]

▸▸ **Answer 3**

Correct answer is A. Mammosomatotroph pitNET[2]

▸▸ **Answer 4**

Correct answer is B. 27%[3]

▸▸ **Answer 5**

Correct answer is A. Left frontal[4]

▸▸ **Answer 6**

Correct answer is B. Left temporal[4]

▸▸ **Answer 7**

Correct answer is A. Astrocytoma[3]

▸▸ **Answer 8**

Correct answer is D. Teratoma[3]

►► Answer 9

Correct answer is B. 6 mg postoperatively 6 hourly[5]

►► Answer 10

Correct answer is C. Temozolamine[6]

►► Answer 11

Correct answer is D. Luxol fast blue[7]

►► Answer 12

Correct answer is B. Epithelial membrane antigen[8]

►► Answer 13

Correct answer is A. G0[9]

►► Answer 14

Correct answer is D. Lungs[9]

►► Answer 15

Correct answer is A. Astrocytomas[10]

►► Answer 16

Correct answer is C. Temporal lobe[4]

►► Answer 17

Correct answer is D. Extreme hypotension resulting from increased ICP[4]

►► Answer 18

Correct answer is B. Lesion of cerebellar hemisphere[11]

►► Answer 19

Correct answer is E. All of the above[11]

►► Answer 20

Correct answer is B. Cerebral metastasis[11]

►► Answer 21

Correct answer is C. Taper off ASM starting 1 week postoperatively[6]

►► Answer 22

Correct answer is E. All of the above[12]

►► Answer 23

Correct answer is E. Both A and B[12]

►► Answer 24

Correct answer is E. All of the above statements are correct[7]

References

[1] Greenberg M, ed. Greenberg's Handbook of Neurosurgery. 10th ed. New York: Thieme; 2023:616
[2] Greenberg M, ed. Greenberg's Handbook of Neurosurgery. 10th ed. New York: Thieme; 2023:620
[3] Greenberg M, ed. Greenberg's Handbook of Neurosurgery. 10th ed. New York: Thieme; 2023:622
[4] Greenberg M, ed. Greenberg's Handbook of Neurosurgery. 10th ed. New York: Thieme; 2023:623
[5] Greenberg M, ed. Greenberg's Handbook of Neurosurgery. 10th ed. New York: Thieme; 2023:626
[6] Greenberg M, ed. Greenberg's Handbook of Neurosurgery. 10th ed. New York: Thieme; 2023:627
[7] Greenberg M, ed. Greenberg's Handbook of Neurosurgery. 10th ed. New York: Thieme; 2023:631
[8] Greenberg M, ed. Greenberg's Handbook of Neurosurgery. 10th ed. New York: Thieme; 2023:635
[9] Greenberg M, ed. Greenberg's Handbook of Neurosurgery. 10th ed. New York: Thieme; 2023:632
[10] Greenberg M, ed. Greenberg's Handbook of Neurosurgery. 10th ed. New York: Thieme; 2023:621
[11] Greenberg M, ed. Greenberg's Handbook of Neurosurgery. 10th ed. New York: Thieme; 2023:625
[12] Greenberg M, ed. Greenberg's Handbook of Neurosurgery. 10th ed. New York: Thieme; 2023:628

36 Genetic Tumor Syndromes Involving CNS

Questions

▸▸ Question 1

The gene locus for von Recklinhausen's disease is on which chromosome?
- A. 17
- B. 22
- C. 25
- D. 19
- E. Chromosome X

▸▸ Question 2

A patient presented with six café au lait spots, each ≥ 15 mm in greatest diameter along with two painful neurofibromas. Lisch nodules in NF1 are present in which of the following?
- A. Nail bed
- B. Scalp hair
- C. Iris
- D. Proximal convoluted renal tubules
- E. Lips

▸▸ Question 3

A patient presented with bilateral hearing loss and seizures. Bilateral vestibular schwannomas and multiple meningiomas are hallmark of which of the following?
- A. NF1
- B. NF2
- C. Tuberous sclerosis
- D. Sturge Weber syndrome
- E. Neurocutaneous melanosis

▸▸ Question 4

Which of the following is a diagnostic criterion of schwannomatosis?
- A. Germline pathogenic NF2 mutation
- B. First-degree relative with NF2 mutation
- C. Pathologically proven meningioma and germline SMARCB1 pathogenic mutation
- D. Schwannomas in previous field of radiation therapy
- E. > 1 pathologically proven schwannoma/meningioma and LOH chromosome 22

▸▸ Question 5

Which of the following is true regarding schwannomatosis versus NF2?
- A. Most NF2 patients have chronic pain
- B. Life expectancy of schwannomatosis is worse than NF2
- C. Surgery may occasionally be associated with worsening of global pain
- D. Pain is localized and associated with the mass

▸▸ Question 6

Subependymal giant cell astrocytoma (SEGA) is associated with tuberous sclerosis (TSC). What is the most common location of SEGA in TSC?
- A. Posterior fossa
- B. Frontal lobe
- C. Sphenoid wing
- D. Foramen of Monro
- E. Torcular Herophili

▸▸ Question 7

Which of the following is not a major diagnostic criterion for tuberous sclerosis (TSC)?
- A. > 3 hypomelanocytic macules > 5 mm diameter
- B. > 3 angiofibromas
- C. > 2 ungual fibroma
- D. > 4 pits in dental enamel
- E. > 2 angiomyolipomas

▸▸ Question 8

Intracerebral calcifications are most frequently associated with which of the following?
- A. NF1
- B. NF2
- C. Tuberous sclerosis
- D. Neurocutaneous melanosis
- E. Von Ricklinghausen's disease

▸▸ Question 9

Infantile myoclonus in tuberous sclerosis respond well to which of the following?
- A. Chemotherapy
- B. Radiotherapy
- C. Mannitol
- D. Steroids
- E. Hormone replacement therapy

▸▸ Question 10

According to diagnostic criteria, von **Hippel-Lindau** (VHL) should be suspected in an individual who has all of the following, except?
- A. Retinal angioma at a young age
- B. Spinal or cerebellar hemangioblastoma

- C. Adrenal or extra-adrenal pheochromocytoma
- D. RCC if the individual is > 47 years old
- E. Endolymphatic sac tumors

▸▸ Question 11

For a patient with or at risk of von Hippel-Lindau (VHL) what is the recommended guideline for retinal examination at 16 + years?

- A. Every 3 months
- B. Every 6 months
- C. Annually
- D. Every 5 years
- E. Every 10 years

▸▸ Question 12

A patient presented with right hemiparesis, hemiatrophy, and homonymous hemianopia along with left port-wine facial nevus. What is the most probable diagnosis?

- A. NF1
- B. NF2
- C. Tuberous sclerosis
- D. Sturge Weber syndrome
- E. Neurocutaneous melanosis

▸▸ Question 13

Neuroectodermal defect during morphogenesis involving melanoblasts of skin and pia mater originating from neural crest cells leads to which of the following?

- A. NF1
- B. NF2
- C. Tuberous sclerosis
- D. Sturge Weber syndrome
- E. Neurocutaneous melanosis

▸▸ Question 14

Which of the following is an autosomal dominant syndrome with benign colonic polyposis, colorectal carcinomas, and tumors of brain with medulloblastoma being the mostly associated brain tumor?

- A. Neurocutaneous melanosis
- B. Brain tumor polyposis syndrome 1
- C. Brain tumor polyposis syndrome 2
- D. Turcot syndrome
- E. Li Fraumeni's syndrome

▸▸ Question 15

Li Fraumeni's syndrome is caused by germ line mutations in which of the following?

- A. TP 53
- B. 17q
- C. 19p
- D. Chromosome X
- E. 22

▸▸ Question 16

An 8-year-old patient presents in neurosurgical OPD with greater than or equal to six café au lait spots (hyperpigmented oval light brown skin macules which are present in greater than 99% cases of NF1), each greater than or equal to 5 mm in greatest dimension on his/her body, greater than or equal to two neurofibromas, and freckling (hyperpigmentation) in the axillary or intertriginous (inguinal) areas. You diagnosed this case as NF1 or Von Recklinghausen's disease. What other abnormalities can lead to diagnosis of this disease?

- A. Optic pathway glioma/pilocytic astrocytoma
- B. More than or equal to two Lisch nodules which are pigmented iris hamartomas that appear as translucent yellow/brown elevations that tend to become more numerous with age
- C. Distinctive osseous abnormalities like sphenoid dysplasia or thinning of long bone cortex with or without pseudarthrosis
- D. A first-degree relative (parent, sibling, or offspring) with NF1 by above criteria
- E. All of the above

▸▸ Question 17

A patient presents to your OPD as diagnosed case of NF1 with optic nerve gliomas. Focal, resectable, and symptomatic lesions should be surgically removed. MEK inhibitors are approved for use in 2 to 18 years of age for symptomatic, inoperable plexiform neurofibromas. How is the patient counselled regarding management of optic nerve gliomas?

- A. Unlike optic gliomas in the absence of NF1, these are rarely chiasmal, are often multiple, and hence have a better prognosis
- B. Most are nonprogressive and should be followed ophthalmologically and with serial imaging (MRI or CT)
- C. Surgical intervention probably does not alter visual impairment
- D. Surgery is reserved for special situations like large disfiguring tumor or pressure on adjacent structures
- E. All of the above

▸▸ Question 18

A patient presents with seizures, multiple intradural spinal tumors, retinal hamartomas, and increased antigenic nerve growth factor. He/she is diagnosed as neurofibromatosis type 2 (NF2) which is also called as MISME syndrome (multiple inherited schwannomas, meningiomas, and ependymomas). All of the following are essential diagnostic criteria of NF2 except?

- A. Unilateral vestibular schwannoma and more than two plexiform neurofibromas
- B. Bilateral vestibular schwannomas on MRI or CT of brain

- C. A first-degree relative (sibling, parent, or offspring) with NF2 and unilateral vestibular schwannomas or any two of meningioma, schwannoma, glioma, or posterior subcapsular opacity
- D. Unilateral vestibular schwannoma and any two of meningioma, schwannoma, glioma, or posterior subcapsular opacity
- E. Multiple meningiomas and unilateral vestibular schwannoma or any two of ependymoma, schwannoma, or posterior subcapsular opacities

▸▸ Question 19

A patient presents with bilateral vestibular schwannomas with intact hearing in both ears. Surgery is planned and MRI of cervical spine is done prior to surgery to rule out any intraspinal tumor. Which statement regarding surgical treatment of this patient is not true?

- A. Smaller tumor is removed first and if hearing is serviceable in the operated side, then the other tumor should be operated
- B. If hearing is not preserved in the operated side, then the other tumor is followed with serial imaging as long as possible
- C. If there is need to operate on the second VS after failure to preserve hearing in the first VS surgery, then subtotal resection is done
- D. If bilateral VS are present and both are asymptomatic then there is no need to operate
- E. Stereotactic radiosurgery is an alternative treatment option

▸▸ Question 20

Schwannomatosis typically presents with multiple schwannomas (spinal, cutaneous or cranial) and less frequently with meningiomas (cranial and spinal) with a propensity for spinal and paraspinal nerves and less frequently for meninges. What is the essential criterion for schwannomatosis?

- A. More than or equal to two schwannomas (nonintradermal and pathologically confirmed) and no bilateral VS on high-quality MRI
- B. One schwannoma or meningioma and one affected first-degree relative
- C. Germline SMAECB1 and LZTR1 mutations
- D. Loss of heterozygosity/deletion of chromosome 22 and two different NF2 mutations
- E. Both A and B

▸▸ Question 21

Schwannomatosis (SWN) presents with chronic pain and pain associated with mass. MRI of entire neuraxis and molecular genetic testing of the biopsied mass should be done. Which statement regarding treatment of SWN is correct?

- A. Surgery should be done for asymptomatic lesions as these can progress to malignant tumor
- B. Surgery for symptomatic schwannomas may relieve local pain
- C. Medical therapy with methotrexate is recommended
- D. There is no chance of worsening of global pain after surgery
- E. Life expectancy is reduced in these patients

▸▸ Question 22

A patient presents with history of myoclonus which converted to generalized tonic clonic seizure. This patient also has facial adenomas which are present since childhood. CT of brain shows intracerebral calcifications primarily located in subependymal region in the walls of lateral ventricles, and these protrude into ventricles causing candle guttering. Treatment of this disease is observation, with surgery (transcallosal or ventriculoscopic approach) reserved for symptomatic lesions like subependymal giant cell astrocytoma (SEGA). What is a major criterion for diagnosis of this condition (tuberous sclerosis complex)?

- A. More than or equal to three hypomelanotic macules more than or equal to 5 mm diameter
- B. More than or equal to three angiofibromas or fibrous cephalic plaque
- C. More than or equal to two ungual fibroma
- D. Shagreen patch
- E. All of the above

▸▸ Question 23

A 60-year-old patient presents to your OPD as diagnosed case of hemangioblastoma of cerebellum, renal cell carcinoma, and pheochromocytoma. Other tumors that are associated with this condition are endolymphatic sac tumors, pancreatic neuroendocrine tumors and cysts, broad ligament cystadenomas, and epididymal cystadenomas. Treatment options for this condition include belzutifan, surgical resection of symptomatic lesion, or stereotactic radiosurgery. What subtype von Hippel-Lindau (VHL) disease is this?

- A. Type 1
- B. Type 2A
- C. Type 2B
- D. Type C
- E. Type D

▸▸ Question 24

Li Fraumeni's syndrome is associated with CNS tumors like primarily SHH activated medulloblastomas, IDH wild-type high-grade gliomas, and choroid plexus carcinomas. Essential criterion for this condition is pathogenic germline alteration in the TP 53 gene. What is the classic criterion for diagnosis of this disease?

- A. Sarcoma before the age of 45 years
- B. A first-degree relative with any cancer before the age of 45 years
- C. A first- or second-degree relative with any cancer before the age of 45 years, sarcoma at any age

- D. All of the above
- E. A first-degree relative with cancer after the age of 55 years with sarcoma as well

▸▸ Question 25

A patient presents with history of seizures, left-sided body weakness, right-sided facial port-wine nevus in the distribution of 1st division of trigeminal nerve, and growth hormone deficiency. On investigations, this patient shows curvilinear double parallel lines or tram tracking on plain skull X-rays, increased intraocular pressure, and leptomeningeal angiomatosis. What is the most probable diagnosis in this case?

- A. Sturge-Weber syndrome
- B. Tuberous sclerosis
- C. Turcot syndrome
- D. Cowden syndrome
- E. Carney syndrome

Answers

▸▸ Answer 1

Correct answer is A. 17[1]

▸▸ Answer 2

Correct answer is C. Iris[2]

▸▸ Answer 3

Correct answer is B. NF2[3]

▸▸ Answer 4

Correct answer is C. Pathologically proven meningioma and germline SMARCB1 pathogenic mutation[4]

▸▸ Answer 5

Correct answer is C. Surgery may occasionally be associated with worsening of global pain[4]

▸▸ Answer 6

Correct answer is D. Foramen of Monro[5]

▸▸ Answer 7

Correct answer is D. > 4 pits in dental enamel[6]

▸▸ Answer 8

Correct answer is C. Tuberous sclerosis[6]

▸▸ Answer 9

Correct answer is D. Steroids[7]

▸▸ Answer 10

Correct answer is D. RCC if the individual is > 47 years old[8]

▸▸ Answer 11

Correct answer is B. Every 6 months[9]

▸▸ Answer 12

Correct answer is D. Sturge Weber syndrome[10]

▸▸ Answer 13

Correct answer is E. Neurocutaneous melanosis[11]

▸▸ Answer 14

Correct answer is C. Brain tumor polyposis syndrome 2[12]

▸▸ Answer 15

Correct answer is A. TP 53[9]

▸▸ Answer 16

Correct answer is E. All of the above[2]

▸▸ Answer 17

Correct answer is E. All of the above[2]

▸▸ Answer 18

Correct answer is A. Unilateral vestibular schwannoma and more than two plexiform neurofibromas[3]

▸▸ Answer 19

Correct answer is D. If bilateral VS are present and both are asymptomatic then there is no need to operate[4]

▸▸ Answer 20

Correct answer is E. Both A and B[13]

▸▸ Answer 21

Correct answer is B. Surgery for symptomatic schwannomas may relieve local pain[6]

▸▸ Answer 22

Correct answer is E. All of the above[6]

▸▸ Answer 23

Correct answer is C. Type 2B[8]

▸▸ Answer 24

Correct answer is D. All of the above[9]

▸▸ **Answer 25**

Correct answer is A. Sturge-Weber syndrome[10]

References

[1] Greenberg M, ed. Greenberg's Handbook of Neurosurgery. 10th ed. New York: Thieme; 2023:638
[2] Greenberg M, ed. Greenberg's Handbook of Neurosurgery. 10th ed. New York: Thieme; 2023:639
[3] Greenberg M, ed. Greenberg's Handbook of Neurosurgery. 10th ed. New York: Thieme; 2023:641
[4] Greenberg M, ed. Greenberg's Handbook of Neurosurgery. 10th ed. New York: Thieme; 2023:642
[5] Greenberg M, ed. Greenberg's Handbook of Neurosurgery. 10th ed. New York: Thieme; 2023:645
[6] Greenberg M, ed. Greenberg's Handbook of Neurosurgery. 10th ed. New York: Thieme; 2023:644
[7] Greenberg M, ed. Greenberg's Handbook of Neurosurgery. 10th ed. New York: Thieme; 2023:646
[8] Greenberg M, ed. Greenberg's Handbook of Neurosurgery. 10th ed. New York: Thieme; 2023:647
[9] Greenberg M, ed. Greenberg's Handbook of Neurosurgery. 10th ed. New York: Thieme; 2023:650
[10] Greenberg M, ed. Greenberg's Handbook of Neurosurgery. 10th ed. New York: Thieme; 2023:652
[11] Greenberg M, ed. Greenberg's Handbook of Neurosurgery. 10th ed. New York: Thieme; 2023:653
[12] Greenberg M, ed. Greenberg's Handbook of Neurosurgery. 10th ed. New York: Thieme; 2023:651
[13] Greenberg M, ed. Greenberg's Handbook of Neurosurgery. 10th ed. New York: Thieme; 2023:643

37 Adult Diffuse Glioma

Questions

▸▸ **Question 1**

Diffuse gliomas are most common primary intra-axial brain tumors. Astrocytes typically appear in the white matter (e.g., centrum semiovale) and traverses through white matter tract. A patient presenting in OPD with history of seizure, his/her CT of brain showing low density lesion, MRI showing abnormal signal on T2WI with no enhancement, and no or very little mass effect is diagnosed as astrocytoma, IDH mutant, grade 2 tumor. Following are the most common locations for this tumor except?

- A. Temporal lobe
- B. Occipital lobe
- C. Posterior frontal lobe
- D. Right anterior parietal lobe
- E. Left anterior parietal lobe

▸▸ **Question 2**

Gliomas can spread through CSF pathways (subarachnoid seeding) in 10 to 25% of high-grade gliomas and rarely may spread systemically. Gliomas can also spread from one part of brain to other part through white matter track. Which of the following statements is incorrect?

- A. Bilateral frontal lobe involvement occurs through genu or body of corpus callosum
- B. Bilateral occipital or parietal lobes involvement occurs through splenium of corpus callosum
- C. Midbrain involvement of tumor occurs through internal capsule
- D. Simultaneous frontal and temporal occurrence of tumor occurs through uncinate fasciculus
- E. Interthalamic adhesions cause bilateral thalamic gliomas

▸▸ **Question 3**

A patient presents in neurosurgical OPD with signs and symptoms of raised ICP. CT of brain was done which showed brain tumor in frontal lobe and solid enhancement on contrast. Microvascular proliferation was seen, and Ki-67 and MIB-1 index was found to be more than 7 to 9% in this tumor on biopsy, which showed it was astrocytoma, IDH mutant, grade 4 tumor. What is the essential diagnostic criterion for IDH mutant tumors?

- A. A diffusely infiltrating tumor *with* IDH1 codon 132 or IDH2 codon 172 missense mutation *with* loss of nuclear ATRX expression or ATRX mutation
- B. A diffusely infiltrating tumor *with* IDH1 codon 132 or IDH2 codon 172 missense mutation *with* exclusion of combined whole arm deletions of 1p and 19q
- C. Astrocytic differentiation by morphology with TP 53 mutation
- D. IDH mutation with Aa and B
- E. A and B

▸▸ **Question 4**

Significant prognosticators for gliomas are postoperative residual tumor volume and preoperative tumor size. Following factors show worse prognosis of glioma except?

- A. Age more than 40 years
- B. No neurologic deficit prior to surgery
- C. Largest tumor diameter of more than or equal to 6 cm
- D. Tumor crossing midline
- E. Subtotal resection

▸▸ **Question 5**

A patient presents with seizure in your clinic for the first time. You advised plain CT of brain which showed hypodense to isodense lesion with calcifications. MRI of brain showed poor demarcation with T1 hypointense lesion and hyperintense on T2 with no enhancement on contrast. The essential diagnostic criteria for diagnosis of oligodendroglioma is a diffusely infiltrating tumor WITH IDH1 codon 132 or IDH2 codon 172 missense mutation WITH combined whole arm deletions of 1p and 19 q. Following features in this patient will characterize this lesion as grade 3 tumor except?

- A. Low mitotic activity
- B. High cellularity
- C. Marked cytological atypia
- D. Pathologically microvascular proliferation
- E. Necrosis with and without palisading

▸▸ **Question 6**

A patient presents with signs of raised ICP in your clinic. You advised urgent MRI which showed lesion with large area of central necrosis and ring enhancement pattern on contrast. Most common locations of these lesions are temporal lobe, parietal lobe, frontal lobe, and occipital lobe in descending order. All of the following are included in essential diagnostic criteria for glioblastoma IDH wildtype except?

- A. DNA methylation of glioblastoma
- B. A diffusely infiltrating astrocytic glioma
- C. IDH wildtype and H3 wildtype
- D. Microvascular proliferation or necrosis
- E. TERT promoter mutation or EGFR gene amplification or +7/−10 chromosome copy number alteration

▸▸ **Question 7**

High grade diffuse gliomas (WHO grades 3 and 4) show improved prognosis with which of the following?

- A. Preoperative performance status, for example, Karnofsky score (KPS) more than 60
- B. Old-aged patients
- C. Nonmethylation of MGMT promotor gene
- D. IDH1 mutation
- E. All of the above

►► Question 8

Gross total resection (GTR) is complete removal of enhancing portions of the tumor and any nonenhancing portion contained within, as verified by postoperative contrast imaging within 48 hours of surgery, or removal of high intensity lesion or very low intensity on T1 MRI in case of nonenhancing lesion. Surgical goals in case of diffuse glioma surgery are to obtain adequate tissue for histological and molecular study and cytoreduction or maximal safe resection with the goal of GTR when feasible. What are relative contraindications of surgery?

- A. Extensive dominant lobe high grade glioma
- B. Lesion with significant bilateral involvement
- C. Karnofsky score less than 70
- D. Multicentric glioma
- E. All of the above

►► Question 9

A patient presents with diffuse astrocytoma grade 2 near eloquent area of brain. The extent of resection of this tumor can be increased or complication can be decreased by using which method?

- A. Image guidance or stereotactic radiosurgery
- B. Preoperative mapping like functional MRI or diffusion tensor imaging
- C. Intraoperative mapping with awake craniotomy
- D. Intraoperative dyes like indocyanine green and 5 amino levulinic acid
- E. All of the above

►► Question 10

Adjuvant radiotherapy or chemotherapy in patients with grade 2 glioma is recommended only if there is subtotal resection or early progression. Which of the following is true regarding Stupp regimen for diffuse glioma patients?

- A. It consists of radiotherapy (fractionated focal radiation) at a dose of 2 Gy per fraction once daily 5 days per week over a period of 6 weeks, for a total dose of 60 Gy
- B. A + Chemotherapy is given such as temozolomide at a dose of 75 g/m^2/d, 7 days per week till end of radiotherapy
- C. B + After first 6 weeks of chemotherapy and radiotherapy 4 weeks gap is given and then chemotherapy is given in 6 cycles each consisting of 5 days of TMZ repeated every 28 days at a dose of 150 mg/m^2/d for first cycle then 200 mg/m^2/d for rest of cycles
- D. C + Cytoreductive surgery
- E. All of the above

►► Question 11

Hypermethylation of the MGMT promoter gene (consists of > 30% methylation) causes reduced levels of MGMT activity. Tumors with reduced levels of MGMT activity are more susceptible to cytotoxic effects of temozolomide. This leads to longer overall survival of these patients from 15.2 months in those without hypermethylation of MGMT to how long?

- A. 20.2 months
- B. 22.2 months
- C. 25.2 months
- D. 28.2 months
- E. 30.2 months

►► Question 12

Pseudoprogression is an increase in contrast enhancing areas on postoperative MRI after giving Stupp regimen due to radiation necrosis or tumor cells killed by chemotherapy. Hence, such enhancing areas within first 6 months of Stupp regimen are considered pseudoprogression. Which of the following studies is helpful with very low specificity and sensitivity to differentiate pseudoprogression from tumor recurrence?

- A. MR perfusion
- B. DWI with higher ADC
- C. MR spectroscopy
- D. PET
- E. All of the above

Answers

►► Answer 1

Correct answer is B. Occipital lobe[1]

►► Answer 2

Correct answer is C. Midbrain involvement of tumor occurs through internal capsule[1]

►► Answer 3

Correct answer is E. A and B[2]

►► Answer 4

Correct answer is B. No neurologic deficit prior to surgery[3]

►► Answer 5

Correct answer is A. Low mitotic activity[3]

►► Answer 6

Correct answer is A. DNA methylation of glioblastoma[4]

▸▸ Answer 7

Correct answer is D. IDH1 mutation[5]

▸▸ Answer 8

Correct answer is E. All of the above[6]

▸▸ Answer 9

Correct answer is E. All of the above[7]

▸▸ Answer 10

Correct answer is C. B + After first 6 weeks of chemotherapy and radiotherapy 4 weeks gap is given and then chemotherapy is given in 6 cycles each consisting of 5 days of TMZ repeated every 28 days at a dose of 150 mg/m²/d for first cycle then 200 mg/m²/d for rest of cycles[8]

▸▸ Answer 11

Correct answer is C. 25.2 months[9]

▸▸ Answer 12

Correct answer is E. All of the above[10]

References

[1] Greenberg M, ed. Greenberg's Handbook of Neurosurgery. 10th ed. New York: Thieme; 2023:658
[2] Greenberg M, ed. Greenberg's Handbook of Neurosurgery. 10th ed. New York: Thieme; 2023:660
[3] Greenberg M, ed. Greenberg's Handbook of Neurosurgery. 10th ed. New York: Thieme; 2023:662
[4] Greenberg M, ed. Greenberg's Handbook of Neurosurgery. 10th ed. New York: Thieme; 2023:665
[5] Greenberg M, ed. Greenberg's Handbook of Neurosurgery. 10th ed. New York: Thieme; 2023:666
[6] Greenberg M, ed. Greenberg's Handbook of Neurosurgery. 10th ed. New York: Thieme; 2023:668
[7] Greenberg M, ed. Greenberg's Handbook of Neurosurgery. 10th ed. New York: Thieme; 2023:670
[8] Greenberg M, ed. Greenberg's Handbook of Neurosurgery. 10th ed. New York: Thieme; 2023:672
[9] Greenberg M, ed. Greenberg's Handbook of Neurosurgery. 10th ed. New York: Thieme; 2023:673
[10] Greenberg M, ed. Greenberg's Handbook of Neurosurgery. 10th ed. New York: Thieme; 2023:674

38 Pediatric Type Diffuse Tumors

Questions

▸▸ Question 1

A young child presents with seizure that is refractory to medication. Histopathology showed monomorphic cells with bland round, ovoid, or spindle nuclei. Which of the following is an essential diagnostic criterion for diffuse astrocytoma, MYB or MYBL1-altered tumors?

- A. Diffuse astrocytoma without histological features of anaplasia *and* no mutation in IDH or H3 genes *and* structural variant of MYB or MYBL1
- B. A or diffuse astrocytoma without anaplasia *and* no mutations in IDH or H3 genes *and* DNA methylation profile aligned with diffuse astrocytoma, MYB or MYBL1 altered
- C. B + absence of LIG2
- D. B + absence of MAP2 expression
- E. All of the above

▸▸ Question 2

A young patient presents with intractable partial epilepsy. On imaging there is nonenhancing cortical based lesion in temporal lobe with total cure with gross total excision. On histopathology, it shows glioma with diffuse growth architecture and a focal angiocentric pattern *and* monomorphic spindled cells with immunophenotypic and/or ultrastructural evidence of astrocytic and ependymal differentiation. What is the most likely diagnosis in this scenario?

- A. Polymorphous low-grade neuroepithelial tumor of the young
- B. Angiocentric glioma
- C. Diffuse glioma MYB- or MYBL1-altered
- D. Diffuse low grade glioma MAPK-pathway altered
- E. None of the above

▸▸ Question 3

A young patient presents with seizure with tumor present in right-sided temporal lobe on imaging. He is diagnosed with polymorphous low-grade neuroepithelial tumor of the young. Following are included in essential diagnostic criteria of this patient except?

- A. Diffuse growth pattern (at least regionally) *and* oligodendroglioma-like components (although these may be minor)
- B. A *and* few (if any) mitotic figure *and* regional CD34 expression by tumor cells and by ramified neural cells in associated cerebral cortex *and* IDH wildtype
- C. B *and* unequivocal expression of BRAF p.V600E on immunohistochemical assessment
- D. C *and* conspicuous calcifications with absence of 1p/19q codeletion
- E. B *and* molecular diagnostic evidence of BRAF p.V600E mutations, FGFR2 or FGFR3 fusions, or potentially other MAPK pathway–driving genetic abnormalities

▸▸ Question 4

Appearance of diffuse low-grade glioma, MAPK pathway altered, may resemble pilocytic astrocytoma complete with cystic elements but these tumors tend to be more extensive on T2 flair images. Which of the following is an essential diagnostic criterion for these tumors?

- A. Diffuse glioma with absence or minimal mitotic activity and neither microvascular proliferation nor necrosis
- B. Genetic alteration in the MAPK pathway
- C. IDH wildtype and H3 wildtype
- D. Absence of homozygous deletion of CDKN2A
- E. All of the above

▸▸ Question 5

Following are correct regarding diffuse midline glioma H3 K27 M altered in children except?

- A. Involvement tends to be in brainstem, pons, or bithalamic
- B. The patient presents with the triad of multiple cranial nerve palsies, long tract signs, and ataxia or obstructive hydrocephalus
- C. Biopsy lacks clinical utility in these patients
- D. Given the high rate of leptomeningeal spread, imaging of the entire neuraxis is recommended
- E. Pontine lesions enlarge pons which is low intensity on T1 and high intensity on T2

▸▸ Question 6

Which of the following is not included in essential diagnostic criteria of diffuse midline glioma, H3 K27M-altered?

- A. A diffuse glioma
- B. Results from molecular analysis enable differentiation of the H3.1 or H3.2 p.K28 (K27)-mutant subtype from the H3.3 p.K28 (K27) mutant type
- C. Loss of H3 p.K28me3 (K27me3) (immunohistochemistry)
- D. Midline location
- E. Presence of a pathogenic mutation or amplification of EGFR (for the EGFR mutant type)

▸▸ Question 7

A young patient presents with seizures and focal neurologic deficit. Imaging shows hemispheric lesion that is typically contrast enhancing and multifocal. The tumor shows to be a cellular infiltrative tumor with mitotic activity AND H3.3 p.G35 R or p.G35 mutation AND hemispheric location AND methylation profile of diffuse hemispheric glioma, H3 G34-mutant. What is most likely diagnosis?

- A. Diffuse pediatric type high-grade glioma, H3 wildtype and IDH wildtype
- B. Infant type hemispheric glioma
- C. Diffuse hemispheric glioma, H3 G34-mutant
- D. Diffuse midline glioma
- E. None of the above

►► Question 8

What is an essential diagnostic criterion for diffuse pediatric type high-grade glioma, H3 wildtype and IDH wildtype?

- A. A diffuse glioma with mitotic activity occurring in a child or a young adult
- B. Absence of mutation in IDH1 or IDH2
- C. Few (if any) mitotic figures
- D. Absence of mutation in H3 genes
- E. Methylation profile aligned with pHGG RTK1, pHGG RTK2, or pHGG MYCN
- F. All of the above

►► Question 9

Following are features of infant type hemispheric glioma except?

- A. Presentation is usually in the first year of life
- B. It presents with agitation, lethargy, and enlarged head circumference
- C. Spine images are not recommended in addition to brain images
- D. Infants with high-grade glioma fare better than older children
- E. Histology consists of well-demarcated cellular tumors involving brain parenchyma and leptomeninges

►► Question 10

What is an essential diagnostic criterion of infant type hemispheric glioma?

- A. Cellular astrocytoma
- B. Presentation in early childhood
- C. Cerebral hemispheric lesions
- D. Presence of typical tyrosine kinase abnormality
- E. All of the above

Answers

►► Answer 1

Correct answer is B. A or diffuse astrocytoma without anaplasia *and* no mutations in IDH or H3 genes *and* DNA methylation profile aligned with diffuse astrocytoma, MYB or MYBL1 altered[1]

►► Answer 2

Correct answer is B. Angiocentric glioma[2]

►► Answer 3

Correct answer is D. C *and* conspicuous calcifications with absence of 1p/19q codeletion[3]

►► Answer 4

Correct answer is E. All of the above[4]

►► Answer 5

Correct answer is C. Biopsy lacks clinical utility in these patients[5]

►► Answer 6

Correct answer is B. Results from molecular analysis enable differentiation of the H3.1 or H3.2 p.K28 (K27)-mutant subtype from the H3.3 p.K28 (K27) mutant type[5]

►► Answer 7

Correct answer is C. Diffuse hemispheric glioma, H3 G34-mutant[6]

►► Answer 8

Correct answer is F. All of the above[7]

►► Answer 9

Correct answer is C. Spine images are not recommended in addition to brain images[8]

►► Answer 10

Correct answer is E. All of the above[8]

References

[1] Greenberg M, ed. Greenberg's Handbook of Neurosurgery. 10th ed. New York: Thieme; 2023:679
[2] Greenberg M, ed. Greenberg's Handbook of Neurosurgery. 10th ed. New York: Thieme; 2023:680
[3] Greenberg M, ed. Greenberg's Handbook of Neurosurgery. 10th ed. New York: Thieme; 2023:681
[4] Greenberg M, ed. Greenberg's Handbook of Neurosurgery. 10th ed. New York: Thieme; 2023:682
[5] Greenberg M, ed. Greenberg's Handbook of Neurosurgery. 10th ed. New York: Thieme; 2023:683
[6] Greenberg M, ed. Greenberg's Handbook of Neurosurgery. 10th ed. New York: Thieme; 2023:685
[7] Greenberg M, ed. Greenberg's Handbook of Neurosurgery. 10th ed. New York: Thieme; 2023:686
[8] Greenberg M, ed. Greenberg's Handbook of Neurosurgery. 10th ed. New York: Thieme; 2023:687

39 Circumscribed Astrocytic Gliomas

Questions

▸▸ **Question 1**

Pilocytic astrocytomas are the most common astrocytic tumors in children which are WHO grade 1 tumor. The most common location for these tumors is cerebellar hemisphere. These are usually cured with complete surgical resection. What is the recommendation for postoperative radiotherapy in such tumors?

- A. It is never indicated
- B. Indicated for all postoperative cases
- C. Indicated for nonresectable recurrence
- D. C + used for malignant recurrence of tumor
- E. Depends on histopathological report

▸▸ **Question 2**

All of the following are differentiating points between pilocytic astrocytoma and pilomyxoid astrocytoma except?

- A. Pilocytic astrocytoma (PCA) shows biphasic compact and loose growth patterns while pilomyxoid astrocytoma (PMA) shows monomorphic pattern with loose cells
- B. PCA shows high proliferative index, while PMA shows low cellularity
- C. PCA may or may not have Rosenthal fibers and eosinophilic granular bodies while PMA often lack Rosenthal fibers and eosinophilic bodies
- D. PMA carries a higher rate of recurrence, worse outcome, and more tendency for CSF dissemination as compared to PCA
- E. PCA most commonly occurs in cerebellar hemisphere, while PMA occurs mostly in hypothalamic and chiasmatic regions

▸▸ **Question 3**

Which of the following statements regarding location of pilocytic astrocytoma (PCA) is incorrect?

- A. 42% of PCAs are found in cerebellum
- B. Percentage of PCAs in cerebral hemisphere is 35% and these most commonly occur in children
- C. Optic gliomas and hypothalamic gliomas constitute 9%
- D. PCAs arising in the optic nerves are called optic gliomas, and they are the most common site in neurofibromatosis type 1
- E. Percentage of brainstem PCAs is 9%

▸▸ **Question 4**

Feature of pilocytic astrocytoma (PCA) on CT or MRI is usually a contrast enhancing mural nodule (especially cerebellar PCAs) with cystic component with little or no surrounding edema. What is the recommended treatment option for PCA?

- A. Excision of nodule along with cyst wall in every case
- B. In tumors with false cyst where cyst wall also enhances, only cyst wall needs to be removed
- C. Both false cyst and mural nodule need to be removed
- D. Cyst wall does not need to be removed in any case
- E. Radiotherapy and chemotherapy are recommended in all postoperative cases

▸▸ **Question 5**

Pilocytic astrocytomas (PCAs) constitute 15% of primary brain tumors in patients aged less than 19 years and 27 to 40% of pediatric posterior fossa tumors. Optic pathway gliomas account for 2% of gliomas in adults and 7% in children. What is the most common location of optic pathway glioma in sporadic cases (other than in NF1)?

- A. Optic nerve
- B. Optic disc
- C. Optic chiasma
- D. Optic nerve with involvement of hypothalamus
- E. Both optic nerves simultaneously

▸▸ **Question 6**

A patient presents with nonspecific visual deficit without proptosis. This patient also has pituitary dysfunction and signs of hydrocephalus. MRI of brain shows mild to moderately enhancing chiasmal tumor. What is the recommended treatment for optic pathway glioma tumors?

- A. Chiasmal tumors are good for biopsy only with CSF shunting and removal of exophytic component
- B. Tumors involving optic nerve are removed using transcranial approach with excision of nerve from the globe all the way back to the chiasma
- C. Transorbital (Kronlein) approach is not appropriate for optic nerve tumors since the tumor may be left in the nerve stump
- D. Radiotherapy and chemotherapy are recommended for chiasmal tumors, multicentric tumors, postoperatively if tumor is found in chiasmal stump end of resected nerve, and malignant tumor
- E. All of the above

▸▸ **Question 7**

A young patient presents with macrocephaly, signs of hydrocephalus, cachexia, and diabetes insipidus. On imaging, a tumor involving the third ventricle and chiasmal region is found. What is the most probable diagnosis in this case?

- A. Chiasmal glioma
- B. Third ventricular tumor
- C. Hypothalamic glioma
- D. Brainstem glioma
- E. Optic nerve glioma

▸▸ **Question 8**

Upper brainstem tumors are usually lower grade tumors and present with cerebellar findings and hydrocephalus while lower brainstem tumors are usually higher grade with signs and symptoms of multiple lower cranial nerve deficits and long tract findings. Following are the patterns that can be identified on MRI in brainstem gliomas except?

- A. Diffuse gliomas, which are midline malignant, H3 k27 mutant, are seen mostly in pediatrics
- B. Cervicomedullary gliomas are mostly low-grade astrocytomas
- C. Ventrally exophytic brainstem gliomas are low-grade gliomas
- D. Focal gliomas are mostly limited to medulla and most are low-grade astrocytomas
- E. Dorsally exophytic gliomas may be low-grade gliomas

▸▸ **Question 9**

Following statements are most appropriate regarding management of brainstem gliomas except?

- A. There is no role of biopsy in nonexophytic infiltrating brainstem gliomas
- B. Exophytic brainstem gliomas with broad attachment to the floor of 4th ventricle precludes complete excision, and survival can be increased in such cases with excision
- C. Surgery in malignant astrocytomas is without benefit; however, biopsy and shunting for hydrocephalus are recommended
- D. Tumors that demonstrate recurrent growth after resection remain histologically benign and are amenable to resection
- E. Radiations are given in 45 to 55 Gy dosage over a 6-week period, 5 days per week, and steroids added to radiotherapy can cause symptomatic improvement in 80% patients

▸▸ **Question 10**

A patient presents with diplopia, visual field deficits, nystagmus, Parinaud's syndrome, ataxia, and seizures along with hydrocephalus. MRI of brain showed a mass projecting dorsally from the quadrigeminal plate. Diagnosis of tectal glioma is made, which is also referred to as the smallest tumor in the body that can lead to death of the patient. What is the management option for these tumors?

- A. VP shunting
- B. Endoscopic third ventriculostomy
- C. Endoscopic aqueductoplasty
- D. Stereotactic radiosurgery
- E. All of the above

▸▸ **Question 11**

A patient presents with history of seizures, and imaging showed a contrast enhancing lesion in temporal region with dural tail. On histopathology, astrocytes with pleomorphic tumor cells were found including large multinucleated cells, spindle cells, xanthomatous cells, and eosinophilic granular bodies. What is the most probable diagnosis in this patient?

- A. Meningioma
- B. Pleomorphic astrocytoma
- C. Pleomorphic xanthoastrocytoma
- D. Subependymal giant cell astrocytoma
- E. None of the above

▸▸ **Question 12**

A young patient presents with signs and symptoms of raised ICP. Imaging showed a tumor arising from the walls of lateral ventricles next to foramen of Monro. Gross total resection of the tumor was done with everolimus given to reduce the tumor size and progression. This tumor has strong association with tuberous sclerosis. What is the most likely diagnosis in this patient?

- A. Choroid plexus papilloma
- B. Intraventricular meningioma
- C. Subependymal giant cell astrocytoma
- D. Chordoid glioma
- E. Astroblastoma

Answers

▸▸ **Answer 1**

Correct answer is D. C + used for malignant recurrence of tumor[1]

▸▸ **Answer 2**

Correct answer is B. PCA shows high proliferative index, while PMA shows low cellularity[2]

▸▸ **Answer 3**

Correct answer is B. Percentage of PCAs in cerebral hemisphere is 35% and these most commonly occur in children[3]

▸▸ **Answer 4**

Correct answer is C. Both false cyst and mural nodule need to be removed[4]

▸▸ **Answer 5**

Correct answer is C. Optic chiasma[5]

▸▸ **Answer 6**

Correct answer is E. All of the above[5]

▸▸ **Answer 7**

Correct answer is C. Hypothalamic glioma[6]

▸▸ Answer 8

Correct answer is C. Ventrally exophytic brainstem gliomas are low-grade gliomas[7]

▸▸ Answer 9

Correct answer is A. There is no role of biopsy in nonexophytic infiltrating brainstem gliomas[7]

▸▸ Answer 10

Correct answer is E. All of the above[8]

▸▸ Answer 11

Correct answer is C. Pleomorphic xanthoastrocytoma[9]

▸▸ Answer 12

Correct answer is C. Subependymal giant cell astrocytoma[10]

References

[1] Greenberg M, ed. Greenberg's Handbook of Neurosurgery. 10th ed. New York: Thieme; 2023:693
[2] Greenberg M, ed. Greenberg's Handbook of Neurosurgery. 10th ed. New York: Thieme; 2023:690
[3] Greenberg M, ed. Greenberg's Handbook of Neurosurgery. 10th ed. New York: Thieme; 2023:691
[4] Greenberg M, ed. Greenberg's Handbook of Neurosurgery. 10th ed. New York: Thieme; 2023:692
[5] Greenberg M, ed. Greenberg's Handbook of Neurosurgery. 10th ed. New York: Thieme; 2023:694
[6] Greenberg M, ed. Greenberg's Handbook of Neurosurgery. 10th ed. New York: Thieme; 2023:695
[7] Greenberg M, ed. Greenberg's Handbook of Neurosurgery. 10th ed. New York: Thieme; 2023:696
[8] Greenberg M, ed. Greenberg's Handbook of Neurosurgery. 10th ed. New York: Thieme; 2023:697
[9] Greenberg M, ed. Greenberg's Handbook of Neurosurgery. 10th ed. New York: Thieme; 2023:699
[10] Greenberg M, ed. Greenberg's Handbook of Neurosurgery. 10th ed. New York: Thieme; 2023:701

40 Glioneuronal and Neuronal Tumors

Questions

▸▸ Question 1

An 11-year-old boy presents with history of seizures. His CT scan shows calcified lesion in temporal lobe. MRI confirms space occupying lesion (SOL) in temporal lobe. The patient underwent surgery and histopathological diagnosis came out to be ganglioglioma. What is the preferred treatment in case of recurrence?

- A. Re-resection
- B. Radiotherapy
- C. Chemotherapy
- D. Observation

▸▸ Question 2

Desmoplastic infantile astrocytoma may recur with anaplastic transformation how long after initial resection?

- A. 3 to 5 years
- B. 8 to 10 years
- C. 12 to15 years
- D. 18 to 20 years

▸▸ Question 3

What is the most common location for dysembryoplastic neuroepithelial tumor (DNET)?

- A. Temporal lobe
- B. Parietal lobe
- C. Occipital lobe
- D. Basal ganglia
- E. Cerebellum

▸▸ Question 4

Which type of rosettes is demonstrated in rosette forming glioneural tumor?

- A. Homer Wright rosettes
- B. Flexner Wintersteiner rosettes
- C. Ependymal rosettes
- D. Neurocyte forming rosette

▸▸ Question 5

Which of the following is not an essential diagnostic criterion for central neurocytoma?

- A. Intraventricular localization
- B. ODG like monomorphic cells
- C. Synaptophysin expression
- D. No sign of malignancy
- E. Methylation profile

▸▸ Question 6

Dysplastic cerebellar gangliocytoma (Lhermitte-Duclos disease) is a cerebellar lesion with features of both a malformation and a low-grade neoplasm, and causes diffuse enlargement of cerebellar folia. It has the propensity to progress and recur after surgery and is strongly associated with which of the following?

- A. Down syndrome
- B. Klinefelter syndrome
- C. Neurofibromatosis I
- D. Li Fraumeni syndrome
- E. Cowden syndrome

▸▸ Question 7

A patient 16 years of age presents with seizure. CT imaging of brain shows hypodense area in temporal lobe with calcifications. T1WI MRI showed hypointense area while T2WI showed hyperintense area. Maximal safe resection of this tumor was done. On histopathology an intra-axial low-grade glioneuronal tumor was noted in combination with neoplastic ganglion and glial cells. Which of the following statements is incorrect regarding ganglioglioma?

- A. The most common location of this tumor is temporal lobe
- B. These are benign tumors with 97% recurrence-free survival of 7.5 years
- C. Radiotherapy is recommended in all postoperative cases
- D. These are slow-growing well-differentiated tumor that primarily affects children and young adults
- E. It is a WHO grade 1 tumor

▸▸ Question 8

On histopathology of a tumor, irregular groups of large, mature ganglion cells were noted WITH matrix resembling normal neuropil sometimes more coarsely fibrillar or vacuolated. Diagnosis of gangliocytoma was made. What is the most common location of this tumor?

- A. Frontal lobe
- B. Hypothalamus
- C. Third ventricle
- D. Temporal lobe
- E. Parietal lobe

▸▸ Question 9

Histopathology of a tumor showed biphasic morphology with dominant desmoplastic leptomeningeal component admixed with a neuroepithelial component containing astrocytic cells only or containing astrocytes or neuronal cells. This lesion is mostly found in cerebral hemisphere of infants often as large cystic lesions frequently attached to the dura. What is the mostly likely diagnosis in this patient?

- A. Gangliocytoma
- B. Desmoplastic infantile ganglioglioma
- C. Desmoplastic infantile astrocytoma
- D. Both A and C
- E. Dysembryoplastic neuroepithelial tumor

▸▸ **Question 10**

A patient 15 years old presents with seizures that are not controlled with medication. CT of brain shows hypodense lesion with distinct margins in the temporal lobe of brain. MRI shows hypointense lesion on T1WI and hyperintense lesion on T2WI with nodular enhancement. Histopathology shows cortical glioneuronal tumor with presence of specific glioneuronal elements. What is the WHO grade of dysembryoplastic neuroepithelial tumor (DNT)?

- A. Grade 1
- B. Grade 2
- C. Grade 3
- D. Grade 4
- E. Grade N/A

▸▸ **Question 11**

Following are essential criteria for diffuse glioneuronal tumor with oligodendroglioma-like features and nuclear clusters (DGONC) (WHO grade N/A) except?

- A. Methylation profile of DGONC
- B. Nuclear clusters of small to medium sized cells exhibiting oligodendroglioma like morphology
- C. Monosomy of chromosome 14
- D. Strong expression of both OLIG2 and synaptophysin
- E. Absence of widespread GFAP expression

▸▸ **Question 12**

A patient presents with dysplastic cerebellar gangliocytoma with gangliocytic lesion enlarging cerebellar folia *and* densely packed ganglion cells of various sizes *and* matrix resembling normal neuropil. What can be the likely presentation of such tumors?

- A. Signs and symptoms of cerebellar mass
- B. Dysmetria
- C. Hydrocephalus
- D. Cranial nerve deficits
- E. All of the above

▸▸ **Question 13**

A patient presents in neurosurgical OPD with complaints of seizure and headache. Biopsy of the tumor showed multinodularity *with* absence of mitotic activity *with* tumor cell/matrix vacuolation *with* tumor cell immunoreactivity for synaptophysin. What is the most common location of multinodular and vacuolating neuronal tumor?

- A. Frontal lobe
- B. Temporal lobe
- C. Parietal lobe
- D. Spinal cord
- E. Occipital lobe

▸▸ **Question 14**

A patient presents in emergency with signs and symptoms of increased intracranial pressure. On CT of brain an intraventricular lesion was found with calcifications and cystic degeneration, heterogeneously isointense on T1 and hyperintense on T2. MR spectroscopy shows high glycine peak. Which of the following is a recommended treatment for central neurocytoma?

- A. Total resection is often curative with no need of postoperative radiotherapy
- B. Subtotal resection can be followed by stereotactic radiosurgery especially if MIB 1 labelling is more than 2 to 4%
- C. Chemotherapy with alkylating agents, platinum-based agents, or vincristine can be done for recurrent or inoperable tumors
- D. After treatment the patient should have long-term follow-up imaging surveillance for recurrence
- E. All of the above

▸▸ **Question 15**

Extraventricular neurocytoma is a variant of central neurocytoma which can be found in all of the following locations except?

- A. Cerebral parenchyma
- B. Brainstem
- C. Thalamus
- D. Corpus callosum
- E. Cerebellum

▸▸ **Question 16**

Cerebellar liponeurocytoma is a WHO grade 2 tumor which was formerly called lipomatous medulloblastoma. Which of the following statements is correct regarding cerebellar neurocytoma prognosis?

- A. These tumors do not have a favorable prognosis
- B. Subtotal resection has a 15% recurrence rate
- C. Postoperative radiation has no effect on progression-free survival
- D. All recurrences were restricted to the posterior fossa
- E. None of the above

Answers

▸▸ **Answer 1**

Correct answer is A. Re-resection[1]

▸▸ **Answer 2**

Correct answer is B. 8 to 10 years[2]

►► Answer 3

Correct answer is A. Temporal lobe[3]

►► Answer 4

Correct answer is D. Neurocyte forming rosette[4]

►► Answer 5

Correct answer is D. No sign of malignancy[5]

►► Answer 6

Correct answer is E. Cowden syndrome[6]

►► Answer 7

Correct answer is C. Radiotherapy is recommended in all postoperative cases[1]

►► Answer 8

Correct answer is D. Temporal lobe[2]

►► Answer 9

Correct answer is D. Both A and C[2]

►► Answer 10

Correct answer is A. Grade 1[3]

►► Answer 11

Correct answer is C. Monosomy of chromosome 14[7]

►► Answer 12

Correct answer is E. All of the above[8]

►► Answer 13

Correct answer is B. Temporal lobe[9]

►► Answer 14

Correct answer is E. All of the above[10]

►► Answer 15

Correct answer is D. Corpus callosum[10]

►► Answer 16

Correct answer is D. All recurrences were restricted to the posterior fossa[11]

References

[1] Greenberg M, ed. Greenberg's Handbook of Neurosurgery. 10th ed. New York: Thieme; 2023:707
[2] Greenberg M, ed. Greenberg's Handbook of Neurosurgery. 10th ed. New York: Thieme; 2023:708
[3] Greenberg M, ed. Greenberg's Handbook of Neurosurgery. 10th ed. New York: Thieme; 2023:709
[4] Greenberg M, ed. Greenberg's Handbook of Neurosurgery. 10th ed. New York: Thieme; 2023:713
[5] Greenberg M, ed. Greenberg's Handbook of Neurosurgery. 10th ed. New York: Thieme; 2023:719
[6] Greenberg M, ed. Greenberg's Handbook of Neurosurgery. 10th ed. New York: Thieme; 2023:651
[7] Greenberg M, ed. Greenberg's Handbook of Neurosurgery. 10th ed. New York: Thieme; 2023:711
[8] Greenberg M, ed. Greenberg's Handbook of Neurosurgery. 10th ed. New York: Thieme; 2023:717
[9] Greenberg M, ed. Greenberg's Handbook of Neurosurgery. 10th ed. New York: Thieme; 2023:718
[10] Greenberg M, ed. Greenberg's Handbook of Neurosurgery. 10th ed. New York: Thieme; 2023:720
[11] Greenberg M, ed. Greenberg's Handbook of Neurosurgery. 10th ed. New York: Thieme; 2023:722

41 Ependymal Tumors

Questions

▸▸ Question 1

Supratentorial ependymomas (WHO grades 2 and 3) are well-circumscribed supratentorial glioma with uniform cells having round nuclei that form focal pseudorosettes or ependymal rosettes embedded in a fibrillary matrix. These are thought to arise from radial glial cells. Which of the following statements is correct regarding treatment of these tumors?

- A. Postoperative radiotherapy has no role in these tumors
- B. WHO grade is the most important prognosticator of survival in adults and children
- C. The outcome is worse for infratentorial than for supratentorial ependymomas in adults
- D. Gross total removal is the most important prognosticator of overall survival in adults and children
- E. Gross total removal cannot be achieved in most of the cases

▸▸ Question 2

Supratentorial tumors with morphological and immunohistochemical features of ependymoma and ZFTA fusion positive are WHO grade 2 or 3 tumors. What is the most common location for these tumors?

- A. Frontal lobe
- B. Parietal lobe
- C. Both A and B
- D. Thalamus
- E. Hypothalamus/third ventricular region

▸▸ Question 3

Supratentorial tumor with morphological and immunohistochemical features of ependymoma with YAP1 fusion positive seem to be restricted to young children. What is the most common location for these tumors?

- A. Thalamus
- B. Hypothalamus
- C. Within or adjacent to the lateral ventricle
- D. Temporal lobe
- E. In spinal cord

▸▸ Question 4

A patient presents in neurosurgical emergency with signs of raised intracranial pressure, diplopia, and facial weakness. MRI of brain was done and posterior fossa ependymoma (WHO grade 2 or 3) was diagnosed radiographically. Following statements are correct regarding this tumor except?

- A. These are mostly found in the floor of the fourth ventricle
- B. Ependymomas have the potential to spread through CSF to the entire neuraxis, a process known as seeding resulting in so-called drop mets
- C. There is no need to do imaging of the entire neuraxis
- D. Extension through the foramina of Luschka or Magendie may be seen
- E. The tumor enhances with IV contrast except for cystic portion or areas of necrosis

▸▸ Question 5

Which of the following statements is incorrect regarding treatment of posterior fossa ependymoma?

- A. The goal of surgery is maximal possible resection of intracranial portion without causing neurological deficit, while gross total resection may not be possible in many cases because of extensive involvement of the floor of the fourth ventricle
- B. Lesions in the fourth ventricle region are approached via midline suboccipital craniectomy
- C. Traditional radiotherapy is 45 to 48 Gy to tumor bed, while for spinal drop mets, 30 Gy is given to the entire spinal axis with boost to regions showing drop mets
- D. There is very small risk of recurrence following subtotal resection
- E. 5-year survival in pediatric population is 20 to 30%, while it is 80% in adults

▸▸ Question 6

Posterior fossa group A (PFA) ependymoma and posterior fossa group B (PFB) ependymoma are both WHO grade 2 or 3 tumors. PFA ependymomas most frequently occurs in preadolescents, while group B ependymoma mostly occurs in adults and adolescents. The prognosis of both these tumors depends on the extent of resection. Which statement is correct regarding location of these tumors?

- A. Both of these tumors arise from the floor of the fourth ventricle
- B. Group B tumors arise from the floor, while group A tumors arise from the roof or lateral wall
- C. Group B tumors arise from the roof or lateral wall, while group A tumors arise from the floor of the fourth ventricle
- D. Both tumors arise from the roof of the fourth ventricle
- E. Location of these tumors is variable in every patient

▸▸ Question 7

Spinal ependymomas are intramedullary spinal gliomas with vast majority of these tumors being grade 2 (grade 3 tumors being rare) and most common location at cervical and cervicothoracic levels. Which of the following are the imaging characteristics of these tumors?

- A. Hypointense on T1 and T2 with no enhancement and often eccentric and poorly demarcated
- B. Hypointense on T1 and hyperintense on T2 with contrast enhancement and often eccentric and poorly demarcated
- C. Hypointense on T1 and hyperintense on T2 with contrast enhancement, and more centrally located and more readily defined
- D. Hypointense on T1 and hypointense on T2 with no contrast enhancement, and more centrally located and more readily defined
- E. Hyperintense on T1 and T2 with contrast enhancement, and more centrally located and more readily defined

▸▸ Question 8

Myxopapillary ependymomas are WHO grade 2 tumors that essentially only occur at conus medullaris or filum terminale and are differentiated from metastatic carcinoma, paragangliomas, schwannomas, chordomas, and myxoid chondrosarcomas by using GFAP staining. Complete excision of these tumors is often not possible due to invasion of the spinal cord parenchyma and/or CSF dissemination. What is the prognosis of these tumors?

- A. Poor prognosis with 10-year survival less than 50%
- B. Unfavorable prognosis with 10-year survival less than 90%
- C. Favorable prognosis with 10-year survival more than 50% in adults and children
- D. Poor prognosis with 10-year survival less than 10%
- E. Favorable prognosis with 10-year survival of more than 90%

▸▸ Question 9

Subependymomas are WHO grade 1 tumors which are mostly incidentally found as nonenhancing, well-demarcated intraventricular mass and are followed up with serial imaging if asymptomatic. What is the most common location for these tumors?

- A. Fourth ventricle
- B. Third ventricle
- C. Lateral ventricles
- D. Sylvian aqueduct
- E. Frontal horn of lateral ventricle

▸▸ Question 10

Spinal ependymoma, MYCN-amplified, is a rare intramedullary tumor, mostly found in cervical and thoracic cord region and shows the same imaging characteristics as other ependymomas. These tumors have poor prognosis and early spread throughout the neuraxis is frequent. What is the recurrence rate of these tumors which are reported up till now?

- A. 100%
- B. 80%
- C. 70%
- D. 60%
- E. 50%

▸▸ Question 11

Ependymomas are believed to arise from bipolar progenitor cells that are thought to be a major source of neurons in the developing nervous system. What are these cells also called?

- A. Radial glial cells
- B. Progenitor cells
- C. Axial cells
- D. Circumferential cells
- E. CD4 positive cells

▸▸ Question 12

All of the following molecular genetic studies are done to subclassify ependymomas except?

- A. ZFTA fusion
- B. YAP1 fusion
- C. P65
- D. L1CAM
- E. BRAF

▸▸ Question 13

Posterior fossa group B ependymomas are mostly WHO grade II/III tumors but have a worse prognosis as they can often be not removed completely due to their propensity to invade which of the following?

- A. Cerebral cortex
- B. Basal cranial nerves
- C. Obex
- D. Mid brain
- E. White matter tracts

▸▸ Question 14

Ependymomas rank 2nd only to medulloblastomas in radiosensitivity. Radiotherapy is administered after surgical excision. What is the dose to tumor bed for cranial lesions?

- A. 30 Gy
- B. 35 to 38 Gy
- C. 3D conformal XRT with 59.4 Gy to tumor bed + 1 cm margin
- D. 62 Gy
- E. 65 Gy

▸▸ Question 15

A young child was operated on for ependymoma. After 2 weeks, CSF cytology was performed that showed evidence of drop mets. What will be the radiotherapy dose to the entire spine in this case?

- A. 30 Gy
- B. 35 to 38 Gy
- C. 45 to 48 Gy
- D. 62 Gy
- E. 65 Gy

▸▸ Question 16

Which of the followings is a distinctive, WHO grade 2 ependymoma variant that essentially only occurs in the filum terminale with the histological features of papillary, with microcystic vacuoles and mucosubstance?

- A. Clear cell
- B. Tanycytic
- C. Myxopapillary
- D. RELA fusion positive
- E. Anaplastic

▸▸ Question 17

When should the first follow-up image be obtained after initial discovery of subependymoma to rule out rapid growth?

- A. 1 month
- B. 3 months
- C. 6 months
- D. 1 year
- E. 5 years

Answers

▸▸ Answer 1

Correct answer is D. Gross total removal is the most important prognosticator of overall survival in adults and children[1]

▸▸ Answer 2

Correct answer is C. Both A and B[2]

▸▸ Answer 3

Correct answer is C. Within or adjacent to the lateral ventricle[2]

▸▸ Answer 4

Correct answer is C. There is no need to do imaging of the entire neuraxis[3]

▸▸ Answer 5

Correct answer is D. There is very small risk of recurrence following subtotal resection[4]

▸▸ Answer 6

Correct answer is B. Group B tumors arise from the floor, while group A tumors arise from the roof or lateral wall[5]

▸▸ Answer 7

Correct answer is C. Hypointense on T1 and hyperintense on T2 with contrast enhancement, and more centrally located and more readily defined[6]

▸▸ Answer 8

Correct answer is E. Favorable prognosis with 10-year survival of more than 90%[7]

▸▸ Answer 9

Correct answer is A. Fourth ventricle[8]

▸▸ Answer 10

Correct answer is A. 100%[6]

▸▸ Answer 11

Correct answer is A. Radial glial cells[9]

▸▸ Answer 12

Correct answer is E. BRAF[1]

▸▸ Answer 13

Correct answer is C. Obex[5]

▸▸ Answer 14

Correct answer is C. 3D conformal XRT with 59.4 Gy to tumor bed + 1 cm margin[10]

▸▸ Answer 15

Correct answer is A. 30 Gy[10]

▸▸ Answer 16

Correct answer is C. Myxopapillary[6]

▸▸ Answer 17

Correct answer is B. 3 months[8]

References

[1] Greenberg M, ed. Greenberg's Handbook of Neurosurgery. 10th ed. New York: Thieme; 2023:725
[2] Greenberg M, ed. Greenberg's Handbook of Neurosurgery. 10th ed. New York: Thieme; 2023:726
[3] Greenberg M, ed. Greenberg's Handbook of Neurosurgery. 10th ed. New York: Thieme; 2023:727
[4] Greenberg M, ed. Greenberg's Handbook of Neurosurgery. 10th ed. New York: Thieme; 2023:728
[5] Greenberg M, ed. Greenberg's Handbook of Neurosurgery. 10th ed. New York: Thieme; 2023:731
[6] Greenberg M, ed. Greenberg's Handbook of Neurosurgery. 10th ed. New York: Thieme; 2023:734

[7] Greenberg M, ed. Greenberg's Handbook of Neurosurgery. 10th ed. New York: Thieme; 2023:735
[8] Greenberg M, ed. Greenberg's Handbook of Neurosurgery. 10th ed. New York: Thieme; 2023:736
[9] Greenberg M, ed. Greenberg's Handbook of Neurosurgery. 10th ed. New York: Thieme; 2023:724
[10] Greenberg M, ed. Greenberg's Handbook of Neurosurgery. 10th ed. New York: Thieme; 2023:729

42 Choroid Plexus Tumors

Questions

▸▸ Question 1

A 2-year-old patient presents with nausea, vomiting, macrocephaly, and seizures. Imaging showed iso- to hyperdense lesion on CT of brain in the ventricle which is hypointense on T1WI and hyperintense on T2WI multilobulated intraventricular mass classically with projecting fronds and densely enhancing. What are the most common locations of this tumor in descending order?

- A. Third ventricle, then fourth ventricle, then lateral ventricles
- B. Lateral ventricles, then third ventricle, then fourth ventricle
- C. Lateral ventricles, then fourth ventricle, then third ventricle
- D. Third ventricle, then lateral ventricle, then fourth ventricle
- E. None of the above

▸▸ Question 2

Atypical choroid plexus papillomas are WHO grade 2 tumors which are located intraventricularly *and* demonstrate choroid plexus differentiation by histopathological and immunophenotypic features *and* are characterized by absence of criteria qualifying for diagnosis of choroid plexus carcinoma *and* which of the following?

- A. More than or equal to 1 mitosis/HPF of 0.23 mm^2
- B. More than or equal to 2 mitosis/HPF of 0.23 mm^2
- C. More than or equal to 3 mitosis/HPF of 0.23 mm^2
- D. More than or equal to 4 mitosis/HPF of 0.23 mm^2
- E. More than or equal to 5 mitosis/HPF of 0.23 mm^2

▸▸ Question 3

Choroid plexus carcinoma is a WHO grade 3 tumor that invades the adjacent brain and primarily occurs in the lateral ventricles of children. These tumors are prone to metastasize through CSF. What is the percentage of these tumors metastasized thorough CSF at the time of diagnosis?

- A. 41%
- B. 31%
- C. 51%
- D. 21%
- E. 11%

▸▸ Question 4

Following are the histopathological features of choroid plexus carcinoma except?

- A. Increased cellularity
- B. Nuclear pleomorphism
- C. Blurring of the papillary pattern with poorly structured sheets of tumor cells
- D. Mitoses usually more than or equal to 2 mitoses/10 HPF of 0.23 mm^2
- E. Necrotic areas

▸▸ Question 5

Imaging of the entire neuraxis is recommended in choroid plexus carcinoma due to high incidence of drop mets. Which of the following are features of choroid plexus carcinoma on MRI?

- A. Heterogenous signals on T1 and T2 with irregular enhancing margins suggesting subependymal invasion
- B. Edema in adjacent brain
- C. Vascular flow voids in 55% of images
- D. Often hydrocephalus is evident
- E. All of the above

▸▸ Question 6

Which of the following statements is correct regarding treatment of choroid plexus carcinoma?

- A. There is no benefit of surgery in malignant choroid plexus tumors
- B. Chemotherapy benefits all of these patients
- C. Radiotherapy was not shown to improve survival in patients undergoing surgery
- D. Adjuvant chemotherapy should be given to all the patients
- E. All of the above

▸▸ Question 7

Atypical choroid plexus papillomas are more likely to recur than their grade 1 counterpart. What is the median age of diagnosis of these tumors?

- A. 6 to 8 months
- B. 8 to 10 months
- C. 10 to 12 months
- D. 12 to 14 months
- E. 14 to 16 months

▸▸ Question 8

Which statement is incorrect regarding treatment and prognosis of grade 1 choroid plexus papilloma?

- A. Choroid plexus papillomas are often cured surgically with total removal
- B. The operation may be difficult because of fragility of the tumor and bleeding from the choroidal arteries
- C. Persistence with second or even third operation is recommended as 5-year survival rate of 84 to 97% can be achieved
- D. Postoperative subdural collections after transcortical tumor excision may occur because of persistent ventriculosubdural fistula which may require subdural peritoneal shunt

- E. Malignant degeneration is common with role of chemotherapy and radiation for these tumors

▸▸ Question 9

What is the common location of choroid plexus papilloma?
- A. Usually infratentorial in adults
- B. A + Supratentorial in children
- C. Supratentorial in adults
- D. C + Infratentorial in children
- E. Equally present supratentorially and infratentorially in adults and children

▸▸ Question 10

Hydrocephalus in choroid plexus papilloma may result from which of the following?
- A. Overproduction of CSF
- B. Obstruction of CSF outflow
- C. Communicating hydrocephalus due to CSF-borne particulates
- D. Does not occur in choroid plexus papilloma
- E. A, B, and C

▸▸ Question 11

A 2-year-old child presented with signs of raised ICP and CT showed hydrocephalus and a densely enhancing multilobulated mass with projecting fronds, within left lateral ventricle. What is the most probable diagnosis?
- A. Ependymoma
- B. Medulloblastoma
- C. Astroblastoma
- D. Choroid plexus papilloma
- E. Ganglioglioma

▸▸ Question 12

What is the usual extraventricular location of choroid plexus papilloma?
- A. Middle fossa
- B. Cribriform plate
- C. CP angle
- D. Ambient cistern
- E. Suprasellar region

▸▸ Question 13

What is the treatment of postoperative ventriculo-subdural collection in choroid plexus papilloma (CPP) surgery?
- A. Craniotomy and evacuation
- B. Subdural drain
- C. Subdural–peritoneal shunting
- D. Subdural–subarachnoid shunting

▸▸ Question 14

About 40% of choroid plexus carcinomas are associated with which syndrome?
- A. Cowden syndrome
- B. von Hippel Lindau syndrome
- C. Li Fraumeni syndrome
- D. Turcot syndrome
- E. Gardner syndrome

▸▸ Question 15

Absence of which mutation is associated with a good prognosis in choroid plexus carcinoma?
- A. TP53
- B. BRAF
- C. ATRX
- D. PTEN
- E. EGFR

Answers

▸▸ Answer 1

Correct answer is C. Lateral ventricles, then fourth ventricle, then third ventricle[1]

▸▸ Answer 2

Correct answer is B. More than or equal to 2 mitosis/HPF of 0.23 mm[22]

▸▸ Answer 3

Correct answer is D. 21%[2]

▸▸ Answer 4

Correct answer is D. Mitoses usually more than or equal to 2 mitoses/10 HPF of 0.23 mm[23]

▸▸ Answer 5

Correct answer is E. All of the above[3]

▸▸ Answer 6

Correct answer is C. Radiotherapy was not shown to improve survival in patients undergoing surgery[3]

▸▸ Answer 7

Correct answer is C. 10 to 12 months[2]

▸▸ Answer 8

Correct answer is E. Malignant degeneration is common with role of chemotherapy and radiation for these tumors[2]

▸▸ Answer 9

Correct answer is B. A + Supratentorial in children[1]

▸▸ Answer 10

Correct answer is E. A, B, and C[4]

▸▸ Answer 11

Correct answer is D. Choroid plexus papilloma[4]

▸▸ Answer 12

Correct answer is C. CP angle[1]

▸▸ Answer 13

Correct answer is C. Subdural–peritoneal shunting[4]

▸▸ Answer 14

Correct answer is C. Li Fraumeni syndrome[3]

▸▸ Answer 15

Correct answer is A. TP53[5]

References

[1] Greenberg M, ed. Greenberg's Handbook of Neurosurgery. 10th ed. New York: Thieme; 2023:739
[2] Greenberg M, ed. Greenberg's Handbook of Neurosurgery. 10th ed. New York: Thieme; 2023:741
[3] Greenberg M, ed. Greenberg's Handbook of Neurosurgery. 10th ed. New York: Thieme; 2023:742
[4] Greenberg M, ed. Greenberg's Handbook of Neurosurgery. 10th ed. New York: Thieme; 2023:740
[5] Greenberg M, ed. Greenberg's Handbook of Neurosurgery. 10th ed. New York: Thieme; 2023:743

43 Embryonal Tumors

Questions

►► Question 1

A 4-year-old patient presents with history of nausea, vomiting, headache, lethargy, and irritability which developed during the course of 6 to 10 weeks. CT of brain showed a hyperdense contrast-enhancing mass in the posterior fossa with calcifications while MRI showed hypo- to isointense lesion on T1, heterogenous lesion on T2. A diagnosis of medulloblastoma (grade 4) tumor is made. Where does this tumor arise in the posterior fossa most commonly?

- A. Floor of the fourth ventricle near fastigium
- B. From the roof of the fourth ventricle
- C. In the cerebellum, they arise in the vermis near the apex of the roof of the fourth ventricle
- D. In the cerebellum, these arise from cerebellar hemisphere
- E. From the floor of the fourth ventricle near the foramen of Magendie

►► Question 2

Medulloblastomas which were formerly called as primitive neuroectodermal tumors (PNET) are now considered under umbrella term embryonal tumors and account for 68% of embryonal tumors. About 10 to 35% of these tumors are seeded to spinal canal at the time of diagnosis and warrants imaging of the entire neuraxis. Which statement is correct regarding treatment of these tumors?

- A. Invasion or attachment to the floor of the fourth ventricle at the brainstem in the region of facial colliculus often limits its excision
- B. Opening of foramen magnum with removal of C1 and C2 arches is often required for midline cerebellar medulloblastomas
- C. 30 to 40% of children require permanent VP shunt postoperatively
- D. Postoperative radiotherapy (54 gray to primary tumor and 18 gray to craniospinal axis) and chemotherapy are needed in almost all patients
- E. All of the above

►► Question 3

Which statement is incorrect regarding poor prognosticators of medulloblastoma?

- A. Poor Karnofsky performance scale score
- B. Inability to perform gross total resection
- C. MDB classification with SHH activated, TP53 wild type with classic histology
- D. Disseminated disease at the time of diagnosis
- E. Younger age of patient for some cell types (< 3 years)

►► Question 4

Which of the following is the most common histologic variant of medulloblastoma which constitutes 72% of medulloblastomas, is predominant in children, is found in all four molecular medulloblastomas, is composed of densely packed undifferentiated small round cells with mild-to-moderate nuclear pleomorphism, and has high mitotic count?

- A. Classic type
- B. Desmoplastic/nodular
- C. MDB with extensive nodularity
- D. Large cell/anaplastic MDB
- E. Both A and B

►► Question 5

A patient is found to have medulloblastoma (MDB) around the foramen of Luschka, arising from the brain stem on imaging. These MDBs account for 15% of adults MDBs with male to female ratio of 1:2 with predominant histologic variant of classic type. In spite of being grade 4, the prognosis for children is excellent with surgery and adjuvant therapy in contrast to poor prognosis in adults. Which molecular type of MDB is this?

- A. WNT activated
- B. SHH activated TP53 wild type
- C. SHH activated TP53 mutant
- D. MDB non-WNT/non-SHH
- E. Group 4 MDB

►► Question 6

Putative cell of origin of SHH activated, TP53 wild type MDB is cerebellar granule neuron cell precursors of the external granule cell layer and cochlear nucleus. What is the predominant histologic variant in SHH activated, TP53 wild type MDB?

- A. Extensive nodularity
- B. Classic
- C. Large cell/anaplastic
- D. Desmoplastic/nodular
- E. Both A and B

►► Question 7

SHH activated, TP 53 mutant MDB is mostly a high-risk tumor. What is the most common histologic variant in these tumors?

- A. Extensive nodularity
- B. Classic
- C. Large cell/anaplastic
- D. Desmoplastic/nodular
- E. Both A and B

▸▸ **Question 8**

Atypical teratoid or rhabdoid tumors are WHO grade 4 embryonal tumors that occur primarily in infants and children. Where in the CNS this tumor can be found?

- A. Cerebral hemispheres
- B. Suprasellar region
- C. Cerebellar hemispheres
- D. Brainstem
- E. Anywhere along the neuraxis

▸▸ **Question 9**

Cribriform neuroepithelial tumors are embryonal tumors that are highly cellular and characterized by presence of cribriform strands and ribbons. What is the location of these tumors?

- A. Brainstem
- B. Cerebellum
- C. Cerebellopontine angle
- D. Near any of the ventricles (third, fourth, or lateral)
- E. Anywhere along the neuraxis

▸▸ **Question 10**

Embryonal tumor with multilayer rosettes is a WHO grade 4 aggressive tumor with mean overall survival of 12 months. This tumor is most commonly found in cerebral hemispheres. Which age group does this tumor affects?

- A. 5 to 10 years
- B. 10 to 14 years
- C. Less than 4 years
- D. After 50 years
- E. None of the above

▸▸ **Question 11**

A child presented with obstructive hydrocephalus. Which of the following is false regarding medulloblastoma?

- A. CT: noncontrast—typically hyperdense and most lesions enhance with contrast
- B. MRI: T1WI—hypo- to isointense
- C. MRI: T2WI—heterogeneous due to tumor cysts, vessels, and calcifications
- D. MRS: decreased choline and elevated NAA
- E. Spinal imaging: MRI with IV gadolinium or CT/myelography with water-soluble contrast should be done to rule out drop mets

▸▸ **Question 12**

What is the 5-year event-free survival (EFS) of very high-risk group of medulloblastoma based on histology and molecular profiling?

- A. > 90%
- B. 75–90%
- C. 50–85%
- D. < 50%

▸▸ **Question 13**

Gross nodular seeding in cerebellar subarachnoid space is designated as which stage in postoperative staging system?

- A. m0
- B. m1
- C. m2
- D. m3
- E. m4

▸▸ **Question 14**

Regarding histological/morphological variants of medulloblastoma, what is the most common variant?

- A. Classic
- B. Large cell
- C. Nodular
- D. With extensive nodularity
- E. Anaplastic

▸▸ **Question 15**

Regarding histologic/morphologic variants of medulloblastoma, which of the following is associated with Gorlin syndrome in early childhood?

- A. Classic
- B. Large cell
- C. Nodular
- D. With extensive nodularity
- E. Anaplastic

▸▸ **Question 16**

Regarding molecular genetics based clusters of medulloblastoma, a midline lesion that is typical in older childhood with male:female = 1:2. Predominant histologic variant is classic. Putative cell of origin is lower rhombic lip progenitor cells and frequently shows genetic mutations in CTNNB1, DDX3X, and TP53. This will be categorized as which of the following?

- A. WNT activated
- B. SHH activated, TP53 mutated
- C. SHH activated, TP53 wild type
- D. Non-WNT, non-SHH group III
- E. Non-WNT, non-SHH group IV

▸▸ **Question 17**

What percentage of children require permanent VP shunt placement following post fossa resection?

- A. 10 to 20%
- B. 20 to 30%
- C. 30 to 40%

- D. 50 to 60%
- E. 60 to 70%

▸▸ Question 18

What is the common location of cribriform neuroepithelial tumors (CRINET)?

- A. Suprasellar
- B. Near the ventricles
- C. CP angle
- D. Subchiasmatic
- E. Pineal region

Answers

▸▸ Answer 1

Correct answer is C. In the cerebellum, they arise in the vermis near the apex of the roof of the fourth ventricle[1]

▸▸ Answer 2

Correct answer is E. All of the above[2]

▸▸ Answer 3

Correct answer is C. MDB classification with SHH activated, TP53 wild type with classic histology[2]

▸▸ Answer 4

Correct answer is A. Classic type[3]

▸▸ Answer 5

Correct answer is B. SHH activated TP53 wild type[4]

▸▸ Answer 6

Correct answer is D. Desmoplastic/nodular[5]

▸▸ Answer 7

Correct answer is C. Large cell/anaplastic[6]

▸▸ Answer 8

Correct answer is E. Anywhere along the neuraxis[7]

▸▸ Answer 9

Correct answer is D. Near any of the ventricles (third, fourth, or lateral)[8]

▸▸ Answer 10

Correct answer is C. Less than 4 years[9]

▸▸ Answer 11

Correct answer is D. MRS: decreased choline and elevated NAA[10]

▸▸ Answer 12

Correct answer is D. < 50%[2]

▸▸ Answer 13

Correct answer is C. m2[2]

▸▸ Answer 14

Correct answer is A. Classic[3]

▸▸ Answer 15

Correct answer is C. Nodular[3]

▸▸ Answer 16

Correct answer is A. WNT activated[4]

▸▸ Answer 17

Correct answer is C. 30 to 40%[2]

▸▸ Answer 18

Correct answer is B. Near the ventricles[8]

References

[1] Greenberg M, ed. Greenberg's Handbook of Neurosurgery. 10th ed. New York: Thieme; 2023:744
[2] Greenberg M, ed. Greenberg's Handbook of Neurosurgery. 10th ed. New York: Thieme; 2023:747
[3] Greenberg M, ed. Greenberg's Handbook of Neurosurgery. 10th ed. New York: Thieme; 2023:749
[4] Greenberg M, ed. Greenberg's Handbook of Neurosurgery. 10th ed. New York: Thieme; 2023:750
[5] Greenberg M, ed. Greenberg's Handbook of Neurosurgery. 10th ed. New York: Thieme; 2023:751
[6] Greenberg M, ed. Greenberg's Handbook of Neurosurgery. 10th ed. New York: Thieme; 2023:752
[7] Greenberg M, ed. Greenberg's Handbook of Neurosurgery. 10th ed. New York: Thieme; 2023:755
[8] Greenberg M, ed. Greenberg's Handbook of Neurosurgery. 10th ed. New York: Thieme; 2023:756
[9] Greenberg M, ed. Greenberg's Handbook of Neurosurgery. 10th ed. New York: Thieme; 2023:757
[10] Greenberg M, ed. Greenberg's Handbook of Neurosurgery. 10th ed. New York: Thieme; 2023:746

44 Pineal Tumors and Pineal Region Lesions

Questions

▸▸ Question 1

Pineal region tumors are relatively rare and are more common in children than in adults. Germinoma is the most common tumor at this location followed by astrocytoma and teratoma. Which of the following is correct regarding the boundaries of pineal region?

- A. Bounded dorsally by the splenium of the corpus callosum and tele choroidea
- B. Bounded ventrally by the quadrigeminal plate and midbrain tectum
- C. Bounded rostrally by the posterior aspect of the third ventricle
- D. Bounded caudally by the cerebellar vermis
- E. All of the above

▸▸ Question 2

Pineal region tumor in an adult of more than 40 years of age is most likely which of the following?

- A. Germinoma
- B. Meningioma or glioma
- C. Teratoma
- D. Ependymoma
- E. Glial cyst (pineal cyst)

▸▸ Question 3

In order to proceed for the management of pineal region mass, MRI of brain with and without contrast is needed. MRI of cervical, thoracic, and lumbar spine with IV contrast is also needed to see any drop metastasis. Which of the following statements is incorrect regarding the treatment of pineal region tumors?

- A. Pineal cyst of less than 2-cm size must be excised with surgery
- B. If there is hydrocephalus, then transventricular biopsy should be taken to see histopathology of tumor
- C. If there is no hydrocephalus, then open biopsy or stereotactic biopsy or navigation-assisted endoscopic biopsy should be taken
- D. If the histopathology comes out to be germinoma, then treatment is radiotherapy and chemotherapy
- E. For all tumors other than germinoma, the option is resection followed by adjuvant therapy

▸▸ Question 4

Two main stereotactic trajectories for pineal region tumors include anterolateral (low frontal) approach below the internal cerebral vein and the second is posterolateral trans-parieto-occipital approach. Which of the following vessels is at risk of damage during pineal region surgery?

- A. Vein of Galen
- B. Basal vein of Rosenthal
- C. Internal cerebral veins
- D. Posterior medial choroidal artery
- E. All of the above

▸▸ Question 5

The pineal gland is a neuroendocrine gland that secretes melatonin in response to photic stimulation of the retina by the bright light, and also regulates secretion of some pituitary hormones. It is outside the blood–brain barrier and is supplied by choroidal branches of the posterior cerebral artery. The tumors which are treated with surgical resection include following except?

- A. Radioresistant tumors like malignant non-germinoma GCTs
- B. Meningiomas and teratomas
- C. Pineacytoma
- D. Germinoma
- E. Well-encapsulated tumors

▸▸ Question 6

Among the following surgical approaches for the pineal region tumors, which is the most common?

- A. Midline infratentorial supracerebellar approach of Horsley and Krause as refined by Stein
- B. Occipital transtentorial approach
- C. Transventricular (requires dilated ventricles and large eccentric lesions)
- D. Lateral paramedian infratentorial
- E. Transcallosal
- F. Paramedian infratentorial supracerebellar approach

▸▸ Question 7

Complications from surgery for pineal region tumors include new visual field deficits, epidural fluid collection, infection, and cerebellar ataxia. What is the surgical mortality rate of pineal region tumor surgery?

- A. 10 to 15%
- B. 15 to 20%
- C. 5 to 10%
- D. 20 to 25%
- E. 25 to 30%

▸▸ Question 8

A patient's biopsy after operation for pineal region tumor shows immature neuroepithelial cells with irregular hyperchromatic nuclei and a high nuclear to cytoplasm ratio, poorly defined cell borders, and a high Ki 67 index (23 to 50%). What is the most likely diagnosis in this case?

- A. Pineoblastoma
- B. Pineocytoma
- C. Parenchymal tumor of intermediate differentiation
- D. Pineoblastomacytoma
- E. All of the above

▸▸ Question 9

What is the WHO grade of papillary tumor of papillary region?

- A. Grade 1
- B. Grade 2
- C. Grade 3
- D. Grade 4
- E. Both grades 1 and 2

▸▸ Question 10

What is the ideal way of getting diagnosis of a pineal region tumor?

- A. Tumor markers
- B. Giving radiation and seeing response
- C. Taking biopsy
- D. Giving chemotherapy
- E. None of the above

▸▸ Question 11

Pineal region is the area of the brain bounded dorsally by the splenium of the corpus callosum and the tela choroidea, ventrally by the quadrigeminal plate and midbrain tectum, rostrally by the posterior aspect of the third ventricle, and caudally by which of the following?

- A. Cerebellar vermis
- B. Pons
- C. Medulla oblongata
- D. Sylvian fissure
- E. Obex

▸▸ Question 12

What is the most common tumor in pineal region in adults (> 40 years)?

- A. Germinoma
- B. Pineal cysts
- C. Meningioma
- D. Paraganglioma

▸▸ Question 13

Pineocytoma is a rare, well-differentiated tumor of the pineal parenchyma consisting of pineocytomatous rosettes of uniform cells and pleomorphic cells having gangliocytic differentiation, and typically affects adults with average age at diagnosis of 43 years. What is the WHO grade for pineocytomas?

- A. I
- B. II
- C. III
- D. IV
- E. Not specified

▸▸ Question 14

Test dose radiation practice for management of pineal region masses was that if a pineal region tumor enhanced uniformly and had the classic appearance of a germinoma on MRI, a test dose of radiation was given, and if the tumor shrank then the diagnosis of germinoma was virtually certain and radiotherapy (XRT) was continued without surgery. What was the XRT dose?

- A. 2 Gy
- B. 3 Gy
- C. 4 Gy
- D. 5 Gy
- E. 10 Gy

▸▸ Question 15

Pineal cysts do not require surgical removal unless they become large enough to cause obstructive hydrocephalus. What is the size at that time usually?

- A. > 2 cm
- B. > 3 cm
- C. > 4 cm
- D. > 5 cm
- E. > 1 cm

▸▸ Question 16

Surgical treatment of pineal region tumors should be limited to all of the following except?

- A. Radioresistant, for example, nongerminomatous GCT
- B. Well-encapsulated tumors
- C. Benign tumors
- D. Pineocytoma
- E. Germinoma

▸▸ Question 17

What is the surgical mortality of pineal region tumors?

- A. 1 to 3%
- B. 3 to 5%
- C. 5 to 10%
- D. 10 to 15%
- E. 15 to 20%

▸▸ Question 18

What is the postoperative 5-year survival rate of pineal tumors?
- A. 65 to 70%
- B. 70 to 86%
- C. 86 to 91%
- D. 91 to 94%
- E. 94 to 98%

▸▸ Question 19

Which of the following computer-assisted cisternal endoscopic approach (CACE) permits visualization of neurovascular structures and avoids traversing brain parenchyma?
- A. Supracerebellar infratentorial
- B. Supracerebellar supratentorial
- C. Infracerebellar infratentorial
- D. Infracerebellar supratentorial
- E. Transtympanic

▸▸ Question 20

Which of the following is the approach to the pineal region tumor extending into corpus callosum and third ventricle?
- A. Occipital transtentorial
- B. Transcallosal
- C. Lateral paramedian infratentorial
- D. Transventricular
- E. Approach of Horsley and Krause

Answers

▸▸ Answer 1

Correct answer is E. All of the above[1]

▸▸ Answer 2

Correct answer is B. Meningioma or glioma[2]

▸▸ Answer 3

Correct answer is A. Pineal cyst of less than 2-cm size must be excised with surgery[3]

▸▸ Answer 4

Correct answer is E. All of the above[3]

▸▸ Answer 5

Correct answer is D. Germinoma[4]

▸▸ Answer 6

Correct answer is A. Midline infratentorial supracerebellar approach of Horsley and Krause as refined by Stein[4]

▸▸ Answer 7

Correct answer is C. 5 to 10%[4]

▸▸ Answer 8

Correct answer is A. Pineoblastoma[5]

▸▸ Answer 9

Correct answer is E. Both grades 1 and 2[6]

▸▸ Answer 10

Correct answer is C. Taking biopsy[1]

▸▸ Answer 11

Correct answer is A. Cerebellar vermis[1]

▸▸ Answer 12

Correct answer is C. Meningioma[2]

▸▸ Answer 13

Correct answer is A. I[7]

▸▸ Answer 14

Correct answer is D. 5 Gy[3]

▸▸ Answer 15

Correct answer is A. > 2 cm[3]

▸▸ Answer 16

Correct answer is E. Germinoma[4]

▸▸ Answer 17

Correct answer is C. 5 to 10%[4]

▸▸ Answer 18

Correct answer is C. 86 to 91%[8]

▸▸ Answer 19

Correct answer is A. Supracerebellar infratentorial[3]

▸▸ Answer 20

Correct answer is B. Transcallosal[4]

References

[1] Greenberg M, ed. Greenberg's Handbook of Neurosurgery. 10th ed. New York: Thieme; 2023:758
[2] Greenberg M, ed. Greenberg's Handbook of Neurosurgery. 10th ed. New York: Thieme; 2023:759
[3] Greenberg M, ed. Greenberg's Handbook of Neurosurgery. 10th ed. New York: Thieme; 2023:760
[4] Greenberg M, ed. Greenberg's Handbook of Neurosurgery. 10th ed. New York: Thieme; 2023:761
[5] Greenberg M, ed. Greenberg's Handbook of Neurosurgery. 10th ed. New York: Thieme; 2023:764
[6] Greenberg M, ed. Greenberg's Handbook of Neurosurgery. 10th ed. New York: Thieme; 2023:765
[7] Greenberg M, ed. Greenberg's Handbook of Neurosurgery. 10th ed. New York: Thieme; 2023:762
[8] Greenberg M, ed. Greenberg's Handbook of Neurosurgery. 10th ed. New York: Thieme; 2023:763

45 Cranial and Paraspinal Nerve Tumors

Questions

▸▸ Question 1

Schwannoma (WHO grade 1) is a benign nerve sheath tumor exclusively or primarily comprised of differentiated neoplastic Schwann cells with peak incidence in the fourth to sixth decades of life. Which statement is correct regarding location of these tumors?

- A. They commonly arise from peripheral nerves in the skin and subcutaneous tissue of the head and neck, or on the flexor surfaces of the limbs
- B. Intracranially they frequently involve the vestibular division of cranial nerve eight
- C. Intracranially these can also arise from cranial nerve five or other cranial nerves
- D. In the spine, these tumors form dumbbell shaped tumors as they extend out through the neural foramen which constricts them
- E. All of the above

▸▸ Question 2

A 10-year-old patient presents with multiple cutaneous lesions that are typically soft, mobile, and asymptomatic. On histopathology, these tumors are found to be composed of neoplastic Schwann cells interspersed with normal cells and infiltrative low cellularity spindle cell neoplasm that is associated with a variably myxoid to collagenous stroma with mixed cell population. What is the most likely diagnosis in this patient?

- A. Schwannomatosis
- B. Neurofibroma
- C. Perineuroma
- D. Neurofibromatosis type 1
- E. Hybrid nerve sheath tumors

▸▸ Question 3

A perineuroma is a benign WHO grade 1 tumor which is comprised exclusively of neoplastic perineural cells. Soft tissue perineuroma arises in deep soft tissues and presents as a soft tissue mass with nonspecific symptoms. Which of the following is not included in the essential diagnostic criteria of perineuroma?

- A. Slender spindle cells with bipolar cytoplasmic processes
- B. Storiform and/or whorled architecture
- C. Positive for at least one perineural antigen (EMA, claudin-1, GLUT1)
- D. Always associated with nerve fiber
- E. Negative for S100

▸▸ Question 4

Hybrid nerve sheath tumors are also known as benign peripheral nerve sheath tumor not otherwise specified (NOS). On histopathology, there are intermingled features of two types of benign nerve sheath tumors and immunohistochemical staining for each component. What is the most common type of hybrid nerve sheath tumor?

- A. Neurofibroma/schwannoma
- B. Schwannoma/perineuroma
- C. Neurofibroma/perineuroma
- D. Schwannoma/meningioma
- E. None of the above

▸▸ Question 5

Malignant melanocytic nerve sheath tumors are aggressive tumors that usually arise from a spinal or autonomic nerve. What neoplastic cells are found in this tumor?

- A. Cells with melanocytic features
- B. A + Schwann cells
- C. A + Neurofibroma cells
- D. A + Astrocytes
- E. A + Meningeal cells

▸▸ Question 6

Malignant peripheral nerve sheath tumors originate from peripheral nerve or a pre-existing benign nerve sheath tumor or in patient with NF-1 (approximately 50% are associated with NF-1). Following are features of this tumor which are associated with a favorable prognosis except?

- A. Smaller tumor size
- B. Female gender and Hispanic white race
- C. No metastasis at presentation
- D. GTR
- E. No association with prior XRT

▸▸ Question 7

A patient presents with low-back pain and radiculopathy. A surgery is performed, and the tumor attached to filum terminale is excised. On preoperative imaging, it showed serpiginous dilated and ectatic blood vessels with a cap sign. On histology, it showed uniform, round or polygonal chief cells congregate in lobules (Zellballen) encompassed by a barely discernible single layer of susentacular (type 2) cells. What is the most probable diagnosis in this patient?

- A. Schwannoma
- B. Myxopapillary ependymoma
- C. Cauda equina neuroendocrine tumor
- D. Neurofibroma
- E. Malignant filum terminale neuroma

▸▸ Question 8

A 35-year-old patient presents with decreasing hearing in right ear, tinnitus in the same ear, difficulty in maintaining balance, abnormal corneal reflex, and nystagmus. Weber test was found lateralizing to the left ear. Further testing showed pure tone audiogram threshold to be less than or equal to 50%, while speech discrimination score was more than or equal to 50% (serviceable hearing). MRI of brain showed oval enhancing tumor centered on IAC and trumpeting sign which was 2.2 cm in size and extended to the brainstem surface without displacing it. What is the Koos grading of this tumor?

- A. Grade 1
- B. Grade 2
- C. Grade 3
- D. Grade 4
- E. Grade 5

▸▸ Question 9

A patient presents with facial nerve palsy. On examination, this patient has obvious but not disfiguring asymmetry of face, slight to moderate motion of forehead, complete closure of eye with effort, and slightly weak mouth with maximal effort. What is the House and Brackmann facial nerve grading in this patient?

- A. Grade 1
- B. Grade 2
- C. Grade 3
- D. Grade 4
- E. Grade 5

▸▸ Question 10

A patient presents with vestibular schwannoma in your clinic. What are the treatment options in this patient?

- A. Surgery through translabyrinthine approach
- B. Surgery through retrosigmoid approach
- C. Surgery through subtemporal approach
- D. Stereotactic radiosurgery
- E. All of the above

▸▸ Question 11

All of the following are desirable for diagnosis of schwannoma except?

- A. Verocay bodies
- B. Subcapsular lymphocytes
- C. Hyalinized blood vessels
- D. Lattice-like pattern of CD34 staining
- E. Loss of SMARCB1 expression

▸▸ Question 12

What is the most common subtype of hybrid nerve sheath tumors?

- A. Schwannoma/perineurioma
- B. Neurofibroma/schwannoma
- C. Neurofibroma/perineurioma

▸▸ Question 13

Which of the following features is not associated with a favorable prognosis for MPNST?

- A. Smaller tumor size
- B. Female gender
- C. GTR
- D. No mets at presentation
- E. No association with prior XRT

▸▸ Question 14

Which of the following tumors of cauda equina demonstrate dilated ectatic blood vessels with a cap sign on T2MRI or GRASS MRI?

- A. Myxopapillary ependymoma
- B. Astrocytoma
- C. Cavernoma
- D. Cauda equina NET
- E. AVM

▸▸ Question 15

A 45-year-old female presented in OPD department with sudden hearing loss (SHL). Treatment options of SHL include all of the following except?

- A. 60-mg prednisone QID × 10 days
- B. Famciclovir 500 mg TID × 10 days
- C. Intravenous heparin
- D. Conservative
- E. Thrombolytic therapy

▸▸ Question 16

On histopathology of vestibular schwannomas along with Antoni A and Antoni B fibers, which of the following can be present?

- A. Psammoma bodies
- B. Verocay bodies
- C. Langerhans cells
- D. Calcifications
- E. Neovascularization

▸▸ Question 17

On the first postoperative day of cerebellopontine angle space occupying lesion (CPA SOL) of a patient, you observed the patient had obvious asymmetry of face, slight to moderate movement of forehead, and complete eye closure with effort. What is the facial nerve palsy grading according to House and Brackmann?

- A. I
- B. II
- C. III
- D. IV
- E. V

▸▸ **Question 18**

For auditory brainstem responses (ABR), which of the following is true?

- A. Diagnosis of hearing loss
- B. Assess the inferior vestibular nerve
- C. Assess the superior vestibular nerve
- D. Prognosticator for hearing preservation
- E. Cannot be assessed in deaf ear

▸▸ **Question 19**

After gross total excision of vestibular schwannoma, when should MRI be done?

- A. Within 72 hours after surgery
- B. At 3 months
- C. At 6 months
- D. At 1 year
- E. At 5 years

▸▸ **Question 20**

In Koos grading system, what is the grade of a vestibular schwannoma (VS) protruding into CPA, not reaching brainstem, with approximate volume of 0.6 cc?

- A. I
- B. II
- C. III
- D. IV
- E. V

▸▸ **Question 21**

What is the normal diameter of IAC?

- A. 0.5 to 0.8 cm
- B. 0.8 to 1 cm
- C. 0.3 to 0.5 cm
- D. 0.4 to 1 cm
- E. 0.1 to 0.5 cm

▸▸ **Question 22**

In which of the following, serviceable hearing is unlikely to be preserved postoperatively?

- A. Preoperative SDS < 75%
- B. Preoperative PTA loss > 25 dB
- C. Preoperative BAER has abnormal wave morphology
- D. Tumor > 2 to 2.5 cm diameter
- E. All of the above

▸▸ **Question 23**

Malignant peripheral nerve sheath tumors are usually associated with which of the following?

- A. NF2
- B. NF1
- C. Li Fraumeni syndrome
- D. Tuberous sclerosis
- E. Terson syndrome

▸▸ **Question 24**

Which of the following structures can be sacrificed in retrosigmoid approach for CPA tumor resection?

- A. Facial nerve
- B. Greater occipital nerve
- C. Petrosal vein
- D. Superior cerebellar artery
- E. PICA

▸▸ **Question 25**

What is the 7th cranial nerve preservation rate in retrosigmoid removal of vestibular schwannoma (VS) when the tumor is > 2 cm?

- A. 26 to 30%
- B. 30 to 50%
- C. 50 to 76%
- D. 70 to 86%
- E. 80 to 96%

Answers

▸▸ **Answer 1**

Correct answer is E. All of the above[1]

▸▸ **Answer 2**

Correct answer is B. Neurofibroma[2]

▸▸ **Answer 3**

Correct answer is D. Always associated with nerve fiber[3]

▸▸ **Answer 4**

Correct answer is B. Schwannoma/perineuroma[4]

▸▸ **Answer 5**

Correct answer is B. A + Schwann cells[5]

▸▸ **Answer 6**

Correct answer is B. Female gender and Hispanic white race[6]

▸▸ **Answer 7**

Correct answer is C. Cauda equina neuroendocrine tumor[7]

▸▸ Answer 8

Correct answer is C. Grade 3[8]

▸▸ Answer 9

Correct answer is C. Grade 3[9]

▸▸ Answer 10

Correct answer is E. All of the above[10]

▸▸ Answer 11

Correct answer is D. Lattice-like pattern of CD34 staining[1]

▸▸ Answer 12

Correct answer is A. Schwannoma/perineurioma[4]

▸▸ Answer 13

Correct answer is B. Female gender[5]

▸▸ Answer 14

Correct answer is D. Cauda equina NET[7]

▸▸ Answer 15

Correct answer is B. Famciclovir 500 mg TID × 10 days[11]

▸▸ Answer 16

Correct answer is B. Verocay bodies[12]

▸▸ Answer 17

Correct answer is C. III[9]

▸▸ Answer 18

Correct answer is D. Prognosticator for hearing preservation[13]

▸▸ Answer 19

Correct answer is D. At 1 year[14]

▸▸ Answer 20

Correct answer is B. II

▸▸ Answer 21

Correct answer is A. 0.5 to 0.8 cm[14]

▸▸ Answer 22

Correct answer is E. All of the above[15]

▸▸ Answer 23

Correct answer is B. NF1[5]

▸▸ Answer 24

Correct answer is C. Petrosal vein[16]

▸▸ Answer 25

Correct answer is C. 50 to 76%[17]

References

[1] Greenberg M, ed. Greenberg's Handbook of Neurosurgery. 10th ed. New York: Thieme; 2023:768
[2] Greenberg M, ed. Greenberg's Handbook of Neurosurgery. 10th ed. New York: Thieme; 2023:771
[3] Greenberg M, ed. Greenberg's Handbook of Neurosurgery. 10th ed. New York: Thieme; 2023:772
[4] Greenberg M, ed. Greenberg's Handbook of Neurosurgery. 10th ed. New York: Thieme; 2023:773
[5] Greenberg M, ed. Greenberg's Handbook of Neurosurgery. 10th ed. New York: Thieme; 2023:774
[6] Greenberg M, ed. Greenberg's Handbook of Neurosurgery. 10th ed. New York: Thieme; 2023:775
[7] Greenberg M, ed. Greenberg's Handbook of Neurosurgery. 10th ed. New York: Thieme; 2023:776
[8] Greenberg M, ed. Greenberg's Handbook of Neurosurgery. 10th ed. New York: Thieme; 2023:784
[9] Greenberg M, ed. Greenberg's Handbook of Neurosurgery. 10th ed. New York: Thieme; 2023:779
[10] Greenberg M, ed. Greenberg's Handbook of Neurosurgery. 10th ed. New York: Thieme; 2023:785
[11] Greenberg M, ed. Greenberg's Handbook of Neurosurgery. 10th ed. New York: Thieme; 2023:778
[12] Greenberg M, ed. Greenberg's Handbook of Neurosurgery. 10th ed. New York: Thieme; 2023:777
[13] Greenberg M, ed. Greenberg's Handbook of Neurosurgery. 10th ed. New York: Thieme; 2023:782
[14] Greenberg M, ed. Greenberg's Handbook of Neurosurgery. 10th ed. New York: Thieme; 2023:783
[15] Greenberg M, ed. Greenberg's Handbook of Neurosurgery. 10th ed. New York: Thieme; 2023:791
[16] Greenberg M, ed. Greenberg's Handbook of Neurosurgery. 10th ed. New York: Thieme; 2023:793
[17] Greenberg M, ed. Greenberg's Handbook of Neurosurgery. 10th ed. New York: Thieme; 2023:797

46 Meningiomas (Intracranial)

Questions

▸▸ Question 1

A patient presents with a long history of headache. MRI shows isointense lesion on T1 while hypointense on T2, signal voids showing calcifications, densely enhancing broad-based attachment to dura, and a dural tail. Hyperostosis of the adjacent bone and homogenously hyperdense lesion on CT of brain are also seen. Meningiomas are the most common primary intracranial tumors in adults, representing 36.4% of CNS tumors that arise from meningothelial cells of arachnoid membrane. Following statements are correct regarding these tumors except?

- A. Most are slow growing benign tumors, with 32% of incidentally discovered meningiomas showing no growth over 3 years follow-up
- B. They are most commonly located along falx, convexity and sphenoid bone
- C. Psammoma bodies are round, microscopic, calcified structures having a concentric laminated appearance
- D. Chordoid and clear cell subtypes have been assigned grade 1 tumor with low rate of recurrence
- E. The most common subtypes of meningioma are meningothelial, fibrous, and transitional

▸▸ Question 2

On histopathology, a meningioma is found to have syncytia-like lobules of epithelioid cells with some nuclei appearing to have holes and pseudoinclusions. Cells resemble arachnoid cap cells mimicking meningothelial hyperplasia which was found adjacent to the optic glioma. Whorls and psammoma bodies are less frequent in this tumor. What is the most likely subtype of this meningioma?

- A. Meningothelial meningioma
- B. Fibrous meningioma
- C. Transitional meningioma
- D. Psammomatous meningioma
- E. Angiomatous meningioma

▸▸ Question 3

The most common locations of meningioma in brain are parasagittal accounting for 20.8%, then convexity (15.2%) and then tuberculum sellae which accounts for 12.8%, and fourth is the sphenoid wing meningioma which accounts for 11.9%. Which of the following statements is correct regarding sphenoid wing meningioma?

- A. It has three basic categories depending on the origin from the sphenoid wing
- B. Behavior and treatment of lateral sphenoid wing (pterional) meningioma are similar to convexity meningioma
- C. Middle third meningiomas are also called as alar meningioma
- D. Medial (clinoidal) meningiomas tend to encase the ICA and the MCA as well as cranial nerves in the region of the superior orbital fissure and the optic nerve. Total removal of this type is often not possible
- E. All of the above are correct

▸▸ Question 4

A patient presents with anosmia, ipsilateral optic atrophy, and contralateral papilledema (Foster Kennedy syndrome). On further evaluation, the patient is found to have apathy, abulia, urinary incontinence, and memory disturbances. Plain MRI of brain and with IV contrast found olfactory groove meningioma. Why is embolization contraindicated in these tumors?

- A. It is very difficult to embolize these tumors
- B. It gets 70 to 80% of blood supply from anterior cerebral artery which is not embolized due to risk of ophthalmic artery embolization and blindness
- C. It gets 70 to 80% of blood supply from anterior ethmoidal artery which is not embolized due to risk of ophthalmic artery embolization and blindness
- D. Embolization of perforating arteries can lead to loss of olfaction in these cases
- E. Wrong embolization poses high risk of brain stem damage

▸▸ Question 5

Parasagittal meningiomas are grouped based on AP direction of the superior sagittal sinus and their location along this direction. Anterior meningiomas are found between ethmoidal plate and coronal suture (44%), middle meningiomas are found between coronal suture and lambdoidal suture accounting for 33%, while posterior meningiomas are found between lambdoid suture and torcular Herophili accounting for 23%. Which of the following statements is not correct regarding Sindou grading system for meningioma invasion of superior sagittal sinus?

- A. Type 1 meningiomas are attached to the lateral wall of sinus
- B. Type 2 meningiomas cause invasion of lateral recess, while type 3 meningiomas cause invasion of lateral wall
- C. Type 4 meningiomas cause invasion of roof of sinus
- D. In type 5, there is incomplete occlusion of sinus with contralateral wall spared
- E. In type 6, there is total sinus occlusion with invasion of contralateral wall

▸▸ Question 6

A patient presents with gradual onset of bitemporal hemianopia, and on examination he is found to have a tumor which originated in the middle cranial fossa, and the site of origin is only 2 cm posterior to that of the olfactory groove meningioma. Which of the following statements is correct regarding these tumors and anatomy of region from where these arise?

- A. This tumor is tuberculum sellae meningioma
- B. Tuberculum sellae is the bony elevation between the chiasmatic sulcus and the sella turcica
- C. Planum sphenoidale, which is the anterior margin of charismatic sulcus, is the demarcation between anterior and middle cranial fossa
- D. Posteriorly growing tuberculum sellae meningioma can mimic pituitary macroadenoma
- E. All of the above

▸▸ **Question 7**

Which of the following is an environmental risk for development of meningioma?

- A. Ionization radiation such as children exposed to ionizing radiation while treating leukemia
- B. Hormonal exposure such as in women receiving hormonal replacement therapy
- C. Mutation of NF2 tumor suppresser gene on chromosome 22q12.2
- D. Those which are associated with NF2 or NF1
- E. Mutations in AKT1, TRAF7, and SMO

▸▸ **Question 8**

Meningiomas characteristically have external carotid artery feeders. What are some notable exceptions where they are fed from the ICA?

- A. Low frontal median meningiomas, for example, olfactory groove, are fed from ethmoidal branches of the ophthalmic artery
- B. Suprasellar meningiomas may also be fed by large branches of the ophthalmic arteries
- C. Parasellar meningiomas tend to be fed from the ICA while secondary vascular supply may be derived from pial branches of the anterior, middle, and posterior cerebral arteries
- D. Petroclival meningiomas are supplied via the artery of tentorium also known as artery of Bernasconi and Cassinari
- E. All of the above

▸▸ **Question 9**

A patient with meningioma is symptomatic, with significant growth on serial imaging (more than 2.5 mm increase in diameter over 1 year) and marked perilesional edema. Excision was done. Postoperative images showed residual tumor with histology report showing anaplastic lesion. Hence, this patient was given postoperative radiotherapy and further treated with MRI-guided laser interstitial thermal therapy. Which of the following is incorrect regarding Simpson grading system for removal of meningioma?

- A. Grade 1 is macroscopically complete removal with excision of dural attachment and abnormal bone, not including sinus resection when involved, with recurrence rate of 9%
- B. Grade 2 is macroscopically complete removal with endothermy coagulation of dural attachment, with recurrence of 19%
- C. Grade 3 is macroscopically complete removal without resection or coagulation of dural attachment or its extradural extension, with recurrence of 29%
- D. Grade 4 is partial removal, removing tumor in situ, with recurrence rate of 44%
- E. Grade 5 is simple decompression with biopsy

▸▸ **Question 10**

Anterior third parasagittal meningiomas can be approached through bicoronal flap with safe division of sinus in this location while posterior to coronal suture, the sinus cannot be divided because of risk of venous drainage compromise. Meningiomas are often very bloody. What is the general principle of meningioma surgery?

- A. Early interruption of arterial blood supply of tumor
- B. Avoid excessive retraction of brain by doing internal decompression of tumor
- C. Dissecting the capsule from the brain
- D. Removal of attached bone and dura when possible
- E. All of the above

▸▸ **Question 11**

Meningiomas are the most common primary intracranial tumors that arise from meningothelial cells of which of the following?

- A. Dura
- B. Arachnoid
- C. Pia
- D. Ependymal lining of ventricles
- E. Radial cells

▸▸ **Question 12**

What are the round, microscopic, calcified structures having concentric, laminated appearance, possibly formed as a tumoricidal defense mechanism, found in meningiomas called?

- A. Psammoma bodies
- B. Mallory bodies
- C. Michaelis Gutmann bodies
- D. Schiller Duval bodies
- E. Verocay bodies

▸▸ **Question 13**

Multiple meningiomas are associated with which of the following?

- A. Neurofibromatosis II
- B. Tuberous sclerosis
- C. Von Hippel Lindau syndrome
- D. Li Fraumeni syndrome
- E. Sturge Weber syndrome

▸▸ **Question 14**

What is the grading criteria for WHO grade 2 meningiomas?

- A. 1–4 mitotic figures in 10 consecutive HPF each of 0.16 mm^2
- B. 4–19 mitotic figures in 10 consecutive HPF each of 0.16 mm^2
- C. 20–25 mitotic figures in 10 consecutive HPF each of 0.16 mm^2
- D. 25–30 mitotic figures in 10 consecutive HPF each of 0.16 mm^2

▸▸ Question 15

What is the most common location of meningiomas?

- A. Parasagittal
- B. CP angle
- C. Olfactory groove
- D. Intrasylvian
- E. Tuberculum sellae

▸▸ Question 16

Which of the sphenoid wing meningiomas tend to encase ICA and MCA frequently?

- A. Clinoidal
- B. Middle
- C. Alar
- D. Pterional
- E. En masse

▸▸ Question 17

What is the Sindou grade of a meningioma with invasion of lateral recess of superior sagittal sinus?

- A. I
- B. II
- C. III
- D. IV
- E. V

▸▸ Question 18

Regarding meningioma surgical excision, what is the Simpson grade of macroscopically complete excision with endothermy coagulation of dural attachment?

- A. I
- B. II
- C. III
- D. IV
- E. V

▸▸ Question 19

Proposed criteria for significant growth of meningiomas includes all of the following except?

- A. 2–5 mm increase in diameter over 1 year
- B. 1 cc increase in volume in 1 year
- C. 15% increase in volume over 1 year
- D. 5 cc increase in volume in 1 year

▸▸ Question 20

Postoperative radiotherapy is not recommended for which of the following?

- A. WHO grade 1 meningiomas with subtotal resection (STR)
- B. Anaplastic meningioma regardless of extent of resection (EOR)
- C. New atypical meningiomas with STR
- D. Recurrent atypical meningioma regardless of EOR

▸▸ Question 21

Which approach provides ideal extended exposure to medial sphenoid wing meningiomas?

- A. Subfrontal approach
- B. Bicoronal approach
- C. Conventional pterional approach
- D. Fronto-temporo-orbito-zygomotomy (FTOZ)
- E. Anterior transpetrosal approach

Answers

▸▸ Answer 1

Correct answer is D. Chordoid and clear cell subtypes have been assigned grade 1 tumor with low rate of recurrence[1]

▸▸ Answer 2

Correct answer is A. Meningothelial meningioma[2]

▸▸ Answer 3

Correct answer is E. All of the above are correct[3]

▸▸ Answer 4

Correct answer is C. It gets 70 to 80% of blood supply from anterior ethmoidal artery which is not embolized due to risk of ophthalmic artery embolization and blindness[4]

▸▸ Answer 5

Correct answer is D. In type 5, there is incomplete occlusion of sinus with contralateral wall spared[5]

▸▸ Answer 6

Correct answer is E. All of the above[5]

▸▸ Answer 7

Correct answer is A. Ionization radiation such as children exposed to ionizing radiation while treating leukemia[6]

▸▸ Answer 8

Correct answer is E. All of the above[7]

▸▸ Answer 9

Correct answer is A. Grade 1 is macroscopically complete removal with excision of dural attachment and abnormal bone, not including sinus resection when involved, with recurrence rate of 9%[8]

▸▸ Answer 10

Correct answer is E. All of the above[8]

▸▸ Answer 11

Correct answer is B. Arachnoid[1]

▸▸ Answer 12

Correct answer is A. Psammoma bodies[1]

▸▸ Answer 13

Correct answer is A. Neurofibromatosis II[6]

▸▸ Answer 14

Correct answer is B. 4–19 mitotic figures in 10 consecutive HPF each of 0.16 mm[29]

▸▸ Answer 15

Correct answer is A. Parasagittal[3]

▸▸ Answer 16

Correct answer is A. Clinoidal[3]

▸▸ Answer 17

Correct answer is B. II[5]

▸▸ Answer 18

Correct answer is B. II[8]

▸▸ Answer 19

Correct answer is D. 5 cc increase in volume in 1 year[10]

▸▸ Answer 20

Correct answer is A. WHO grade 1 meningiomas with subtotal resection (STR)[11]

▸▸ Answer 21

Correct answer is D. Fronto-temporo-orbito-zygomotomy (FTOZ)[12]

References

[1] Greenberg M, ed. Greenberg's Handbook of Neurosurgery. 10th ed. New York: Thieme; 2023:803
[2] Greenberg M, ed. Greenberg's Handbook of Neurosurgery. 10th ed. New York: Thieme; 2023:804
[3] Greenberg M, ed. Greenberg's Handbook of Neurosurgery. 10th ed. New York: Thieme; 2023:807
[4] Greenberg M, ed. Greenberg's Handbook of Neurosurgery. 10th ed. New York: Thieme; 2023:808
[5] Greenberg M, ed. Greenberg's Handbook of Neurosurgery. 10th ed. New York: Thieme; 2023:809
[6] Greenberg M, ed. Greenberg's Handbook of Neurosurgery. 10th ed. New York: Thieme; 2023:810
[7] Greenberg M, ed. Greenberg's Handbook of Neurosurgery. 10th ed. New York: Thieme; 2023:812
[8] Greenberg M, ed. Greenberg's Handbook of Neurosurgery. 10th ed. New York: Thieme; 2023:815
[9] Greenberg M, ed. Greenberg's Handbook of Neurosurgery. 10th ed. New York: Thieme; 2023:806
[10] Greenberg M, ed. Greenberg's Handbook of Neurosurgery. 10th ed. New York: Thieme; 2023:813
[11] Greenberg M, ed. Greenberg's Handbook of Neurosurgery. 10th ed. New York: Thieme; 2023:814
[12] Greenberg M, ed. Greenberg's Handbook of Neurosurgery. 10th ed. New York: Thieme; 2023:817

47 Mesenchymal, Nonmeningothelial Tumors

Questions

▸▸ **Question 1**

A patient presented in neurosurgery OPD with brain imaging showing meningioma-like features. Surgery was done and histopathology showed variably cellular tumor composed of spindled to ovoid cells arranged around a branching and hyalinized vasculature *and* variable stromal collagen deposition *and* STAT6 nuclear expression. This tumor has a high rate of recurrence as late as decades. What is the most likely diagnosis?

- A. Atypical meningioma
- B. Pleomorphic astrocytoma
- C. Solitary fibrous tumor
- D. Carcinomatous fibrous tumor
- E. None of the above

▸▸ **Question 2**

A patient is found to have tumor with tightly packed capillary-sized and cavernous vessels with a single layer of benign epithelial cells. This tumor is found most commonly in the spine followed by skull and uncommonly in the brain parenchyma, nerve roots, and cauda equina with a predilection for thoracic and lumbar region (often multiple). Following are the imaging findings in a patient with hemangioma except?

- A. Polka-dot sign is found on axial images
- B. Corduroy pattern is found on longitudinal images
- C. Calcifications are very rare in these tumors
- D. T2 MRI shows mixed signal internally
- E. The surrounding hemosiderin ring is low density on T2 with blooming artifact

▸▸ **Question 3**

A patient presents with nausea, vomiting, headache, cerebellar signs, and obstructive hydrocephalus. CT of brain showed low density cystic lesion with contrast enhancing nodule in the posterior fossa, MRI showed serpentine vascular signal voids with cystic lesion, and blood workup showed polycythemia. These tumors are most common primary intra-axial tumors in the adult posterior fossa and 30% of these occur as part of Von Hippel Lindau (VHL) disease. What is the most likely diagnosis in this patient?

- A. Hemangioma
- B. Pilocytic astrocytoma
- C. Epidermoid tumor
- D. Hemangioblastoma
- E. Dermoid tumor

▸▸ **Question 4**

Which of the following statements is incorrect regarding treatment of hemangioblastoma?

- A. Gross total resection with removal of mural nodule and leaving cyst wall is optimal treatment (unless there is evidence of thickened wall cysts with tumor on MRI or direct visualization during surgery)
- B. Preoperative embolization may help reduce the vascularity
- C. Prognosis is excellent following GTR and is better for cases with VHL than for sporadic cases
- D. In case of cystic brainstem hemangioblastoma, solid tumor of the nodule is removed under microscope
- E. Radiotherapy is helpful for multiple small deep lesions, inoperable brainstem hemangioblastomas, for patients who are not surgical candidate, although it does not prevent regrowth following subtotal excision

▸▸ **Question 5**

A 50-year-old male patient presents with backache, pain in legs, sphincter disturbance, and nerve root symptoms. CT and MRI show centrally located bony destruction with an anterior soft tissue mass (with small calcifications) which is confined anteriorly by soft presacral fascia. This lesion is hypointense on T1, hyperintense on T2, and contrast enhancing. A firm fixed mass is palpable between rectum and sacrum on rectal examination. What is the most likely diagnosis in this patient?

- A. Spinal chordoma
- B. Chondrosarcoma
- C. Osteosarcoma
- D. Osteochondroma
- E. Osteoblastoma

▸▸ **Question 6**

Chordomas are rare tumors which arise from remnant of the primitive notochord (which normally differentiates into the nucleus pulposus of the intervertebral disks). Histologically these tumors are considered low grade but still why are these primary malignant tumors?

- A. Difficulty of total removal
- B. A high recurrence rate of 85% following surgery
- C. They metastasize in 5 to 20% of cases
- D. Locally aggressive and osteo-destructive
- E. All of the above

▸▸ **Question 7**

Four types of chordomas have been identified, namely, conventional, chondroid, dedifferentiated, and poorly differentiated. Which statement is incorrect regarding location of chordoma?

- A. Chordoma can arise anywhere along entire the neuraxis where there is remnant of notochord
- B. 35% occur cranially in the spheno-occipital region (clivus)
- C. 53% occur in the spine at the sacrococcygeal region

- D. 3% are intracranial tumors while 1% are primary spine tumors
- E. Less commonly, these may occur in the spine above sacrum

▸▸ Question 8

What is the most appropriate management options regarding chordomas?

- A. For chordomas caudal to the third sacral segment, a posterior approach with wide en block excision and postoperative radiation is usually the best option
- B. Decompression is best avoided because entering the mass serves to spread the tumor (surgically induced metastasis) which will then regrow
- C. Chordomas located in the C2 are usually not amenable to en bloc resection
- D. If s2 nerve roots are the most caudal nerve roots spared, there is 50% chance of normal bladder and bowel function while above this, most will have impaired bladder control and bowel problems
- E. All of the above

▸▸ Question 9

Which statement is correct regarding radiotherapy in chordoma patients?

- A. Radiotherapy does prevent recurrence when done in conjunction with palliative or debulking surgery
- B. It is indicated only for residual, recurrent, or inoperable cases
- C. Best results are obtained only with en bloc excision combined with high dose radiotherapy
- D. Proton beam therapy alone or combined with high-energy X-ray photon therapy is more effective than conventional radiotherapy and is readily available
- E. Early radiation has no effect on longer survival

▸▸ Question 10

Chemotherapeutic agent imatinib (a tyrosine kinase inhibitor) has some antitumor effect in chordoma. Which subtype of chordoma has worse prognosis?

- A. Dedifferentiated
- B. Poorly differentiated
- C. Conventional
- D. Chondroid
- E. Both A and B

▸▸ Question 11

Radiologically, a solitary fibrous tumor may be mistaken for which tumor?

- A. Astrocytoma
- B. Meningioma
- C. Osteosarcoma
- D. Fibrous dysplasia
- E. Oligodendroglioma

▸▸ Question 12

What is the characteristic of WHO grade 3 solitary fibrous tumor?

- A. Hypocellular tumor, < 2.5 mitosis/10 HPF
- B. Dense tumor, > 2.5 mitosis/mm^2 (> 5 mitosis/10 HPF)
- C. Dense tumor, > 5 mitosis/mm^2 (> 10 mitosis/10 HPF)
- D. > 2.5 mitosis/mm^2 (> 5 mitosis/10 HPF) with tumoral necrosis
- E. Dense tumor, > 5 mitosis/mm^2 (> 10 mitosis/10 HPF) with tumoral necrosis

▸▸ Question 13

Which of the following is the most common site of hemangiomas?

- A. Skull
- B. Spine
- C. Brain parenchyma
- D. Nerve roots
- E. Cauda equina

▸▸ Question 14

Which of the following is the most common primary intra-axial tumor in the adult posterior fossa?

- A. Pilocytic astrocytoma
- B. Ependymoma
- C. Choroid plexus papilloma
- D. Hemangioblastoma
- E. Medulloblastoma

▸▸ Question 15

If the cases of intracerebral hemorrhage (ICH) are carefully examined, which tumor is likely to be found as an underlying cause?

- A. AVM
- B. Hemangiomas
- C. Hemangioblastoma
- D. Cavernoma
- E. Hemangioblastoma

▸▸ Question 16

Which of the following is the most common cyst pattern seen in hemangioblastoma?

- A. No associated cyst
- B. Peritumoral cyst alone
- C. Intratumoral cyst
- D. Peritumoral and intratumoral cysts

►► **Question 17**

Which of the following is not an angiographic pattern seen in hemangioblastoma?
- A. Vascular mural nodule on side of avascular cyst
- B. Vascular lesion surrounding avascular cyst
- C. Solid vascular mass
- D. Multiple, separate vascular nodules
- E. Avascular cyst surrounding vascular lesion

►► **Question 18**

Chordoma originates from which of the following layers?
- A. Notochord
- B. Neural crest cells
- C. Mesoderm
- D. Ectoderm
- E. Endoderm

►► **Question 19**

A patient underwent sacrectomy for chordoma. The s2 nerve root was spared. What is the chance of preservation of bladder and bowel control?
- A. 10%
- B. 20%
- C. 30%
- D. 40%
- E. 50%

Answers

►► **Answer 1**

Correct answer is C. Solitary fibrous tumor[1]

►► **Answer 2**

Correct answer is C. Calcifications are very rare in these tumors[2]

►► **Answer 3**

Correct answer is D. Hemangioblastoma[3]

►► **Answer 4**

Correct answer is C. Prognosis is excellent following GTR and is better for cases with VHL than for sporadic cases[4]

►► **Answer 5**

Correct answer is A. Spinal chordoma[5]

►► **Answer 6**

Correct answer is E. All of the above[6]

►► **Answer 7**

Correct answer is D. 3% are intracranial tumors while 1% are primary spine tumors[6]

►► **Answer 8**

Correct answer is E. All of the above[5]

►► **Answer 9**

Correct answer is C. Best results are obtained only with en bloc excision combined with high dose radiotherapy[7]

►► **Answer 10**

Correct answer is E. Both A and B[7]

►► **Answer 11**

Correct answer is B. Meningioma[1]

►► **Answer 12**

Correct answer is D. > 2.5 mitosis/mm^2 (> 5 mitosis/10 HPF) with tumoral necrosis[1]

►► **Answer 13**

Correct answer is B. Spine[1]

►► **Answer 14**

Correct answer is D. Hemangioblastoma[2]

►► **Answer 15**

Correct answer is C. Hemangioblastoma[8]

►► **Answer 16**

Correct answer is B. Peritumoral cyst alone[3]

►► **Answer 17**

Correct answer is E. Avascular cyst surrounding vascular lesion[3]

►► **Answer 18**

Correct answer is A. Notochord[6]

►► **Answer 19**

Correct answer is E. 50%[5]

References

[1] Greenberg M, ed. Greenberg's Handbook of Neurosurgery. 10th ed. New York: Thieme; 2023:821
[2] Greenberg M, ed. Greenberg's Handbook of Neurosurgery. 10th ed. New York: Thieme; 2023:822
[3] Greenberg M, ed. Greenberg's Handbook of Neurosurgery. 10th ed. New York: Thieme; 2023:824
[4] Greenberg M, ed. Greenberg's Handbook of Neurosurgery. 10th ed. New York: Thieme; 2023:825
[5] Greenberg M, ed. Greenberg's Handbook of Neurosurgery. 10th ed. New York: Thieme; 2023:827
[6] Greenberg M, ed. Greenberg's Handbook of Neurosurgery. 10th ed. New York: Thieme; 2023:826
[7] Greenberg M, ed. Greenberg's Handbook of Neurosurgery. 10th ed. New York: Thieme; 2023:828
[8] Greenberg M, ed. Greenberg's Handbook of Neurosurgery. 10th ed. New York: Thieme; 2023:823

48 Melanocytic Tumors and CNS Germ Cell Tumors

Questions

▸▸ Question 1

A patient presents to neurosurgical OPD with MRI showing hyperintensity of leptomeninges with subarachnoid spaces on T1WI and same lesions hypointense on T2WI, with multifocal nodularity and invasion of Virchow-Robin (perivascular) spaces. On histology, there are diffuse, multifocal, primary meningeal melanocytic lesion with invasion of CNS parenchyma, marked cytological atypia, absence of mitotic activity, and necrosis. What is the location of diffuse meningeal melanocytic neoplasms in the brain?

- A. Temporal lobes
- B. Cerebellum
- C. Pons
- D. Medulla
- E. All of the above

▸▸ Question 2

A well-developed, solid, noninfiltrating tumor arises from the leptomeninges, characterized by epithelioid, fusiform, polyhedral, or spindled melanocytes with no evidence of anaplasia, necrosis, or increased mitoses. These lesions are most commonly found in cervical and thoracic spine. What is the most likely diagnosis in this scenario?

- A. Meningeal melanoma
- B. Meningeal melanocytoma
- C. Meningeal melanomatosis
- D. Meningeal melanocytosis
- E. None of the above

▸▸ Question 3

All of the following are included in the essential diagnostic criteria of meningeal melanoma except?

- A. Circumscribed/localized primary melanocytic neoplasm in the meninges
- B. Mitotic count more than 1.5 mitosis/mm^2
- C. Demonstration of GNAQ, GNA11, PLCB4, or CYSLTR2 mutation
- D. Necrosis
- E. Marked cytological atypia

▸▸ Question 4

Meningeal melanomas are pleomorphic, anaplastic, mitotically active, and often invade CNS tissue and may demonstrate necrosis. These tumors may spread through CSF pathways, and occasionally systemic metastases outside the CNS do occur. Which statement regarding management of these tumors is correct?

- A. These are not aggressive tumors
- B. With GTR, prognosis is better than with cutaneous melanoma metastatic to the CNS
- C. These tumors respond well to radiotherapy
- D. Peak age of these tumors is in 4th decade
- E. All of the above

▸▸ Question 5

Germ cell tumors primarily affect children and adolescents with peak age of 10 to 14 years. Which of the following statements is incorrect regarding these tumors?

- A. 80 to 90% of these tumors occur in the midline usually in the suprasellar and pineal region
- B. These tumors are not sensitive to radiotherapy
- C. Simultaneous suprasellar and pineal region lesions is diagnostic of so-called synchronous germ cell tumors which constitutes 13% of germ cell tumors
- D. In the pineal region, these tumors occur predominantly in males while in females germ cell tumors are more common in the suprasellar region
- E. All intracranial germ cell tumors are malignant and may metastasize via CSF and systemically

▸▸ Question 6

Germ cell tumors can (but not always) give rise to tumor markers in the CSF. Which of the following statements is correct?

- A. Choriocarcinoma and 50% of germinoma show elevated levels of beta human chorionic gonadotropin levels in the CSF
- B. Yolk sac tumors, embryonal carcinoma, and occasionally teratoma show elevated levels of alpha-fetoprotein
- C. Intracranial germinomas show elevated serum or CSF levels of placental alkaline phosphate
- D. Many of these tumors are mixed cell type and many pineal region tumors do not give rise to markers
- E. All of the above

▸▸ Question 7

A patient presents with tumor that has germ cell tumor with components exhibiting differentiation along at least two of the three somatic tissue lines (ectoderm, endoderm, mesoderm) and fully differentiated adult type histology and absence of germ cell tumor components. What is the most likely diagnosis in this patient?

- A. Mature teratoma
- B. Immature teratoma
- C. Teratoma with somatic type malignancy
- D. Germinoma
- E. Embryonal carcinoma

▸▸ **Question 8**

Which statement is incorrect regarding germinoma?

- A. These contain large undifferentiated-appearing cells resembling primordial germ cells with ample glycogen-rich clear cytoplasm containing round, vesicular, and centrally placed nuclei
- B. Necrosis is common in these tumors
- C. Mitotic activity is variable
- D. The cells are arranged in sheets, lobules, or cords with trabeculae
- E. Some may have syncytiotrophoblastic giant cells

▸▸ **Question 9**

Which of the following is not included in the essential diagnostic criteria of embryonal carcinoma?

- A. A germ cell tumor with large epithelioid cells
- B. Cytokeratin expression
- C. CD30 or OCT4 expression
- D. Absent or only focal nonmembranous KIT expression
- E. Absence of hCG expression, absence of AFP expression, and absence of other germ cell tumor components

▸▸ **Question 10**

Which of the following is a feature if choriocarcinoma?

- A. Only syncytiotrophoblasts are seen
- B. Only cytotrophoblastic elements are visible
- C. Both syncytiotrophoblasts and cytotrophoblasts are seen
- D. It shows APD expression
- E. There is CD30 expression

▸▸ **Question 11**

How are primary CNS melanocytic tumors distinguished from other pigmented CNS neoplasms like melanotic nerve sheath tumors?

- A. Location
- B. Negri bodies
- C. Tissue histology
- D. Molecular analysis
- E. Alkylation profiling

▸▸ **Question 12**

What is the most common location of germ cell tumors in females?

- A. Suprasellar
- B. Pineal region
- C. CP angle
- D. Cisterna magna
- E. Interpeduncular cistern

▸▸ **Question 13**

Regarding germ cell tumors, which CSF tumor marker is expressed in almost 100% of choriocarcinomas?

- A. Beta HCG
- B. ALP
- C. PLAP
- D. AFP
- E. INF

▸▸ **Question 14**

What is the diagnostic criterion for mature teratoma?

- A. A germ cell tumor with components exhibiting differentiation along all three somatic tissue lines
- B. Fully differentiated
- C. Dedifferentiated
- D. Fetal histology
- E. Presence of embryonal germ cell components

▸▸ **Question 15**

Absence of all of the following is essential for diagnosis of choriocarcinoma except?

- A. KIT
- B. AFP
- C. CD30
- D. OCT4
- E. β-HCG

Answers

▸▸ **Answer 1**

Correct answer is E. All of the above[1]

▸▸ **Answer 2**

Correct answer is B. Meningeal melanocytoma[2]

▸▸ **Answer 3**

Correct answer is C. Demonstration of GNAQ, GNA11, PLCB4, or CYSLTR2 mutation[3]

▸▸ **Answer 4**

Correct answer is B. With GTR, prognosis is better than with cutaneous melanoma metastatic to the CNS[3]

▸▸ **Answer 5**

Correct answer is B. These tumors are not sensitive to radiotherapy[3]

▸▸ Answer 6

Correct answer is E. All of the above[4]

▸▸ Answer 7

Correct answer is A. Mature teratoma[5]

▸▸ Answer 8

Correct answer is B. Necrosis is common in these tumors[6]

▸▸ Answer 9

Correct answer is B. Cytokeratin expression[7]

▸▸ Answer 10

Correct answer is C. Both syncytiotrophoblasts and cytotrophoblasts are seen[8]

▸▸ Answer 11

Correct answer is D. Molecular analysis[1]

▸▸ Answer 12

Correct answer is A. Suprasellar[4]

▸▸ Answer 13

Correct answer is A. Beta HCG[4]

▸▸ Answer 14

Correct answer is B. Fully differentiated[5]

▸▸ Answer 15

Correct answer is E. β-HCG[8]

References

[1] Greenberg M, ed. Greenberg's Handbook of Neurosurgery. 10th ed. New York: Thieme; 2023:829
[2] Greenberg M, ed. Greenberg's Handbook of Neurosurgery. 10th ed. New York: Thieme; 2023:830
[3] Greenberg M, ed. Greenberg's Handbook of Neurosurgery. 10th ed. New York: Thieme; 2023:831
[4] Greenberg M, ed. Greenberg's Handbook of Neurosurgery. 10th ed. New York: Thieme; 2023:832
[5] Greenberg M, ed. Greenberg's Handbook of Neurosurgery. 10th ed. New York: Thieme; 2023:833
[6] Greenberg M, ed. Greenberg's Handbook of Neurosurgery. 10th ed. New York: Thieme; 2023:835
[7] Greenberg M, ed. Greenberg's Handbook of Neurosurgery. 10th ed. New York: Thieme; 2023:836
[8] Greenberg M, ed. Greenberg's Handbook of Neurosurgery. 10th ed. New York: Thieme; 2023:838

49 Hematolymphoid Tumors Involving the CNS

Questions

▸▸ **Question 1**

A 50-year-old patient presents in OPD with symptoms of mental status changes, increased ICP, generalized seizure, and multiple cranial palsies. Risk factors for CNS lymphomas are immunosuppression (AIDS, transplants), Epstein-Barr virus, and collagen vascular disease. What is the best statement regarding management of these tumors?

- A. Treatment is usually with radiotherapy and steroids with very good response initially to steroids (short-lived disappearance also known as "Ghost Tumors")
- B. There can be a need for placement of ventricular access reservoir for chemotherapy
- C. Biopsy should be taken prior to commencement of treatment to confirm the diagnosis
- D. Debulking of extremely large tumors causing symptoms should be done
- E. All of the above

▸▸ **Question 2**

The essential diagnostic criteria for primary diffuse large B-cell lymphoma of the CNS are biopsy-proven mature large B-cell lymphoma confined to the CNS at presentation *and* expression of one or more B-cell markers (CD20, CD19, CD22, CD79a, PAX5). Which of the following are other types of CNS lymphoma?

- A. Immunodeficiency-associated CNS lymphoma (AIDS related, EBV related, lymphomatoid granulomatosis)
- B. Intravascular large B-cell lymphoma
- C. Miscellaneous rare lymphomas in the CNS (low grade B-cell lymphomas, T-cell and NK/T-cell lymphomas, anaplastic large lymphoma)
- D. Extranodal marginal zone lymphoma of mucosa-associated lymphoid tissue (MALT lymphoma) of the dura
- E. All of the above

▸▸ **Question 3**

Following are the conditions with increased risk of CNS lymphoma except?

- A. Collagen vascular disease (SLE, Sjogren's syndrome, rheumatoid arthritis)
- B. Organ transplant recipients (post-transplant lymphoproliferative disease) and AIDS patient
- C. Low incidence in elderly due to good immune system in these patients
- D. Severe congenital immunodeficiency syndrome
- E. Epstein-Barr virus related

▸▸ **Question 4**

What are the common sites of primary CNS lymphomas (PCNSL)?

- A. Temporal and occipital lobes of brain
- B. Corpus callosum, basal ganglia, periventricular region, and cerebellum
- C. Brainstem, leptomeninges, and spinal cord
- D. Suprasellar region and pineal region
- E. None of the above

▸▸ **Question 5**

A patient presents with painful skin nodules and plaques in the abdomen and lower extremities, fever, cranial neuropathies, and multifocal cerebrovascular events. Biopsy showed malignant lymphoid cells in the small arteries, veins, and capillaries with little or no parenchymal extension. What is the most likely diagnosis in this patient?

- A. Fungal infection of CNS blood vessels
- B. Inflammation of CNS blood vessels due to chronic infection
- C. Intravascular lymphomatosis or angioendotheliomatosis
- D. B cell lymphoma of CNS vasculature
- E. T cell lymphoma of the CNS

▸▸ **Question 6**

Following are the investigations and their findings in PCNSL except?

- A. Multiple hyperdense lesions on CT of brain which are contrast enhancing and shows as fluffy cotton balls
- B. Bright on DWI and isointense to hypointense on ADC map
- C. Low levels of serum lactate dehydrogenase indicates rapid cell turnover and is an independent poor prognosticator
- D. Sensitivity of CSF analysis is higher when more than 10.5 mL of CNS is taken with up to 3 LPs
- E. Immunoglobulin analysis shows a single elevated immunoglobulin heavy chain band with lymphoma

▸▸ **Question 7**

Radiation therapy for PCNSL consists of whole brain radiation after biopsy with 40 to 50 gray total dose in 1.8 to 3 gray daily fraction while chemotherapeutic agents are methotrexate, which is given through intraventricular access device with 6 doses of 12 mg twice a week combined with IV leucovorin, and rituximab. What is the management for overdosage of methotrexate?

- A. Ventricular lumbar perfusion over several hours with 240 mL of warm saline, 2000 U of carboxypeptidase G2 intrathecally with IV dexamethasone and IV leucovorin
- B. Stopping the drug and start draining CSF through LP
- C. Draining the CSF and IV steroids
- D. Stopping the drug and giving IV steroids with intrathecal (IT) leucovorin
- E. None of the above

▸▸ Question 8

With no treatment of PCNLS, median survival is 1.8 to 3.3 months following diagnosis. Which statement is correct regarding median survival after radiotherapy?

- A. There is no effect of radiotherapy on median survival
- B. Median survival is 10 months with 47% at 1 year, 16% at 2 years, 8% at 3 years, and 3 to 4% at 5 years
- C. Median survival is 87% at 1 year, 47% at 2 years, 16% at 3 years, 8% at 5 years
- D. Increase in median survival is according to the age of the patient
- E. There is no role of chemotherapeutic agent on recurrence of the tumor

▸▸ Question 9

The essential diagnostic criteria of immunodeficiency-associated CNS lymphomas are a B cell lymphoma confined to the CNS at presentation, in an immunodeficient patient *and* EBV positivity of tumor cells. What is the median survival of patients with this disease?

- A. 1 to 3 months
- B. 3 to 5 months
- C. 5 to 7 months
- D. 7 to 9 months
- E. 9 to 11 months

▸▸ Question 10

A patient presents with tender enlarging skull mass. Skull X-ray shows round or oval, sclerotic, punched-out skull lesion with sharply defined margins, involving both inner and outer tables (the disease begins in the diploic space) often with beveled edges, and a central bone density is occasionally noted. CT of brain showed characteristic appearance of a soft tissue mass within area of bony destruction having a central density. What is the location of Langerhans cell histiocytosis?

- A. Craniofacial bones and skull base favoring the parietal and frontal bones
- B. Hypothalamic pituitary region
- C. Meninges
- D. Choroid plexus
- E. All of the above

▸▸ Question 11

What is the pathologic difference between primary and secondary CNS lymphomas?

- A. N/C ratio
- B. Mitotic activity
- C. Ki67 index
- D. Hyper-/hypochromasia
- E. No difference

▸▸ Question 12

What is the most common supratentorial location of PCNSL?

- A. Frontal lobe
- B. Temporal lobe
- C. Parietal lobe
- D. Occipital lobe
- E. Cerebellum

▸▸ Question 13

Which virus is most frequently associated with PCNSL in AIDS patient?

- A. Epstein Barr
- B. *H. influenzae*
- C. Human papilloma virus
- D. Norovirus
- E. Respiratory syncytial virus

▸▸ Question 14

What is the histopathologic workup to differentiate B-cell from T-cell variant of PCNSL?

- A. Gram staining
- B. Light microscopy
- C. Frozen section
- D. Electron microscopy
- E. Immunohistochemical stains

▸▸ Question 15

A patient presented with PCNSL. He was sent to ophthalmologist for visual problems and an intra-ocular lymphoma was diagnosed. At what dose of radiotherapy the ocular lymphoma can be managed?

- A. 5 Gy
- B. 7 Gy
- C. 15 Gy
- D. 45 Gy
- E. 54 Gy

▸▸ Question 16

Regarding CSF examination in PCNSL, proteomics may show elevated CSF levels of which of the following?

- A. Antithrombin III
- B. IgG bands
- C. LDH
- D. Lactate
- E. Wide bands

▸▸ Question 17

The standard treatment after tissue biopsy of PCNSL is whole-brain radiation therapy with total dose of how much?

- A. 4 to 5 Gy
- B. 30 to 40 Gy

- C. 40 to 50 Gy
- D. 54 Gy
- E. 50 to 60 Gy

▸▸ **Question 18**

Regarding chemotherapy for PCNSL, the addition of intraventricular methotrexate delivered through a ventricular access device may result in better survival. What is the rescue drug given intravenously with this regime?

- A. Dexamethasone
- B. Methotrexate
- C. Leucovorin
- D. Avil
- E. Acetaminophen

▸▸ **Question 19**

What is the most common location of Langerhans cell histiocytosis?

- A. Craniofacial bones and skull base
- B. Hypothalamic pituitary region
- C. Occipital bone
- D. Meninges
- E. Choroid plexus

Answers

▸▸ **Answer 1**

Correct answer is E. All of the above[1]

▸▸ **Answer 2**

Correct answer is E. All of the above[2]

▸▸ **Answer 3**

Correct answer is C. Low incidence in elderly due to good immune system in these patients[3]

▸▸ **Answer 4**

Correct answer is B. Corpus callosum, basal ganglia, periventricular and cerebellum[3]

▸▸ **Answer 5**

Correct answer is C. Intravascular lymphomatosis or angioendotheliomatosis[4]

▸▸ **Answer 6**

Correct answer is C. Low levels of serum lactate dehydrogenase indicates rapid cell turnover and is an independent poor prognosticator[5]

▸▸ **Answer 7**

Correct answer is A. Ventricular lumbar perfusion over several hours with 240 mL of warm saline, 2000 U of carboxypeptidase G2 intrathecally with IV dexamethasone and IV leucovorin[5]

▸▸ **Answer 8**

Correct answer is B. Median survival is 10 months with 47% at 1 year, 16% at 2 years, 8% at 3 years, and 3 to 4% at 5 years[6]

▸▸ **Answer 9**

Correct answer is B. 3 to 5 months[6]

▸▸ **Answer 10**

Correct answer is E. All of the above[7]

▸▸ **Answer 11**

Correct answer is E. No difference[1]

▸▸ **Answer 12**

Correct answer is A. Frontal lobe[2]

▸▸ **Answer 13**

Correct answer is A. Epstein Barr[1]

▸▸ **Answer 14**

Correct answer is E. Immunohistochemical stains[3]

▸▸ **Answer 15**

Correct answer is B. 7 Gy[4]

▸▸ **Answer 16**

Correct answer is A. Antithrombin III[5]

▸▸ **Answer 17**

Correct answer is C. 40 to 50 Gy[5]

▸▸ **Answer 18**

Correct answer is C. Leucovorin[5]

▸▸ **Answer 19**

Correct answer is A. Craniofacial bones and skull base[7]

References

[1] Greenberg M, ed. Greenberg's Handbook of Neurosurgery. 10th ed. New York: Thieme; 2023:840
[2] Greenberg M, ed. Greenberg's Handbook of Neurosurgery. 10th ed. New York: Thieme; 2023:841
[3] Greenberg M, ed. Greenberg's Handbook of Neurosurgery. 10th ed. New York: Thieme; 2023:842
[4] Greenberg M, ed. Greenberg's Handbook of Neurosurgery. 10th ed. New York: Thieme; 2023:843
[5] Greenberg M, ed. Greenberg's Handbook of Neurosurgery. 10th ed. New York: Thieme; 2023:844
[6] Greenberg M, ed. Greenberg's Handbook of Neurosurgery. 10th ed. New York: Thieme; 2023:845
[7] Greenberg M, ed. Greenberg's Handbook of Neurosurgery. 10th ed. New York: Thieme; 2023:846

50 Tumors of the Sellar Region

Questions

▸▸ Question 1

Craniopharyngiomas are thought to develop from residual cells of Rathke's pouch (craniopharyngeal duct) in the sellar region. These constitute 5 to 11% of pediatric brain tumors, which makes them the most common non-neuroepithelial intracerebral tumor in children. These tumors are considered benign in histology and malignant in behavior. Why these tumors are malignant in behavior?

- A. Because of distant metastasis of these tumors
- B. Because of extensive damage to the bone in sellar region
- C. Due to involvement of neural tissue which makes them difficult to cure
- D. Because it often involves the floor of the third ventricle with resultant hydrocephalus
- E. Because of damage to optic apparatus

▸▸ Question 2

Craniopharyngiomas, with bimodal age distribution (childhood peak age 5–15 years, adult peak age 45–60 years), and solid and cystic squamous epithelial tumor with stellate reticulum, wet keratin, and basal palisades, tend to arise from the superior anterior margin of pituitary. Which statement is incorrect regarding location and imaging of adamantinomatous craniopharyngiomas?

- A. Most occur in the region of sella turcica and pituitary infundibulum
- B. Most are purely sellar lesions, with rare extension into the suprasellar region
- C. Pure involvement of the third ventricle is more common with the papillary craniopharyngiomas
- D. 90% of adamantinomas exhibit at least two of the following C features: cyst formation, prominent calcifications, contrast enhancement in the cyst wall
- E. Fluid in the cyst varies but usually contains cholesterol crystals

▸▸ Question 3

Papillary craniopharyngioma (CP) constitutes 10% of all CPs and occurs almost exclusively in adults with a mean age of 40 to 55 years. These are less frequently cystic than adamantinomas and are most commonly located at which of the following?

- A. Intrasellar region
- B. Infundibular recess and tuber cinereum of the floor of the third ventricle
- C. Invade extensively into sphenoid sinus
- D. Cause destruction of surrounding bones and grow into these
- E. These extend extensively into the parasellar region

▸▸ Question 4

Arterial feeders that supply the craniopharyngiomas arise from which artery?

- A. Anterior cerebral artery
- B. Anterior communicating artery
- C. Internal carotid artery
- D. Posterior communicating artery
- E. All of the above

▸▸ Question 5

Which of the following statements is incorrect regarding treatment of craniopharyngioma?

- A. With microscope possible approaches through subfrontal and frontotemporal regions include: subchiasmatic (between optic nerves and anterior to chiasma), opticocarotid region, lamina terminalis, transfrontal–transsphenoidal with drilling of tuberculum sellae
- B. Alternatives to frontotemporal approaches include: pure transsphenoidal, transcallosal, combined subfrontal pterional approach and extended transnasal transsphenoidal endoscopic resection
- C. Postoperative radiotherapy (XRT) has no role in preventing regrowth when residual is left behind and also it does not cause endocrine dysfunction, optic neuritis, and dementia
- D. Steroids are given in physiologic doses in all patients as all of these are considered hypoadrenal
- E. Diabetes insipidus often shows up early may be as a part of triphasic response and treated initially with fluid replacement

▸▸ Question 6

In most series, 5-year survival after craniopharyngioma (CP) operation is 55 to 85% with 5 to 10% mortality. What is the most cause of mortality in these patients?

- A. From injury to brain stem which causes long tract signs and cranial nerve palsies
- B. Damage to hypothalamus bilaterally which may lead to hyperthermia, somnolence, and loss of thirst sensation
- C. Postoperative malignant hydrocephalus
- D. Postoperative sudden brain herniation
- E. All of the above

▸▸ Question 7

A patient presents with bitemporal hemianopia, hypopituitarism, headache, and diabetes insipidus. Imaging characteristics of these tumors are similar to that of adenomas with cure requiring gross total resection with a higher recurrence rate. These tumors include pituicytoma, granular cell tumor of the sellar region, and spindle cell oncocytoma. Where do these low-grade tumors originate from?

- A. Pituicytes of the neurohypophysis (posterior pituitary)

- B. Infundibulum/pituitary stalk
- C. Pituicytes of anterior pituitary
- D. Remnants of Rathke's pouch
- E. Both A and B

▸▸ Question 8

Pituitary adenoma is a clonal neoplasm of anterior pituitary hormone producing cells which are also called as pituitary neuroendocrine tumors (PitNET). Following are included in the essential diagnostic criteria of pituitary adenoma/PitNET tumors except?

- A. Reticular fiber disruption
- B. Sellar suprasellar location
- C. Histologic features of low-grade neuroendocrine tumors that display destruction of the normal anterior gland acinar structure
- D. Subclassified based on immunoreactivity for pituitary hormones
- E. Subclassified on the basis of lineage-specific transcription factors

▸▸ Question 9

A patient presents with progressive blindness, ophthalmoplegia, CSF rhinorrhea, and hyperprolactinemia in blood. On MRI pituitary tumor with invasion of the surrounding structures was seen with encasement of internal carotid artery and noncontiguous metastasis was seen categorizing this tumor as pituitary carcinoma. What are the suggested management options for invasive pituitary tumors?

- A. Initial surgery by a surgeon with extensive experience in pituitary surgery
- B. If Ki67 index comes out to be more than 3 then p53 immunodetection and mitotic count should be evaluated as potential predictors of tumor's aggressiveness
- C. Repeat surgery should be considered for residual or recurrent tumors while XRT can also be given for clinically relevant tumor remnant with markers that suggest aggressive behavior
- D. Chemotherapy for tumors showing continued growth on Stupp regimen (temozolomide 150–200 mg/m^2 for 5 consecutive days for 28 days with XRT and continued for 6 months if clinical response is evident)
- E. All of the above

▸▸ Question 10

Which of the following is not included in the Hardy's classification (anatomic classification) of invasive pituitary tumors?

- A. Extension includes suprasellar extension (0, A, B, and C) and parasellar extension (D and E)
- B. 0, A, B, and C denote no tumor extension, extension into suprasellar cistern, extension into anterior recess of the third ventricle, and extension into the floor of the third ventricle, respectively
- C. Invasion/spread includes spread into the floor, into the sphenoid sinus, and distant metastasis
- D. Spread/invasion is classified as 1, 2, 3, 4, and 5 which indicate no sellar expansion with tumor < 10 mm, sellar expansion with tumor > 10 mm, localized perforation of sellar floor, diffuse destruction of sellar floor, and spread via CSF or blood, respectively
- E. All of the above statements are correct

▸▸ Question 11

Which craniopharyngioma with epithelium that forms stellate reticulum, wet keratin, and basal palisades and frequently shows CTNNB1 mutations and aberrant nuclear expression of beta-catenin is now considered a distinct tumor differentiated by gene mutation?

- A. Adamantinomatous
- B. Papillary
- C. Pseudopapillary
- D. Xanthochromic
- E. Malignant

▸▸ Question 12

In contrast to adamantinomatous craniopharyngioma which of the following is a part of the diagnostic criteria of papillary craniopharyngioma?

- A. Absence of BRAF p. V600E mutation
- B. Immunoreactivity for BRAF p. V600E
- C. Presence of nuclear beta-catenin immunoreactivity
- D. Presence of CTNNB1 mutation
- E. Keratinizing mature squamous epithelium covering fibrovascular cores or a cyst wall

▸▸ Question 13

All of the following vessels supply blood to craniopharyngioma except?

- A. ACA
- B. A-comm
- C. ICA
- D. P-comm
- E. Basilar artery (BA) bifurcation

▸▸ Question 14

Which of the following is the most common presenting symptom of infundibular tumors?

- A. Hypopituitarism
- B. Headache
- C. Visual field defect
- D. Diabetes insipidus
- E. Secondary amenorrhea

▸▸ Question 15

According to Wilson's anatomic classification for invasive pituitary tumors, what is the grade for localized perforation of the sellar floor?

- A. 1
- B. A

- C. B
- D. 3
- E. C

▸▸ Question 16

If Ki-67 index of an invasive pituitary tumor comes out to be > 3%, then which further investigation is warranted for decision of XRT?

- A. p53 immunodetection
- B. BRAF immunodetection
- C. EGFR immunodetection
- D. PTCH immunodetection
- E. Rb immunodetection

Answers

▸▸ Answer 1

Correct answer is C. Due to involvement of neural tissue which makes them difficult to cure[1]

▸▸ Answer 2

Correct answer is B. Most are purely sellar lesions, with rare extension into the suprasellar region[2]

▸▸ Answer 3

Correct answer is B. Infundibular recess and tuber cinereum of the floor of the third ventricle[3]

▸▸ Answer 4

Correct answer is E. All of the above[3]

▸▸ Answer 5

Correct answer is C. Postoperative radiotherapy (XRT) has no role in preventing regrowth when residual is left behind and also it does not cause endocrine dysfunction, optic neuritis, and dementia[4]

▸▸ Answer 6

Correct answer is B. Damage to hypothalamus bilaterally which may lead to hyperthermia, somnolence, and loss of thirst sensation[5]

▸▸ Answer 7

Correct answer is E. Both A and B[6]

▸▸ Answer 8

Correct answer is A. Reticular fiber disruption[7]

▸▸ Answer 9

Correct answer is E. All of the above[8]

▸▸ Answer 10

Correct answer is E. All of the above statements are correct[9]

▸▸ Answer 11

Correct answer is A. Adamantinomatous[2]

▸▸ Answer 12

Correct answer is B. Immunoreactivity for BRAF p. V600E[3]

▸▸ Answer 13

Correct answer is E. Basilar artery (BA) bifurcation[3]

▸▸ Answer 14

Correct answer is C. Visual field defect[10]

▸▸ Answer 15

Correct answer is D. 3[9]

▸▸ Answer 16

Correct answer is A. p53 immunodetection[8]

References

[1] Greenberg M, ed. Greenberg's Handbook of Neurosurgery. 10th ed. New York: Thieme; 2023:849
[2] Greenberg M, ed. Greenberg's Handbook of Neurosurgery. 10th ed. New York: Thieme; 2023:850
[3] Greenberg M, ed. Greenberg's Handbook of Neurosurgery. 10th ed. New York: Thieme; 2023:851
[4] Greenberg M, ed. Greenberg's Handbook of Neurosurgery. 10th ed. New York: Thieme; 2023:852
[5] Greenberg M, ed. Greenberg's Handbook of Neurosurgery. 10th ed. New York: Thieme; 2023:854
[6] Greenberg M, ed. Greenberg's Handbook of Neurosurgery. 10th ed. New York: Thieme; 2023:855
[7] Greenberg M, ed. Greenberg's Handbook of Neurosurgery. 10th ed. New York: Thieme; 2023:856
[8] Greenberg M, ed. Greenberg's Handbook of Neurosurgery. 10th ed. New York: Thieme; 2023:858
[9] Greenberg M, ed. Greenberg's Handbook of Neurosurgery. 10th ed. New York: Thieme; 2023:857
[10] Greenberg M, ed. Greenberg's Handbook of Neurosurgery. 10th ed. New York: Thieme; 2023:853

51 PitNET/Adenomas—Clinical Consideration

Questions

▸▸ Question 1

Most primary pituitary tumors are benign and arise from anterior pituitary gland (adenohypophysis). About 50% of pituitary tumors are less than 50 mm at the time of diagnosis, and these may be difficult to find at the time of surgery. What is the size of microadenomas?

- A. Less than 5 mm
- B. Less than 1 cm
- C. Less than or equal to 1 cm
- D. Less than 8 mm
- E. Any size with no mass effects

▸▸ Question 2

PitNETs arise from the six adenohypophyseal cell types. These comprise 10% of intracranial tumors and peak incidence is in the 3rd and 4th decades of life. What are the most common pituitary tumors?

- A. Prolactinomas
- B. Cortisol producing pituitary tumors
- C. Nonfunctioning PitNETs
- D. Lactotroph tumors
- E. Somatotroph tumors

▸▸ Question 3

A PitNET without cell type specific differentiation based on immunohistochemistry, transcription factors, and negative PAS stain constitutes of 5 to 30% of surgically resected adenomas. These account for 5 to 30% of surgically resected adenomas and typically occur after the age of 60 years. What are these tumors called?

- A. Null cell tumor
- B. Nonfunctioning adenomas
- C. Undifferentiated adenomas
- D. Acidophil stem cell tumor
- E. Mature PIT1-lineage tumor

▸▸ Question 4

Most PitNET/adenomas are sporadic and arise from a somatic mutation of single progenitor cells. However, PitNET may also occur as part of syndromes including which of the following?

- A. Multiple endocrine adenomatosis or neoplasia
- B. Carney complex
- C. Familial isolated pituitary adenoma
- D. McCune-Albright syndrome
- E. All of the above

▸▸ Question 5

A patient presents with bitemporal hemianopia, hydrocephalus, ptosis, facial pain, diplopia, CSF rhinorrhea, and headache (possibly because of increased intrasellar pressure). On imaging, it comes out to be pituitary macroadenoma causing mass effects and panhypopituitarism on investigations. Which pituitary hormone becomes decreased first in this case?

- A. Growth hormone
- B. Gonadotropins (LH, FSH)
- C. TSH
- D. ACTH
- E. Prolactin

▸▸ Question 6

A patient presents with sudden onset of headache, visual disturbance, and loss of consciousness. A plain CT of the brain was done which showed hemorrhagic mass in sella turcica. CTA was done to rule out aneurysmal bleed which came out to be positive. MRI showed it to be a case of pituitary apoplexy. What is the recommended management for this condition?

- A. Hydrocortisone 100 to 200 mg IV bolus followed by 2 to 5 mg/h IV bolus
- B. Rapid decompression within 7 days with transcranial or transsphenoidal approach
- C. Complete removal of tumor is usually not necessary
- D. Ventricular drainage for hydrocephalus is generally required
- E. All of the above

▸▸ Question 7

A women presents with amenorrhea-galactorrhea syndrome (also known as Forbes-Albright syndrome, also known as Ahumadadel Castillo syndrome), infertility, and bones mass loss. What is the most common secretory adenoma?

- A. Gonadotropin secreting tumor
- B. Prolactinoma
- C. Growth hormone secreting tumor
- D. Cortisol secreting tumor
- E. None of the above

▸▸ Question 8

A patient presents with increasing hand and foot size, frontal bossing, prognathism, cardiac arrythmias, hypertension, glucose intolerance, peripheral nerve entrapment syndrome, joints pain, and sleep apnea. Brain imaging with endocrine tests, cardiology consult, and colonoscopy was done in this patient, and surgery is planned for removal of tumor. What is the suggested criteria for biochemical cure of acromegalic patient?

- A. Normal IGF1 level
- B. Growth hormone level less than 5 ng/mL
- C. Growth hormone nadir less than 1 ng/mL after OGST
- D. No residual tumor on MRI of brain
- E. A, B, and C

▸▸ Question 9

A patient presents with buffalo hump like shape, striae over lower abdomen, hyperpigmentation, osteoporosis, and generalized muscle wasting. On lab findings, there was elevated 24-hour urine free cortisol, failure to suppress cortisol with low dose (1 mg) dexamethasone test, normal or elevated ACTH, and hyperglycemia. These tumors constitute 10 to 12% of pituitary adenomas. What is the most likely tumor?

- A. Gonadotrophins
- B. Growth hormone producing tumor
- C. Prolactinomas
- D. ACTH secreting tumor
- E. TSH secreting tumor

▸▸ Question 10

Nonfunctioning pituitary tumors present with mass effect and constitute 15 to 30% pituitary tumors (most common pituitary tumors). These tumors are mostly derived from which cells?

- A. Gonadotroph cells
- B. Lactotroph cells
- C. Somatotroph cells
- D. Thyrotroph cells
- E. Acidophil stem cells

▸▸ Question 11

Predominant secretion of prolactin over GH is seen in which of the following subtype of PIT1 lineage tumors?

- A. Mammosomatotroph tumor
- B. Mature PIT1 lineage tumor
- C. Lactotroph tumor
- D. Immature PIT1 lineage tumor
- E. Acidophil stem cell tumor

▸▸ Question 12

Pituitary tumors represent what percentage of intracranial tumors?

- A. 2%
- B. 5%
- C. 10%
- D. 20%
- E. 30%

▸▸ Question 13

A 40-year-old male presented with sudden severe headache, visual disturbance, and loss of consciousness. A better improvement in ophthalmoplegia can be achieved in pituitary apoplexy if surgery is performed within what time?

- A. 7 days
- B. 10 days
- C. 14 days
- D. 21 days
- E. 1 month

▸▸ Question 14

A 35-year-old female presents with amenorrhea and decreasing vision. Radiology shows pituitary macroadenoma with gross destruction of sellar floor. What is the modified Hardy's (Wilson's) classification grade?

- A. I
- B. II
- C. III
- D. IV
- E. V

▸▸ Question 15

A 30-year-old female with amenorrhea was referred by endocrinologist to your clinic. What is the most common cause of secondary amenorrhea in women of reproductive potential?

- A. Prolactinoma
- B. OCPs
- C. Pregnancy
- D. Forbes Albright syndrome
- E. Ovarian cysts

▸▸ Question 16

A 40-year-old depressive male with centripetal obesity, hypertension, hirsutism, and acne was referred by physician for neurosurgical opinion. Available laboratory reports show decreased ACTH levels. What is the probable source of hypercortisolism in this patient?

- A. Pituitary
- B. Lung/Pancreas tumor
- C. Adrenals
- D. Hypothalamus
- E. Medullary thyroid cancer

▸▸ Question 17

A 50-year-old hypertensive male complains of headache, excessive perspiration, joint pains, sleep apnea, and fatigue. What should an acromegalic patient be screened for?

- A. Thyroid cancer
- B. Colon cancer
- C. Seminomas
- D. Uterine fibroids
- E. Chronic pancreatitis

▸▸ Question 18

A 35-year-old female with visual field defects was referred by ophthalmologist. Which of the following hormones is least

prone to be reduced due to compression of pituitary gland by a macroadenoma?
- A. GH
- B. FSH
- C. LH
- D. Prolactin
- E. TSH

▸▸ Question 19

Simmond's cachexia is associated with which of the following?
- A. Chronic panhypopituitarism
- B. Autoimmune hypophysitis
- C. Acromegaly
- D. Decreased growth hormone levels
- E. Prolactinoma

▸▸ Question 20

What is the most common cause of Cushing syndrome?
- A. Iatrogenic
- B. Transsphenoidal excision of pituitary tumor
- C. Pituitary macroadenoma
- D. Adrenal adenoma
- E. Parathyroid gland tumors

Answers

▸▸ Answer 1

Correct answer is B. Less than 1 cm[1]

▸▸ Answer 2

Correct answer is C. Nonfunctioning PitNETs[1]

▸▸ Answer 3

Correct answer is A. Null cell tumor[1]

▸▸ Answer 4

Correct answer is E. All of the above[2]

▸▸ Answer 5

Correct answer is A. Growth hormone[3]

▸▸ Answer 6

Correct answer is E. All of the above[4]

▸▸ Answer 7

Correct answer is B. Prolactinoma[5]

▸▸ Answer 8

Correct answer is E. A, B, and C[6]

▸▸ Answer 9

Correct answer is D. ACTH secreting tumor[7]

▸▸ Answer 10

Correct answer is A. Gonadotroph cells[8]

▸▸ Answer 11

Correct answer is E. Acidophil stem cell tumor[9]

▸▸ Answer 12

Correct answer is C. 10%[1]

▸▸ Answer 13

Correct answer is A. 7 days[5]

▸▸ Answer 14

Correct answer is D. IV[10]

▸▸ Answer 15

Correct answer is C. Pregnancy[8]

▸▸ Answer 16

Correct answer is B. Lung/Pancreas tumor[8]

▸▸ Answer 17

Correct answer is B. Colon cancer[6]

▸▸ Answer 18

Correct answer is D. Prolactin[3]

▸▸ Answer 19

Correct answer is A. Chronic panhypopituitarism[3]

▸▸ Answer 20

Correct answer is A. Iatrogenic[8]

References

[1] Greenberg M, ed. Greenberg's Handbook of Neurosurgery. 10th ed. New York: Thieme; 2023:861
[2] Greenberg M, ed. Greenberg's Handbook of Neurosurgery. 10th ed. New York: Thieme; 2023:863

[3] Greenberg M, ed. Greenberg's Handbook of Neurosurgery. 10th ed. New York: Thieme; 2023:864
[4] Greenberg M, ed. Greenberg's Handbook of Neurosurgery. 10th ed. New York: Thieme; 2023:865
[5] Greenberg M, ed. Greenberg's Handbook of Neurosurgery. 10th ed. New York: Thieme; 2023:866
[6] Greenberg M, ed. Greenberg's Handbook of Neurosurgery. 10th ed. New York: Thieme; 2023:870
[7] Greenberg M, ed. Greenberg's Handbook of Neurosurgery. 10th ed. New York: Thieme; 2023:868
[8] Greenberg M, ed. Greenberg's Handbook of Neurosurgery. 10th ed. New York: Thieme; 2023:867
[9] Greenberg M, ed. Greenberg's Handbook of Neurosurgery. 10th ed. New York: Thieme; 2023:862
[10] Greenberg M, ed. Greenberg's Handbook of Neurosurgery. 10th ed. New York: Thieme; 2023:857

53 PitNET/Adenomas—General Management

Questions

▸▸ Question 1

Prolactinoma is the only pituitary tumor for which medical therapy (dopamine agonist) is the primary treatment modality (in certain cases). Which of the following statements is incorrect regarding hormone replacement therapy in patients with pituitary hormone deficits?

- A. Indication of corticosteroids administration is inadequate cortisol reserve as demonstrated by failing a cosyntropin stimulation test (failure to achieve peak cortisol level of more than 18 µg/dL in response to cosyntropin)
- B. Physiologic replacement dose of cortisol is 20 mg PO every a.m. and 10 mg PO every 4 p.m. and stress doses may be needed
- C. Thyroid replacement is done before giving cortisol in patients with adrenal deficiency
- D. Hypothyroid patients frequently undergo surgery without adequate replacement with no untoward effect
- E. Testosterone replacement can promote tumor growth and should be waited until stabilization of tumor

▸▸ Question 2

What is the recommended treatment option for tumors secreting growth hormone or ACTH?

- A. An aggressive surgical approach is needed because the secretion product is harmful and effective medical adjuvants are lacking
- B. Growth hormone secreting tumors are pretreated with somatostatin analog therapy to reduce surgical risks
- C. In elderly patients or in tumors more than 4-cm diameter, the tumor is debulked transsphenoidally and then adjuvant radio- or chemotherapy is given
- D. In younger age and tumor size less than 4 cm, radical surgery to remove the whole tumor is done (may utilize cranio-orbito-zygomatic skull base approach)
- E. All of the above

▸▸ Question 3

What is the primary treatment modality for nonfunctioning pituitary adenomas?

- A. Surgical resection
- B. Treatment with dopamine agonists (bromocriptine) and somatostatin analog (octreotide)
- C. Radiotherapy
- D. Only observation
- E. A combination of surgery, radiotherapy, and chemotherapy is needed in all cases

▸▸ Question 4

All of the following are included in the surgical indications of nonfunctioning pituitary macroadenomas except?

- A. Tumors causing symptoms by mass effect, for example, visual field deficits
- B. Tumors with no symptoms of endocrine or visual field deficit but elevated chiasma never need surgical intervention at this point of time
- C. Acute or rapid visual or other neurologic deterioration
- D. To obtain tissue for pathological diagnosis
- E. Nelson's syndrome

▸▸ Question 5

Prolactinomas are essentially the only pituitary adenomas for which medical therapy is sometimes the primary treatment modality. If prolactin levels are more than 500 ng/mL with no acute progression, an initial attempt at purely medical control should be made as the chances of normalizing prolactin surgically with preoperative level more than 500 ng/mL are very low, and these tumors may shrink dramatically with bromocriptine. What are the surgical indications in patients with prolactinomas?

- A. Prolactin levels less than 500 ng/mL in tumors that are not extensively invasive
- B. If there is no significant decrease in prolactin levels in 4 to 6 weeks after medical therapy
- C. If there is no decrease in visual deficits in 4 to 6 weeks after medical therapy
- D. No shrinkage in tumor size on MRI in 4 to 6 weeks after medical therapy
- E. All of the above

▸▸ Question 6

Bromocriptine (Parlodel) is a drug that binds to dopamine receptors (dopamine agonist) on normal and tumor lactotrophs, inhibiting synthesis and secretion of prolactin and other cell processes resulting in decreased cell division and growth. It has side effects of nausea, headache, fatigue, orthostatic hypotension, psychosis, and vasospasm. Following statements regarding bromocriptine therapy are true except?

- A. It frequently reduces the tumor size in 6 to 8 weeks in 75% of patients with macroadenomas
- B. Parlodel is supplied in 2.5 mg scored tablets and 5 mg capsules
- C. Starting dose is 1.25 mg PO every hour, adding 2.5 mg/d as necessary and making dosage change every 2 to 4 weeks for microadenomas and every 3 to 4 days for macroadenomas causing mass effect

- D. To shrink large tumors or for very high prolactin levels, 7.5 mg TID for approximately 6 months is needed, then after that maintenance dose of 5 to 7.5 mg daily is given with initial recheck in about 4 weeks
- E. There is no improvement in tolerance of this medicine with bedtime dosing, with food, or slow dose escalation

▸▸ Question 7

Cabergoline (Dostinex) is a selective D2 dopamine agonist with which control of prolactin and resumption of ovulatory cycles may be better than with bromocriptine. It has side effects of headache, GI symptoms, and cardiac valve disease while it is contraindicated in uncontrolled hypertension or in eclampsia or preeclampsia patients. Which statement regarding its dosage is correct?

- A. It is started at 0.25 mg PO twice weekly and each dose is increased by 0.25 mg every 4 weeks with typical dosage of 0.5 to 1 mg twice weekly
- B. It is started at 0.5 mg PO twice weekly and each dose is increased by 0.25 mg every 4 weeks with typical dosage of 0.5 to 1 mg twice weekly
- C. It is started at 0.25 mg PO twice weekly and each dose is increased by 0.5 mg every 4 weeks with typical dosage of 0.5 to 1 mg twice weekly
- D. It is started at 0.25 mg PO twice weekly and each dose is increased by 0.25 mg every 4 weeks with typical dosage of 5 to 10 mg twice weekly
- E. It is started at 0.25 mg PO twice weekly and each dose is increased by 0.25 mg every 8 weeks with typical dosage of 0.5 to 1 mg twice weekly

▸▸ Question 8

If response to dopamine agonist therapy is satisfactory then treatment is given for 1 to 4 years. What is the indication of discontinuation of this drug?

- A. Decrease in size of prolactinoma to the point with no mass effect and prolactin levels to normal
- B. Microadenomas or macroadenomas that are no longer visible on MRI
- C. Prolactin levels less than 20 ng/mL
- D. Decreasing symptoms of mass effect or prolactin levels
- E. None of the above

▸▸ Question 9

Asymptomatic elderly patients do not require surgery while for other patients, surgery (transsphenoidal) is currently the best initial therapy, providing more rapid reduction in GH levels and decompression. Which of the following statements is correct regarding medical management of acromegaly?

- A. Medical therapy is reserved for patients who are not cured by surgery or who cannot tolerate surgery
- B. Bromocriptine (Parlodel) decreases GH level to less than 10 ng/mL in 54% of cases and to less than 5 ng/mL in only 5% of cases while tumor shrinkage occurs only in 20% of cases
- C. Octreotide (Sandostatin) is a somatostatin analog that reduces GH levels in 71% of cases, reduces IGF 1 level in 93% of cases, while tumor volume is reduced in only 30% of cases
- D. Pegvisomant (Somavert) reduces IGF 1 levels in 97% of cases with treatment for more than 12 months and is given in case of failure of somatostatin therapy
- E. All of the above

▸▸ Question 10

Which of the following is not included in the medical management of Cushing's disease?

- A. If pituitary MRI shows a mass, then transsphenoidal surgery is indicated
- B. If pituitary MRI is negative and IPS sampling is positive, surgery is recommended to look for source and its removal
- C. If pituitary surgery is performed but biochemical cure could not be obtained, then re-exploration is never considered
- D. Stereotactic radiosurgery or medical therapy is indicated in case of failure of surgery to remove the whole tumor
- E. Adrenalectomy can also be considered in patients with failure of all options to remove the pituitary source

▸▸ Question 11

Corticosteroid replacement therapy is indicated when cosyntropin stimulation test fails to achieve a peak cortisol level of what?

- A. > 10 µg/dL
- B. > 12 µg/dL
- C. > 15 µg/dL
- D. > 18 µg/dL
- E. > 20 µg/dL

▸▸ Question 12

After cosyntropin test for cortisol reserves, hormone replacement therapy was advised. What is the physiologic replacement dose?

- A. 20 mg a.m., 20 mg 4 p.m.
- B. 20 mg a.m., 10 mg 4 p.m.
- C. 10 mg a.m., 10 mg 4 p.m.
- D. 10 mg a.m., 20 mg 4 p.m.
- E. 0.5 mg PO at 11 p.m.

▸▸ Question 13

What is the recommended treatment in an elderly patient or > 4-cm size tumor secreting GH/ACTH?

- A. Radical surgery via FTOZ
- B. Transsphenoidal debulking
- C. Medical treatment only
- D. SRS + somatostatin
- E. Pretreatment with somatostatin followed by transsphenoidal debulking

►► Question 14

What is the typical maintenance dose of Parlodel for prolactinoma?
- A. 1.25 mg
- B. 2.5 to 15 mg
- C. 20 mg
- D. 30 mg in divided doses
- E. 50 mg/wk in divided doses

►► Question 15

For medical management of acromegaly, Sandostatin long acting release (LAR) depot injections are given initially at 20 mg intramuscularly at what interval?
- A. Alternative days
- B. Twice weekly
- C. Fortnightly
- D. Every month
- E. After 6 months

►► Question 16

What is the initial dose of ketoconazole for Cushing's disease?
- A. 100 mg OD
- B. 100 mg BID
- C. 200 mg BID
- D. 500 mg BID
- E. 1 g OD

►► Question 17

What is the conventional external beam radiotherapy (EXBRT) for pituitary adenomas?
- A. 12 Gy
- B. 40 to 50 Gy
- C. 59.4 Gy
- D. 60 Gy
- E. 30 Gy with 45 Gy to tumor bed

►► Question 18

A patient is incidentally discovered to have a pituitary macroadenoma which is asymptomatic and nonfunctional. When should the patient undergo first surveillance scan to document rapid growth?
- A. 1 month
- B. 3 months
- C. 6 months
- D. 8 months
- E. 12 months

Answers

►► Answer 1

Correct answer is C. Thyroid replacement is done before giving cortisol in patients with adrenal deficiency[1]

►► Answer 2

Correct answer is E. All of the above[1]

►► Answer 3

Correct answer is A. Surgical resection[2]

►► Answer 4

Correct answer is B. Tumors with no symptoms of endocrine or visual field deficit but elevated chiasma never need surgical intervention at this point of time[2]

►► Answer 5

Correct answer is E. All of the above[3]

►► Answer 6

Correct answer is E. There is no improvement in tolerance of this medicine with bedtime dosing, with food, or slow dose escalation[3]

►► Answer 7

Correct answer is A. It is started at 0.25 mg PO twice weekly and each dose is increased by 0.25 mg every. 4 weeks with typical dosage of 0.5 to 1 mg twice weekly[3]

►► Answer 8

Correct answer is B. Microadenomas or macroadenomas that are no longer visible on MRI[4]

►► Answer 9

Correct answer is E. All of the above[5]

►► Answer 10

Correct answer is C. If pituitary surgery is performed but biochemical cure could not be obtained, then re-exploration is never considered[5]

►► Answer 11

Correct answer is D. > 18 μg/dL[6]

▸▸ Answer 12

Correct answer is B. 20 mg a.m., 10 mg 4 p.m.[1]

▸▸ Answer 13

Correct answer is E. Pretreatment with somatostatin followed by transsphenoidal debulking[1]

▸▸ Answer 14

Correct answer is B. 2.5 to 15 mg[3]

▸▸ Answer 15

Correct answer is D. Every month[5]

▸▸ Answer 16

Correct answer is C. 200 mg BID[7]

▸▸ Answer 17

Correct answer is B. 40 to 50 Gy[8]

▸▸ Answer 18

Correct answer is C. 6 months[2]

References

[1] Greenberg M, ed. Greenberg's Handbook of Neurosurgery. 10th ed. New York: Thieme; 2023:886
[2] Greenberg M, ed. Greenberg's Handbook of Neurosurgery. 10th ed. New York: Thieme; 2023:887
[3] Greenberg M, ed. Greenberg's Handbook of Neurosurgery. 10th ed. New York: Thieme; 2023:888
[4] Greenberg M, ed. Greenberg's Handbook of Neurosurgery. 10th ed. New York: Thieme; 2023:889
[5] Greenberg M, ed. Greenberg's Handbook of Neurosurgery. 10th ed. New York: Thieme; 2023:891
[6] Greenberg M, ed. Greenberg's Handbook of Neurosurgery. 10th ed. New York: Thieme; 2023:881
[7] Greenberg M, ed. Greenberg's Handbook of Neurosurgery. 10th ed. New York: Thieme; 2023:892
[8] Greenberg M, ed. Greenberg's Handbook of Neurosurgery. 10th ed. New York: Thieme; 2023:893

54 PitNET/Adenomas—Surgical Management, Outcome, and Recurrence Management

Questions

▸▸ Question 1

Surgery for pituitary adenomas require medical management just before and after surgery. Which of the following statements regarding medical management of pituitary adenomas undergoing surgery is incorrect?

- A. A hypothyroid patient cannot tolerate surgery until thyroid replacement is done for at least 4 weeks before surgery
- B. For transsphenoidal surgery, polysporin ointment should be applied in both nostrils a night before surgery
- C. 1 g ampicillin + 0.5 g sulbactam should be given IV at midnight and 6 a.m. before surgery
- D. Hydrocortisone sodium succinate (Solu-Cortef) should be given 50 mg IM at 11 p.m. and 6 a.m. before surgery
- E. On call to OR a drip of dextrose 5% lactated ringer with 20 mEq KCL/L plus 50 mg of Solu-Cortef at 75 mL/h is hung and intraoperative 100 mg hydrocortisone IV every 8 hours is given

▸▸ Question 2

What are the indications of transcranial approaches for the surgery of pituitary adenomas?

- A. Minimal enlargement of the sella with a large suprasellar mass, especially if the diaphragma sellae is tightly constricting the tumor (producing a cottage loaf tumor), and the suprasellar component is causing chiasmal compression
- B. Extrasellar extension into the middle fossa that is larger than the intrasellar component
- C. Unrelated pathology that may complicate a transsphenoidal approach, for example, a parasellar aneurysm
- D. Usually fibrous tumor that could not be completely removed on a previous transsphenoidal approach or a recurrent tumor following a previous transsphenoidal surgery
- E. All of the above

▸▸ Question 3

Which of the following statements are correct regarding surgical approaches for pituitary adenomas?

- A. Transsphenoidal approach is indicated for microadenomas, macroadenomas without significant extension laterally beyond the confines of sella turcica, patients with CSF rhinorrhea, and tumors with extension into sphenoid air sinus
- B. Subfrontal approach provides access to both the optic nerves and it may be more difficult in patients with prefixed chiasma
- C. Frontotemporal (pterional) approach places optic nerve and sometimes carotid artery in line of vision of tumor. There is also limited access to intrasellar components using this approach while it provides good access to tumors with significant unilateral extrasellar extension
- D. Subtemporal approach is usually not a viable choice with poor visualization of optic nerve, chiasma, and carotid artery. It also does not allow total removal of intrasellar component
- E. All of the above

▸▸ Question 4

Transsphenoidal surgery can lead to intraoperative disasters which include injury to carotid artery in the lateral aspect of opening. It needs to be packed with fat, fascia, and woven surgical, which can lead to pseudoaneurysm and needs postoperative detection through CT angiography. This pseudoaneurysm is treated endoscopically or with surgical application of clips above and below the pseudoaneurysm. Other intraoperative disaster is injury to the pons which can occur through which of the following?

- A. Opening through the floor of the frontal fossa
- B. Opening through the clivus
- C. By reaching deep through the sella and rongeuring blindly
- D. Opening the floor of sella to extreme laterally
- E. Opening through the inferior clinoid

▸▸ Question 5

Following are the steps in the transsphenoidal surgery to remove pituitary tumor except?

- A. Endoscope is used to locate the middle concha and it is followed posteriorly to identify sphenoid ostium, which is located slightly above the posterior extent of middle concha
- B. Posterior part of the septum is broken and the sphenoid sinus is reached by breaking through the vomer bone
- C. Floor of the sella is opened in the middle using the nasal septum as the midline, using bayoneted chisel or high-speed diamond burr
- D. Dura is opened in plus pattern using bipolar cautery
- E. Tumor is brought into the field using ring curettes and removed with pituitary rongeurs or aspirated with suction

▸▸ Question 6

What is the most common complication after removal of pituitary adenoma?

- A. Transient alteration in ADH levels with diabetes insipidus
- B. Secondary empty sella syndrome
- C. Hydrocephalus with coma
- D. Pituitary abscess or meningitis
- E. CSF rhinorrhea

▸▸ Question 7

In using frontotemporal (pterional) approach for removal of pituitary tumor, right-sided approach is usually employed because of less risk to dominant hemisphere with the exception of which of the following?

- A. When the left eye is the side of worsening
- B. If there is dominant left-sided tumor extension
- C. If there is another pathology on the left side (aneurysm)
- D. If there is some other pathology at that side
- E. All of the above

▸▸ Question 8

Diagnostic criteria for diabetes insipidus is urine output of more than 250 mL/h for 2 hours and urine specific gravity of less than 1.005. Patients after pituitary tumor surgery are placed on DI watch which includes strict intake, output monitoring every 1 hour, urine specific gravity every 4 hour or any time urine output is more than 250 mL/h, and serum electrolytes every 6 hours. Which statement is incorrect regarding postoperative management of these patients?

- A. Basal IV fluid is 5% dextrose with ½ normal saline plus 20 mEq KCL/L at appropriate rate of 75 to 100 mL/h
- B. If urine output is above the basal, then excess is replaced mL to mL with ½ normal saline
- C. If the urine output is too high (more than 300 mL/h for 4 hours or more than 500 mL/h for 2 hours) and urine specific gravity is also less than 1.005, then vasopressin is started with 5 u aqueous vasopressin IV/IM every 6 hours or desmopressin injection SQ or IV in 0.5 to 1 mL (2–4 µg) in two divided doses
- D. Electrolytes with osmolarity every 6 hours are done
- E. Nasal packing is removed on the second postoperative day

▸▸ Question 9

After pituitary surgery, hydrocortisone is tapered in 24 to 48 hours postoperatively. 6 a.m. cortisol level is checked after discontinuing hydrocortisone. Which level of cortisol indicates continuation of hydrocortisone?

- A. Less than 12 µg/dL
- B. Less than 15 µg/dL
- C. Less than 9 µg/dL
- D. Less than 18 µg/dL
- E. Less than 21 µg/dL

▸▸ Question 10

What are the biochemical cure criteria for acromegalic patients after surgery?

- A. IGF 1 levels within age-matched reference range
- B. Basal (morning) serum GH level less than 5 ng/mL
- C. Growth hormone nadir less than 1 ng/mL in OGST
- D. No detectable growth hormone after OGST
- E. A, B, and C

▸▸ Question 11

A 40-year-old male presented with features of hypothyroidism. Thyroid function tests showed decreased TSH and T4 levels while MRI showed a pituitary adenoma. Hormone replacement to correct hypothyroidism usually takes how long?

- A. 3 days
- B. 7 days
- C. 10 days
- D. 4 weeks
- E. 3 months

▸▸ Question 12

Which of the following transcranial approaches is usually not a viable choice due to poor visualization of optic nerve/chiasm and carotids?

- A. Unifrontal
- B. Subfrontal
- C. Bifrotal
- D. Frontotemporal
- E. Subtemporal

▸▸ Question 13

What is the recommended dural opening in endonasal transsphenoidal surgery?

- A. C shaped
- B. Z shaped
- C. Horseshoe shaped
- D. X shaped
- E. + Shaped

▸▸ Question 14

After endonasal transsphenoidal excision of pituitary adenoma, what is the recommended duration for antibiotic cover?

- A. Till nasal pack is removed
- B. Till DI is managed
- C. 24 hours
- D. 7 days
- E. 10 days

▸▸ Question 15

Regarding diagnostic criteria for diabetes insipidus, urinary specific gravity is which of the following?

- A. > 1.030
- B. > 1.020
- C. > 1.010
- D. < 1.030
- E. < 1.005

▸▸ Question 16

For treatment of diabetes insipidus, what is the usual dose of intranasal DDAVP?

- A. 10 to 40 µg BID
- B. 10 mg TDS

- C. 50 μg BID
- D. 50 μg TDS
- E. 20 μg q 06 hours

▸▸ Question 17

Following transsphenoidal excision of pituitary adenoma, MRI to be used as baseline for assessment of recurrence should be obtained after how long?

- A. 24 hours
- B. 48 hours
- C. 72 hours
- D. 3 weeks
- E. 3 months

▸▸ Question 18

After pituitary adenoma excision and initial 48 hours surveillance, when should serum sodium levels be re-checked to avoid symptomatic postoperative hyponatremia?

- A. After 72 hours
- B. Daily for 5 days
- C. Every third day
- D. Days 7 to 8
- E. Weekly for 1 month

▸▸ Question 19

What is the recommended management for tumors demonstrating significant regrowth or symptoms following initial resection?

- A. Surgery
- B. Chemotherapy
- C. Radiotherapy
- D. Chemotherapy with radiotherapy
- E. Watchful waiting

▸▸ Question 20

Following effective treatment of Cushing disease, when does hypertension usually improve?

- A. Does not improve
- B. Within 48 hours
- C. Within a week
- D. Within 6 months
- E. Over a year

Answers

▸▸ Answer 1

Correct answer is A. A hypothyroid patient cannot tolerate surgery until thyroid replacement is done for at least 4 weeks before surgery[1]

▸▸ Answer 2

Correct answer is E. All of the above[2]

▸▸ Answer 3

Correct answer is E. All of the above[2]

▸▸ Answer 4

Correct answer is B. Opening through the clivus[3]

▸▸ Answer 5

Correct answer is D. Dura is opened in plus pattern using bipolar cautery[3]

▸▸ Answer 6

Correct answer is A. Transient alteration in ADH levels with diabetes insipidus[4]

▸▸ Answer 7

Correct answer is E. All of the above[5]

▸▸ Answer 8

Correct answer is E. Nasal packing is removed on the second postoperative day[6]

▸▸ Answer 9

Correct answer is C. Less than 9 μg/dL[6]

▸▸ Answer 10

Correct answer is E. A, B, and C[7]

▸▸ Answer 11

Correct answer is D. 4 weeks[1]

▸▸ Answer 12

Correct answer is E. Subtemporal[2]

▸▸ Answer 13

Correct answer is D. X shaped[3]

▸▸ Answer 14

Correct answer is A. Till nasal pack is removed[5]

▸▸ Answer 15

Correct answer is E. < 1.005[5]

▸▸ **Answer 16**

Correct answer is A. 10 to 40 μg BID[5]

▸▸ **Answer 17**

Correct answer is E. 3 months[7]

▸▸ **Answer 18**

Correct answer is D. Days 7 to 8[5]

▸▸ **Answer 19**

Correct answer is A. Surgery[8]

▸▸ **Answer 20**

Correct answer is E. Over a year[9]

References

[1] Greenberg M, ed. Greenberg's Handbook of Neurosurgery. 10th ed. New York: Thieme; 2023:896
[2] Greenberg M, ed. Greenberg's Handbook of Neurosurgery. 10th ed. New York: Thieme; 2023:897
[3] Greenberg M, ed. Greenberg's Handbook of Neurosurgery. 10th ed. New York: Thieme; 2023:898
[4] Greenberg M, ed. Greenberg's Handbook of Neurosurgery. 10th ed. New York: Thieme; 2023:900
[5] Greenberg M, ed. Greenberg's Handbook of Neurosurgery. 10th ed. New York: Thieme; 2023:901
[6] Greenberg M, ed. Greenberg's Handbook of Neurosurgery. 10th ed. New York: Thieme; 2023:902
[7] Greenberg M, ed. Greenberg's Handbook of Neurosurgery. 10th ed. New York: Thieme; 2023:903
[8] Greenberg M, ed. Greenberg's Handbook of Neurosurgery. 10th ed. New York: Thieme; 2023:906
[9] Greenberg M, ed. Greenberg's Handbook of Neurosurgery. 10th ed. New York: Thieme; 2023:904

Part XIII

Other Tumors and Tumor-Like Conditions

XIII

55 Metastasis to the CNS

Questions

▸▸ Question 1

Cerebral metastases are the most common brain tumors seen clinically. Increasing incidence of cerebral metastasis is due to which factor?

- A. Increasing length of survival of cancer patients as a result of improvement in treatment of primary cancer
- B. Enhanced ability to diagnose CNS tumors due to availability of CT and MRI
- C. Many chemotherapeutic agents do not cross blood–brain barrier providing a heaven for tumor growth there
- D. Some chemotherapeutic agents may transiently weaken the blood–brain barrier and allow CNS seeding with tumor
- E. All of the above

▸▸ Question 2

All of the following tumors spread commonly through the CNS pathways except?

- A. Oligodendroglioma
- B. High-grade gliomas
- C. Embryonal tumors like medulloblastomas
- D. Ependymomas
- E. Pineal region tumors like pineocytoma, germ cell tumor, and pineoblastoma

▸▸ Question 3

A solitary lesion in the posterior fossa of an adult is considered metastasis until proven otherwise. What is the most common location of cerebral metastasis in the supratentorial region parenchyma?

- A. Occipital lobe
- B. Parietal lobe
- C. Temporal lobe
- D. Behind sylvian fissure near the junction of occipital, parietal, and temporal lobe
- E. Near internal capsule

▸▸ Question 4

The most common source of cerebral metastasis in an adult is lungs (44%), which is followed by breast (10%), kidney (7%), and GI (6%). All of the following are sources of cerebral metastasis in pediatric patients except?

- A. Melanoma
- B. Neuroblastoma
- C. Rhabdomyosarcoma
- D. Wilm's tumor
- E. There is zero incidence of cerebral metastasis in pediatric patients

▸▸ Question 5

Small cell lung cancer is more likely to produce cerebral metastasis than any other bronchogenic cell type. Which of the following statements is incorrect regarding management of these tumors?

- A. These are radioresistant tumors
- B. Prophylactic cranial irradiation with whole brain irradiation reduces the incidence of symptomatic brain metastasis and increases survival with 25 Gy in 10 fractions
- C. Surgical resection is considered for immediately life-threatening large lesions
- D. For multiple small cell lung carcinoma brain lesions, 30 Gy radiotherapy in 10 fractions plus chemotherapy is given
- E. For recurrent brain metastasis after failure of initial treatment, radiotherapy with 20 Gy in 10 fractions is given

▸▸ Question 6

Non–small cell lung cancer includes adenocarcinoma, and large cell, squamous cell, and bronchoalveolar tumors. What are the staging studies for known primary lung cancer?

- A. PET scan
- B. Chest scan
- C. Bone scan
- D. Brain CT or MRI
- E. All of the above

▸▸ Question 7

What are the surgical indications in a patient with metastatic melanoma to the brain?

- A. Patients with one to four CNS metastases that can be completely resected when systemic disease is absent or slowly progressive
- B. For symptomatic relief, for example, lesion causing painful pressure
- C. Life-threatening lesion, for example, large posterior fossa lesion causing painful pressure
- D. For hemorrhagic lesions causing symptoms by mass effect due to clot
- E. All of the above

▸▸ Question 8

Following are the predictors of poor outcome in a patient with metastatic melanoma of brain except?

- A. Less than three metastatic lesions within the brain
- B. Development of brain metastasis after the diagnosis of extracranial disease
- C. Elevated lactate dehydrogenase by more than twice the normal
- D. Presence of bone metastasis
- E. Multiple brain metastasis and extensive visceral disease

▸▸ **Question 9**

A patient presents with brain metastasis in neurosurgical OPD. What metastatic workup is needed in this patient?
- A. CT of the chest, abdomen, and pelvis
- B. Radionuclide bone scan
- C. Mammogram in women
- D. Prostate-specific antigen in men and PET scan in all patients with metastasis
- E. All of the above

▸▸ **Question 10**

Which of the following is a highly radioresistant brain metastasis?
- A. Small cell lung cancer
- B. Germ cell tumors
- C. Thyroid cancer
- D. Lymphoma
- E. Leukemia

▸▸ **Question 11**

What is the most common primary CNS tumor responsible for extraneural spread mostly to lung, bone marrow, lymph nodes, and abdomen?
- A. Medulloblastoma
- B. Ependymoma
- C. Butterfly tumor
- D. Teratoma
- E. GBM

▸▸ **Question 12**

Which of the following has the highest incidence of parenchymal cerebral metastases?
- A. Corpus callosum
- B. Posterior to sylvian fissure
- C. Middle frontal gyrus
- D. Gyrus rectus
- E. Hypophysis

▸▸ **Question 13**

What is the most common source of cerebral metastases in adults?
- A. Lung carcinoma
- B. Breast carcinoma
- C. Renal cell carcinoma
- D. Melanoma
- E. Prostate adenoma

▸▸ **Question 14**

Small-cell lung cancer (SCLC) was established as the primary source for a patient admitted with cerebral metastases. He was treated with chemotherapy and radiotherapy with total radiotherapy dose of 25 Gy. Recurrent brain metastases after failure of this initial treatment will be treated with how much total radiotherapy dose?
- A. 20 Gy
- B. 30 Gy
- C. 50 Gy
- D. 54 Gy
- E. 60 Gy

▸▸ **Question 15**

What is the upper limit of number of melanoma mets that can be surgically removed in patients without systemic disease?
- A. 4
- B. 6
- C. 8
- D. 10
- E. Number is irrelevant

▸▸ **Question 16**

Melanoma is quite radioresistant but responds well to chemotherapy with which of the following?
- A. Alkylating agents
- B. Antimetabolites
- C. Microtubule inhibitors
- D. Bleomycin
- E. Doxorubicin

▸▸ **Question 17**

When multiple lesions are present on CT or MRI of brains with multiple metastases, "Whoever counts the most metastases is right" is?
- A. Chamber's rule
- B. Collin's law
- C. Rule of Spence
- D. Steel's rule of thirds
- E. Chief's doctrine

▸▸ **Question 18**

How should a solitary, symptomatic, large, and accessible metastasis in a patient with stable systemic disease and KPS > 70 be treated?
- A. Surgical excision
- B. Whole brain radiation
- C. Stereotactic radiosurgery
- D. Surgery and chemotherapy
- E. Surgery and whole brain radiation

▸▸ **Question 19**

Which of the following cerebral metastases is highly radioresistant to WBXRT?

- A. Small cell lung carcinoma
- B. Germ cell tumors
- C. Lymphoma
- D. Renal cell carcinoma
- E. Multiple myeloma

▸▸ Question 20

Regarding the treatment of spinal epidural metastases, which procedure reduces pain associated with pathologic fractures and is associated with an increase in functional outcome?

- A. Transpedicular screw fixation
- B. Transthoracic costotransverectomy
- C. Transthoracic transpedicular facet sparing
- D. Kyphoplasty
- E. Lumbar interbody fusion

▸▸ Question 21

Urinary kappa Bence-Jones proteins are associated with which of the following?

- A. Leptomeningeal carcinomatosis
- B. Multiple myeloma
- C. Primary CNS lymphoma
- D. Wilm's tumor
- E. Neuroblastoma

▸▸ Question 22

What is spinal metastatic lesion that scores 8 on SINS considered as?

- A. Stable
- B. Impending instability
- C. Unstable
- D. Not applicable

Answers

▸▸ Answer 1

E. All of the above[1]

▸▸ Answer 2

A. Oligodendroglioma[1]

▸▸ Answer 3

Correct answer is D. Behind sylvian fissure near the junction of occipital, parietal, and temporal lobe[2]

▸▸ Answer 4

Correct answer is A. Melanoma[2]

▸▸ Answer 5

Correct answer is A. These are radioresistant tumors[3]

▸▸ Answer 6

Correct answer is E. All of the above[4]

▸▸ Answer 7

Correct answer is E. All of the above[5]

▸▸ Answer 8

Correct answer is A. Less than three metastatic lesions within the brain[5]

▸▸ Answer 9

Correct answer is E. All of the above[6]

▸▸ Answer 10

Correct answer is C. Thyroid cancer[7]

▸▸ Answer 11

Correct answer is A. Medulloblastoma[2]

▸▸ Answer 12

Correct answer is B. Posterior to sylvian fissure[2]

▸▸ Answer 13

Correct answer is A. Lung carcinoma[2]

▸▸ Answer 14

Correct answer is A. 20 Gy[3]

▸▸ Answer 15

Correct answer is A. 4[8]

▸▸ Answer 16

Correct answer is A. Alkylating agents[5]

▸▸ Answer 17

Correct answer is A. Chamber's rule[9]

▸▸ Answer 18

Correct answer is E. Surgery and whole brain radiation[10]

▸▸ Answer 19

Correct answer is D. Renal cell carcinoma[7]

▸▸ **Answer 20**

Correct answer is D. Kyphoplasty[11]

▸▸ **Answer 21**

Correct answer is B. Multiple myeloma[12]

▸▸ **Answer 22**

Correct answer is B. Impending instability[13]

References

[1] Greenberg M, ed. Greenberg's Handbook of Neurosurgery. 10th ed. New York: Thieme; 2023:908
[2] Greenberg M, ed. Greenberg's Handbook of Neurosurgery. 10th ed. New York: Thieme; 2023:909
[3] Greenberg M, ed. Greenberg's Handbook of Neurosurgery. 10th ed. New York: Thieme; 2023:911
[4] Greenberg M, ed. Greenberg's Handbook of Neurosurgery. 10th ed. New York: Thieme; 2023: 911
[5] Greenberg M, ed. Greenberg's Handbook of Neurosurgery. 10th ed. New York: Thieme; 2023:913
[6] Greenberg M, ed. Greenberg's Handbook of Neurosurgery. 10th ed. New York: Thieme; 2023:915
[7] Greenberg M, ed. Greenberg's Handbook of Neurosurgery. 10th ed. New York: Thieme; 2023:917
[8] Greenberg M, ed. Greenberg's Handbook of Neurosurgery. 10th ed. New York: Thieme; 2023:912
[9] Greenberg M, ed. Greenberg's Handbook of Neurosurgery. 10th ed. New York: Thieme; 2023:914
[10] Greenberg M, ed. Greenberg's Handbook of Neurosurgery. 10th ed. New York: Thieme; 2023:916
[11] Greenberg M, ed. Greenberg's Handbook of Neurosurgery. 10th ed. New York: Thieme; 2023:926
[12] Greenberg M, ed. Greenberg's Handbook of Neurosurgery. 10th ed. New York: Thieme; 2023:930
[13] Greenberg M, ed. Greenberg's Handbook of Neurosurgery. 10th ed. New York: Thieme; 2023:927

56 Other Tumors, Cysts, and Tumor-Like Lesions

Questions

▸▸ **Question 1**

What is the modified Kadish grade of an esthesioneuroblastoma extending to paranasal sinus?

- A. A
- B. B
- C. C
- D. D
- E. E

▸▸ **Question 2**

What is the system used to define all upper respiratory tract carcinomas and describe nuclear pleomorphism, mitotic activity, rosette presence, and necrosis?

- A. Modified Kadish
- B. Biller's
- C. Dulguerov's
- D. Calcattera's
- E. Hyam's

▸▸ **Question 3**

Regarding differences between craniopharyngioma and Rathke's cleft cyst, the former has a thicker cyst wall, contains cholesterol crystals within the cyst, and is lined by which epithelium?

- A. Single layer cuboidal
- B. Three-layered cuboidal
- C. Stratified squamous
- D. Parietal and chief cells
- E. Tall columnar

▸▸ **Question 4**

Which of the following is not associated with higher rates of recurrence in Rathke's cleft cyst?

- A. Grade of lesion
- B. Purely suprasellar location
- C. Reactive metaplasia in the cyst wall
- D. Infection in the cyst
- E. Use of a fat graft within the cyst cavity

▸▸ **Question 5**

Which of the following is associated with the risk of sudden death?

- A. Craniopharyngioma
- B. Rathke's cleft cyst
- C. Colloid cyst
- D. GBM
- E. Small cell tumors

▸▸ **Question 6**

Which of the following approaches to the third ventricle can only be done in the presence of hydrocephalus and is not suitable with slit ventricles?

- A. Transcallosal
- B. Transcortical
- C. Subfrontal
- D. Subchiasmatic
- E. Lamina terminalis

▸▸ **Question 7**

Regarding differences between epidermoid and dermoid cysts, the former is associated with which of the following?

- A. Also includes hair follicles and sebaceous glands
- B. More commonly near midline
- C. More frequently associated with other congenital anomalies
- D. Repeated bouts of bacterial meningitis
- E. Chemical meningitis

▸▸ **Question 8**

All of the following are options for treatment of pineal cysts except?

- A. Watchful waiting
- B. Endoscopic third ventriculostomy
- C. Aspiration only (stereotactic or endoscopic): may not get enough tissue for diagnosis
- D. Cyst excision
- E. Chemotherapy

▸▸ **Question 9**

Visual deterioration due to empty sella syndrome may be treated with which of the following?

- A. Chiasmapexy
- B. Bromocriptine
- C. Fat graft placement
- D. Binoculars
- E. Visual rehab programs

▸▸ **Question 10**

Which of the following is a major indication for surgery in primary empty sella syndrome?

- A. CSF leak
- B. Hyperprolactinemia

- C. Hydrocephalus
- D. Headache
- E. Trauma

▸▸ **Question 11**

Which of the following is *not* the cause of secondary empty sella syndrome?

- A. Trauma
- B. Successful surgery for pituitary adenoma
- C. Radiotherapy for pituitary adenoma
- D. Pseudotumor cerebri
- E. Hypothalamic glioma

▸▸ **Question 12**

Regarding pheochromocytoma, investigations may include genetic testing, plasma metanephrines, 24-hour urinary catecholamines and metanephrines, and CT and MRI of adrenal glands. In the setting of raised urinary markers, which test can be used to differentiate between essential hypertension and pheochromocytoma?

- A. Serum ionized and free sodium levels
- B. Renal arteriogram
- C. Ankle brachial index
- D. Clonidine suppression test
- E. Low-dose steroids test

▸▸ **Question 13**

In the modified Jackson classification, what is the class for a glomus tumor extending into the petrous apex?

- A. I
- B. II
- C. III
- D. IV
- E. V

Answers

▸▸ **Answer 1**

Correct answer is B. B[1]

▸▸ **Answer 2**

Correct answer is E. Hyam's[1]

▸▸ **Answer 3**

Correct answer is C. Stratified squamous[2]

▸▸ **Answer 4**

Correct answer is A. Grade of lesion[3]

▸▸ **Answer 5**

Correct answer is C. Colloid cyst[4]

▸▸ **Answer 6**

Correct answer is B. Transcortical[5]

▸▸ **Answer 7**

Correct answer is E. Chemical meningitis[6]

▸▸ **Answer 8**

Correct answer is E. Chemotherapy[7]

▸▸ **Answer 9**

Correct answer is A. Chiasmapexy[8]

▸▸ **Answer 10**

Correct answer is A. CSF leak[8]

▸▸ **Answer 11**

Correct answer is E. Hypothalamic glioma[8]

▸▸ **Answer 12**

Correct answer is D. Clonidine suppression test[9]

▸▸ **Answer 13**

Correct answer is C. III[10]

References

[1] Greenberg M, ed. Greenberg's Handbook of Neurosurgery. 10th ed. New York: Thieme; 2023:935
[2] Greenberg M, ed. Greenberg's Handbook of Neurosurgery. 10th ed. New York: Thieme; 2023:949
[3] Greenberg M, ed. Greenberg's Handbook of Neurosurgery. 10th ed. New York: Thieme; 2023:951
[4] Greenberg M, ed. Greenberg's Handbook of Neurosurgery. 10th ed. New York: Thieme; 2023:944
[5] Greenberg M, ed. Greenberg's Handbook of Neurosurgery. 10th ed. New York: Thieme; 2023:947
[6] Greenberg M, ed. Greenberg's Handbook of Neurosurgery. 10th ed. New York: Thieme; 2023:937
[7] Greenberg M, ed. Greenberg's Handbook of Neurosurgery. 10th ed. New York: Thieme; 2023:948
[8] Greenberg M, ed. Greenberg's Handbook of Neurosurgery. 10th ed. New York: Thieme; 2023:952
[9] Greenberg M, ed. Greenberg's Handbook of Neurosurgery. 10th ed. New York: Thieme; 2023:940
[10] Greenberg M, ed. Greenberg's Handbook of Neurosurgery. 10th ed. New York: Thieme; 2023:942

57 Pseudotumor Cerebri Syndrome (PTCS)

Questions

▸▸ Question 1

Pseudotumor cerebri syndrome is a group of conditions characterized by increased intracranial pressure with no evidence of intracranial mass, hydrocephalus, infection, or hypertensive encephalopathy. What is the ICP?
- A. ≥ 3 cm CSF
- B. ≥ 5 cm CSF
- C. ≥ 10 cm CSF
- D. ≥ 15 cm CSF
- E. ≥ 25 cm CSF

▸▸ Question 2

Secondary pseudotumor cerebri is commonly associated with which of the following?
- A. Spontaneous subarachnoid hemorrhage
- B. Dural sinus thrombosis
- C. Sudden hearing loss
- D. Horner syndrome
- E. CSF pleocytosis

▸▸ Question 3

Which of the following is not included in the modified Dandy's criteria for pseudotumor cerebri?
- A. Signs and symptoms of increased ICP
- B. No localizing signs
- C. Increased CSF pressure without chemical or cytological abnormalities
- D. Ventriculomegaly
- E. No intracranial mass

▸▸ Question 4

Vision in pseudotumor cerebri should be followed with which of the following?
- A. Perimetry
- B. Optic coherence test
- C. Visual evoked potentials
- D. Measuring intraocular pressures
- E. MRI of globe

▸▸ Question 5

What is the treatment for improvement of vision in a patient of pseudotumor cerebri with visual loss without headache?
- A. Lumboperitoneal shunt
- B. Cisterna magna shunt
- C. VP shunt
- D. Optic nerve sheath fenestration
- E. Furosemide

▸▸ Question 6

What is the duration of fulminant PTCS defined as time between onset of symptoms and severe loss of acuity or visual field?
- A. < 2 weeks
- B. < 4 weeks
- C. < 6 weeks
- D. < 8 weeks

▸▸ Question 7

Which of the following drugs is not recommended in PTCS because of associated exacerbation of weight gain and risk of venous thrombosis?
- A. Acetazolamide
- B. Furosemide
- C. Steroids
- D. Topiramate
- E. Methazolamide

▸▸ Question 8

Pseudotumor cerebri is characterized by absence of intracranial mass or infection and presence of papilledema and symptomatic ICP elevation of more than 20 cm H_2O?
- A. 3
- B. 5
- C. 10
- D. 15
- E. 25

▸▸ Question 9

Pseudotumor cerebri is commonly associated with which of the following?
- A. Spontaneous subarachnoid hemorrhage
- B. Dural sinus thrombosis
- C. Sudden hearing loss
- D. Horner syndrome
- E. CSF pleocytosis

▸▸ Question 10

Which of the following is not included in the modified Dandy's criteria for pseudotumor cerebri?
- A. Signs and symptoms of increased ICP
- B. No localizing signs

- C. Increased CSF pressure without chemical or cytological abnormalities
- D. Ventriculomegaly
- E. No intracranial mass

Answers

▸▸ Answer 1

Correct answer is E. ≥ 25 cm CSF[1]

▸▸ Answer 2

Correct answer is B. Dural sinus thrombosis[1]

▸▸ Answer 3

Correct answer is D. Ventriculomegaly[2]

▸▸ Answer 4

Correct answer is A. Perimetry[3]

▸▸ Answer 5

Correct answer is D. Optic nerve sheath fenestration[4]

▸▸ Answer 6

Correct answer is B. < 4 weeks[5]

▸▸ Answer 7

Correct answer is C. Steroids[4]

▸▸ Answer 8

Correct answer is E. 25[1]

▸▸ Answer 9

Correct answer is B. Dural sinus thrombosis[1]

▸▸ Answer 10

Correct answer is D. Ventriculomegaly[2]

References

[1] Greenberg M, ed. Greenberg's Handbook of Neurosurgery. 10th ed. New York: Thieme; 2023:955
[2] Greenberg M, ed. Greenberg's Handbook of Neurosurgery. 10th ed. New York: Thieme; 2023:959
[3] Greenberg M, ed. Greenberg's Handbook of Neurosurgery. 10th ed. New York: Thieme; 2023:961
[4] Greenberg M, ed. Greenberg's Handbook of Neurosurgery. 10th ed. New York: Thieme; 2023:965
[5] Greenberg M, ed. Greenberg's Handbook of Neurosurgery. 10th ed. New York: Thieme; 2023:967

58 Tumor and Tumor-Like Lesions of the Skull

Questions

▸▸ Question 1

Osteoma, hemangioma, dermoid, epidermoid, chondroma, meningioma, and aneurysmal bone cyst are benign tumors of the skull. Malignancy of skull is suggested by a single large lesion or multiple > 6 osteolytic lesions of the skull. These tumors are ragged, undermined, and lack sclerosis. Which of the following are malignant tumors of the skull?

- A. Bone metastasis to the skull like prostate, breast, lung, kidney, thyroid, and lymphoma
- B. Chondrosarcoma
- C. Osteogenic sarcoma
- D. Fibrosarcoma
- E. All of the above

▸▸ Question 2

A 55-year-old female patient presents with a swelling on cranial vault which she noticed was slow growing. On skull X-ray, it comes out as round, sclerotic, well-demarcated, homogenous dense projection arising from the outer table of the skull. On nuclear bone scan it comes out to be hot spot. Osteomas are asymptomatic lesions requiring surgery only for cosmetic reasons or pressure on adjacent structures. Which of the following is not included in the triad of Gardner's syndrome?

- A. Increased density or hyperostosis of calvaria
- B. Multiple cranial osteomas of calvaria, sinuses, or mandible
- C. Colonic polyposis
- D. Soft tissue tumors
- E. None of the above is related to the triad of Gardner's syndrome

▸▸ Question 3

Hemangiomas are benign tumors which commonly occur in the skull and spine and constitute 7% of the skull tumors. These are of two types, namely, cavernous (common) and capillary (rare). Which of the following is the imaging characteristics of these tumors?

- A. X-rays show a circular lucency with honeycomb or trabecular pattern (seen in 50% of cases) or radial trabeculations producing a sunburst pattern (seen in 11% of cases), while sclerotic margins are evident in only 33% of cases
- B. CT of brain shows hypodense lesion with sclerotic spaced trabeculations
- C. This lesion is nonenhancing on brain CT
- D. Bone scan is typically hot
- E. All of the above

▸▸ Question 4

The gross appearance of hemangioma is a hard tumor with blue doomed mass beneath the pericranium. What is the recommended treatment option for these tumors?

- A. En block excision or curettage with radiation considered for inaccessible tumors
- B. Radiation has no role in these tumors
- C. These tumors require no treatment and resolve on their own
- D. Partial excision is adequate for these tumors
- E. The goal of surgery is decompression only

▸▸ Question 5

A patient presents with a mass over the calvarium. On X-ray, there appears to be an osteolytic lesion with well-defined and sclerotic margins. CT of brain shows nonenhancing hypodense lesion and on MRI, these are like CSF low intensity on T1 and high signal intensity on T2 but unlike CSF they are high signal intensity on DWI. What could be the most likely diagnosis in this patient?

- A. Epidermoid tumor of the skull
- B. Dermoid tumors of the skull
- C. Osteoma of brain
- D. Osteosarcoma
- E. Both A and B

▸▸ Question 6

Epidermoid or dermoid occurs when ectodermal rests are entrapped in the development of skull which causes these tumors to arise from the diploe and expand into both inner and outer tables. What is the recommended option for these tumors?

- A. Radiotherapy
- B. Chemotherapy
- C. Surgical treatment with curettage
- D. Endoscopic treatment
- E. All of the above

▸▸ Question 7

Which of the following is not a non-neoplastic skull lesion?

- A. Osteopetrosis
- B. Paget's disease
- C. Hyperostosis frontalis interna
- D. Fibrous dysplasia
- E. Hemangioma

▸▸ Question 8

A patient presents with hypertension, seizures, headache, dementia, and irritability. Plain skull X-ray shows thickening of the frontal bone with characteristic sparing of the midline. CT demonstrates a 10-mm bony thickening, and bone scan shows up moderate uptake. What are the most likely conditions associated with hyperostosis frontalis interna?

- A. Morgagni's syndrome, which includes headache, obesity, virilism and neuropsychiatric disorders
- B. Endocrine abnormalities like acromegaly or hyperprolactinemia
- C. Metabolic abnormalities like hyperphosphatemia and obesity
- D. Diffuse idiopathic skeletal hyperostosis (DISH)
- E. All of the above

▸▸ Question 9

Fibrous dysplasia is a non-neoplastic benign condition in which normal bone is replaced with fibrous connective tissue. Most lesion occurs in ribs, proximal femur, and craniofacial bones?

- A. Cystic, sclerotic, or mixed
- B. Monostotic fibrous dysplasia which is most common
- C. Polyostotic fibrous dysplasia
- D. Polyostotic fibrous dysplasia as part of McCune Albright syndrome (which include the triad of cafe au lait spots, endocrinopathy, and polyostotic fibrous dysplasia)
- E. B, C, and D

▸▸ Question 10

A patient presents with local swelling with pain and tenderness over it. He/she also has pathological fracture, decreasing hearing function, seizures, and darkened hair pigmentation. Management includes which of the following?

- A. Removal of dysplastic bone, curettage, and cranioplasty
- B. Acute visual deterioration is treated with high dose glucocorticosteroids and decompression
- C. Involvement of multidisciplinary team for skull base lesions
- D. Copious amount of irrigation during drilling to avoid thermal injury
- E. All of the above

▸▸ Question 11

Which of the following is not a benign tumor of skull?

- A. Osteoma
- B. Hemangioma
- C. Chondroma
- D. Osteogenic sarcoma
- E. Meningioma

▸▸ Question 12

What is the most common primary bone tumor of the calvaria?

- A. Osteoma
- B. Hemangioma
- C. Chordoma
- D. Osteogenic sarcoma
- E. Meningioma

▸▸ Question 13

Skull X-ray showing circular lucency with honeycomb, trabecular, or sunburst pattern is most commonly seen with which of the following?

- A. Osteoma
- B. Hemangioma
- C. Chordoma
- D. Osteogenic sarcoma
- E. Meningioma

▸▸ Question 14

Which of the following is a primary malignant tumor of clivus or sacrum showing physaliphorous cells on histopathology?

- A. Osteoma
- B. Hemangioma
- C. Chordoma
- D. Osteogenic sarcoma
- E. Meningioma

▸▸ Question 15

Fibrous dysplasia is associated with which of the following?

- A. MISME syndrome
- B. McCune-Albright syndrome
- C. Post traumatic
- D. X-linked inheritance
- E. Autosomal dominant inheritance

▸▸ Question 16

Which of the following is the most frequent site of involvement in the monostotic fibrous dysplasia (MFD)?

- A. Proximal femur
- B. Distal tibia
- C. Zygomatic-maxillary complex
- D. Frontal air sinuses
- E. Skull foramina

►► **Question 17**

Pain is a common presentation of fibrous dysplasia and in cases of widespread lesions and raised alkaline phosphatase, it responds well to which of the following?

- A. Calcitonin
- B. RANK ligands
- C. Steroids
- D. Radiotherapy
- E. Chemotherapy

►► **Question 18**

In fibrous dysplasia, acute visual deterioration associated with an expansile lesion near the optic canal should be treated with surgical decompression and what?

- A. Calcitonin
- B. RANK ligands
- C. Steroids
- D. Radiotherapy
- E. Chemotherapy

Answers

►► **Answer 1**

Correct answer is E. All of the above[1]

►► **Answer 2**

Correct answer is A. Increased density or hyperostosis of calvaria[1]

►► **Answer 3**

Correct answer is E. All of the above[2]

►► **Answer 4**

Correct answer is A. En block excision or curettage with radiation considered for inaccessible tumors[3]

►► **Answer 5**

Correct answer is E. Both A and B[4]

►► **Answer 6**

Correct answer is C. Surgical treatment with curettage[5]

►► **Answer 7**

Correct answer is E. Hemangioma[6]

►► **Answer 8**

Correct answer is E. All of the above[6]

►► **Answer 9**

Correct answer is E. B, C, and D[7]

►► **Answer 10**

Correct answer is E. All of the above[8]

►► **Answer 11**

Correct answer is D. Osteogenic sarcoma[3]

►► **Answer 12**

Correct answer is A. Osteoma[3]

►► **Answer 13**

Correct answer is B. Hemangioma[5]

►► **Answer 14**

Correct answer is C. Chordoma[9]

►► **Answer 15**

Correct answer is B. McCune-Albright syndrome[10]

►► **Answer 16**

Correct answer is C. Zygomatic-maxillary complex[10]

►► **Answer 17**

Correct answer is A. Calcitonin[11]

►► **Answer 18**

Correct answer is C. Steroids[8]

References

[1] Greenberg M, ed. Greenberg's Handbook of Neurosurgery. 10th ed. New York: Thieme; 2023:969

[2] Greenberg M, ed. Greenberg's Handbook of Neurosurgery. 10th ed. New York: Thieme; 2023:970

[3] Greenberg M, ed. Greenberg's Handbook of Neurosurgery. 10th ed. New York: Thieme; 2023:972

[4] Greenberg M, ed. Greenberg's Handbook of Neurosurgery. 10th ed. New York: Thieme; 2023:971–972

[5] Greenberg M, ed. Greenberg's Handbook of Neurosurgery. 10th ed. New York: Thieme; 2023:973
[6] Greenberg M, ed. Greenberg's Handbook of Neurosurgery. 10th ed. New York: Thieme; 2023:974
[7] Greenberg M, ed. Greenberg's Handbook of Neurosurgery. 10th ed. New York: Thieme; 2023:976
[8] Greenberg M, ed. Greenberg's Handbook of Neurosurgery. 10th ed. New York: Thieme; 2023:978
[9] Greenberg M, ed. Greenberg's Handbook of Neurosurgery. 10th ed. New York: Thieme; 2023:825
[10] Greenberg M, ed. Greenberg's Handbook of Neurosurgery. 10th ed. New York: Thieme; 2023:975
[11] Greenberg M, ed. Greenberg's Handbook of Neurosurgery. 10th ed. New York: Thieme; 2023: 978

59 Tumors of the Spine and Spinal Cord

Questions

▸▸ **Question 1**

About 15% of primary CNS tumors are intraspinal and most spinal tumors are benign presenting with compression rather than invasion. Which of the following statements regarding these tumors is not true?

- A. Metastasis is only found in the extradural compartment
- B. 55% are extradural tumors
- C. 40% are intradural extramedullary tumors and arise mostly from leptomeninges or roots
- D. Only 5% are intramedullary spinal cord tumors
- E. Lymphoma may occur in all three compartments and are divided into primary or secondary (metastasis)

▸▸ **Question 2**

Most of the extradural tumors are metastasis which can be osteolytic like lymphoma, lung, breast, or prostate or these can be osteoblastic like prostate carcinoma (CA) which is most common in men while in females breast CA is most common. Other extradural tumors include the following except?

- A. Chordomas and osteoid osteoma
- B. Osteoblastoma and aneurysmal bone cyst
- C. Chondrosarcoma and osteochondroma
- D. Vertebral hemangioma and giant cell tumors
- E. Meningioma and neurofibromas

▸▸ **Question 3**

Intradural extramedullary tumors include meningiomas, neurofibromas, lipomas, or rarely metastasis. Which of the following are the most common intramedullary spinal cord tumors?

- A. Astrocytoma and ependymoma including myxopapillary ependymoma
- B. Malignant glioblastoma and dermoid
- C. Epidermoid and teratoma
- D. Lipoma and hemangioblastoma
- E. Neuroma and syringomyelia

▸▸ **Question 4**

A patient presents with an intradural extramedullary spinal cord tumor, which occurs mostly in 40 to 70 years of age and affects females 4 times more than males. These are mostly found in the thoracic region and in 68% of cases, these tumors are lateral to the spinal cord, in 15% they are anterior, while in 18% they are posterior. Which tumor fulfills all these characteristics?

- A. Neurofibroma
- B. Schwannoma
- C. Meningioma
- D. Lipoma
- E. Lymphoma

▸▸ **Question 5**

Spinal schwannomas are intradural extramedullary spinal tumors that are mostly slow growing benign tumors and arise mostly (75%) from dorsal (sensory) rootlets with early symptoms of radicular pain. All of the following statements regarding Asazuma et al classification of dumbbell spinal schwannomas are correct except?

- A. Type 1 tumors are intradural and extradural tumors and are restricted to the spinal canal. These can be operated through posterior approach
- B. Type 2 tumors are all extradural and are subclassified as 2a (do not extend beyond the neural foramina), 2b (inside the spinal canal and paravertebral), and 2c (foraminal and paravertebral). Tumors 2a and 2b can be operated posteriorly
- C. Type 3a tumors are intradural and extradural foraminal, and 3b tumors are intradural and extradural paravertebral, with only 3a and some upper cervical 3b operable posteriorly
- D. Type 4 tumors are extradural intravertebral tumors and can be operated posteriorly
- E. Type 5 tumors are extradural, extralaminar with laminar invasion while type 6 tumors are multidirectional with bone erosion

▸▸ **Question 6**

Ependymomas are the intradural spinal cord tumors that require MRI of the entire neuraxis because of potential for seeding. These are slow-growing benign tumors with male predominance and mostly occur in the 3rd to 6th decades of life. These are mostly found in conus medullaris, filum terminale, or cauda equina where these are called as what?

- A. Papillary tumors
- B. Myxopapillary ependymomas
- C. End spinal cord tumors
- D. Ependymomas at conus
- E. None of the above

▸▸ **Question 7**

What is the most common presentation of an intramedullary spinal cord tumor?

- A. Pain which can be radicular (increases with Valsalva maneuver and spine movements, especially consider SCT if dermatome is unusual for disk herniation), local (pain during recumbency or nocturnal pain is classic for spinal cord tumors), or medullary (dysesthetic, nonradicular, and often bilateral)
- B. Motor disturbances
- C. Nonpainful sensory disturbances

- D. Sphincters disturbances
- E. Scoliosis or torticollis

▸▸ Question 8

It is usually difficult to distinguish intramedullary spinal cord tumors from intradural extramedullary or extradural tumors on clinical grounds. How schwannomas can be distinguished from intramedullary tumors on clinical grounds?

- A. Schwannomas often start with radicular pain that later progress to cord involvement
- B. Most intramedullary spinal cord tumors are located posteriorly in the cord which may cause sensory findings to predominate
- C. Intramedullary spinal cord tumors cause dissociative type of sensory loss with decreased pain and temperature and preserved light touch as in Brown-Sequard syndrome
- D. Urogenital symptoms like difficulty evacuating, retention, and incontinence are early signs in conus or cauda equina lesions
- E. All of the above

▸▸ Question 9

Mainstay of diagnosis for intramedullary tumors is MRI in which ependymoma enhance intensely, often associated with hemorrhage and cysts. While plain radiographs show vertebral body destruction, there is enlarged intervertebral foramina or increased interpedicular distance with fusiform cord widening on myelography. What is the technical consideration while doing surgery on these tumors?

- A. These tumors should be debulked internally using ultrasonic aspirator and laser
- B. An attempt should be made to make a plane between the tumor and the cord
- C. Total excision is must in all these tumors
- D. No radiotherapy is needed for residual tumors
- E. If cystic component is evident, an attempt should be made to aspirate the whole cyst at the start of surgery

▸▸ Question 10

A patient presents with pain localized to one point on back. MRI shows vertebral body lesion, which is focal, round, hyperintense on T1 and T2 with enhancement on contrast. CT of spine shows multiple, high-density dots on axial images (polka dot sign), while plain radiograph shows vertically oriented striations (corduroy pattern) or honeycomb appearance. What are the management options for these tumors?

- A. Radiotherapy
- B. Embolization
- C. Vertebroplasty
- D. Surgery (which can be through posterior approach if only posterior elements are involved or if there is VB involvement with no expansion, and anterior corpectomy with strut graft if VB is involved with anterior canal compression or extensive anterior and posterior elements and soft tissue involvement)
- E. All of the above

▸▸ Question 11

Which of the following is the most common extradural tumor of spine?

- A. Neurofibroma
- B. Ependymoma
- C. Aneurysmal bone cyst
- D. Chordoma
- E. Metastases

▸▸ Question 12

Which of the following is the most common intradural extramedullary tumor of spine?

- A. Neurofibroma
- B. Ependymoma
- C. Aneurysmal bone cyst
- D. Chordoma
- E. Metastases

▸▸ Question 13

Which of the following is the most common intradural intramedullary tumor of spine?

- A. Neurofibroma
- B. Ependymoma
- C. Aneurysmal bone cyst
- D. Chordoma
- E. Metastases

▸▸ Question 14

Which of the following is the most common location of spinal meningioma?

- A. Upper cervical
- B. Subaxial cervical
- C. Thoracic
- D. Lumbar
- E. Sacral

▸▸ Question 15

According to Asazuma classification system for dumbbell spinal schwannomas, what is the type of a tumor that is totally extradural?

- A. 1
- B. 2
- C. 3
- D. 4
- E. 5

▸▸ Question 16

About 90% of intramedullary spinal cord tumors in pediatric age group are ependymoma and which of the following?
- A. Neurofibroma
- B. Astrocytoma
- C. Meningioma
- D. Metastases
- E. Lymphoma

▸▸ Question 17

Where are myxopapillary ependymomas located?
- A. Craniocervical junction
- B. Upper thoracic spine
- C. Lower thoracic spine
- D. Ilium
- E. Filum terminale

▸▸ Question 18

What is a classic symptom for spinal cord tumor?
- A. Nocturnal pain
- B. Morning stiffness
- C. Burning hands syndrome
- D. Spinothalamic tract deficit
- E. Corticospinal tract deficit

▸▸ Question 19

For the investigation of spinal cord tumor, CSF xanthochromia and clotting due to fibrinogen occur in which of the following?
- A. Queckenstedt's test
- B. Froin's syndrome
- C. Wada test
- D. Factor V laden activity
- E. Halo ring sign

▸▸ Question 20

During intraoperative electrophysiological monitoring which of the following is continuously measured and can alert the surgeon immediately when deterioration starts to occur?
- A. MEP
- B. SSEP
- C. BIS
- D. EMG
- E. D waves

Answers

▸▸ Answer 1

Correct answer is A. Metastasis is only found in the extradural compartment[1]

▸▸ Answer 2

Correct answer is E. Meningioma and neurofibromas[2]

▸▸ Answer 3

Correct answer is A. Astrocytoma and ependymoma including myxopapillary ependymoma[2]

▸▸ Answer 4

Correct answer is C. Meningioma[3]

▸▸ Answer 5

Correct answer is D. Type 4 tumors are extradural intravertebral tumors and can be operated posteriorly[4]

▸▸ Answer 6

Correct answer is B. Myxopapillary ependymomas[5]

▸▸ Answer 7

Correct answer is A. Pain which can be radicular (increases with Valsalva maneuver and spine movements, especially consider SCT if dermatome is unusual for disk herniation), local (pain during recumbency or nocturnal pain is classic for spinal cord tumors), or medullary (dysesthetic, nonradicular, and often bilateral)[6]

▸▸ Answer 8

Correct answer is E. All of the above[6]

▸▸ Answer 9

Correct answer is A. These tumors should be debulked internally using ultrasonic aspirator and laser[7]

▸▸ Answer 10

Correct answer is E. All of the above[8]

▸▸ Answer 11

Correct answer is E. Metastases[1]

▸▸ Answer 12

Correct answer is A. Neurofibroma[2]

▸▸ Answer 13

Correct answer is B. Ependymoma[2]

▸▸ Answer 14

Correct answer is C. Thoracic[3]

▸▸ Answer 15

Correct answer is B. 2[9]

▸▸ **Answer 16**

Correct answer is B. Astrocytoma[10]

▸▸ **Answer 17**

Correct answer is E. Filum terminale[5]

▸▸ **Answer 18**

Correct answer is A. Nocturnal pain[11]

▸▸ **Answer 19**

Correct answer is B. Froin's syndrome[6]

▸▸ **Answer 20**

Correct answer is E. D waves[7]

References

[1] Greenberg M, ed. Greenberg's Handbook of Neurosurgery. 10th ed. New York: Thieme; 2023:979

[2] Greenberg M, ed. Greenberg's Handbook of Neurosurgery. 10th ed. New York: Thieme; 2023:980

[3] Greenberg M, ed. Greenberg's Handbook of Neurosurgery. 10th ed. New York: Thieme; 2023:981

[4] Greenberg M, ed. Greenberg's Handbook of Neurosurgery. 10th ed. New York: Thieme; 2023: 982

[5] Greenberg M, ed. Greenberg's Handbook of Neurosurgery. 10th ed. New York: Thieme; 2023:985

[6] Greenberg M, ed. Greenberg's Handbook of Neurosurgery. 10th ed. New York: Thieme; 2023:987

[7] Greenberg M, ed. Greenberg's Handbook of Neurosurgery. 10th ed. New York: Thieme; 2023:988

[8] Greenberg M, ed. Greenberg's Handbook of Neurosurgery. 10th ed. New York: Thieme; 2023:995

[9] Greenberg M, ed. Greenberg's Handbook of Neurosurgery. 10th ed. New York: Thieme; 2023:982

[10] Greenberg M, ed. Greenberg's Handbook of Neurosurgery. 10th ed. New York: Thieme; 2023:984

[11] Greenberg M, ed. Greenberg's Handbook of Neurosurgery. 10th ed. New York: Thieme; 2023:986

Part XIV

Head Trauma

XIV

60 Head Trauma: General Information, Grading, and Initial Management

Questions

▸▸ Question 1

Brain injury from trauma results from two distinct processes which are primary brain injury and secondary brain injury. Focus is on prevention of secondary injuries which requires good general medical care and an understanding of intracranial pressure. Which of the following are included in the secondary brain injury?

- A. Intracranial hematomas and edema
- B. Hypoxemia
- C. Ischemia (primarily due to elevated intracranial pressure or from shock)
- D. Vasospasm
- E. All of the above

▸▸ Question 2

A patient is being transferred to a neurosurgery facility and is consulted with a neurosurgeon prior to transfer about the possible factors that should be assessed and stabilized. What factors need to be stabilized and kept in mind before transfer of the patient?

- A. Hypoxia or hypoventilation
- B. Hypotension or hypertension
- C. Anemia and seizures
- D. Infection or hyperthermia and spinal stability
- E. All of the above

▸▸ Question 3

A patient with GCS 14 or GCS 15 plus brief loss of consciousness for less than 15 minutes or impaired alertness is categorized as mild head injury. When a patient will be categorized as moderate head injury?

- A. A patient with GCS 9–13
- B. A patient with loss of consciousness for more than 5 minutes
- C. A patient with focal neurologic deficit
- D. A, B, and C
- E. A patient with GCS 3–8

▸▸ Question 4

Hypotension, BP less than 90 mmHg, doubles the mortality while hypoxia (apnea or cyanosis or PaO_2 less than 60 mmHg on ABG) also increases the mortality. The combination of both increases the risk of bad outcome and increases mortality by how much?

- A. Two times
- B. Three times
- C. Four times
- D. The patient cannot survive for more than a few hours with this combination
- E. None of the above

▸▸ Question 5

Sedatives and paralytics may lead to higher incidence of pneumonia, longer ICU stays, and possible sepsis. These agents also impair neurologic assessment and are reserved for cases with clinical evidence of intracranial hypertension. All of the following are clinical signs of intracranial hypertension except?

- A. Pupillary dilation (unilateral or bilateral)
- B. Asymmetric pupillary reaction to light
- C. Absence of corneal reflex
- D. Decerebrate or decorticate posturing
- E. Progressive deterioration of neurologic examination not attributable to extracranial factors

▸▸ Question 6

A patient who is unable to maintain airway or who is hypoxic despite supplemental O_2 needs to be intubated. What are the other indications for intubation?

- A. Depressed level of consciousness with GCS less than or equal to 8
- B. Need for hyperventilation
- C. Severe maxillofacial trauma
- D. Need for pharmacologic paralysis for evaluation or management like for irritable patient to send him/her for plain CT of brain
- E. All of the above

▸▸ Question 7

Hyperventilation and mannitol (0.25–1 g/kg over less than 20 minutes) (after adequate volume resuscitation) are reserved in the acute setting for patients with signs of transtentorial herniation or progressive neurologic deterioration not attributable to extracranial causes. Hyperventilation ($PaCO_2$ less than or equal to 25 mmHg) is not recommended prophylactically as it may exacerbate cerebral ischemia or may cause hypocalcemia with tetany. What are the indications of mannitol in emergency?

- A. Evidence of intracranial hypertension (clinical signs of intracranial hypertension)
- B. Evidence of mass effect (focal deficit or hemiparesis)
- C. Sudden deterioration prior to CT of brain (including pupillary dilatation)
- D. After CT of brain that identifies the lesion which is causing raised ICP or after CT of brain if going to the OR
- E. All of the above

▸▸ **Question 8**

Routine use of prophylactic antiseizure medications in traumatic brain injury is ineffective in preventing the late development of post-traumatic seizures, that is, epilepsy. ASMs (e.g., phenytoin, valproate, or carbamazepine) may be used to decrease the incidence of early post-traumatic seizures (within 7 days of TBI). Conditions with increased risk of post-traumatic seizures and require ASMs include which of the following?

- A. Acute subdural, epidural, and intracerebral hematoma
- B. Open depressed fracture with parenchymal injury
- C. Seizure within the first 24 hours after injury or GCS less than 10
- D. Penetrating brain injury or cortical contusion on CT or history of alcohol abuse
- E. All of the above

▸▸ **Question 9**

A patient with head trauma needs neurologic examination which includes cranial nerve examination (second, sixth, and seventh), level of consciousness (GCS), motor examination, sensory examination, and reflexes. A patient presents with racoon eye (periorbital ecchymoses), battles sign (postauricular ecchymoses), CSF rhinorrhea, and hemotympanum (laceration of external auditory canal). Where is the suspected injury in this patient?

- A. Frontal bone fracture of skull
- B. Fracture of occiput and frontal bone
- C. Fracture of base of skull
- D. Fracture of facial bones
- E. Fracture of frontal, parietal, and occipital bones of skull

▸▸ **Question 10**

Brain CT is needed for the initial evaluation in traumatic brain injury patients with which of the following risk factors?

- A. GCS less than or equal to 14 or unresponsiveness
- B. Coagulopathy including antiplatelet and anticoagulants drugs and seizure
- C. Penetrating skull trauma or focal neurologic deficit
- D. Polytrauma, suspected nonaccidental trauma (child abuse), or deteriorating neurologic status
- E. All of the above

▸▸ **Question 11**

All of the following are true regarding Marshall CT classification of traumatic brain injury severity score except?

- A. Category 1 is diffuse injury with no visible pathology and mortality of 6.4%
- B. Category 2 is diffuse injury with midline shift of 0 to 5 mm, no high or mixed density lesion of more than 25 mL, and mortality in this case is 11%
- C. Category 3 is diffuse injury (swelling) with midline shift of 0 to 5 mm, basal cisterns compressed or completely effaced with no high density or mixed density lesion of more than 25 mL, and mortality of 29%
- D. Category 4 is diffuse injury (shift) with midline shift of more than 5 mm and no high or mixed density lesion of more than 25 mL and mortality of 30%
- E. Category 5 is evacuated mass lesion with mortality of 30%

▸▸ **Question 12**

Rotterdam scores 2, 3, 4, and 5 have mortality of 6.8, 16, 26, and 53%, respectively. Which of the following statements is correct regarding Rotterdam score?

- A. Midline shift of more than 5 mm has 1 point
- B. Presence of epidural mass has 1 point
- C. Basal cisterns compressed has 1 point while absence has 2 points
- D. Presence of intraventricular blood or traumatic SAH has 1 point
- E. All of the above

▸▸ **Question 13**

What is the criterion for observation at home for a head injury patient?

- A. Head CT is not indicated or it is normal if indicated
- B. Initial GCS more than or equal to 14
- C. Patient is now neurologically intact
- D. Patient is accompanied by responsible, sober adult and has reasonable access to return to the hospital
- E. All of the above

▸▸ **Question 14**

Indirect optic nerve injury during trauma injury can cause transient visual loss. Mega dose steroids can be used as an adjunct to diagnosis and treatment. What is the most common segment of the optic nerve which is damaged during optic nerve injury?

- A. Intraocular (1 mm in length)
- B. Intracranial (10 mm in length)
- C. Intraorbital (25–30 mm)
- D. Intracanalicular (10 mm)
- E. None of the above

▸▸ **Question 15**

Where should the first burr hole be placed in case of emergency exploratory burr hole placement?

- A. Temporal burr hole ipsilateral to the side of pupillary dilatation
- B. Frontal burr hole toward ipsilateral burr hole
- C. Parietal burr hole
- D. Occipital burr hole
- E. Temporal burr hole opposite to the side of pupillary dilatation

▸▸ Question 16

An adult male presented in the emergency with history of roadside accident. He was conscious and oriented with main complaints of headache and neck pain. What are the most common spine fractures associated with significant head trauma?

- A. C1–C3
- B. Subaxial spine
- C. Cervicothoracic junction
- D. Thoracolumbar junction
- E. Coccygeal

▸▸ Question 17

A female presented in the emergency after fall from bike. She was tachypneic and hypotensive. What is the resuscitation target for systolic blood pressure after head injury?

- A. > 60 mmHg
- B. > 70 mmHg
- C. > 80 mmHg
- D. > 85 mmHg
- E. > 90 mmHg

▸▸ Question 18

During resuscitation after head injury, oxygenation should be maintained and hypoxia avoided. What should be the minimal goal?

- A. $PaO_2 = 40$ and $SpO_2 = 60$
- B. $PaO_2 > 40$ and $SpO_2 > 60$
- C. $PaO_2 > 50$ and $SpO_2 > 80$
- D. $PaO_2 > 60$ and $SpO_2 > 90$
- E. $PaO_2 = 100$ and $SpO_2 = 100$

▸▸ Question 19

An adult patient was brought to the emergency after head trauma with GCS score of 7 that indicates need for endotracheal intubation. What is the role of peri-procedural antibiotics?

- A. Reduces pneumonia
- B. Reduces ICU stay
- C. Reduces hospital stay
- D. Reduces mortality
- E. No role

▸▸ Question 20

What is the target $PaCO_2$ for hyperventilation for intracranial hypertension after traumatic brain injury?

- A. < 30
- B. 30 to 35
- C. 35 to 40
- D. 40
- E. 40 to 45

▸▸ Question 21

A middle-aged man was admitted in the emergency with head injury. Plain CT of brain reveals midline shift of 3 cm, effacement of basal cisterns, but no mass lesion. According to Marshall CT classification of traumatic brain injury, what category is this?

- A. I
- B. II
- C. III
- D. IV
- E. V

▸▸ Question 22

A middle-aged man was admitted in the emergency with head injury. Plain CT of brain reveals midline shift of 3 cm, effacement of basal cisterns, traumatic subarachnoid hemorrhage, but no mass lesion. What is the sum score according to the Rotterdam score for CT findings in traumatic brain injury?

- A. 0
- B. 1
- C. 2
- D. 3
- E. 4

▸▸ Question 23

A middle-aged man was brought to the emergency room. He is unconscious and not maintaining vital signs. Diagnostic peritoneal lavage was positive. What is the next step in management?

- A. Resuscitate in emergency room with double IV lines
- B. Transfuse blood
- C. Shift to operation room for laparotomy
- D. Get plain CT of brain along with cervical spine X-rays
- E. Get plain CT of brain, cervical spine and chest X-rays

▸▸ Question 24

Regarding exploratory burr holes for traumatic brain injury but with no localizing signs, where should the first burr hole be done?

- A. Frontal
- B. Temporal
- C. Parietal
- D. Occipital
- E. Posterior fossa

▸▸ Question 25

Regarding exploratory burr holes for traumatic brain injury but with no localizing signs, where should the last burr hole be done?

- A. Frontal
- B. Temporal

- C. Parietal
- D. Occipital
- E. Posterior fossa

Answers

►► Answer 1

Correct answer is E. All of the above[1]

►► Answer 2

Correct answer is E. All of the above[2]

►► Answer 3

Correct answer is D. A, B, and C[2]

►► Answer 4

Correct answer is B. Three times[3]

►► Answer 5

Correct answer is C. Absence of corneal reflex[4]

►► Answer 6

Correct answer is E. All of the above[4]

►► Answer 7

Correct answer is E. All of the above[5]

►► Answer 8

Correct answer is E. All of the above[6]

►► Answer 9

Correct answer is C. Fracture of base of skull[7]

►► Answer 10

Correct answer is E. All of the above[8]

►► Answer 11

Correct answer is D. Category 4 is diffuse injury (shift) with midline shift of more than 5 mm and no high or mixed density lesion of more than 25 mL and mortality of 30%[9]

►► Answer 12

Correct answer is E. All of the above[10]

►► Answer 13

Correct answer is E. All of the above[10]

►► Answer 14

Correct answer is D. Intracanalicular (10 mm)[11]

►► Answer 15

Correct answer is A. Temporal burr hole ipsilateral to the side of pupillary dilatation[11]

►► Answer 16

Correct answer is A. C1–C3[1]

►► Answer 17

Correct answer is E. > 90 mmHg[12]

►► Answer 18

Correct answer is D. $PaO_2 > 60$ and $SpO_2 > 90$[4]

►► Answer 19

Correct answer is A. Reduces pneumonia[4]

►► Answer 20

Correct answer is B. 30 to 35[4]

►► Answer 21

Correct answer is C. III[13]

►► Answer 22

Correct answer is D. 3[13]

►► Answer 23

Correct answer is C. Shift to operation room for laparotomy[14]

►► Answer 24

Correct answer is B. Temporal[11]

►► Answer 25

Correct answer is E. Posterior fossa[11]

References

[1] Greenberg M, ed. Greenberg's Handbook of Neurosurgery. 10th ed. New York: Thieme; 2023:1000
[2] Greenberg M, ed. Greenberg's Handbook of Neurosurgery. 10th ed. New York: Thieme; 2023:1001
[3] Greenberg M, ed. Greenberg's Handbook of Neurosurgery. 10th ed. New York: Thieme; 2023: 1002

[4] Greenberg M, ed. Greenberg's Handbook of Neurosurgery. 10th ed. New York: Thieme; 2023:1003
[5] Greenberg M, ed. Greenberg's Handbook of Neurosurgery. 10th ed. New York: Thieme; 2023:1004
[6] Greenberg M, ed. Greenberg's Handbook of Neurosurgery. 10th ed. New York: Thieme; 2023:1005
[7] Greenberg M, ed. Greenberg's Handbook of Neurosurgery. 10th ed. New York: Thieme; 2023:1006
[8] Greenberg M, ed. Greenberg's Handbook of Neurosurgery. 10th ed. New York: Thieme; 2023:1008
[9] Greenberg M, ed. Greenberg's Handbook of Neurosurgery. 10th ed. New York: Thieme; 2023:1011
[10] Greenberg M, ed. Greenberg's Handbook of Neurosurgery. 10th ed. New York: Thieme; 2023:1012
[11] Greenberg M, ed. Greenberg's Handbook of Neurosurgery. 10th ed. New York: Thieme; 2023:1016
[12] Greenberg M, ed. Greenberg's Handbook of Neurosurgery. 10th ed. New York: Thieme; 2023:1002
[13] Greenberg M, ed. Greenberg's Handbook of Neurosurgery. 10th ed. New York: Thieme; 2023:1010
[14] Greenberg M, ed. Greenberg's Handbook of Neurosurgery. 10th ed. New York: Thieme; 2023:1013

61 Concussion, High Altitude Cerebral Edema, Cerebrovascular Injuries

Questions

▸▸ Question 1

All of the following are correct regarding concussion injury except?

- A. It is considered mild because it is not life-threatening itself
- B. It is a complex pathophysiological process resulting in alteration of the brain function
- C. There is identifiable abnormality in standard structural imaging
- D. It is usually rapid, short lived, and resolves spontaneously
- E. It may include transient deficits in balance, coordination, memory, cognition, strength, and alertness

▸▸ Question 2

How a patient with concussion injury is diagnosed?

- A. Abnormal finding in the imaging studies
- B. Self-reporting of abnormal functions like vacant stare, dazed or stunned, headache, nausea, vomiting, fatigue, seeing stars, photophobia, phonophobia, speech alterations or incoordination
- C. Observed physiological abnormalities or assessment of cognitive functions like slow to answer, easy distractibility, disorientation, memory deficits, and unaware of the date, time, and place
- D. Both B and C
- E. With blood tests and LP studies

▸▸ Question 3

Diffusion tensor imaging, functional MRI, positron emission tomography (PET), single photon emission CT, MR spectroscopy, and quantitative EEG are being used for research purposes for evaluation of concussive injuries. What is the acute pathophysiology of concussion injury?

- A. Potassium efflux and sodium/calcium influx
- B. Unrestricted hyperacute glutamate release from lipid membranes at cellular level
- C. Cortical spread of depression like state by voltage/ligand gated ion channels
- D. Widespread intracellular energy reserve depletion with increase in ADP
- E. All of the above

▸▸ Question 4

Most symptoms from concussion resolve within 7 to 10 days and do not require treatment. About 10 to 15% of concussed individuals can develop postconcussive syndrome with symptoms beginning within 4 weeks of injury and remaining for more than 1 month after onset of symptoms. Which of the following statements is most appropriate regarding second impact syndrome?

- A. Injury occurring within few days of concussion injury
- B. Second injury when the patient is still symptomatic from the earlier one
- C. Second injury when the patient is still symptomatic with no further sequalae
- D. Second injury leading to malignant cerebral edema due to vascular engorgement which is refractory to all treatment and leads to death in 50 to 100% of cases
- E. Second injury leading to severe symptoms with no significant mortality

▸▸ Question 5

Diffuse axonal injury is a primary injury of rotational acceleration/deceleration head injury. Which of the following statements is not correct regarding grading of diffuse axonal injury?

- A. Mild clinical grade is coma for 6 to 24 hours followed by mild-to-moderate memory impairment and mild to moderate disabilities
- B. Moderate clinical grade is coma for more than 24 hours followed by confusion and long-lasting amnesia, mild-to-severe memory, and behavioral and cognitive deficits
- C. Severe clinical grade is coma lasting for months with flexor and extensor posturing, cognitive, memory, speech, sensory motor, and personal deficits
- D. Grade 1 histological grade is axonal injury in the white matter of cerebral hemisphere, corpus callosum, brain stem, and less commonly cerebellum
- E. Grade 2 histologic grading is focal lesion in the corpus callosum in addition to the above while grade 3 histologic grade does not exist

▸▸ Question 6

Post-traumatic conductive hearing loss classically occurs due to which of the following?

- A. Longitudinal temporal bone fracture with disruption of the ossicular chain and hemotympanum
- B. Injury to the cochlea with temporal bone fracture or cochlear concussion
- C. Injury to the cranial nerve 8
- D. Injury to the brain stem like inferior colliculi, superficial siderosis of the brain stem, injury to bilateral frontal lobe or middle temporal gyrus
- E. Injury to pinna

▸▸ Question 7

A patient presented with headache, insomnia, fatigue, shortness of breath, and edema of hands, feet, lungs, and cerebrum after having rapid ascent to 15,000 feet. On examination, he is found to have retinal hemorrhages, papilledema, and vitreous hemorrhages. What does tight fit hypothesis postulate about the development of this acute mountain sickness?

- A. It occurs because of dilatation of the ventricles and CSF spaces
- B. Because of tight brain spaces
- C. Because of tight CSF spaces like small ventricles and subarachnoid CSF spaces
- D. Because of rapid loss of water content due to developing edema
- E. None of the above

▸▸ Question 8

A patient after head trauma presented with blunt cerebrovascular injury. Signs and symptoms of this injury include arterial hemorrhage from neck/nose/mouth (immediately needs to be taken to OR), cervical bruit in patients less than 50 years old, expanding cervical hematoma, focal neurologic deficit, neurologic deficit inconsistent with head CT, or stroke on CT or MRI of brain. 16 MD CTA (16 slice multidetector CT angiography) or catheter arteriogram is used for diagnosis of this condition. What are the traumatic factors with high risk of BCVI?

- A. Severe cervical hyperextension with rotation or hyperflexion
- B. High energy transfer mechanism with displaced midface fracture or basilar skull fracture
- C. TBI consistent with DAI and GCS less than 6
- D. Cervical vertebral body or transverse foramen fracture or any fracture involving c1 and c3
- E. All of the above

▸▸ Question 9

Which of the following is the treatment for blunt cerebrovascular injuries according to the grade (Denver grading scale)?

- A. Grade 1 is luminal irregularity with less than 25% stenosis which is treated with aspirin only
- B. Grade 2 is more than equal to 25% stenosis or intraluminal thrombus or raised intimal flap which is treated with aspirin only
- C. Garde 3 is pseudoaneurysm which is treated with anticoagulation with heparin (heparin and aspirin are roughly equivalent for grade 3; however, most will need to be studied for 7 to 10 days and heparin is easier to stop for an angiography and if the lesion does not heal then endovascular stenting is considered)
- D. Grade 4 is occlusion and needs endovascular occlusion to prevent embolization
- E. Grade 5 is transection with free extravasation which is a lethal injury needing urgent surgical repair if accessible or endovascular stenting with concurrent thrombosis
- F. All of the above

▸▸ Question 10

Which of the following are the trauma contraindications to anticoagulation?

- A. Active bleeding
- B. Potential for bleeding
- C. In whom the consequences of bleeding are severe like liver or spleen injuries or major pelvic fractures
- D. All of the above
- E. There is no contraindication to anticoagulation after trauma

▸▸ Question 11

A patient presented with complaints of headache, photophobia, and tinnitus after a fall from bicycle. There was no history of loss of consciousness. What is the expected CT finding for the diagnosis of concussion?

- A. Midline shift
- B. Hematoma
- C. Effacement of basal cisterns
- D. Intraventricular hemorrhage
- E. Normal CT of brain

▸▸ Question 12

Functional MRI consists of two types: task-based and resting. What is it based on?

- A. Blood oxygen level dependent effect
- B. Blood carbon dioxide level dependent effect
- C. Voxel analysis
- D. Tractography
- E. Histogram analysis

▸▸ Question 13

A student athlete who had concussion during a football match is able to do moderate activity with increased heart rate. According to 5-step return-to-play progression scale, this athlete is at what step?

- A. Baseline
- B. Step 1
- C. Step 2
- D. Step 3
- E. Step 4

▸▸ Question 14

A comatosed patient was brought to emergency department after roadside accident and was managed in ICU with mechanical ventilation. He improved partially after 1 day but suffered confusion and long-lasting amnesia along with mild-to-severe memory, behavioral, and cognitive deficits. There had been no evidence of mass lesion or ischemia on CT scans. What is the clinical grade of diffuse axonal injury in this case?

- A. Minor
- B. Mild
- C. Moderate
- D. Severe
- E. Critical

▸▸ Question 15

What is the histological grading for diffuse axonal injury with axonal injury in the white matter of the cerebral hemisphere, corpus callosum, brain stem, and cerebellum?
- A. I
- B. II
- C. III
- D. IV
- E. V

▸▸ Question 16

There is 1 to 2% incidence of blunt cerebrovascular injuries with head injury, and 16 slice multidetector CTA or catheter angiogram is used for diagnosis and Denver grading of such injuries. If CTA shows pseudoaneurysm, what is the Denver grade?
- A. I
- B. II
- C. III
- D. IV
- E. V

▸▸ Question 17

Traumatic risk factors with high risk for BCVI include all of the following except?
- A. Severe cervical hyperextension with rotation or hyperflexion
- B. TBI consistent with DAI and GCS < 6
- C. c4 fracture
- D. Near hanging with anoxic brain injury
- E. Clothesline type injury

▸▸ Question 18

What is the recommended management for Denver grade 4 injury?
- A. Rx with aspirin
- B. Endovascular occlusion
- C. Anticoagulation with heparin
- D. Most resolve own their own
- E. Urgent surgical repair

Answers

▸▸ Answer 1

Correct answer is C. There is identifiable abnormality in standard structural imaging[1]

▸▸ Answer 2

Correct answer is D. Both B and C[2]

▸▸ Answer 3

Correct answer is E. All of the above[3]

▸▸ Answer 4

Correct answer is D. Second injury leading to malignant cerebral edema due to vascular engorgement which is refractory to all treatment and leads to death in 50 to 100% of cases[4]

▸▸ Answer 5

Correct answer is E. Grade 2 histologic grading is focal lesion in the corpus callosum in addition to the above while grade 3 histologic grade does not exist[5]

▸▸ Answer 6

Correct answer is A. Longitudinal temporal bone fracture with disruption of the ossicular chain and hemotympanum[6]

▸▸ Answer 7

Correct answer is C. Because of tight CSF spaces like small ventricles and subarachnoid CSF spaces[6]

▸▸ Answer 8

Correct answer is E. All of the above[7]

▸▸ Answer 9

Correct answer is F. All of the above[8]

▸▸ Answer 10

Correct answer is D. All of the above[8]

▸▸ Answer 11

Correct answer is E. Normal CT of brain[1]

▸▸ Answer 12

Correct answer is A. Blood oxygen level dependent effect[3]

▸▸ Answer 13

Correct answer is C. Step 2[9]

▸▸ Answer 14

Correct answer is C. Moderate[5]

▸▸ Answer 15

Correct answer is A. I[5]

▸▸ **Answer 16**

Correct answer is C. III[10]

▸▸ **Answer 17**

Correct answer is C. c4 fracture[7]

▸▸ **Answer 18**

Correct answer is B. Endovascular occlusion[8]

References

[1] Greenberg M, ed. Greenberg's Handbook of Neurosurgery. 10th ed. New York: Thieme; 2023:1019

[2] Greenberg M, ed. Greenberg's Handbook of Neurosurgery. 10th ed. New York: Thieme; 2023:1020

[3] Greenberg M, ed. Greenberg's Handbook of Neurosurgery. 10th ed. New York: Thieme; 2023:1023

[4] Greenberg M, ed. Greenberg's Handbook of Neurosurgery. 10th ed. New York: Thieme; 2023:1025

[5] Greenberg M, ed. Greenberg's Handbook of Neurosurgery. 10th ed. New York: Thieme; 2023:1027

[6] Greenberg M, ed. Greenberg's Handbook of Neurosurgery. 10th ed. New York: Thieme; 2023:1028

[7] Greenberg M, ed. Greenberg's Handbook of Neurosurgery. 10th ed. New York: Thieme; 2023:1029

[8] Greenberg M, ed. Greenberg's Handbook of Neurosurgery. 10th ed. New York: Thieme; 2023:1031

[9] Greenberg M, ed. Greenberg's Handbook of Neurosurgery. 10th ed. New York: Thieme; 2023:1024

[10] Greenberg M, ed. Greenberg's Handbook of Neurosurgery. 10th ed. New York: Thieme; 2023:1030

62 Neuromonitoring in Head Trauma

Questions

▸▸ Question 1

Monro–Kellie doctrine states that the sum of the intracranial volumes (CBV, brain, CSF, and other constituents like tumor or hematoma) is constant and that an increase in any one of these must be offset by an equal decrease in another as these volumes are contained in an inelastic and completely closed container (skull). The increased ICP will act to force one or more of the other constituents out through the foramen magnum. Which of the following will be displaced first?

- A. Cerebrospinal fluid (total volume is 150 mL in brain and spinal canal)
- B. Intravenous blood (total cerebral blood volume is 150 mL)
- C. Arterial blood
- D. Brain parenchyma (total volume is 1,400 mL)
- E. Hematoma or any tumor which is causing the increase in ICP

▸▸ Question 2

A patient after head trauma presents with hypertension, bradycardia, and respiratory irregularity (Cushing's triad). His intracranial pressure is 25 mmHg (normal intracranial pressure is 10–15 mmHg in adults or older children, 3–7 mmHg in young children, and 1.5–6 mmHg in term infants), while his cerebral perfusion pressure (CPP) is 60 mmHg (normal CPP is more than 50 mmHg). His plain CT of the brain is normal. What are the risk factors for intracranial hypertension with a normal brain CT?

- A. Age more than 40 years
- B. Systolic blood pressure less than 90 mmHg
- C. Decerebrate posturing on motor examination
- D. Decorticate posturing on motor examination
- E. All of the above

▸▸ Question 3

Following are the indications for ICP monitoring except?

- A. Patients who cannot follow command (patients with GCS less than equal to 8) or patients who do not localize
- B. Patients with multiple systems injuries with altered level of consciousness (especially where therapies for other injuries may have deleterious effects on ICP like high levels of PEEP or the need for large volumes of IV fluids or the need for heavy sedation)
- C. Patients with coagulopathy in which coagulopathy cannot be corrected
- D. Patients with traumatic intracranial mass like EDH, SDH, or depressed skull fracture
- E. Patients with fulminant liver failure with INR more than 1.5 and grade 3 or 4 coma; a subarachnoid bolt is inserted after administration of factor seven 40 μg/kg IV over 1 to 2 minutes

▸▸ Question 4

Complications of ICP monitors include infection, hemorrhage, malfunction or obstruction, and malposition. Identified risk factors for infection include which of the following?

- A. ICH or SDH or IVH or ICP more than 20 mmHg
- B. Neurosurgical operation or irrigation of system
- C. Leakage around IVCs or open skull fractures
- D. Other infections like septicemia or pneumonia OR duration of monitoring more than 5 days
- E. All of the above

▸▸ Question 5

Which of the following is the most accurate method of monitoring ICP?

- A. Intraventricular catheter
- B. Intraparenchymal monitor
- C. Subarachnoid screw (bolt)
- D. Subdural bolt
- E. Epidural bolt

▸▸ Question 6

Normal ICP waveforms are due to arterial pulsations and respirations. Arterial systolic blood pressure wave is a 1 to 2 mmHg peak with a small dicrotic notch which is followed by smaller less distinct peaks and it is followed by a peak corresponding to the central venous A wave from the right atrium. ICP elevations of more than or equal to 50 mmHg for 5 to 20 minutes cause a pathological waveform which is called as what?

- A. Lundberg A waves or plateau waves
- B. Lundberg B waves
- C. Pressure pulses
- D. Lundberg C waves
- E. Traube-Hering waves

▸▸ Question 7

Indications for jugular venous oxygen monitoring (SjVOs) and brain oxygen tension monitoring ($PbtO_2$) include the need for augmented hyperventilation (pCO_2 equal to 20–25 mmHg). Normal value of jugular venous oxygen saturation is more than 60% (less than 50% suggest ischemia) or arterial jugular venous oxygen content difference of more than 9 mL/dL indicates global cerebral ischemia while its value less than 4 mL/dL indicate cerebral hyperemia. Normal value for brain oxygen content is more than 25 mmHg while values less than 15 mmHg demonstrates ischemia and increases the likelihood of death. What is the management suggestion for brain tissue oxygen content value less than 15 to 20 mmHg?

- A. Cerebral blood flow study should be done to determine generalizability of brain oxygen content monitor reading

- B. Tier one includes keeping body temperature less than 37.5 °C while increasing CPP to more than 60 mmHg
- C. Tier two includes increasing FiO_2 to 60%, increasing $paCO_2$ to 45 to 50 mmHg, and transfusion of PRBCs until Hgb is more than 10 g/dL
- D. Tier three is increasing FiO_2 to 100%, increasing PEEP and decreasing ICP to less than 10 mmHg by draining CSF, and giving mannitol and sedatives
- E. All of the above

▸▸ Question 8

Normal white matter blood flow is 18 to 25 mL/100 g-mint (values less than 15 may indicate vasospasm or ischemia while values less than 10 may indicate infarction), while normal gray matter blood is 67 to 80 mL/100 g-mint. K value of probe tip less than 4.9 indicates which of the following?

- A. Probe tip is probably out of the brain
- B. Probe tip is probably too deep
- C. Probe tip is in abnormal position
- D. Probe tip damage to some brain tissue
- E. All of the above

▸▸ Question 9

Goal of IC hypertension include keeping ICP less than 22 mmHg and CPP more than 60 to 70 mmHg. What are the general measures which should be utilized routinely for ICP control?

- A. Elevation of head of bed to 30 to 45 degrees, keeping neck straight and avoiding neck constrictions, avoiding arterial hypotension (as hypotension reduces CBF), controlling hypertension (by using nicardipine if not tachycardic and beta blocker if tachycardic), avoiding hypoxia (PaO_2 less than 60 mmHg or O_2 set less than 90%), ventilation to normocarbia ($PaCO_2$ 35–40 mmHg), light sedation (codeine 30–60 mg IM every 4 hours), plain CT of brain
- B. Heavy sedation (fentanyl 1–2 mL or MSO4 2–4 mg IV every 1 hour), draining 3 to 5 mL CSF if IVC is present, hyperventilation ($PaCO_2$ 30–35 mmHg), mannitol 0.25 to 1 g/kg, bolus of 10 to 20 mL of 23.4% of hypertonic saline, augmented hyperventilation ($PaCO_2$ to 25–30 mmHg)
- C. Be sure the patient is sedated and paralyzed, draining of 3 to 5 mL CSF, mannitol 1 g/kg IV bolus, hyperventilate ($PaCO_2$ less than 25 mmHg), pentobarbital 100 mg slow IV or thiopental 2.5 mg/kg IV over 10 minutes
- D. Decompressive craniectomy
- E. All of the above

▸▸ Question 10

Longer periods of hyperventilation are needed in patients with documented intracranial hypertension unresponsive to sedation and paralysis and for intracranial hypertension that results from hyperemia. Which of the following are the caveats of hyperventilation?

- A. It is avoided during the first 5 days of injury if possible
- B. It is not used prophylactically without proper indications
- C. If documented IC HTN is unresponsive to other therapies, hyperventilate $PaCO_2$ only to 30 to 35 mmHg
- D. If $PaCO_2$ of 25 to 30 mmHg is necessary, then monitoring of jugular venous oxygen content or cerebral blood flow should be done
- E. $PaCO_2$ should not be reduced below 25 mmHg
- F. All of the above

▸▸ Question 11

Rapidly developing hyperemia following head injury is due to loss of autoregulation. What is the mortality associated with malignant cerebral edema?

- A. 50%
- B. 70%
- C. 80%
- D. 90%
- E. Almost 100%

▸▸ Question 12

Of the following methods for ICP monitoring, which is both diagnostic and offers a benefit in treatment for intracranial hypertension?

- A. Intraventricular
- B. Dural
- C. Subdural
- D. Subarachnoid bolt
- E. Parenchymal

▸▸ Question 13

Of the following methods for ICP monitoring, which is the most accurate?

- A. Intraventricular
- B. Dural
- C. Subdural
- D. Subarachnoid bolt
- E. Parenchymal

▸▸ Question 14

Which of the following is not a risk factor for intracranial hypertension (IC-HTN) with a normal CT?

- A. Age > 40 years
- B. SBP > 90 mmHg
- C. SBP < 90 mmHg
- D. Decerebrate posturing
- E. Decorticate posturing

▸▸ Question 15

ICP monitoring can be discontinued how many hours after cessation of ICP therapy?

- A. 6 to 12 hours
- B. 12 to 18 hours

- C. 18 to 24 hours
- D. 24 to 48 hours
- E. 48 to 72 hours

▸▸ Question 16

What is the jugular venous oxygen saturation ($SjVO_2$) level that is suggestive of ischemia?

- A. < 90
- B. < 80
- C. < 70
- D. < 60
- E. < 50

▸▸ Question 17

Thermal diffusion flowmetry permits regional cerebral blood flow monitoring in the white matter. What is the value that is suggestive of infarction?

- A. < 90
- B. < 50
- C. < 40
- D. < 20
- E. < 10

▸▸ Question 18

A patient with traumatic brain injury was brought to emergency department. Vital check showed hypertension. Hypertension with normal pulse rate secondary to head injury should be treated with which of the following?

- A. Beta blocker
- B. Calcium channel blocker
- C. Alpha blockers
- D. Angiotensin receptor blockers
- E. Hold fluids

▸▸ Question 19

For acute management of raised ICP after traumatic brain injury, 20% mannitol was instituted at 1.4 g/kg over 20 minutes and followed by 20 mg of furosemide. What is the serum osmolarity level at which further osmotic therapy is rendered nonbeneficial?

- A. > 120 mOsm/L
- B. > 180 mOsm/L
- C. > 250 mOsm/L
- D. > 280 mOsm/L
- E. > 320 mOsm/L

▸▸ Question 20

In case of intracranial hypertension refractory to sedation, hyperventilation, and osmotic therapy, what is the desired $PaCO_2$ level for augmented hyperventilation?

- A. 20 to 25 mmHg
- B. 25 to 30 mmHg
- C. 30 to 35 mmHg
- D. 35 mmHg
- E. > 40 mmHg

▸▸ Question 21

The goal of ICP management is to keep cerebral perfusion pressure (CPP) within what range?

- A. > 50 to 60 mmHg
- B. > 60 to 70 mmHg
- C. > 70 to 80 mmHg
- D. > 80 to 90 mmHg
- E. > 90 to 100 mmHg

Answers

▸▸ Answer 1

Correct answer is A. Cerebrospinal fluid (total volume is 150 mL in brain and spinal canal)[1]

▸▸ Answer 2

Correct answer is E. All of the above[2]

▸▸ Answer 3

Correct answer is C. Patients with coagulopathy in which coagulopathy cannot be corrected[3]

▸▸ Answer 4

Correct answer is E. All of the above[4]

▸▸ Answer 5

Correct answer is A. Intraventricular catheter[5]

▸▸ Answer 6

Correct answer is A. Lundberg A waves or plateau waves[6]

▸▸ Answer 7

Correct answer is E. All of the above[7]

▸▸ Answer 8

Correct answer is A. Probe tip is probably out of the brain[7]

▸▸ Answer 9

Correct answer is A. Elevation of head of bed to 30 to 45 degrees, keeping neck straight and avoiding neck constrictions, avoiding arterial hypotension (as hypotension reduces CBF), controlling hypertension (by using nicardipine if not

tachycardic and beta blocker if tachycardic), avoiding hypoxia (PaO_2 less than 60 mmHg or O_2 set less than 90%), ventilation to normocarbia ($PaCO_2$ 35–40 mmHg), light sedation (codeine 30–60 mg IM every 4 hours), plain CT of brain[8]

►► Answer 10

Correct answer is F. All of the above[9]

►► Answer 11

Correct answer is E. Almost 100%[10]

►► Answer 12

Correct answer is A. Intraventricular[4]

►► Answer 13

Correct answer is A. Intraventricular[4]

►► Answer 14

Correct answer is B. SBP > 90 mmHg[2]

►► Answer 15

Correct answer is E. 48 to 72 hours[3]

►► Answer 16

Correct answer is E. < 50[6]

►► Answer 17

Correct answer is E. < 10[7]

►► Answer 18

Correct answer is B. Calcium channel blocker[11]

►► Answer 19

Correct answer is E. > 320 mOsm/L[12]

►► Answer 20

Correct answer is B. 25 to 30 mmHg[11]

►► Answer 21

Correct answer is B. > 60 to 70 mmHg[13]

References

[1] Greenberg M, ed. Greenberg's Handbook of Neurosurgery. 10th ed. New York: Thieme; 2023:1037

[2] Greenberg M, ed. Greenberg's Handbook of Neurosurgery. 10th ed. New York: Thieme; 2023:1038

[3] Greenberg M, ed. Greenberg's Handbook of Neurosurgery. 10th ed. New York: Thieme; 2023:1039

[4] Greenberg M, ed. Greenberg's Handbook of Neurosurgery. 10th ed. New York: Thieme; 2023:1040

[5] Greenberg M, ed. Greenberg's Handbook of Neurosurgery. 10th ed. New York: Thieme; 2023:1041

[6] Greenberg M, ed. Greenberg's Handbook of Neurosurgery. 10th ed. New York: Thieme; 2023:1045

[7] Greenberg M, ed. Greenberg's Handbook of Neurosurgery. 10th ed. New York: Thieme; 2023:1046

[8] Greenberg M, ed. Greenberg's Handbook of Neurosurgery. 10th ed. New York: Thieme; 2023:1050

[9] Greenberg M, ed. Greenberg's Handbook of Neurosurgery. 10th ed. New York: Thieme; 2023:1053

[10] Greenberg M, ed. Greenberg's Handbook of Neurosurgery. 10th ed. New York: Thieme; 2023:1026

[11] Greenberg M, ed. Greenberg's Handbook of Neurosurgery. 10th ed. New York: Thieme; 2023:1048

[12] Greenberg M, ed. Greenberg's Handbook of Neurosurgery. 10th ed. New York: Thieme; 2023:1054

[13] Greenberg M, ed. Greenberg's Handbook of Neurosurgery. 10th ed. New York: Thieme; 2023:1036

63 Skull Fractures

Questions

▸▸ Question 1

About 90% of pediatric skull fractures are linear and involve the calvaria. Linear skull fractures over the convexity rarely require surgical intervention. How can linear skull fractures be differentiated from normal plain film findings?

- A. Density of linear skull fracture is dark black while that in case of vessel groove and suture line it is gray in color
- B. Linear skull fractures are straight in course while vessel groove is more like curve and suture line follows course of known suture lines
- C. Linear skull fractures are usually nonbranching while vessel groove is often branching and suture line joins other suture lines
- D. Linear skull fractures are very thin while vessel groove is thicker than fracture line and suture line is jagged and wide
- E. All of the above are correct

▸▸ Question 2

Surgery is considered for depressed skull fractures with deficit referable to underlying brain and for fractures depressed more than the thickness of calvaria. Nonsurgical management of depressed skull fracture may be considered in the following situations except?

- A. Fractures overlying a major dural sinus always needs to be operated
- B. No evidence (clinical or CT) of dural penetration
- C. No significant intracranial hematoma
- D. Depression is less than 1 cm
- E. No frontal sinus involvement and no wound infection or gross contamination
- F. No gross cosmetic deformity

▸▸ Question 3

Following are the technical considerations during the surgery for depressed skull fracture except?

- A. Debridement of skin edges
- B. Elevation of bone fragments
- C. Dural laceration is never repaired
- D. Debridement of devitalized brain
- E. Reconstruction of the skull

▸▸ Question 4

A patient presents in the emergency with a lateral blow to the head. The fracture line passes though the petrosquamosal suture parallel to and through the EAC. It may cause a conductive hearing loss by disrupting the ossicular chain and/or by producing hemotympanum. What type of fracture produces this kind of deficit?

- A. Longitudinal fracture
- B. Anterior posterior fracture
- C. Transverse fracture
- D. Multiple basal skull fractures
- E. None of the above

▸▸ Question 5

What is the management option for post-traumatic facial palsy?

- A. Steroids are often utilized
- B. Consult with ENT surgeon
- C. Surgical nerve 7th decompression
- D. Surgical decompression
- E. All of the above

▸▸ Question 6

Which of the following are the clinical signals for basal skull fracture?

- A. CSF otorrhea or rhinorrhea
- B. Hemotympanum or laceration of the external auditory meatus
- C. Postauricular ecchymoses (battle's sign)
- D. Periorbital ecchymoses (raccoon's eye)
- E. All of the above

▸▸ Question 7

Which of the following conditions may be associated with basal skull fractures that may require specific management?

- A. Traumatic aneurysm
- B. Post-traumatic cavernous carotid fistula
- C. Meningitis or cerebral abscess
- D. Cosmetic deformities
- E. CSF fistula
- F. All of the above

▸▸ Question 8

In the presence of a frontal sinus fracture, intracranial air on CT must be presumed to be due to dural laceration. Risks of posterior wall fractures include brain abscess, CSF leak, and cyst or mucocele formation. At what age, frontal sinus becomes radiographically evident?

- A. At 6 years
- B. At 8 years
- C. At 10 years
- D. At 11 years
- E. None of the above

►► Question 9

How is a fracture of the frontal air sinus dealt with?

- A. The rear wall of the sinus is removed
- B. Mucosa is then stripped off from the wall of the sinus down to the nasofrontal duct
- C. Temporalis muscle plugs are then packed into the frontonasal ducts
- D. Bony wall of the sinus is drilled and removed
- E. All of the above are steps in dealing with a frontal sinus fracture

►► Question 10

Which of the following is an etiology of pneumocephalus?

- A. Skull defects including postneurosurgical procedures, post traumatic, congenital, or neoplastic
- B. Infection with gas-producing organism or mastoiditis
- C. Post invasive procedures like lumbar puncture, ventriculostomy, or spinal anesthesia
- D. Spinal trauma or barotrauma
- E. All of the above

►► Question 11

When can nonsurgical management be considered for open, depressed skull fracture?

- A. There is evidence of dural penetration
- B. Significant intracranial hematoma
- C. Depression is < 1 cm
- D. Frontal sinus involvement
- E. No gross cosmetic deformity

►► Question 12

Sensorineural hearing loss is caused by what type of temporal bone fractures?

- A. Transverse
- B. Longitudinal
- C. Oblique
- D. Axial
- E. Parallel to IAC axis

►► Question 13

Clivus fracture may be associated with injury to which cranial nerve?

- A. I
- B. II
- C. VI
- D. IX

►► Question 14

The frontal sinus is lined with respiratory epithelium, the mucous secretion of which drains through the frontonasal duct medially and inferiorly into which of the following?

- A. Inferior nasal meatus
- B. Middle nasal meatus
- C. Superior nasal meatus
- D. Lateral nasal meatus
- E. Anterior nasal meatus

►► Question 15

Cranialization of frontal air sinus refers to which of the following?

- A. Removal of rear wall
- B. Stripping off the mucosa
- C. Packing with gelfoam
- D. Packing with temporalis muscle
- E. Obliteration of frontonasal duct

►► Question 16

Craniofacial dislocation is classified as which Le Fort fracture?

- A. I
- B. II
- C. III
- D. IV
- E. Mixed

►► Question 17

CT of brain after head injury showed pneumocephalus. Air appears darker than CSF and has a Hounsfield coefficient of what?

- A. −500
- B. −1,000
- C. −2,000
- D. 5,000
- E. 10,000

►► Question 18

100% O_2 is given for symptomatic or significant postoperative pneumocephalus. For how long can 100% FiO_2 be tolerated?

- A. 6 to 12 hours
- B. 12 to 24 hours
- C. 24 to 48 hours
- D. 48 to 72 hours
- E. 72 to 96 hours

Answers

►► Answer 1

Correct answer is E. All of the above are correct[1]

►► Answer 2

Correct answer is A. Fractures overlying a major dural sinus always needs to be operated[1]

▸▸ Answer 3

Correct answer is C. Dural laceration is never repaired[2]

▸▸ Answer 4

Correct answer is A. Longitudinal fracture[2]

▸▸ Answer 5

Correct answer is E. All of the above[3]

▸▸ Answer 6

Correct answer is E. All of the above[3]

▸▸ Answer 7

Correct answer is F. All of the above[4]

▸▸ Answer 8

Correct answer is B. At 8 years[4]

▸▸ Answer 9

Correct answer is E. All of the above are steps in dealing with a frontal sinus fracture[5]

▸▸ Answer 10

Correct answer is E. All of the above[6]

▸▸ Answer 11

Correct answer is C. Depression is < 1 cm[1]

▸▸ Answer 12

Correct answer is A. Transverse[7]

▸▸ Answer 13

Correct answer is C. VI[3]

▸▸ Answer 14

Correct answer is B. Middle nasal meatus[5]

▸▸ Answer 15

Correct answer is A. Removal of rear wall[5]

▸▸ Answer 16

Correct answer is C. III[5]

▸▸ Answer 17

Correct answer is B. −1,000[6]

▸▸ Answer 18

Correct answer is C. 24 to 48 hours[8]

References

[1] Greenberg M, ed. Greenberg's Handbook of Neurosurgery. 10th ed. New York: Thieme; 2023:1062

[2] Greenberg M, ed. Greenberg's Handbook of Neurosurgery. 10th ed. New York: Thieme; 2023:1063

[3] Greenberg M, ed. Greenberg's Handbook of Neurosurgery. 10th ed. New York: Thieme; 2023:1065

[4] Greenberg M, ed. Greenberg's Handbook of Neurosurgery. 10th ed. New York: Thieme; 2023:1066

[5] Greenberg M, ed. Greenberg's Handbook of Neurosurgery. 10th ed. New York: Thieme; 2023:1067

[6] Greenberg M, ed. Greenberg's Handbook of Neurosurgery. 10th ed. New York: Thieme; 2023:1068

[7] Greenberg M, ed. Greenberg's Handbook of Neurosurgery. 10th ed. New York: Thieme; 2023:1064

[8] Greenberg M, ed. Greenberg's Handbook of Neurosurgery. 10th ed. New York: Thieme; 2023:1069

64 Traumatic Hemorrhagic Conditions

Questions

▸▸ Question 1

A patient presenting with refractory intracranial hypertension due to diffuse parenchymal injury with clinical and radiographic evidence for impending transtentorial herniation should have decompressive craniectomy. While a patient presenting with medically refractory posttraumatic cerebral edema and associated intracranial hypertension should have which of the following?

- A. Bifrontal decompressive craniectomy within 24 hours
- B. Bifrontal decompressive craniectomy within 48 hours
- C. Treatment with hyperventilation
- D. Decompressive bifrontal craniectomy within 4 hours
- E. None of the above

▸▸ Question 2

Nonoperative management of traumatic intracerebral hemorrhage (TICH) with intensive monitoring and serial imaging is used in patients without neurologic compromise, no significant mass effect on CT, and controlled ICP. What are the indications for surgical evacuation of TICH?

- A. Progressive neurologic deterioration referable to TICH
- B. Medically refractory intracranial hypertension or signs of mass effect on CT
- C. TICH volume more than 50 mL
- D. GCS equal to 6 to 8 with frontal or temporal TICH volume more than 20 mL with midline shift of more than 5 mm and/or compressed basal cisterns on CT
- E. All of the above

▸▸ Question 3

Incidence of delayed traumatic intracerebral hemorrhage (DTICH) in patients with GCS less than 9 is almost 10%. When does most DTICH occur?

- A. Within 24 hours of injury
- B. Within 5 days of injury
- C. Within 72 hours of injury
- D. Within 7 days of injury
- E. Within 9 days of injury

▸▸ Question 4

A patient after road traffic accident (RTA) presents with brief period of LOC followed by a lucid interval of few hours in which he remained conscious and then deteriorated suddenly. On CT of the brain, there is a biconvex hyperdense area on right parietal area with possible rupture of middle meningeal artery. The patient is also showing ipsilateral dilated pupil and contralateral hemiparesis on examination. What are the indications of surgical evacuation of this lesion?

- A. EDH volume of more than 30 mL
- B. EDH thickness of more than 15 mm
- C. Midline shift of more than 5 mm
- D. GCS less than 8
- E. Focal neurologic deficit
- F. All of the above

▸▸ Question 5

Subdural hematoma is typically more diffuse, less uniform, usually crescentic over brain surface, often less dense as compared to extradural hematoma (EDH), and cannot cross intradural barriers like falx or tentorium whereas an EDH can. Which of the following statements is correct regarding acute subdural hematoma (ASDH) density changes with time?

- A. Acute SDH is from 1 to 3 days and is hyperdense on CT relative to brain
- B. Subacute SDH is from 4 days to 2 or 3 weeks and it is isodense to brain
- C. Chronic SDH is from 3 weeks to 3 or 4 months and it is hypodense (approaching density of CSF)
- D. After about 1 to 2 months, it may become lenticular in shape with density more than CSF but less than fresh blood
- E. All of the above

▸▸ Question 6

According to the 4-hour rule, patients operated within 4 hours of injury had 30% mortality compared to 90% mortality if surgery was delayed for more than 4 hours. Also, functional survival (Glasgow outcome scale more than or equal to 4) rate of 65% could be achieved with surgery within 4 hours. What are the indications of surgery for ASDH?

- A. Thickness greater than 10 mm
- B. Midline shift more than 5 mm
- C. ASDH with thickness less than 10 mm and midline shift less than 5 mm should undergo surgery if GCS drops by more than 2 points from the time of injury to admission or the pupils are asymmetric, fixed, and dilated or ICP is more than 20 mmHg
- D. A, B, and C
- E. Patient presenting after 4 hours of injury should never be evacuated

▸▸ Question 7

Mortality rate of ASDH is 50 to 90%. The variables which strongly influence outcome in patients with ASDH includes mechanism of injury, age, neurologic condition on admission, and postoperative ICP. Which statement is correct regarding admission GCS, mortality, and functional survival in these patients?

- A. Patients with admission GCS 3 has 90% mortality and functional survival of only 5%
- B. Patients with admission GCS 4 has 76% mortality and functional survival of only 10%
- C. Patients with admission GCS 5 has 62% mortality and functional survival of only 18%
- D. Patients with admission GCS 3 has 51% mortality and functional survival of only 44%
- E. All of the above

▸▸ Question 8

A young child presents with history of backwards fall from standing position after which the child cried and then developed a generalized seizure. On CT of the brain, ASDH is found with hyperdense blood, and the patient is diagnosed as case of infantile acute subdural hematoma. What is the most appropriate management in this patient?

- A. Percutaneous subdural tap
- B. Craniotomy and evacuation of clot
- C. Subdural peritoneal shunt
- D. Burr hole and drainage of clot
- E. None of the above

▸▸ Question 9

Many chronic subdural hematoma (CSDH) start out as acute subdurals in which fibroblasts invade due to an inflammatory response. These fibroblasts form neomembranes on the inner and outer surface of the clot which is followed by neocapillaries, enzymatic fibrinolysis, and liquefaction of blood clot. Which of the following is incorrect regarding Markwalder neurologic grading scale for CSDH?

- A. Grade 0 is neurologically intact patients
- B. Grade 1 is alert and oriented patient with mild symptoms (H/A) and no or minimal neurologic deficit
- C. Grade 2 is drowsy or disoriented and variable neurologic deficit (hemiparesis)
- D. Grade 3 is stuporous but responds appropriately to noxious stimulus and severe focal signs (hemiplegia)
- E. Grade 4 is noncomatose patient with motor response to noxious stimuli

▸▸ Question 10

Management step for CSDH includes seizure prophylaxis, coagulopathies reversal, and treatment of hematoma if symptomatic (focal deficit, mental status change, seizure, and severe headache). A patient with CSDH shows improvement after approximately 20% removal of collection. Postoperatively, CT shows persistent fluid in 78% of cases on postoperative day 10 and in 15% on postoperative day 40. Hence, it is recommended not to treat persistent fluid collections evident on CT within 20 days postoperatively. What are the surgical options in patients with CSDH?

- A. Placing two subdural burr holes
- B. Single large burr hole with irrigation and aspiration
- C. Single burr hole drainage with placement of a subdural drain
- D. Twist drill craniostomy
- E. Craniotomy with excision of subdural membrane
- F. All of the above

▸▸ Question 11

For medically refractory IC-HTN and post-traumatic edema, bifrontal decompressive craniectomy should be done within what time?

- A. 6 hours
- B. 12 hours
- C. 24 hours
- D. 36 hours
- E. 48 hours

▸▸ Question 12

Which of the following is an indication for surgical evacuation of TICH?

- A. Volume > 10 cm^3
- B. Volume > 20 cm^3
- C. Volume > 15 cm^3
- D. Volume > 30 cm^3
- E. Volume > 50 cm^3

▸▸ Question 13

A middle-aged male presented to emergency department after roadside accident with GCS 7, right dilated pupil, and left hemiparesis. CT of brain shows left-sided traumatic lesion. What is Kernohan's notch phenomenon?

- A. Stalk effect
- B. Talk and die syndrome
- C. Long tract sign
- D. False localizing sign
- E. Radiological error

▸▸ Question 14

Mottling of density on brain CT in extradural hematoma is described in which of the following?

- A. Chronic
- B. Delayed
- C. Acute
- D. Subacute
- E. Hyperacute

▸▸ Question 15

A small volume extradural hematoma was managed medically without surgery. The patient remained clinically stable and a follow-up scan was done 1 week later and the patient was discharged. If the patient remains asymptomatic, when

should the next follow-up CT scan to document resolution be performed?
- A. 2 weeks
- B. 4 weeks
- C. 6 months
- D. 1 year
- E. 5 years

▸▸ **Question 16**

The mortality associated with acute subdural hematoma can be reduced from 90 to 30% if surgery is performed within what time?
- A. 4 hours
- B. 6 hours
- C. 8 hours
- D. 12 hours
- E. 3 days

▸▸ **Question 17**

ICP monitoring should be instituted in all patients with acute subdural hematoma with what GCS score?
- A. 15
- B. 13
- C. 12
- D. 10
- E. < 9

▸▸ **Question 18**

After burr hole drainage for chronic subdural hematoma, clinical improvement is expected after evacuation of how much volume?
- A. 1% of volume
- B. 2% of volume
- C. 5% of volume
- D. 10% of volume
- E. 20% of volume

▸▸ **Question 19**

Which of the following is not a treatment option for chronic subdural hematoma?
- A. Single burr hole
- B. Two burr holes
- C. Twist drill craniostomy
- D. Craniotomy and evacuation
- E. Decompressive craniectomy

▸▸ **Question 20**

EDH with all of the following characteristics can be managed conservatively except?
- A. Volume < 30 cm^3
- B. Thickness > 15 mm
- C. Midline shift < 5 mm
- D. GCS > 8
- E. No focal neurological deficit

▸▸ **Question 21**

A patient who is drowsy and has right hemiparesis has what grade according to Markwalder scale for CSDH?
- A. 0
- B. 1
- C. 2
- D. 3
- E. 4

▸▸ **Question 22**

What is the definitive treatment for recurrent subdural hygroma?
- A. Burr hole evacuation
- B. Arachnoid repair
- C. Craniotomy and evacuation
- D. Subdural-peritoneal shunt
- E. Sudural-cisternal shunt

Answers

▸▸ **Answer 1**

Correct answer is B. Bifrontal decompressive craniectomy within 48 hours[1]

▸▸ **Answer 2**

Correct answer is E. All of the above[2]

▸▸ **Answer 3**

Correct answer is C. Within 72 hours of injury[2]

▸▸ **Answer 4**

Correct answer is F. All of the above[3]

▸▸ **Answer 5**

Correct answer is E. All of the above[4]

▸▸ **Answer 6**

Correct answer is D. A, B, and C[4]

▸▸ **Answer 7**

Correct answer is E. All of the above[5]

▸▸ **Answer 8**

Correct answer is B. Craniotomy and evacuation of clot[6]

▸▸ Answer 9

Correct answer is E. Grade 4 is noncomatose patient with motor response to noxious stimuli[7]

▸▸ Answer 10

Correct answer is F. All of the above[8]

▸▸ Answer 11

Correct answer is E. 48 hours[1]

▸▸ Answer 12

Correct answer is E. Volume > 50 cm^3[1]

▸▸ Answer 13

Correct answer is D. False localizing sign[2]

▸▸ Answer 14

Correct answer is E. Hyperacute[3]

▸▸ Answer 15

Correct answer is B. 4 weeks[3]

▸▸ Answer 16

Correct answer is A. 4 hours[4]

▸▸ Answer 17

Correct answer is E. < 9[4]

▸▸ Answer 18

Correct answer is E. 20% of volume[8]

▸▸ Answer 19

Correct answer is E. Decompressive craniectomy[8]

▸▸ Answer 20

Correct answer is B. Thickness > 15 mm[3]

▸▸ Answer 21

Correct answer is C. 2[7]

▸▸ Answer 22

Correct answer is D. Subdural-peritoneal shunt[9]

References

[1] Greenberg M, ed. Greenberg's Handbook of Neurosurgery. 10th ed. New York: Thieme; 2023:1071

[2] Greenberg M, ed. Greenberg's Handbook of Neurosurgery. 10th ed. New York: Thieme; 2023:1072

[3] Greenberg M, ed. Greenberg's Handbook of Neurosurgery. 10th ed. New York: Thieme; 2023:1074

[4] Greenberg M, ed. Greenberg's Handbook of Neurosurgery. 10th ed. New York: Thieme; 2023:1078

[5] Greenberg M, ed. Greenberg's Handbook of Neurosurgery. 10th ed. New York: Thieme; 2023:1079

[6] Greenberg M, ed. Greenberg's Handbook of Neurosurgery. 10th ed. New York: Thieme; 2023:1081

[7] Greenberg M, ed. Greenberg's Handbook of Neurosurgery. 10th ed. New York: Thieme; 2023:1082

[8] Greenberg M, ed. Greenberg's Handbook of Neurosurgery. 10th ed. New York: Thieme; 2023:1083

[9] Greenberg M, ed. Greenberg's Handbook of Neurosurgery. 10th ed. New York: Thieme; 2023:1086

65 Gunshot Wounds and Nonmissile Penetrating Brain Injuries

Questions

▸▸ Question 1

Primary injury from gunshot wound of head results from which factor?

- A. Injury to the soft tissue (direct scalp or facial injury, soft tissue and bacteria dragged intracranially, and pressure waves of gas combustion)
- B. Comminuted fracture of bone (may injure subjacent vascular or cortical tissue)
- C. Cerebral injuries from missile (from fragmentation of bullet, ricochet off the bone)
- D. Coup + contrecoup injury from missile impact on head
- E. All of the above

▸▸ Question 2

Secondary injury from gunshot wound of head (GSWH) includes cerebral edema which may cause rapid rise in ICP within minutes. Cardiac output also falls initially which together with high ICP adversely affects cerebral perfusion pressure. Other complicating factors may include DIC and intracranial hemorrhage from lacerated blood and vessels. Which of the following statements is incorrect regarding late complications of this injury?

- A. Cerebral abscess
- B. Typically aneurysm which is rare in distal ACA
- C. Seizures
- D. Fragment migration (migration into the ventricles may cause hydrocephalus)
- E. Lead toxicity

▸▸ Question 3

Entry gunshot wound is typically smaller than the exit wound due to bullet mushrooming. Also, at the surgery or autopsy, entry wound would typically show beveling of the inner table while exit wound has a beveled outer table. A salvageable patient after some time of gunshot wound of head (GSWH) developed delayed hemorrhage and the trajectory of the bullet on investigations is found to be through the named vessels. What investigation does this patient need to determine vascular status?

- A. Doppler ultrasound
- B. CT of brain with bone window
- C. CT angiography
- D. Bone scan
- E. Dexa scan

▸▸ Question 4

A patient with gunshot wound injury of head needs initial control of bleeding, measures to lower ICP including head of bed (HOB) elevation, steroids, hyperventilation, and mannitol. What is the goal of surgery in these patients?

- A. Debridement of devitalized tissue and evacuation of hematoma
- B. Removal of accessible bone fragments and retrieval of bullet fragment
- C. Obtaining hemostasis and watertight dural closure
- D. Separation of intracranial compartment from air sinuses traversed by the bullet and identification of entry and exit wound for forensic purpose
- E. All of the above

▸▸ Question 5

The level of consciousness is the most important prognosticator after gunshot wound of head (GSWH). Especially poor prognosis is associated with which of the following?

- A. Bullet that crosses the midline
- B. Bullet that passes through the geographic center of the brain
- C. Bullet that enters and traverses the ventricles
- D. More lobes traversed by the bullet
- E. All of the above

▸▸ Question 6

What are the indications of preoperative angiography in a patient with gunshot wound of head (GSWH)?

- A. Object passes in the region of large named artery
- B. Object passes near dural sinus
- C. Visible evidence of arterial bleeding
- D. Unexpected delayed hemorrhage
- E. All of the above

▸▸ Question 7

What is the surgical technique for removal of foreign body in a patient with nonmissile penetrating injury (injury from knives, arrows, and lawn darts)?

- A. Empiric antibiotic coverage before surgery
- B. Optimal control by performing craniotomy
- C. Dura is opened before removing the object
- D. Removal of the object ideally should follow the entry trajectory
- E. Debridement of any easily accessible impacted bone and other extracranial tissue and material along the track
- F. All of the above

▸▸ Question 8

AP and lateral skull X-rays provide useful information in case of gunshot injury to head as they are less susceptible to artifact from the bullet than the CT scan. It also helps to localize metal

and bone fragments and entrance and exit wounds. What information can we get with brain CT of the patient?
- A. It demonstrates location of bone and metal
- B. It delineates the bullet trajectory
- C. It assess the passage of the bullet through ventricles and how many quadrants of the hemisphere have been traversed by the bullet
- D. It shows amount of blood within the brain and assesses intracranial hematomas
- E. All of the above

▸▸ **Question 9**

Bullet injury can cause explosive intracranial injury that is uniformly fatal. It can also cause laceration and maceration along the path of the trajectory. Shock waves and temporary cavitation are produced by the bullet at what velocity?
- A. More than 100 m/s
- B. More than 250 m/s
- C. More than 1000 m/s
- D. At 600 to 750 m/s
- E. None of the above

▸▸ **Question 10**

Which one of the following is incorrect regarding initial management of a patient with gunshot wound injury of head?
- A. Controlling of bleeding and shaving of skull to see entry and exit wounds
- B. Initiating the medical therapy including HOB elevation, mannitol, hyperventilation, and steroids
- C. Prophylaxis against GI ulcers and antiseizure medication
- D. There is no need of tetanus toxoid administration in this patient
- E. Administration of antibiotics

▸▸ **Question 11**

What is the most lethal type of head injury?
- A. Motor vehicle accident
- B. Gunshot wounds to head
- C. Acute subdural hematoma
- D. Extradural hematoma
- E. Posterior fossa hemorrhagic contusions

▸▸ **Question 12**

A postoperative CSF fistula after surgery for gunshot wound to head should be repaired if it persists more than how long?
- A. Always repair immediately
- B. 1 day
- C. 3 days
- D. 1 week
- E. 14 days

▸▸ **Question 13**

Most organisms are sensitive to penicillinase resistant agents, for example, nafcillin, and it is recommended for how long to prevent meningitis and abscess formation?
- A. Single shot
- B. 24 hours
- C. 3 days
- D. 5 days
- E. 2 weeks

▸▸ **Question 14**

What is the usual location for traumatic aneurysm?
- A. Distal ACA
- B. Proximal MCA
- C. Middle MCA
- D. Vertebral artery
- E. Basilar apex

▸▸ **Question 15**

What is the most important prognostic factor in the outcome for gunshot wound of head (GSWH)?
- A. Level of consciousness
- B. Path of bullet
- C. Hematoma seen on CT
- D. Suicide attempt
- E. CSF leak

▸▸ **Question 16**

Which of the following is an indication of preoperative angiography in penetrating injuries?
- A. Object traverses the ventricle
- B. Active uncontrolled hemorrhage
- C. Object passes near dural sinus
- D. Object passes near a vein
- E. Presence of extradural hematoma

Answers

▸▸ **Answer 1**

Correct answer is E. All of the above[1]

▸▸ **Answer 2**

Correct answer is B. Typically aneurysm which is rare in distal ACA[2]

▸▸ **Answer 3**

Correct answer is C. CT angiography[2]

▸▸ Answer 4

Correct answer is E. All of the above[3]

▸▸ Answer 5

Correct answer is E. All of the above[4]

▸▸ Answer 6

Answer:E. All of the above[2]

▸▸ Answer 7

Correct answer is F. All of the above[5]

▸▸ Answer 8

Correct answer is E. All of the above[3]

▸▸ Answer 9

Correct answer is D. At 600 to 750 m/s[1]

▸▸ Answer 10

Correct answer is D. There is no need of tetanus toxoid administration in this patient[3]

▸▸ Answer 11

Correct answer is B. Gunshot wounds to head[1]

▸▸ Answer 12

Correct answer is E. 14 days[4]

▸▸ Answer 13

Correct answer is D. 5 days[3]

▸▸ Answer 14

Correct answer is A. Distal ACA[2]

▸▸ Answer 15

Correct answer is A. Level of consciousness[4]

▸▸ Answer 16

Correct answer is C. Object passes near dural sinus[4]

References

[1] Greenberg M, ed. Greenberg's Handbook of Neurosurgery. 10th ed. New York: Thieme; 2023:1093
[2] Greenberg M, ed. Greenberg's Handbook of Neurosurgery. 10th ed. New York: Thieme; 2023:1094
[3] Greenberg M, ed. Greenberg's Handbook of Neurosurgery. 10th ed. New York: Thieme; 2023:1095
[4] Greenberg M, ed. Greenberg's Handbook of Neurosurgery. 10th ed. New York: Thieme; 2023:1096
[5] Greenberg M, ed. Greenberg's Handbook of Neurosurgery. 10th ed. New York: Thieme; 2023:1097

66 Pediatric Head Injury

Questions

▸▸ **Question 1**

The overall mortality for all pediatric head injuries requiring hospitalization has been reported between 10 and 13%. Which of the following are injuries peculiar to pediatric patients?

- A. Birth injuries like skull fractures, cephalhematoma, epidural and subdural hematomas, brachial plexus injuries
- B. Perambulator/walker injuries, nonaccidental injuries (formerly called child abuse), for example, shaken baby syndrome, and injuries from skateboarding, scooters
- C. Injuries related to the easier penetrability of the pediatric skull like recreational lawn darts, cephalhematoma
- D. Leptomeningeal cyst also known as growing skull fracture or retroclival hematoma
- E. All of the above

▸▸ **Question 2**

CT is recommended in a patient below 2 years of age with less than or equal to 14 or other signs of altered mental status. Which of the following is another condition in which CT of brain is a must?

- A. Occipital, parietal, or temporal scalp hematoma
- B. Palpable skull fracture
- C. History of loss of consciousness for more than or equal to 5 seconds
- D. Severe mechanism of injury
- E. Not acting normally according to the parents

▸▸ **Question 3**

A child with GCS 14 or 15 and normal CT scan can be considered for home observation if neurologically stable. What is the risk of these patients to have an occult brain injury?

- A. 0%
- B. 2%
- C. 4%
- D. 6%
- E. 8%

▸▸ **Question 4**

Cephalhematoma are of two types. One is subgaleal hematoma in which bleeding separates galea from periosteum while the other is subperiosteal hematoma (some refer to this as cephalhematoma) which is most commonly found in the newborn. What is the recommended treatment for these?

- A. Aspiration of the blood as soon as possible
- B. If the lesion is calcified then there is no need of surgery for cosmetic reason
- C. Treatment beyond analgesics is almost never required and almost usually resolve within 2 to 3 weeks
- D. There is no need to follow hematocrit or hematoma in large lesions
- E. Percutaneous aspiration of cystic component

▸▸ **Question 5**

A young child after a fall from height develops scalp mass with head pain alone. Radiography shows progressive widening of fracture and scalloping or saucering of edges. Mean age at injury is less than 1 year and over 90% occur before the age of 3 years. Post-traumatic leptomeningeal cysts rarely occur after more than 6 months of the injury. Which of the following are surgical steps are necessary for post-traumatic leptomeningeal cysts?

- A. Wide craniotomy around the fracture
- B. Repair of the dural defect
- C. Replacement of the bone
- D. Pseudo growing fractures should be followed with X-rays and operated only if expansion persists beyond several months
- E. All of the above

▸▸ **Question 6**

Most common skull fractures in pediatric age group is frontal and parietal regions. In young children, remodeling of the skull occurs as a result of brain growth as it tends to smooth out the deformity. What are the indications of surgery in case of simple skull fractures?

- A. Definitive evidence of dural penetration
- B. Persistent cosmetic defect in the older child after the swelling has subsided
- C. Focal neurologic deficits related to the fracture
- D. All of the above

▸▸ **Question 7**

Ping pong fracture is a green stick type of fracture in which caving of focal area of bone occurs as in a crushed area of a ping pong ball. It is usually seen in only newborn due to plasticity of the skull. Which one of the following is not an indication of surgery in these patients?

- A. When fracture is in the temporoparietal region in the absence of underlying brain injury
- B. Radiographic evidence of intraparenchymal bone fragments
- C. Associated neurologic deficit and signs of increased ICP
- D. Signs of CSF leak deep to the galea
- E. Situations in which the patient is unable to come for long-term follow-up

▸▸ Question 8

Dural sinus thrombosis (DST) or compression may occur if fracture of skull bone occurs in the vicinity of dural sinuses. Anticoagulation is recommended in children with DST. What are the advantages of giving anticoagulation in these patients?

- A. Reduction in the incidence of thrombus propagation
- B. Decreases venous infarction
- C. Reduces poor outcome incidence
- D. All of the above

▸▸ Question 9

Retroclival hematoma has a propensity for children with high-speed motor vehicle accident and is mostly managed conservatively with brace. This can be associated with 2, 3, 4, 5, 7, 9, 11, and 12 cranial injuries, while it can be associated with atlantooccipital dislocation, occipital condyle fracture, disruption of the apical odontoid ligament, fracture of clivus, or odontoid fracture. What are indications of surgery in these patients?

- A. Ligamentous instability
- B. Cranial nerve deficits
- C. For evacuation of hematoma
- D. For hydrocephalus
- E. All of the above

▸▸ Question 10

Vigorous shaking of a child produces violent whiplash like angular acceleration decelerations of the head which may lead to significant head injury. All of the following are findings in a shaken baby syndrome child except?

- A. Epidural hematoma
- B. Subdural hematoma
- C. Subarachnoid hematoma
- D. Retinal hemorrhages
- E. Marks on chest, multiple ribs fracture, or pulmonary contusion

▸▸ Question 11

According to the PECARN algorithm for children < 2 years of age, if the patient has parietal scalp hematoma and history of LOC for > 5 seconds, what is the guideline for CT scan?

- A. Recommended
- B. CT versus observation based on physician's experience
- C. Parental preference
- D. CT not recommended

▸▸ Question 12

Subperiosteal hematoma seen in newborn babies absorbs on its own in what percentage of patients?

- A. 50%
- B. 60%
- C. 70%
- D. 80%
- E. 90%

▸▸ Question 13

What is the treatment for a true post-traumatic leptomeningeal cyst?

- A. Analgesics
- B. Observation
- C. Serial imaging
- D. Surgery
- E. No treatment indicated

▸▸ Question 14

In temporoparietal ping pong fractures, surgery is not indicated in which of the following?

- A. Radiographic evidence of intraparenchymal bone fragments
- B. Associated neurological deficit
- C. Signs of raised ICP
- D. CSF leak deep to galea
- E. Patient can have long-term follow-up

▸▸ Question 15

What is the investigation of choice for retroclival hematoma?

- A. Plain CT of brain
- B. Plain MRI of brain
- C. CT angiography
- D. MR angiography
- E. Duplex scan

▸▸ Question 16

Which of the following is a green-stick type of fracture typically seen in pediatric patients resulting in caving in of a focal area of the skull as a crushed area due to the plasticity of the skull?

- A. Ping pong
- B. Stellate
- C. Residual
- D. Bilateral
- E. Tripod

▸▸ Question 17

Which of the following is the most common hematoma associated with shaken baby syndrome?

- A. Bilateral subdural
- B. Extradural
- C. Subarachnoid
- D. Extradural
- E. Intraparenchymal

Answers

▸▸ Answer 1

Correct answer is E. All of the above[1]

▸▸ Answer 2

Correct answer is B. Palpable skull fracture[1]

▸▸ Answer 3

Correct answer is A. 0%[2]

▸▸ Answer 4

Correct answer is C. Treatment beyond analgesics is almost never required and almost usually resolve within 2 to 3 weeks[3]

▸▸ Answer 5

Correct answer is E. All of the above[3]

▸▸ Answer 6

Correct answer is D. All of the above[4]

▸▸ Answer 7

Correct answer is A. When fracture is in the temporoparietal region in the absence of underlying brain injury[4]

▸▸ Answer 8

Correct answer is D. All of the above[5]

▸▸ Answer 9

Correct answer is E. All of the above[5]

▸▸ Answer 10

Correct answer is A. Epidural hematoma[6]

▸▸ Answer 11

Correct answer is B. CT versus observation based on physician's experience[1]

▸▸ Answer 12

Correct answer is D. 80%[2]

▸▸ Answer 13

Correct answer is D. Surgery[3]

▸▸ Answer 14

Correct answer is E. Patient can have long-term follow-up[4]

▸▸ Answer 15

Correct answer is B. Plain MRI of brain[7]

▸▸ Answer 16

Correct answer is A. Ping pong[4]

▸▸ Answer 17

Correct answer is A. Bilateral subdural[6]

References

[1] Greenberg M, ed. Greenberg's Handbook of Neurosurgery. 10th ed. New York: Thieme; 2023:1098
[2] Greenberg M, ed. Greenberg's Handbook of Neurosurgery. 10th ed. New York: Thieme; 2023:1099
[3] Greenberg M, ed. Greenberg's Handbook of Neurosurgery. 10th ed. New York: Thieme; 2023:1100
[4] Greenberg M, ed. Greenberg's Handbook of Neurosurgery. 10th ed. New York: Thieme; 2023:1101
[5] Greenberg M, ed. Greenberg's Handbook of Neurosurgery. 10th ed. New York: Thieme; 2023:1103
[6] Greenberg M, ed. Greenberg's Handbook of Neurosurgery. 10th ed. New York: Thieme; 2023:1104
[7] Greenberg M, ed. Greenberg's Handbook of Neurosurgery. 10th ed. New York: Thieme; 2023:1102

67 Head Injury: Long-Term Management, Complications, and Outcome

Questions

▸▸ Question 1

The risk of developing DVT is 20% in untreated severe traumatic brain injury. Hence, unless contraindicated, graduated compression stockings or intermittent compression boots are recommended until patients are ambulatory. Low molecular weight heparin (LMWH) or low dose unfractionated heparin in conjunction with mechanical measures lowers the DVT risk but increases the risk for which of the following?

- A. Drug reaction
- B. Longer hospital stay for administration of heparin
- C. Expansion of intracranial hemorrhage
- D. Infection of the wound
- E. None of the above

▸▸ Question 2

Nutritional replacement should begin within 72 hours of head injury in order to achieve 140% of predicted basal energy expenditure (BEE) in nonparalyzed patients while 100% of predicted BEE in paralyzed patients by which post trauma day (mortality is reduced in patients who receive full caloric replacement by that day)?

- A. 7
- B. 9
- C. 11
- D. 13
- E. 15

▸▸ Question 3

Isotonic solutions should be used at full strength starting at 30 mL/h along with enteral or parenteral feeding. Gastric residual is checked every 4 hours and feedings is held if residuals exceed what volume?

- A. 400 mL in an adult
- B. 300 mL in an adult
- C. 200 mL in an adult
- D. 125 mL in an adult
- E. 50 mL in an adult

▸▸ Question 4

What percentage of daily calories should be provided as protein daily?

- A. 10
- B. 15
- C. 20
- D. 25
- E. 30

▸▸ Question 5

Incidence of clinically symptomatic hydrocephalus within 3 months of traumatic subarachnoid hemorrhage is approximately 12%. Which of the following are the factors which increase the risk of hydrocephalus after traumatic subarachnoid hemorrhage?

- A. Older age
- B. Intraventricular hemorrhage
- C. Blood thickness more than or equal to 5 mm
- D. Diffuse distribution of blood versus focal distribution
- E. All of the above

▸▸ Question 6

All of the following are factors favoring shunt placement in a patient with post traumatic hydrocephalus except?

- A. Elevated pressure on one or more LPs
- B. Papilledema on fundoscopy is not present
- C. Symptoms of head/pressure
- D. Finding of transependymal absorption on CT of T2WI MRI
- E. Patients whose neurologic recovery seems worse than expected

▸▸ Question 7

The status of basal cisterns is evaluated on axial CT scan at the level of the midbrain where they are divided into three limbs. One posterior limb which is called as quadrigeminal cistern and two lateral limbs which are posterior portions of ambient cisterns. Which of the following options are correct regarding status of basal cisterns compression with Glasgow outcome scale 5 (good outcome)?

- A. Normal—35%
- B. Compressed—19%
- C. Absent—11%
- D. Nonvisualized—12%
- E. All of the above statements are correct

▸▸ Question 8

Midline shift is defined at the level of foramen of Monro and is calculated by dividing biparietal diameter (the width of intracranial compartment at this level) by 2 and subtracting SP (the distance from the inner table to the septum pellucidum on the side of the shift). Midline shift may be most probably associated with which one of the following?

- A. Severe headache
- B. Persistent vomiting
- C. Diplopia
- D. Altered level of consciousness
- E. Ophthalmoplegia

▸▸ **Question 9**

Apolipoprotein (apoE-4) presence portends a worse prognosis following traumatic brain injury. Which of the following are the late complications from traumatic brain injury?
- A. Post-traumatic seizures
- B. Communicating hydrocephalus
- C. Post-traumatic concussive syndrome
- D. Hypogonadotropic hypogonadism
- E. Chronic traumatic encephalopathy or Alzheimer's disease
- F. All of the above

▸▸ **Question 10**

A patient after some time of traumatic head injury presents with headache, dizziness, visual disturbances, difficulty concentrating, dementia, emotional difficulties, and personality changes. Supportive and reassuring counselling of this patient is done. What tests can be performed if symptoms from minor head trauma persist for more than 3 months?
- A. Head CT
- B. MRI
- C. BAER
- D. Neuropsychological battery
- E. All of the above

▸▸ **Question 11**

What is the advantage of early tracheostomy in severe head injury?
- A. Reduces duration for mechanical ventilation
- B. Reduces pneumonia
- C. Reduces mortality
- D. Reduces duration for antibiotics
- E. Reduces ICP

▸▸ **Question 12**

Establishment of full caloric requirement should not be delayed beyond what post-trauma day?
- A. 1
- B. 3
- C. 7
- D. 10
- E. 14

▸▸ **Question 13**

Rested comatose patients with isolated head injury have how much metabolic expenditure compared to normal for that patient?
- A. 100%
- B. 140%
- C. 300%
- D. 350%
- E. 500%

▸▸ **Question 14**

Regarding nutritional requirement in head trauma patient, caloric requirement provided with proteins should be how much?
- A. 1%
- B. 5%
- C. 7%
- D. ≥ 15%
- E. 50%

▸▸ **Question 15**

Following are the factors favoring hydrocephalus for which shunt should be considered except?
- A. Elevated pressure on LP
- B. Papilledema
- C. Symptom of headache
- D. Transependymal absorption on CT/T2WI MRI
- E. Good neurological recovery than expected

▸▸ **Question 16**

Midline shift is defined at what level?
- A. Frontal horn
- B. Basal cisterns
- C. Foramen of Monro
- D. Temporal tip
- E. Brain stem

▸▸ **Question 17**

Which genotype is associated with poor prognosis after head injury?
- A. ApoE ε4 allele
- B. 1p-19q codeletion
- C. Chromosome 4
- D. Loss of heterozygosity on long arm of chromosome 22
- E. XXYY

▸▸ **Question 18**

How can post-traumatic dementia be differentiated from chronic traumatic encephalopathy?
- A. It occurs after single closed head injury
- B. Specific CT scan features
- C. Blood pathology reports
- D. Genotype studies
- E. Chromosomal abnormalities

▸▸ **Question 19**

A patient is in persistent vegetative state after traumatic brain injury. What is the Glasgow outcome score?
- A. I
- B. II

- C. III
- D. IV
- E. V

▸▸ **Question 20**

NG tube feeding may interfere with absorption of which of the following?

- A. Phenytoin
- B. Phenobarbital
- C. Antituberculous therapy
- D. Steroids
- E. Omeprazole

▸▸ **Question 21**

In addition to periprocedural antibiotics for endotracheal intubation, ICP rise may be decreased by giving which of the following intravenously?

- A. Lidocaine
- B. Omeprazole
- C. Phenytoin
- D. Valproic acid
- E. Carbamazepine

Answers

▸▸ **Answer 1**

Correct answer is C. Expansion of intracranial hemorrhage[1]

▸▸ **Answer 2**

Correct answer is A. 7[1]

▸▸ **Answer 3**

Correct answer is D. 125 mL in an adult[2]

▸▸ **Answer 4**

Correct answer is B. 15[3]

▸▸ **Answer 5**

Correct answer is E. All of the above[3]

▸▸ **Answer 6**

Correct answer is B. Papilledema on fundoscopy is not present[3]

▸▸ **Answer 7**

Correct answer is E. All of the above statements are correct[4]

▸▸ **Answer 8**

Correct answer is D. Altered level of consciousness[4]

▸▸ **Answer 9**

Correct answer is F. All of the above[5]

▸▸ **Answer 10**

Correct answer is E. All of the above[6]

▸▸ **Answer 11**

Correct answer is A. Reduces duration for mechanical ventilation[1]

▸▸ **Answer 12**

Correct answer is C. 7[1]

▸▸ **Answer 13**

Correct answer is B. 140%[2]

▸▸ **Answer 14**

Correct answer is D. ≥ 15%[2]

▸▸ **Answer 15**

Correct answer is E. Good neurological recovery than expected[3]

▸▸ **Answer 16**

Correct answer is C. Foramen of Monro[4]

▸▸ **Answer 17**

Correct answer is A. ApoE ε4 allele[5]

▸▸ **Answer 18**

Correct answer is A. It occurs after single closed head injury[6]

▸▸ **Answer 19**

Correct answer is D. II[7]

▸▸ **Answer 20**

Correct answer is A. Phenytoin[2]

▸▸ **Answer 21**

Correct answer is A. Lidocaine[8]

References

[1] Greenberg M, ed. Greenberg's Handbook of Neurosurgery. 10th ed. New York: Thieme; 2023:1106
[2] Greenberg M, ed. Greenberg's Handbook of Neurosurgery. 10th ed. New York: Thieme; 2023:1107
[3] Greenberg M, ed. Greenberg's Handbook of Neurosurgery. 10th ed. New York: Thieme; 2023:1108
[4] Greenberg M, ed. Greenberg's Handbook of Neurosurgery. 10th ed. New York: Thieme; 2023:1110
[5] Greenberg M, ed. Greenberg's Handbook of Neurosurgery. 10th ed. New York: Thieme; 2023:1111
[6] Greenberg M, ed. Greenberg's Handbook of Neurosurgery. 10th ed. New York: Thieme; 2023:1113
[7] Greenberg M, ed. Greenberg's Handbook of Neurosurgery. 10th ed. New York: Thieme; 2023:1641
[8] Greenberg M, ed. Greenberg's Handbook of Neurosurgery. 10th ed. New York: Thieme; 2023:1050

Part XV

Spine Trauma

XV

68 Spine Injuries—General Information, Neurologic Assessment, Whiplash and Sports-Related Injuries, Pediatric Spine Injuries

Questions

▸▸ Question 1

"The ability of the spine under physiologic loads to limit displacement so as to prevent injury or irritation of the spinal cord and nerve roots (including cauda equina) and to prevent incapacitating pain or deformity or pain due to structural changes" is the conceptual definition of clinical stability of spine from White and Punjabi. The level of injury is defined as the most caudal segment with motor function that is at least 3 out of 5 and if pain and temperature sensations are intact. Which of the following is true representation of incomplete spinal cord injury?

- A. Any residual motor or sensory function more than three segments below the level of the injury
- B. Sensation (including position sense) or voluntary movement in the LEs in the presence of a cervical or thoracic spinal cord injury
- C. Sacral sparing which is preserved sensation around the anus, voluntary rectal sphincter contraction, or voluntary toe flexion
- D. An injury does not qualify as incomplete with preserved sacral reflexes alone (bulbocavernous)
- E. All of the above

▸▸ Question 2

Complete spinal cord injury is lack of preservation of any motor and/or sensory function more than three segments below the level of the injury in the absence of spinal shock. Spinal shock is often used in two completely different senses. Which of the following statements is true regarding the second sense of spinal shock?

- A. It is the hypotension due to interruption of sympathetics (which implies spinal cord injury above T1)
- B. It is the hypotension due to unopposed parasympathetics, loss of muscle tone due to skeletal muscle paralysis below the level of injury, and loss of blood from associated wounds
- C. It is the transient loss of all neurologic functions (including segmental and polysynaptic reflex activity and autonomic function) below the level of spinal cord injury which leads to flaccid paralysis and areflexia but may abate in as little as 72 hours but typically persists for 1 to 2 weeks, occasionally several months
- D. This is not accompanied by loss of bulbocavernosus reflex
- E. Spinal cord reflexes immediately above the level of injury are never depressed

▸▸ Question 3

Whiplash-associated disorder (WAD) is defined as a traumatic injury to the soft tissue structures in the region of the cervical spine due to hyperflexion, hyperextension, or rotational injury in the absence of fractures, dislocations, or intervertebral disk herniations. Which of the following is true regarding grading of whiplash-associated injury?

- A. Grade 1 (neck pain or stiffness or tenderness with no signs) is managed with range of motion exercises and these should be started immediately with early return to daily activities encouraged immediately
- B. Grade 2 (neck pain or stiffness or tenderness with reduced range of motion or point tenderness) is treated with range of motion exercises started immediately, return to regular activities ASAP, cervical collar and rest for no more than 72 hours, passive modality therapies like heat, ice, TENS, ultrasound, relaxation, etc., are optional if symptoms last for more than 3 weeks and with NSAIDs and non-narcotic analgesics
- C. Grade 3 (pain, tenderness, stiffness, reduced range of motion, point tenderness and symptoms with increased weakness, sensory deficit with absent deep tendon reflex) is treated with all of the above except that the cervical collar is used for no more than 96 hours; occasional narcotics may also be given or surgery only for progressive neurologic deficit and persisting neck pain
- D. Surgery is needed for all other grades of WAD

▸▸ Question 4

Which of the following statements is correct regarding pediatric spine injuries?

- A. A retroclival hematoma should raise the index of suspicion for AOD
- B. When AOD is a consideration, cervical CT is the imaging modality of choice to measure the condyle C1 interval
- C. Most stable fractures and ligamentous injuries may be treated nonsurgically, and C2 synchondrosis fractures are usually managed with halo traction
- D. SCIWORA, synchondrosis fractures (os odontoideum, C2 synchondrosis) and atlanto-axial rotatory fixation/subluxation are somewhat unique to pediatric population
- E. All of the above

▸▸ Question 5

Pseudospread of atlas is defined as more than 2 mm total overlap of the two C1 lateral masses on C2 on AP open mouth view (which may be diagnosed as Jefferson fracture), while pseudosubluxation is anterior displacement or significant angulation usually of c3 and c4. True subluxation in children may occur because of which of the following?

- A. Fractures like hangman's fracture
- B. Injury to the c2–c3 disk and posterior elements
- C. Jefferson fracture
- D. Odontoid tip fracture
- E. None of the above

▸▸ Question 6

Which of the following is correct regarding pediatric c spine injuries?

- A. Children less than 8 months of age when restrained, immobilization with thoracic elevation or an occipital recess allows more neutral alignment due to the relatively large head
- B. In children less than 7 years old, c2 synchondrosis is treated with closed reduction and halo immediately
- C. Acute atlanto-axial rotatory subluxation does not reduce spontaneously and require closed reduction and halo immobilization
- D. All of the above

▸▸ Question 7

Which of the following statements regarding sports-related spinal spine injury is correct?

- A. Type one is permanent spinal cord injury
- B. Type two is transient SCI without radiologic abnormality
- C. Type three is radiologic abnormality without neurologic deficit
- D. All of the above

▸▸ Question 8

Which of the following are the characteristics of spear tackler's spine?

- A. Cervical spinal stenosis
- B. Loss of normal cervical lordosis
- C. Evidence of pre-existing cervical abnormality
- D. Documented spear tackler's technique
- E. All of the above

▸▸ Question 9

After injury to the spinal cord, disproportionately greater motor deficit in the upper extremity than the lower ones usually results from hyperextension injuries in the presence of osteophytic spur. What is the most probable diagnosis?

- A. Central cord syndrome
- B. Brown Sequard syndrome
- C. Left right dissociative loss
- D. Gerstmann syndrome
- E. None of the above

▸▸ Question 10

A patient presents with pain, and paresthesias in the neck, upper arms, and torso. Long tract findings are minimal with mild paresis of the upper extremity. What is this condition called?

- A. Central cord syndrome
- B. Posterior cord syndrome
- C. Gerstmann syndrome
- D. None of the above

▸▸ Question 11

A patient presented to the emergency after roadside accident. He was conscious, oriented, and mobile. He complained of neck pain and on examination, there were only reduced range of motion and point tenderness. What is the whiplash-associated disorder grade?

- A. 0
- B. 1
- C. 2
- D. 3
- E. 4

▸▸ Question 12

About 70% of patients with whiplash-associated disorder (WAD) recover within how long?

- A. 1 month
- B. 3 months
- C. 6 month
- D. 12 months
- E. 24 months

▸▸ Question 13

Odontoid epiphysiolysis is a fracture through the neurocentral synchondrosis. It might mimic which of the following?

- A. Hangman type I
- B. Hangman type II
- C. Jefferson type
- D. Odontoid type I
- E. Odontoid type II

▸▸ Question 14

According to NEXUS criteria, X-ray of the cervical spine is recommended in which of the following?

- A. GCS 15
- B. Neurologically intact
- C. Posterior midline cervical tenderness and distracting pain
- D. Not hypotensive without explanation
- E. Not intoxicated

▸▸ Question 15

Pseudospread of the atlas is defined as > 2 mm total overlap of the two C1 lateral masses on C2 on AP open-mouth view. It might mimic which of the following?

- A. Hangman type I
- B. Hangman type II
- C. Jefferson type
- D. Odontoid type I
- E. Odontoid type II

▸▸ **Question 16**

Regarding cervicothoracic orthosis, which of the following is most effective for bracing against flexion–extension and rotation?

- A. Miami J
- B. Poster brace
- C. Guilford
- D. SOMI
- E. Yale brace

▸▸ **Question 17**

In American Spinal Injury Association (ASIA) scoring system, what is the label for a complete spinal cord injury?

- A. A
- B. B
- C. C
- D. D
- E. E

▸▸ **Question 18**

What is Beevor's sign test used for?

- A. Meningismus
- B. Abdominal cutaneous reflex
- C. Ankle plantar flexion
- D. Wrist extensors
- E. Plantars

▸▸ **Question 19**

A patient presented after roadside accident. He had an open wound and abrasions on the forehead and suffered from quadriparesis after injury with upper limbs worse than lower limbs. What will be the most common condition?

- A. Brown Sequard syndrome
- B. Central cord syndrome
- C. Anterior spinal syndrome
- D. Posterior spinal syndrome
- E. Cauda equina syndrome

▸▸ **Question 20**

A patient presented after roadside accident. On examination, there was paraplegia along with loss of pain and temperature sensation but preserved two-point discrimination, joint position sense, and deep pressure sensation. What is the most probable diagnosis?

- A. Brown Sequard syndrome
- B. Central cord syndrome
- C. Anterior spinal syndrome
- D. Posterior spinal syndrome
- E. Cauda equina syndrome

▸▸ **Question 21**

A patient presented with penetrating spine trauma. On examination, there was ipsilateral motor paralysis and loss of proprioception and vibratory sense and contralateral loss of pain and temperature sensation. This is classical for which of the following?

- A. Brown Sequard syndrome
- B. Central cord syndrome
- C. Anterior spinal syndrome
- D. Posterior spinal syndrome
- E. Cauda equina syndrome

Answers

▸▸ **Answer 1**

Correct answer is E. All of the above[1]

▸▸ **Answer 2**

Correct answer is D. This is not accompanied by loss of the bulbocavernosus reflex[3]

▸▸ **Answer 3**

Correct answer is D. Surgery is needed for all other grade of WAD[4]

▸▸ **Answer 4**

Correct answer is E. All of the above[5]

▸▸ **Answer 5**

Correct answer is A. Fractures like hangman's fracture[6]

▸▸ **Answer 6**

Correct answer is D. All of the above[7]

▸▸ **Answer 7**

Correct answer is D. All of the above[8]

▸▸ **Answer 8**

Correct answer is E. All of the above[9]

▸▸ **Answer 9**

Correct answer is B. Brown Sequard syndrome[10]

▸▸ **Answer 10**

Correct answer is B. Posterior cord syndrome[11]

▸▸ **Answer 11**

Correct answer is C. 2[12]

▸▸ **Answer 12**

Correct answer is C. 6 month[4]

▸▸ **Answer 13**

Correct answer is E. Odontoid type II[5]

▸▸ **Answer 14**

Correct answer is C. Posterior midline cervical tenderness and distracting pain[13]

▸▸ **Answer 15**

Correct answer is C. Jefferson type[14]

▸▸ **Answer 16**

Correct answer is E. Yale brace[7]

▸▸ **Answer 17**

Correct answer is A. A[15]

▸▸ **Answer 18**

Correct answer is B. Abdominal cutaneous reflex[16]

▸▸ **Answer 19**

Correct answer is B. Central cord syndrome[17]

▸▸ **Answer 20**

Correct answer is C. Anterior spinal syndrome[18]

▸▸ **Answer 21**

Correct answer is A. Brown Sequard syndrome[10]

References

[1] Greenberg M, ed. Greenberg's Handbook of Neurosurgery. 10th ed. New York: Thieme; 2023:1118
[2] White AA, Panjabi MM. The problem of clinical instability in the human spine: a systematic approach. In: Clinical Biomechanics of the Spine. 2nd ed. Philadelphia: J.B. Lippincott; 1990:277–378
[3] Greenberg M, ed. Greenberg's Handbook of Neurosurgery. 10th ed. New York: Thieme; 2023:119
[4] Greenberg M, ed. Greenberg's Handbook of Neurosurgery. 10th ed. New York: Thieme; 2023:1120
[5] Greenberg M, ed. Greenberg's Handbook of Neurosurgery. 10th ed. New York: Thieme; 2023:1121
[6] Greenberg M, ed. Greenberg's Handbook of Neurosurgery. 10th ed. New York: Thieme; 2023:1112
[7] Greenberg M, ed. Greenberg's Handbook of Neurosurgery. 10th ed. New York: Thieme; 2023:1124
[8] Greenberg M, ed. Greenberg's Handbook of Neurosurgery. 10th ed. New York: Thieme; 2023:1125
[9] Greenberg M, ed. Greenberg's Handbook of Neurosurgery. 10th ed. New York: Thieme; 2023:1126
[10] Greenberg M, ed. Greenberg's Handbook of Neurosurgery. 10th ed. New York: Thieme; 2023:1136
[11] Greenberg M, ed. Greenberg's Handbook of Neurosurgery. 10th ed. New York: Thieme; 2023:1137
[12] Greenberg M, ed. Greenberg's Handbook of Neurosurgery. 10th ed. New York: Thieme; 2023:1119
[13] Greenberg M, ed. Greenberg's Handbook of Neurosurgery. 10th ed. New York: Thieme; 2023:1122
[14] Greenberg M, ed. Greenberg's Handbook of Neurosurgery. 10th ed. New York: Thieme; 2023:1123
[15] Greenberg M, ed. Greenberg's Handbook of Neurosurgery. 10th ed. New York: Thieme; 2023:1132
[16] Greenberg M, ed. Greenberg's Handbook of Neurosurgery. 10th ed. New York: Thieme; 2023:1130
[17] Greenberg M, ed. Greenberg's Handbook of Neurosurgery. 10th ed. New York: Thieme; 2023:1133
[18] Greenberg M, ed. Greenberg's Handbook of Neurosurgery. 10th ed. New York: Thieme; 2023:1135

69 Management of Spinal Cord Injury

Questions

▸▸ Question 1

The major causes of death in a spinal cord injury patient are aspiration and shock. Initial survey of a trauma patient should be done according to the ATLS protocol in which airway, breathing, and circulation should be assessed. Which of the following are the management steps in the field?

- A. Spine immobilization (by placing the patient on board, placing sandbags on both sides or using a rigid collar)
- B. Blood pressure is maintained for which dopamine is the agent of choice and is preferred over fluids but fluids are also given as necessary
- C. Oxygenation is maintained for which intubation may be needed and chin lift is done for intubation without neck extension
- D. Brief motor examination should be done to identify deficits in a conscious patient by asking him/her to move legs or arms or hands or toes
- E. All of the above

▸▸ Question 2

Which of the following are the management steps of a patient at hospital with suspected spinal injury?

- A. NG intubation and Foley catheterization
- B. DVT prophylaxis and temperature regulation
- C. Checking electrolytes
- D. More detailed neurological examination, radiographic evaluation, and medical management which includes methylprednisolone and other experimental drugs
- E. All of the above

▸▸ Question 3

Methylprednisolone for the treatment of acute spinal cord injury is not recommended and high dose steroids can be associated with harmful effects and even death. Following are the management options for the management and prophylaxis of deep vein thrombosis except?

- A. LMW heparin, rotating beds, adjusted dose of heparin, or some combination of these
- B. LMW heparin (titrating dose of SQ heparin every 12 hours to a PTT of 1.5 times control or 5,000 units SQ every 12 hours) plus pneumatic compression stockings or electrical stimulation
- C. Low-dose heparin and oral anticoagulation should not be used alone
- D. Vena cava interruption filters should be used as routine prophylaxis in all the patients
- E. Duplex Doppler ultrasound, impedance plethysmography, venography, and clinical examination are recommended as diagnostic tests for DVT in patients with SCI

▸▸ Question 4

Radiographic studies are not needed in a patient with no mental status change with no neck pain or posterior midline tenderness (with no distracting pain), no focal neurologic deficit and with no associated significant injuries that would detract or distract from the evaluation. Following are the criteria that should be met before removal of the cervical collar except?

- A. Asymptomatic patients who are alert with no neck pain or tenderness with full range of motion and without neurologic deficit or distracting pain
- B. Penetrating brain trauma unless the trajectory suggests direct cervical spinal cord injury
- C. In an obtunded patient with normal cervical CT scan and gross movement of all four extremities, there is strong recommendation to get flexion–extension X-rays
- D. Patients who are awake with neck pain or tenderness and normal cervical CT scan after either normal and adequate dynamic flexion and extension cervical spine X-rays and normal cervical MRI
- E. If MRI is normal, the collar may be safely removed

▸▸ Question 5

What are the indicators that should alert a surgeon that there may be significant spinal cord injury?

- A. Retropharyngeal space more than 7 mm and retrotracheal space more than 14 or 22 mm in children
- B. Displaced paravertebral fat stripe
- C. Tracheal deviation and laryngeal dislocation
- D. Loss of lordosis or acute kyphotic angulation or torticollis
- E. All of the above

▸▸ Question 6

Flexion–extension X-rays help to identify ligamentous injuries. Which of the following are the contraindications of these X-rays?

- A. Noncooperative patient with some mental impairment
- B. Subluxation of more than 3.5 mm at any level on neutral lateral c spine X-ray which is a marker for possible instability
- C. The patient is not neurologically intact
- D. In obtunded patients
- E. All of the above

▸▸ Question 7

After a suspected spinal cord injury, MRI should be done within what time?

- A. 48 to 72 hours
- B. 24 hours
- C. 12 hours

- D. 5 days
- E. 8 hours

▸▸ Question 8

Traction is used in a patient to reduce fracture dislocations, maintain normal alignment, and immobilize the cervical spine to prevent further spinal cord injury. Following are the contraindications of traction except?

- A. Atlanto-occipital dislocation
- B. Very elderly patients or patients with demineralized skull can undergo cervical traction without any problem
- C. Type 2A or 3 hangman's fracture
- D. Skull defect at anticipated pin site or if age is less than 3 years
- E. Patients with an additional rostral injury or patient with movement disorders

▸▸ Question 9

Which of the following tongs can be used for applying traction?

- A. Crutch filed tongs
- B. Gardner Wells tongs
- C. Screw ring tongs
- D. Halo ring
- E. Halo vest

▸▸ Question 10

After spinal cord injury, surgical decompression should be done within what time?

- A. 12 hours
- B. 24 hours
- C. 36 hours
- D. 48 hours
- E. 72 hours

▸▸ Question 11

Deep venous thrombosis (DVT) prophylaxis is indicated in spinal cord injury patients because the incidence of DVT in spinal cord injury might be up to what percent?

- A. 5%
- B. 10%
- C. 25%
- D. 50%
- E. 100%

▸▸ Question 12

Regarding radiographic imaging in trauma patients who are obtunded or unevaluable, what is the imaging modality of choice?

- A. AP/Lateral X-ray
- B. Open mouth odontoid view
- C. Dynamic X-rays
- D. CT scan
- E. MRI of spine

▸▸ Question 13

For evaluation of traumatic cervical spine injury, cervical spine must be cleared radiographically from the cranio-cervical junction up to C7–T1 junction. Which view can be used to evaluate cervicothoracic junction if it is being missed on lateral view?

- A. AP view
- B. Oblique view
- C. Open mouth odontoid view
- D. Swimmer's view
- E. Pillar's view

▸▸ Question 14

Neural foramina are well demonstrated on which view?

- A. AP view
- B. Oblique view
- C. Open mouth odontoid view
- D. Swimmer's view
- E. Pillar's view

▸▸ Question 15

One of the radiographic signs of C-spine trauma is the status of soft tissues and retropharyngeal space. In adults when is it considered a sign of injury?

- A. > 1 mm
- B. > 2 mm
- C. > 3 mm
- D. > 5 mm
- E. > 7 mm

▸▸ Question 16

All of the following are contraindications to cervical skull traction except?

- A. Atlantooccipital dislocation
- B. Type IIA or III hangman's fracture
- C. Skull fracture at anticipated pin site
- D. Age > 4 years
- E. Patients with movement disorders

▸▸ Question 17

For locked facets, how are Gardener Wells tongs applied?

- A. Neutral
- B. Flexion
- C. Extension
- D. Contraindicated

▸▸ Question 18

Surgery for ongoing compression in spinal cord injury should ideally be done within what time?

- A. 1 hour
- B. 4 hours
- C. 6 hours
- D. 12 hours
- E. 24 hours

Answers

▸▸ Answer 1

Correct answer is E. All of the above[1]

▸▸ Answer 2

Correct answer is E. All of the above[2]

▸▸ Answer 3

Correct answer is D. Vena cava interruption filters should be used as routine prophylaxis in all the patients[3]

▸▸ Answer 4

Correct answer is C. In an obtunded patient with normal cervical CT scan and gross movement of all four extremities, there is strong recommendation to get flexion–extension X-rays[4]

▸▸ Answer 5

Correct answer is E. All of the above[3]

▸▸ Answer 6

Correct answer is E. All of the above[5]

▸▸ Answer 7

Correct answer is A. 48 to 72 hours[5]

▸▸ Answer 8

Correct answer is B. Very elderly patients or patients with demineralized skull can undergo cervical traction without any problem[6]

▸▸ Answer 9

Correct answer is C. Screw ring tongs[7]

▸▸ Answer 10

Correct answer is B. 24 hours[8]

▸▸ Answer 11

Correct answer is E. 100%[9]

▸▸ Answer 12

Correct answer is D. CT scan[4]

▸▸ Answer 13

Correct answer is D. Swimmer's view[10]

▸▸ Answer 14

Correct answer is B. Oblique view[10]

▸▸ Answer 15

Correct answer is E. > 7 mm[10]

▸▸ Answer 16

Correct answer is D. Age > 4 years[6]

▸▸ Answer 17

Correct answer is B. Flexion[11]

▸▸ Answer 18

Correct answer is E. 24 hours[7]

References

[1] Greenberg M, ed. Greenberg's Handbook of Neurosurgery. 10th ed. New York: Thieme; 2023:1139
[2] Greenberg M, ed. Greenberg's Handbook of Neurosurgery. 10th ed. New York: Thieme; 2023:1140
[3] Greenberg M, ed. Greenberg's Handbook of Neurosurgery. 10th ed. New York: Thieme; 2023:1142
[4] Greenberg M, ed. Greenberg's Handbook of Neurosurgery. 10th ed. New York: Thieme; 2023:1143
[5] Greenberg M, ed. Greenberg's Handbook of Neurosurgery. 10th ed. New York: Thieme; 2023:1146
[6] Greenberg M, ed. Greenberg's Handbook of Neurosurgery. 10th ed. New York: Thieme; 2023:1147
[7] Greenberg M, ed. Greenberg's Handbook of Neurosurgery. 10th ed. New York: Thieme; 2023:1149
[8] Greenberg M, ed. Greenberg's Handbook of Neurosurgery. 10th ed. New York: Thieme; 2023:1150
[9] Greenberg M, ed. Greenberg's Handbook of Neurosurgery. 10th ed. New York: Thieme; 2023:1141
[10] Greenberg M, ed. Greenberg's Handbook of Neurosurgery. 10th ed. New York: Thieme; 2023:1144
[11] Greenberg M, ed. Greenberg's Handbook of Neurosurgery. 10th ed. New York: Thieme; 2023:1148

70 Occipitoatlantoaxial Injuries

Questions

▸▸ Question 1

Occipitoatlantal injuries are twice more common in children than in adults because of flatter condyles, higher ratio of cranium to body weight, and ligament laxity. Which of the following methods are devised radiographically to diagnose atlanto-occipital dislocation (AOD)?

- A. Basion axial interval is the distance between the basion and rostral extension of posterior axial line (which is posterior cortical margin of body of C2). It should be from 4 to 12 mm in adults and 0 to 12 mm in children on X-rays
- B. Basion to dental interval (BDI) which is the distance from the basion to the closest point on the tip of dens should be less than 8.5 mm (range 1.4–8.5 mm) on CT, while it should be less than 10.5 mm in children
- C. Atlantooccipital interval also known as condyle–C1 interval which should be less than 1.4 mm in adults and less than 2.5 mm in children
- D. Power's ratio or Dublin measure which is ratio between BC (basion to posterior arch of C1) and AO (anterior arch of C1 to opisthion) should be less than 1 in adults and less than 0.9 in children
- E. All of the above

▸▸ Question 2

Power's ratio of more than one encompasses all the cases of AOD. According to the Traynelis classification of atlanto-occipital dislocation normal alignment of clivus and dens is that inferior tip of clivus should point directly to the tip of dens, while types I, II, and III are anterior dislocation of foramen magnum, longitudinal dislocation, or posterior dislocation of foramen magnum. According to grading and management of AOD, which of the following statements is correct?

- A. Grade 1 AOD is no abnormal CT criteria and only moderately abnormal MRI (high signal in posterior ligament or occipitoatlantal joint)
- B. Grade 1 needs only external orthosis
- C. Grade 2 includes more than or equal to one abnormal criteria on CT and gross abnormal MRI findings on occipitoatlantal joints, tectorial membrane, or alar or cruciate ligament
- D. Grade 2 requires surgical stabilization
- E. All of the above

▸▸ Question 3

A patient presents after blunt trauma with high energy with occipital pain or tenderness, impaired cervical movement, lower cranial nerve palsies, and retropharyngeal soft tissue swelling. Which statement is not correct about the Anderson and Montesano classification of occipital condyle fractures and their treatment?

- A. Type I is comminuted from impact which may occur with axial loading and treated with or without external immobilization (collar or halo)
- B. Type II is extension of linear basilar skull fracture treated with or without external immobilization
- C. Type III is avulsion of condyle fragment which may occur during rotation, lateral bending, or a combination of mechanisms, and it is treated with external immobilization for 6 to 8 weeks
- D. There is difference in outcome between surgically treated patients or patients with only external immobilization

▸▸ Question 4

A young child after head trauma presents with cock robins head position with head in 20-degree rotation to one side, 20-degree rotation to the other, and slight 10-degree flexion with reduced range of motion. X-ray of cervical spine shows frontal projection of C2 with simultaneous oblique projection of C1. Which of the following is true regarding Fielding and Hawkins classification of rotatory atlantoaxial subluxation and its management?

- A. Type I is intact TAL, bilateral facet injury with AD less than or equal to 3 and it is treated with soft collar
- B. Type II is injured TAL and unilateral facet injury with AD 3.1 to 5 and it is treated with SOMI or rigid collar
- C. Type III is injured TAL with bilateral facet joint disruption and AD more than 5 and it is treated with halo
- D. Type IV is incompetence of odontoid because of fracture or erosion with posterior displacement of C1
- E. After 6 to 8 weeks of immobilization, stability with flexion–extension X-rays is done and surgical fusion is never done with residual instability with posterior lateral mass fixation

▸▸ Question 5

A patient after head injury presents in neurosurgical emergency in which total overhang of both C1 lateral masses on C2 is more than or equal to 7 and MRI shows loss of continuity of TAL and high signal within TAL. Dickman type is anatomic disruption of TAL without osseous component with possible findings in type IA of loss of continuity of TAL with high signal within the TAL and type IB with osteoperiosteal TAL disruption. All type I Dickman injuries are fused while in case of Dickman type II which is physiologic disruption of TAL with detachment of C1 tubercle from C1 lateral mass what is the treatment?

- A. Treat with immobilization only
- B. Immobilization with fusion in all cases
- C. Fusion is done only in cases that are still unstable after 3 to 4 months of immobilization
- D. Fusion is not recommended in irreducible subluxation
- E. None of the above

▸▸ Question 6

Jefferson type I is anterior arch of C1 fracture or posterior arch fracture, type II is anterior and posterior arch fracture, while type III is lateral mass fracture. All are treated with rigid immobilization for 10 to 12 weeks except?

- A. Cases with TAL disrupted are treated with surgical stabilization and fusion
- B. Cases with type III fracture
- C. Cases with instability
- D. Cases with neurologic deficit
- E. None of the above

▸▸ Question 7

According to Levine classification of hangman's fracture (modified Effendi system), traction is contraindicated in which fractures?

- A. In type I (vertical pars fracture just posterior to VB)
- B. In type IA (fracture lines on each side are not parallel and fracture may pass through foramen transversarium on one side)
- C. Type II (vertical fracture through pars with disruption of C2–C3 disk and posterior longitudinal ligament)
- D. Type IIA oblique fracture usually anterior–inferior to posterior–superior with little subluxation of less than 3 mm but more angulation of more than 15 degrees
- E. Type III which is type II plus C2 and C3 facet capsule disruption
- F. Both type IIA and type III

▸▸ Question 8

Indications for surgery of hangman's fracture are inability to reduce the fracture, failure of external immobilization to prevent movement at the fracture site, traumatic C2–C3 disk herniation with compromise of the spinal cord, and established nonunion. Which of the following is hangman's fracture requiring surgery?

- A. Levine types II and III
- B. Francis grades 2, 4, and 5
- C. Anterior displacement of C2 by more than 50% of the AP diameter of C3 VB
- D. If angulation produces widening of either the anterior or posterior border of the C2–C3 disk space more than the height of C3–C4 disk below
- E. All of the above

▸▸ Question 9

According to the Anderson and D'Alonzo classification of odontoid fractures, type I is through the tip, type II is through the base of the neck, type IIA is similar to type II but with large bone chips, and type III is through the body. Following are the indications of surgical management of these fractures except?

- A. Isolated type II odontoid fractures in adults more than 50 years of age should be considered for surgical stabilization and fusion
- B. Types II and III with dens displacement of more than or equal to 5 mm
- C. Type IIA fracture
- D. Inability to maintain or achieve alignment with external immobilization
- E. Nondisplaced type I, II, and III fractures

▸▸ Question 10

A patient presents with occipitocervical neck pain and myelopathy. On investigation, there is a separate bone ossicle of variable size with smooth cortical borders separated from a foreshortened odontoid peg. Type I is orthotopic in which ossicle moves with anterior arch of C1 while type II is dystopic in which ossicle is functionally fused to the basion. Which of the following are true regarding management of these fractures?

- A. Patients without neurologic signs and symptoms may be followed with clinical or radiographic surveillance or with posterior C1–C2 fusion
- B. Patients with neurologic signs and symptoms or C1–C2 instability are treated with posterior C1–C2 internal fixation and fusion
- C. If surgery is done and rigid internal immobilization is not done, then postoperative halo immobilization is done
- D. For patients with irreducible cervicomedullary compression and/or evidence of associated occipito-atlantal instability, occipital cervical fusion with or without C1 laminectomy should be done
- E. For patients with irreducible cervicomedullary compression, consider ventral decompression
- F. All of the above

▸▸ Question 11

In Traynelis classification, anterior dislocation of occiput relative to the atlas is what type?

- A. I
- B. II
- C. III
- D. IV
- E. V

▸▸ Question 12

In pediatric patients, the highest sensitivity and specificity for AOD is CT measurement of which of the following?

- A. Condyle–C1 interval (CCI)
- B. Basion–axial interval (BAI)
- C. Basion–dental interval (BDI)
- D. Power's ratio
- E. X-line method

▸▸ **Question 13**

According to Anderson and Montesano classification, avulsion of condyle fragment in occipital condyle fracture is what type?
- A. I
- B. II
- C. III
- D. IV
- E. V

▸▸ **Question 14**

In Fielding and Hawkins classification of rotatory atlantoaxial subluxation, an anterior displacement of > 5 mm and injury to bilateral facets and transverse atlantal ligament is what type?
- A. I
- B. II
- C. III
- D. IV
- E. V

▸▸ **Question 15**

What is the treatment of Grisel's syndrome?
- A. Steroids
- B. Antibiotics
- C. Calcitonin
- D. Surgery
- E. Observation

▸▸ **Question 16**

According to Dickman classification of transverse atlantal ligament disruption, detachment of the C1 tubercle from the C1 lateral mass is what type?
- A. IA
- B. IB
- C. II
- D. III
- E. IV

▸▸ **Question 17**

Jefferson fracture involving posterior arch alone or anterior arch alone is what Landell's class?
- A. I
- B. II
- C. III
- D. IV
- E. V

▸▸ **Question 18**

A vertical fracture through pars with disruption of C2–C3 disk and posterior longitudinal ligament along with subluxation of C2 on C3 of > 3 mm and angulation is what hangman type?
- A. I
- B. II
- C. III
- D. IV
- E. V

▸▸ **Question 19**

According to Anderson and D'Alonzo classification, odontoid fractures through the base of neck of odontoid is what type?
- A. I
- B. II
- C. III
- D. IV
- E. V

▸▸ **Question 20**

What is the best management option for combined C1 and type III odontoid fracture?
- A. Steroids
- B. Surgery
- C. Crutchfield traction
- D. Halo
- E. Muscle relaxants

Answers

▸▸ **Answer 1**

Correct answer is E. All of the above[1]

▸▸ **Answer 2**

Correct answer is E. All of the above[2]

▸▸ **Answer 3**

Correct answer is D. There is difference in outcome between surgically treated patients or patients with only external immobilization[3]

▸▸ **Answer 4**

Correct answer is E. After 6 to 8 weeks of immobilization, stability with flexion–extension X-rays is done and surgical fusion is never done with residual instability with posterior lateral mass fixation[4]

▸▸ Answer 5

Correct answer is C. Fusion is done only in cases that are still unstable after 3 to 4 months of immobilization[5]

▸▸ Answer 6

Correct answer is A. Cases with TAL disrupted are treated with surgical stabilization and fusion[6]

▸▸ Answer 7

Correct answer is F. Both type IIA and type III[7]

▸▸ Answer 8

Correct answer is E. All of the above[8]

▸▸ Answer 9

Correct answer is E. Nondisplaced type I, II, and III fractures[9]

▸▸ Answer 10

Correct answer is F. All of the above[10]

▸▸ Answer 11

Correct answer is A. I[11]

▸▸ Answer 12

Correct answer is A. Condyle–C1 interval (CCI)[1]

▸▸ Answer 13

Correct answer is C. III[3]

▸▸ Answer 14

Correct answer is C. III[3]

▸▸ Answer 15

Correct answer is B. Antibiotics[12]

▸▸ Answer 16

Correct answer is C. II[5]

▸▸ Answer 17

Correct answer is A. I[6]

▸▸ Answer 18

Correct answer is B. II[7]

▸▸ Answer 19

Correct answer is B. II[13]

▸▸ Answer 20

Correct answer is D. Halo[14]

References

[1] Greenberg M, ed. Greenberg's Handbook of Neurosurgery. 10th ed. New York: Thieme; 2023:1153
[2] Greenberg M, ed. Greenberg's Handbook of Neurosurgery. 10th ed. New York: Thieme; 2023:1156
[3] Greenberg M, ed. Greenberg's Handbook of Neurosurgery. 10th ed. New York: Thieme; 2023:1157
[4] Greenberg M, ed. Greenberg's Handbook of Neurosurgery. 10th ed. New York: Thieme; 2023:1159
[5] Greenberg M, ed. Greenberg's Handbook of Neurosurgery. 10th ed. New York: Thieme; 2023:1161
[6] Greenberg M, ed. Greenberg's Handbook of Neurosurgery. 10th ed. New York: Thieme; 2023:1163
[7] Greenberg M, ed. Greenberg's Handbook of Neurosurgery. 10th ed. New York: Thieme; 2023:1167
[8] Greenberg M, ed. Greenberg's Handbook of Neurosurgery. 10th ed. New York: Thieme; 2023:1168
[9] Greenberg M, ed. Greenberg's Handbook of Neurosurgery. 10th ed. New York: Thieme; 2023:1173
[10] Greenberg M, ed. Greenberg's Handbook of Neurosurgery. 10th ed. New York: Thieme; 2023:1176
[11] Greenberg M, ed. Greenberg's Handbook of Neurosurgery. 10th ed. New York: Thieme; 2023:1155
[12] Greenberg M, ed. Greenberg's Handbook of Neurosurgery. 10th ed. New York: Thieme; 2023:1158
[13] Greenberg M, ed. Greenberg's Handbook of Neurosurgery. 10th ed. New York: Thieme; 2023:1172
[14] Greenberg M, ed. Greenberg's Handbook of Neurosurgery. 10th ed. New York: Thieme; 2023:1178

71 Subaxial (C3 through C7) Injuries/Fractures

Questions

▸▸ Question 1

Subaxial cervical spine injury classification (SLIC) is used to assess injuries to the diskoligamentous complex, in addition to neurologic and bony injuries. Which of the following is correct regarding SLIC?

- A. According to the morphology, scores of 0, 1, 2, 3, and 4 are given to no abnormality, simple compression, burst fracture, distraction and rotation, and translation, respectively
- B. According to diskoligamentous complex, scores of 0, 1, and 2 are given to intact, intermediate, and disrupted
- C. According to the neurologic status, scores of 0, 1, 2, 3, and + 1 are given to intact, complete spinal cord injury, incomplete spinal cord injury, and continuous cord compression with neuro deficit
- D. Only patients with score of 5 or more are treated with surgical management
- E. All of the above

▸▸ Question 2

Flexion injury acting alone will produce unilateral or bilateral facet dislocation. Flexion injury with compression will produce which type of injury?

- A. Anterior VB fracture with kyphosis, disruption of interspinous ligament, and teardrop fracture
- B. Torn posterior ligaments and dislocated and locked facets
- C. Fractured spinous process and possible lamina
- D. Burst fracture
- E. Fracture through lateral mass or facet including horizontalization of facet

▸▸ Question 3

In general, compromise of anterior elements produces more instability in extension, while compromise of posterior elements produces more instability in flexion. Which of the following is correct regarding White and Panjabi model of subaxial cervical spine stability?

- A. Anterior elements destroyed or unable to function, posterior elements destroyed or unable to function, positive stretch test or spinal cord damage are given the score of 2
- B. Nerve root damage, abnormal disk narrowing, developmentally narrow canal with either sagittal diameter less than 13 mm or Pavlov ratio less than 0.8 and dangerous loading anticipated are given a score of 1
- C. In neutral position cervical spine, sagittal displacement of more than 3.5 mm or 20% while in flexion–extension cervical X-rays sagittal plane translation of more than 3.5 mm or 20% are given point 2
- D. Relative sagittal plane angulation more than 11 degrees in neutral position cervical spine X-rays and sagittal plane angulation more than 20 degrees in flexion–extension cervical spine X-rays are given point 2
- E. Cervical spine is considered unstable if total score is more than or equal to 5
- F. All of the above

▸▸ Question 4

Clay shoveler's fracture is avulsion of spinous process of which vertebra?

- A. C6
- B. C7
- C. C8
- D. T1
- E. T2

▸▸ Question 5

Teardrop fracture is a type of flexion injury which results from axial loading at the vertex of the skull with neck flexed or from hyperflexion. Following are findings in this type of fracture except?

- A. A small chip of bone just beyond the anterior inferior edge of the involved vertebral body on the lateral cervical spine film
- B. Often associated with a fracture through the sagittal plane of the VB which can almost always be seen on AP view
- C. A large triangular fragment of the anterior inferior VB
- D. Fractured vertebra is usually displaced posteriorly
- E. Other fractures through the vertebral body never occur

▸▸ Question 6

Which of the following patients with subluxation are treated with conservative approach only?

- A. Subluxation on plain radiograph is less than or equal to 3.5 mm with no neurological deficit
- B. A + No abnormal movement on flexion–extension views
- C. Angulation more than 11 degrees with neurological deficit
- D. Subluxation of less than 3.5 mm with neurological deficit
- E. All of the above

▸▸ Question 7

Unilateral locked facet is produced with flexion plus rotation while hyperflexion injury produces bilateral locked facet. Which of the following are the signs that are visible in case of locked facet?

- A. Naked facet sign on axial CT in which the articulating surface of the facet will be seen with appropriate articulating mate either absent or on the wrong side
- B. Bow tie sign on lateral X-ray which would be seen as left and right facets at the level of injury side by side instead of the normal superimposed position

- C. Oblique X-ray may depict blocking of the neural foramen
- D. All of the above

▸▸ **Question 8**

Traction is applied in pounds 3 times the cervical vertebral level and increased by 5 to 10 pounds increments at 10 to 15 minutes interval until desired alignment is achieved (under SSEP or MEP monitoring or using lateral c spine X-ray or fluoroscopy). Following are the end points of traction application except?

- A. 10 pounds per vertebral level is not increased or some say up to 5 pounds
- B. If distraction of perched/locked facet or desired reduction is achieved
- C. If occipital cervical instability develops
- D. If any disk space height exceeds 5 mm
- E. If any neurologic deterioration occurs

▸▸ **Question 9**

Classification of cervical lateral mass and facet fracture includes following except?

- A. Separation fracture is fracture through lamina and ipsilateral pedicle which permits horizontalization of facet
- B. Comminuted fracture is multiple fracture often associated with lateral angulation deformity
- C. Split fracture is coronally oriented vertical fracture in one lateral mass with invagination of one articular facet of level below
- D. Traumatic spondylosis is bilateral horizontal fracture through pars interarticularis
- E. Pars fracture with isthmic subtype is also included in this

▸▸ **Question 10**

Indications of anterior approach in cervical spine are fractured vertebral body with bone retropulsed into the spinal canal, most extensive injuries, severe fracture of posterior elements that preclude posterior stabilization and fusion, most extension injuries, and in traumatic subluxation of cervical spine. Following are the complications of anterior approach except?

- A. Anterior cage problems like cage displacement or extrusion, cage subsidence/telescoping into the end plate and vertebral body fracture
- B. Problems with plating like screw pull out, loosening or breakage, fatigue fracture of plate, screw injury of nerve root spinal cord or vertebral artery
- C. Nonunion of graft
- D. Improper surgical approach or failure to incorporate all unstable levels
- E. Injury to subclavian vessels

▸▸ **Question 11**

A patient presented with subaxial C spine injury. He sustained a compression fracture with indeterminate diskoligamentous complex status and root injury. What is the total score according to the SLIC?

- A. 1
- B. 2
- C. 3
- D. 4
- E. 5

▸▸ **Question 12**

Surgical management for subaxial C spine injury is indicated with an SLIC score of how much?

- A. 1
- B. 2
- C. 3
- D. 4
- E. 5

▸▸ **Question 13**

Burst fracture of subaxial cervical spine is associated with which of the following?

- A. Compression in neutral position
- B. Flexion with compression
- C. Extension with compression
- D. Flexion with distraction
- E. Extension with distraction

▸▸ **Question 14**

Teardrop fracture of subaxial cervical spine is associated with which of the following?

- A. Compression in neutral position
- B. Flexion with compression
- C. Extension with compression
- D. Flexion with distraction
- E. Extension with distraction

▸▸ **Question 15**

A score of 1 point in White and Panjabi scheme for stability of subaxial spine is given to which of the following?

- A. Anterior elements destroyed or unable to function
- B. Posterior elements destroyed or unable to function
- C. Positive stretch test
- D. Spinal cord damage
- E. Pavlov ratio < 0.8

▸▸ **Question 16**

Clay shoveler's fracture is the avulsion of spinous process. It usually involves which of the following?

- A. C4
- B. C5
- C. C6

- D. C7
- E. T1

▸▸ **Question 17**

Lateral CT scan in unilateral locked facet depicts visualization of left and right facets at the level of the injury instead of the normal superimposed position. What is this called?

- A. Bow tie sign
- B. Naked facets
- C. Quadrangular
- D. Teardrop
- E. Seat belt

▸▸ **Question 18**

In cervical skull traction for closed reduction locked facets, one of the end points of the procedure is when the disk space height exceeds what distance?

- A. 1 mm
- B. 3 mm
- C. 5 mm
- D. 7 mm
- E. 10 mm

▸▸ **Question 19**

According to the classification of cervical lateral mass and facet fractures, bilateral horizontal fractures through pars interarticularis, separating anterior spinal elements from posterior, is what?

- A. Separation fracture
- B. Comminuted fracture
- C. Split fracture
- D. Traumatic spondylosis
- E. Rule of Steele

▸▸ **Question 20**

SCIWORA is best managed with which of the following?

- A. Antibiotics
- B. Steroids
- C. Immobilization
- D. Surgery
- E. Laminectomy

Answers

▸▸ **Answer 1**

Correct answer is E. All of the above[1]

▸▸ **Answer 2**

Correct answer is A. Anterior VB fracture with kyphosis, disruption of interspinous ligament and teardrop fracture[2]

▸▸ **Answer 3**

Correct answer is F. All of the above[3]

▸▸ **Answer 4**

Correct answer is B. C7[3]

▸▸ **Answer 5**

Correct answer is E. Other fractures through the vertebral body never occur[4]

▸▸ **Answer 6**

Correct answer is E. All of the above[5]

▸▸ **Answer 7**

Correct answer is D. All of the above[6]

▸▸ **Answer 8**

Correct answer is D. If any disk space height exceeds 5 mm[7]

▸▸ **Answer 9**

Correct answer is E. Pars fracture with isthmic subtype is also included in this[8]

▸▸ **Answer 10**

Correct answer is E. Injury to subclavian vessels[9]

▸▸ **Answer 11**

Correct answer is C. 3[1]

▸▸ **Answer 12**

Correct answer is E. 5[2]

▸▸ **Answer 13**

Correct answer is A. Compression in neutral position[2]

▸▸ **Answer 14**

Correct answer is B. Flexion with compression[2]

▸▸ **Answer 15**

Correct answer is E. Pavlov ratio < 0.8[3]

▸▸ **Answer 16**

Correct answer is D. C7[3]

▸▸ **Answer 17**

Correct answer is A. Bow tie sign[6]

▸▸ **Answer 18**

Correct answer is E. 10 mm[7]

▸▸ **Answer 19**

Correct answer is D. Traumatic spondylosis[8]

▸▸ **Answer 20**

Correct answer is C. Immobilization[10]

References

[1] Greenberg M, ed. Greenberg's Handbook of Neurosurgery. 10th ed. New York: Thieme; 2023:1181
[2] Greenberg M, ed. Greenberg's Handbook of Neurosurgery. 10th ed. New York: Thieme; 2023:1182
[3] Greenberg M, ed. Greenberg's Handbook of Neurosurgery. 10th ed. New York: Thieme; 2023:1183
[4] Greenberg M, ed. Greenberg's Handbook of Neurosurgery. 10th ed. New York: Thieme; 2023:1184
[5] Greenberg M, ed. Greenberg's Handbook of Neurosurgery. 10th ed. New York: Thieme; 2023:1186
[6] Greenberg M, ed. Greenberg's Handbook of Neurosurgery. 10th ed. New York: Thieme; 2023:1187
[7] Greenberg M, ed. Greenberg's Handbook of Neurosurgery. 10th ed. New York: Thieme; 2023:1190
[8] Greenberg M, ed. Greenberg's Handbook of Neurosurgery. 10th ed. New York: Thieme; 2023:1192
[9] Greenberg M, ed. Greenberg's Handbook of Neurosurgery. 10th ed. New York: Thieme; 2023:1196
[10] Greenberg M, ed. Greenberg's Handbook of Neurosurgery. 10th ed. New York: Thieme; 2023:1197

72 Thoracic, Lumbar, and Sacral Spine Fracture

Questions

▸▸ Question 1

Denis three-column model of spine attempts to identify CT criteria of instability of thoracolumbar spine fractures. Which of the following statements is incorrect regarding this model?

- A. Anterior column consist of anterior half of vertebral body, anterior half of disk, and the anterior longitudinal ligament
- B. Middle column consist of posterior half of disk and vertebral body including posterior longitudinal ligament
- C. Posterior column consist of posterior bony complex (posterior arch) with interposed posterior ligamentous complex (supraspinous and interspinous ligament, facet joints and capsule, and ligamentum flavum)
- D. Injury to posterior column alone does cause instability in flexion

▸▸ Question 2

Minor spinal injuries involve only a part of column and do not lead to acute instability (when not accompanied by major injuries). These injuries include which of the following?

- A. Fracture of transverse process except in two areas (L4–L5 which can cause lumbosacral plexus injury and T1–T2 which can cause brachial plexus injury)
- B. Fracture of articular process or pars interarticularis
- C. Isolated fracture of spinous process
- D. Isolated laminar fracture
- E. All of the above

▸▸ Question 3

McAfee classification describes six main types of fractures. A simplified system with four categories includes the following except?

- A. Compression fracture which includes anterior column compression and posterior distraction if severe
- B. Burst fracture which includes compression of both anterior and middle columns
- C. Seat belt fracture in which there is middle and posterior column distraction with intact or mild compression of anterior column
- D. Fracture dislocation which includes compression, rotation, and shear of anterior column along with distraction, rotation, and shear of middle and posterior columns
- E. All of the above

▸▸ Question 4

Pure axial load can cause compression of vertebral body and compression failure of anterior and middle columns. Five subtypes of L5 burst fracture are fracture of both end plates, fracture of superior end plate, fracture of inferior end plate, burst rotation, and burst lateral flexion. Which the following is a radiographic picture of this type of fracture?

- A. On lateral X-ray, there can be cortical fracture of posterior vertebral body wall, loss of VB height and retropulsion of bone fragment from end plate into the canal
- B. AP X-ray can show increase in interpediculate distance, vertical fracture of lamina, and splaying of facet joints
- C. CT can demonstrate break in the posterior body wall with retropulsion of bone into the spinal canal
- D. MRI may show possible cord compression anteriorly with possible cord compression usually with fragments occupying more than 50% of the canal diameter
- E. All of the above

▸▸ Question 5

Denis categorized spine injuries as 1st degree, 2nd degree, and 3rd degree causing mechanical instability, neurologic instability, and both mechanical and neurological instability, respectively. Following are included in the unstable compression fracture except?

- A. Single compression fracture with loss of more than 50% height with angulation or excessive kyphotic angulation at one segment
- B. Three or more contiguous compression fracture
- C. Neurologically intact patient
- D. Disrupted posterior column or more than the minimal middle column fracture
- E. Progressive kyphosis (risk of kyphosis increases when loss of height of anterior vertebral body is more than 75%)

▸▸ Question 6

Which of the following is incorrect regarding thoracolumbar injury classification and severity score (TLICS)?

- A. Compression fracture, burst component or lateral angulation more than 15 degrees, translational/rotational injuries, and distraction injuries are given numbers 1, 2, 3, and 4, respectively
- B. Intact neurologic status, root injury, complete spinal cord injury, incomplete spinal cord injury, and cauda equina syndrome are given numbers 0, 2, 2, 3, and 3, respectively
- C. Intact posterior ligamentous complex, undetermined status, and definite injury to posterior ligamentous complex are given numbers 0, 2, and 3, respectively
- D. Patients with a score of more than or equal to 4 are surgical candidates

▸▸ Question 7

Postoperative wound infection with spinal instability is due to which organism?

- A. *Staphylococcus aureus*
- B. *Staphylococcus epidermidis*
- C. *E. coli*

- D. *Pseudomonas aeruginosa*
- E. Pneumococcal organisms

▸▸ Question 8

Risk factors for osteoporosis include cigarette smoking, drugs (like heavy alcohol consumption, phenytoin, warfarin, chronic heparin use, steroids use), postmenopausal female, physical inactivity, low calcium intake, and low serum levels of vitamin D. Diagnosis of osteoporosis can be made using DEXA scan which measures bone mineral density at proximal femur, lumbosacral spine, and forearm. Which of the following are the treatment options for osteoporosis?

- A. Drugs that increase bone formation, for example, parathyroid hormone analogues and sodium fluoride
- B. Drugs that reduce bone resorption like estrogen, calcium and vitamin D analogues, calcitonin, bisphosphonates, estrogen analogues, and RANK ligand
- C. Percutaneous vertebroplasty
- D. Kyphoplasty
- E. All of the above

▸▸ Question 9

Indications for kyphoplasty include painful osteoporotic compression fractures, for affected levels from T5 to L5, some symptomatic vertebral hemangiomas, osteolytic metastasis and multiple myeloma, and pathologic compression fracture. Following are the contraindications of kyphoplasty except?

- A. Coagulopathy
- B. No focal neurologic deficit
- C. Spinal instability
- D. Completely healed fractures
- E. Active infections

▸▸ Question 10

Which of the following is correct regarding sacral fractures?

- A. Zone I is fracture of region of ala sparing the central canal and neural foramina
- B. Zone II is fracture through the region of sacral foramina
- C. Zone III is vertical fracture through the region of central canal
- D. Zone IV is transverse fracture through the region of central canal
- E. All of the above

▸▸ Question 11

According to three-column model of spine by Denis, which of the following is not included in the middle column?

- A. Posterior half of disk
- B. Posterior wall of vertebral body
- C. Posterior annulus fibrosus
- D. Posterior longitudinal ligament (PLL)
- E. Posterior arch

▸▸ Question 12

Burst fracture has five subtypes. Which of the following is the most common?

- A. Fracture of both end plates
- B. Fracture of superior end plate
- C. Fracture of inferior end plate
- D. Burst rotation
- E. Burst lateral flexion

▸▸ Question 13

Chance fracture is a subtype of which of the following?

- A. Compression
- B. Burst
- C. Seat belt
- D. Three-column failure
- E. Fracture-dislocation

▸▸ Question 14

Surgery is indicated in burst fracture when kyphotic angle is greater than what?

- A. 5
- B. 7
- C. 10
- D. 15
- E. 20

▸▸ Question 15

Cushing's disease is a risk factor for osteoporosis if the disease persists for how long?

- A. 1 month
- B. 3 months
- C. 6 months
- D. 1 year
- E. 2 years

▸▸ Question 16

Bone mineral density measurement is the best predictor for future fractures if done at what level?

- A. Proximal femur
- B. Distal tibia
- C. Lumbosacral spine
- D. Ribs
- E. Mid radius

▸▸ Question 17

Findings in dual energy X-ray absorptiometry for norms of subjects of same age and sex as the patient are what?

- A. B score
- B. T score

- C. Z score
- D. Alpha score
- E. Beta score

►► Question 18

Kyphoplasty gives additional benefit over vertebroplasty because it might provide which of the following?
- A. Pain relief
- B. Height restoration
- C. More minimal invasive approach
- D. Paraspinal muscle strength
- E. Extra bone mineral density

►► Question 19

A sacral fracture in the region of sacral foramina sparing the central canal involves which sacral zone?
- A. I
- B. II
- C. III
- D. IV
- E. V

►► Question 20

A neurologically intact patient with lumbar burst fracture presents to the emergency. Integrity of PLC is undetermined. What is the recommended management based on his TLICS score?
- A. Nonoperative candidate
- B. Gray zone, may be considered for operative/nonoperative management
- C. Surgical candidate
- D. Not applicable

Answers

►► Answer 1

Correct answer is D. Injury to posterior column alone does cause instability in flexion[1]

►► Answer 2

Correct answer is E. All of the above[2]

►► Answer 3

Correct answer is E. All of the above[2]

►► Answer 4

Correct answer is E. All of the above[3]

►► Answer 5

Correct answer is C. Neurologically intact patient[4]

►► Answer 6

Correct answer is D. Patients with a score of more than or equal to 4 are surgical candidates[5]

►► Answer 7

Correct answer is A. *Staphylococcus aureus*[6]

►► Answer 8

Correct answer is E. All of the above[7]

►► Answer 9

Correct answer is C. Spinal instability[8]

►► Answer 10

Correct answer is E. All of the above[9]

►► Answer 11

Correct answer is E. Posterior arch[1]

►► Answer 12

Correct answer is B. Fracture of superior end plate[2]

►► Answer 13

Correct answer is C. Seat belt[3]

►► Answer 14

Correct answer is E. 20[10]

►► Answer 15

Correct answer is E. 2 years[11]

►► Answer 16

Correct answer is A. Proximal femur[11]

►► Answer 17

Correct answer is C. Z score[11]

►► Answer 18

Correct answer is B. Height restoration[8]

►► Answer 19

Correct answer is B. II[9]

▸▸ Answer 20

Correct answer is B. Gray zone, may be considered for operative/nonoperative management[5]

References

[1] Greenberg M, ed. Greenberg's Handbook of Neurosurgery. 10th ed. New York: Thieme; 2023:1200
[2] Greenberg M, ed. Greenberg's Handbook of Neurosurgery. 10th ed. New York: Thieme; 2023:1201
[3] Greenberg M, ed. Greenberg's Handbook of Neurosurgery. 10th ed. New York: Thieme; 2023:1202
[4] Greenberg M, ed. Greenberg's Handbook of Neurosurgery. 10th ed. New York: Thieme; 2023:1205
[5] Greenberg M, ed. Greenberg's Handbook of Neurosurgery. 10th ed. New York: Thieme; 2023:1207
[6] Greenberg M, ed. Greenberg's Handbook of Neurosurgery. 10th ed. New York: Thieme; 2023:1208
[7] Greenberg M, ed. Greenberg's Handbook of Neurosurgery. 10th ed. New York: Thieme; 2023:1214
[8] Greenberg M, ed. Greenberg's Handbook of Neurosurgery. 10th ed. New York: Thieme; 2023:1213
[9] Greenberg M, ed. Greenberg's Handbook of Neurosurgery. 10th ed. New York: Thieme; 2023:1216
[10] Greenberg M, ed. Greenberg's Handbook of Neurosurgery. 10th ed. New York: Thieme; 2023:1206
[11] Greenberg M, ed. Greenberg's Handbook of Neurosurgery. 10th ed. New York: Thieme; 2023:1209

73 Penetrating Spine Injuries and Long-Term Complications of Spine Injuries

Questions

▸▸ Question 1

What are the indications for surgery in case of gunshot wound injury?

- A. Injury to cauda equina or neurologic deterioration
- B. Compression of a nerve root or CSF leak
- C. Spinal instability or to remove a copper jacket bullet
- D. Incomplete lesion or need for debridement or vascular injuries
- E. For late complications like migrant bullet, lead toxicity, or late spinal instability
- F. All of the above

▸▸ Question 2

Penetrating injuries to neck are divided into three zones which are the following except?

- A. Zone 1 is inferior from the head of the clavicle to the thoracic outlet
- B. Zone 2 is from the clavicle to the angle of mandible
- C. Zone 3 is from angle of mandible to base of skull
- D. Zone 4 is from base of skull to the level of foramen of Monro

▸▸ Question 3

Penetrating injury of neck may cause which of the following?

- A. Shock or hypoxemia due to asphyxiation
- B. Cranial nerve injury
- C. Nerve root or brachial plexus involvement
- D. Spinal cord involvement with complete or incomplete spinal cord injury or spinal shock
- E. All of the above

▸▸ Question 4

Extravasation of blood or intimal dissection of a vessel can be diagnosed with help of which of the following?

- A. Cervical X-ray
- B. Cervical CT with bone window
- C. MRI with MRV
- D. CT angiography of neck vessels
- E. DEXA scan

▸▸ Question 5

Surgical exploration for neck injuries is indicated for which of the following?

- A. Penetrating injury piercing the platysma and anterior triangle of neck
- B. Penetrating injury in posterior triangle of neck
- C. Penetrating injury in lateral triangle of neck
- D. Penetrating injury below angle of mandible
- E. All of the above

▸▸ Question 6

ICA ligation is recommended for injuries in which bleeding cannot be controlled, and it is associated with worse outcome. Endovascular technique is also suitable for select cases. Open carotid repair is recommended in which of the following patients?

- A. With major neurologic deficit
- B. With no or minor neurologic deficit
- C. With poor neurologic outcome patients
- D. In brain dead patients
- E. None of the above

▸▸ Question 7

VA can be ligated in case of iatrogenic injury. In case of elective procedure, what is the prerequisite for VA ligation?

- A. Knowledge of the patency of contralateral VA
- B. Ability of fill of the ipsilateral PICA from retrograde flow from BA
- C. Knowledge of patency of ICA on both sides
- D. A and B

▸▸ Question 8

Delayed deterioration following spinal cord injury can occur because of which of the following?

- A. Post-traumatic syringomyelia or subacute ascending progressive myelopathy
- B. Unrecognized spinal instability or tethered spinal cord
- C. Delayed spinal epidural hematoma or apoptosis of neurons
- D. Glial scar formation
- E. All of the above

▸▸ Question 9

Autonomic hyperreflexia can occur due to spinal cord injury which can lead to pounding headache, flushing, or diaphoresis above the lesion. It occurs only in patients with lesion above which of the following?

- A. T12
- B. T9
- C. T6
- D. T2
- E. Can occur at any level injury

▸▸ **Question 10**

Treatment options for autonomic hyperreflexia include which of the following?

- A. Immediate HOB elevation
- B. Making sure that bladder is empty and that tight apparels are removed
- C. Control of hypertension
- D. IV diazepam
- E. All of the above

▸▸ **Question 11**

Which of the following is a late complication of gunshot wound to spine causing anemia, encephalopathy, motor neuropathy, nephropathy, and abdominal colic?

- A. Cauda equina syndrome
- B. Lead toxicity
- C. Brown Sequard syndrome
- D. CSF fistula
- E. Catheter tip granuloma

▸▸ **Question 12**

Injury in the neck from the clavicle to the angle of the mandible is an injury of which zone?

- A. I
- B. II
- C. III
- D. IV
- E. V

▸▸ **Question 13**

Which of the following is the most commonly injured artery in penetrating neck trauma?

- A. ICA
- B. ECA
- C. CCA
- D. Vertebral artery
- E. Transverse cervical artery

▸▸ **Question 14**

A patient with penetrating spine injury had a delayed deterioration. There were signal changes extending to four levels above the original injury and was labeled as subacute progressive ascending myelopathy (SPAM). What is the median time of occurrence post injury?

- A. 1 day
- B. 3 days
- C. 13 days
- D. 1 month
- E. 3 months

▸▸ **Question 15**

In patients with spinal cord injury above T6, pounding headache, flushing, and diaphoresis above the lesion may occur due to autonomic hyperreflexia which is due to release of which of the following?

- A. Epinephrine
- B. Norepinephrine
- C. Dopamine
- D. Serotonin
- E. Bradykinin

Answers

▸▸ **Answer 1**

Correct answer is F. All of the above[1]

▸▸ **Answer 2**

Correct answer is D. Zone 4 is from base of skull to the level of foramen of Monro[2]

▸▸ **Answer 3**

Correct answer is E. All of the above[2]

▸▸ **Answer 4**

Correct answer is E. DEXA scan[2]

▸▸ **Answer 5**

Correct answer is E. All of the above[2]

▸▸ **Answer 6**

Correct answer is B. With no or minor neurologic deficit[3]

▸▸ **Answer 7**

Correct answer is D. A and B[3]

▸▸ **Answer 8**

Correct answer is E. All of the above[3]

▸▸ **Answer 9**

Correct answer is C. T6[4]

▸▸ **Answer 10**

Correct answer is E. All of the above[5]

▸▸ **Answer 11**

Correct answer is B. Lead toxicity[1]

▸▸ **Answer 12**

Correct answer is B. II[2]

▸▸ **Answer 13**

Correct answer is C. CCA[2]

▸▸ **Answer 14**

Correct answer is C. 13 days[3]

▸▸ **Answer 15**

Correct answer is B. Norepinephrine[4]

References

[1] Greenberg M, ed. Greenberg's Handbook of Neurosurgery. 10th ed. New York: Thieme; 2023:1219
[2] Greenberg M, ed. Greenberg's Handbook of Neurosurgery. 10th ed. New York: Thieme; 2023:1220
[3] Greenberg M, ed. Greenberg's Handbook of Neurosurgery. 10th ed. New York: Thieme; 2023:1221
[4] Greenberg M, ed. Greenberg's Handbook of Neurosurgery. 10th ed. New York: Thieme; 2023:1222
[5] Greenberg M, ed. Greenberg's Handbook of Neurosurgery. 10th ed. New York: Thieme; 2023:1223

Part XVI

Nontraumatic Spine and Spinal Cord Conditions

XVI

74 Low-Back Pain

Questions

►► Question 1

Conservative treatment for low-back pain consists of therapy for first 4 to 6 weeks which includes physiotherapy, analgesics (NSAIDS), and sometimes epidural steroid injections (only in acute radiculopathy cases). Which of the following are the indications for MRI of lumbosacral spine in patients with backache with subsequent surgical treatment of identified problem appropriately?

- A. Progressive neurologic deficit (e.g., weakness)
- B. Cauda equina syndrome (includes bladder issues, saddle anesthesia)
- C. Intractable pain
- D. Failure of medical treatment
- E. All of the above

►► Question 2

Generalized displacement of disk material is defined as displacement of more than 50% or 180 degrees beyond the peripheral limit of disk space. On the other hand, herniation is localized displacement of disk material less than 50% or 180 degrees beyond the limits of the intervertebral disk space. Following statements are true regarding herniation of disk except?

- A. Focal herniation is less than 25% of disk space
- B. Broad based disk herniation is 20 to 25% of the disk herniation
- C. Schmorl's node is not a type of disk herniation
- D. Protrusion is a type of disk herniation in which the fragment does not have a neck
- E. Extrusion is a type of disk herniation in which the fragment has a neck which is further subdivided into sequestration and migration

►► Question 3

Dysfunction of nerve root, which may include pain in the distribution of the nerve root or dermatomal sensory disturbances or weakness of the muscle innervated by that nerve root or hypoactive muscle reflexes of the same muscles or a combination of these, is termed as?

- A. Myelopathy
- B. Mechanical low-back pain
- C. Sciatica
- D. Radiculopathy
- E. None of the above

►► Question 4

Diminished sensations over medial malleolus plus medial foot, dorsum of foot, and lateral malleolus plus lateral foot suggests L4, L5, and S1 nerve root involvement, respectively. A patient presenting with history of fever with vertebral tenderness and very limited range of spinal motion has most likely which of the following?

- A. Spinal tumor
- B. Spinal osteoarthritis
- C. Spinal infection
- D. Spinal degenerative disease
- E. Spinal instability

►► Question 5

Abnormal disk morphology on MRI is loss of T2WI signal intensity (black disk), disk space collapse, Modic changes, and high intensity zones (these findings also frequently occur in asymptomatic patients). Diskography (injection of water-soluble contrast agent directly into the nucleus pulposus of the intervertebral disk) is done through the Kambin's triangle to find out pathologic disk. Following are included in the boundaries of Kambin's triangle except?

- A. Exiting nerve root
- B. Superior end plate of inferior vertebral body
- C. Thecal sac
- D. Inferior facet of superior vertebral body
- E. All are included in the boundaries of Kambin's triangle

►► Question 6

To see dynamic instability in spine, which of the following tests is done?

- A. Flexion–extension lumbar spine X-rays
- B. Oblique X-rays
- C. Standing scoliosis X-rays
- D. Lateral spine X-rays
- E. Anteroposterior spine X-rays

►► Question 7

Following are the advantages of CT scan over MRI except?

- A. Excellent bony detail
- B. Less expensive
- C. Outpatient evaluation
- D. More claustrophobic
- E. Faster scanning

►► Question 8

Following are included in the conservative treatment of low-back pain except?

- A. Bed rest for the first 2 to 3 days, activity modification (like prolonged sitting, bending or twisting, limiting lifting objects)
- B. Exercise starting from walking in the first 2 weeks then conditioning exercises for the trunk muscles

- C. NSAIDs and paracetamol
- D. Epidural injection for short-term relief of radicular pain
- E. Oral steroids

▸▸ Question 9

Which of the following is an indication of lumbar fusion in case of disk herniation?

- A. Evidence of preoperative lumbar spinal deformity or instability
- B. In patients with chronic axial low-back pain associated with radiculopathy
- C. Both A and B
- D. Spondylolisthesis grade 1 without degenerative changes
- E. None of the above

▸▸ Question 10

Which of the following statements is correct regarding surgical option for low-back problems?

- A. Routine HLD or initial recurrence of HLD is treated with standard diskectomy or with microdiskectomy
- B. Foraminal or far-lateral HLD can be treated with partial or total facetectomy, extra canal approach or endoscopic techniques
- C. Only lumbar spinal stenosis can be treated with simple decompression laminectomy
- D. Patients with degenerative spondylolisthesis, stenosis and radiculopathy, adult degenerative scoliosis, or instability are treated with laminectomy plus fusion
- E. All of the above

▸▸ Question 11

Failure to satisfactorily improve low-back pain or radiculopathy following back surgery is called as failed back surgery syndrome. Which of the following are the causes of "failed back surgery syndrome"?

- A. Incorrect initial diagnosis or continued compression caused by residual disk, epidural hematoma, or pseudomeningocele
- B. Permanent nerve root injury preoperatively or after surgery
- C. Adhesive arachnoiditis or diskitis
- D. Spondylosis
- E. All of the above

▸▸ Question 12

Surgery for failed back syndrome is recommended only for recurrent or residual disk, instability, or a pseudomeningocele. Following are true regarding MRI study of patients after operation for back pain except?

- A. MRI study done after surgery is always done with contrast if there is no contraindication
- B. Scar enhances on post-contrast MRI study
- C. Disk does not enhance on contrast MRI
- D. MRI is done only without contrast in all cases

▸▸ Question 13

Myelographic classification of arachnoiditis includes which of the following?

- A. Unilateral focal filling defect centered on nerve root sleeve adjacent to disk space
- B. Circumferential constriction around thecal sac
- C. Complete obstruction with stalactites or candle guttering
- D. Infundibular cul de sac with loss of radicular striations
- E. All of the above

▸▸ Question 14

In disk herniation, sequestration is when the fragment has lost continuity with the disk of origin. It is a subtype of which of the following?

- A. Disk bulge
- B. Extrusion
- C. Focal
- D. Broad based
- E. Extrusion

▸▸ Question 15

Bone marrow edema associated with acute or subacute inflammation showing hypointensity on T1WI and hyperintensity on T2WI is what Modic type?

- A. I
- B. II
- C. III
- D. IV
- E. V

▸▸ Question 16

What is the score of bed-bound patients according to Oswestry disability index?

- A. 0 to 20
- B. 21 to 30
- C. 41 to 60
- D. 61 to 80
- E. 81 to 100

▸▸ Question 17

Diminished Achilles reflex suggests dysfunction of root of which of the following?

- A. L2
- B. L3
- C. L4
- D. L5
- E. S1

▸▸ Question 18

For diskography, injection of water-soluble contrast agent directly into the nucleus pulposus of the intervertebral disk being studied is performed by percutaneous needle access through which of the following?
- A. Pedicle
- B. Facet
- C. Kambin's triangle
- D. Anterolateral quadrant
- E. Transforaminal

▸▸ Question 19

For nonspecific lower backache, for how long bed rest should be allowed?
- A. Not recommended
- B. Few hours
- C. 1 day
- D. 2 days
- E. 4 days

▸▸ Question 20

Patients with disabling low-back pain due to two-level degenerative disease without stenosis or spondylolisthesis for ≥ 2 years with radiological evidence of disk degeneration at L4–L5, L5–S1, or both and failed best medical management, should be treated with which of the following?
- A. Thoracolumbar spinal orthosis
- B. Physical therapy
- C. Steroid
- D. Facet capsule injections
- E. Lumbar fusion

▸▸ Question 21

First-time recurrence after diskectomy should be treated with which of the following?
- A. Same as first-time presenting herniated disk
- B. Steroids
- C. Epidural injections
- D. Physical therapy
- E. Anterior lumbar interbody fusion

▸▸ Question 22

Arachnoiditis is an inflammatory condition of the lumbar nerve roots and may present as three different patterns on MRI. What is the pattern where roots adhere to meninges around periphery?
- A. Empty thecal sac
- B. Candle dripping
- C. Guttering
- D. Two central cords
- E. Central adhesion

▸▸ Question 23

What is the myelographic classification of arachnoiditis type for unilateral focal filling defect centered on the nerve root sleeve adjacent to disk space?
- A. I
- B. II
- C. III
- D. IV
- E. V

Answers

▸▸ Answer 1

Correct answer is E. All of the above[1]

▸▸ Answer 2

Correct answer is C. Schmorl's node is not a type of disk herniation[2]

▸▸ Answer 3

Correct answer is D. Radiculopathy[2]

▸▸ Answer 4

Correct answer is C. Spinal infection[3]

▸▸ Answer 5

Correct answer is D. Inferior facet of superior vertebral body[4]

▸▸ Answer 6

Correct answer is A. Flexion–extension lumbar spine X-rays[5]

▸▸ Answer 7

Correct answer is D. More claustrophobic[5]

▸▸ Answer 8

Correct answer is E. Oral steroids[6]

▸▸ Answer 9

Correct answer is C. Both A and B[7]

▸▸ Answer 10

Correct answer is E. All of the above[7]

▸▸ Answer 11

Correct answer is E. All of the above[8]

►► Answer 12

Correct answer is D. MRI is done only without contrast in all cases[9]

►► Answer 13

Correct answer is E. All of the above[10]

►► Answer 14

Correct answer is B. Extrusion[2]

►► Answer 15

Correct answer is A. I[7]

►► Answer 16

Correct answer is E. 81 to 100[11]

►► Answer 17

Correct answer is E. S1[3]

►► Answer 18

Correct answer is C. Kambin's triangle[4]

►► Answer 19

Correct answer is E. 4 days[12]

►► Answer 20

Correct answer is E. Lumbar fusion[13]

►► Answer 21

Correct answer is A. Same as first-time presenting herniated disk[7]

►► Answer 22

Correct answer is A. Empty thecal sac[10]

►► Answer 23

Correct answer is A. I[10]

References

[1] Greenberg M, ed. Greenberg's Handbook of Neurosurgery. 10th ed. New York: Thieme; 2023:1226
[2] Greenberg M, ed. Greenberg's Handbook of Neurosurgery. 10th ed. New York: Thieme; 2023:1227
[3] Greenberg M, ed. Greenberg's Handbook of Neurosurgery. 10th ed. New York: Thieme; 2023:1230
[4] Greenberg M, ed. Greenberg's Handbook of Neurosurgery. 10th ed. New York: Thieme; 2023:1235
[5] Greenberg M, ed. Greenberg's Handbook of Neurosurgery. 10th ed. New York: Thieme; 2023:1232
[6] Greenberg M, ed. Greenberg's Handbook of Neurosurgery. 10th ed. New York: Thieme; 2023:1238
[7] Greenberg M, ed. Greenberg's Handbook of Neurosurgery. 10th ed. New York: Thieme; 2023:1240
[8] Greenberg M, ed. Greenberg's Handbook of Neurosurgery. 10th ed. New York: Thieme; 2023:1243
[9] Greenberg M, ed. Greenberg's Handbook of Neurosurgery. 10th ed. New York: Thieme; 2023:1245
[10] Greenberg M, ed. Greenberg's Handbook of Neurosurgery. 10th ed. New York: Thieme; 2023:1244
[11] Greenberg M, ed. Greenberg's Handbook of Neurosurgery. 10th ed. New York: Thieme; 2023:1228
[12] Greenberg M, ed. Greenberg's Handbook of Neurosurgery. 10th ed. New York: Thieme; 2023:1237
[13] Greenberg M, ed. Greenberg's Handbook of Neurosurgery. 10th ed. New York: Thieme; 2023:1239

75 Lumbar Disk Herniation and Radiculopathy

Questions

▸▸ Question 1

The nerve root en passant is the nerve in lateral recess that passes through the neural foramen of the level below; for example, for L4–L5 level, it would be L5 nerve root while exiting nerve root at this level would be L4 nerve root. Most of the herniated lumbar disks are paramedian which cause compression on which of the following?

- A. Exiting nerve root
- B. Traversing nerve root
- C. Both A and B
- D. It causes thecal sac compression only
- E. None of the above

▸▸ Question 2

Which of the following statements is incorrect regarding clinical findings with herniated lumbar disk?

- A. Symptoms may start off with back pain, which after days or weeks gradually or sometimes suddenly yields to radicular pain often with reduction of the back pain
- B. Pain is relieved upon flexing the knee and thigh (e.g., with a pillow under the knees)
- C. Remaining in any position (sitting, standing, or lying) for too long may also exacerbate the pain, sometimes necessitating position changes at intervals that range from every few minutes to 10 to 20 minutes
- D. Pain is increased with coughing, sneezing, or straining at the stool
- E. Bladder symptoms are never present with a herniated lumbar disk

▸▸ Question 3

Which of the following signs are used to test tension on nerve roots in case of radiculopathy?

- A. Lasegue's sign also known as straight leg raise sign (with the patient supine, the afflicted limb is raised by the ankle until pain is solicited, which should occur at angle less than 60 degrees and consists of leg pain or paresthesias in the distribution of pain)
- B. Cram test (with the patient supine, the symptomatic leg is raised with the knee slightly flexed and then extending the knee will produce pain similar to Lasegue's sign)
- C. Crossed straight leg raising test also known as Fajersztajn's sign (SLR on the painless leg cause contralateral limb pain)
- D. Femoral stretch test also known as reverse straight leg raising, which is positive with L2, L3, or L4 nerve root compression
- E. All of the above

▸▸ Question 4

The most common level of herniated lumbar disk is L5–S1 which is 45 to 50%, the second most common level is L4–L5 which is 40 to 45%, while L3–L4 is involved in only 3 to 10% of cases. Which of the following are the symptoms caused by the S1 nerve root compression?

- A. Diminished ankle jerk (Achilles)
- B. Motor weakness of gastrocnemius causing weak plantar flexion
- C. Decreased sensations in the area of lateral malleolus and lateral foot
- D. Pain distribution in the posterior lower extremity often up to the ankle
- E. All of the above

▸▸ Question 5

Cauda equina syndrome causes urinary retention, saddle anesthesia, significant motor weakness, and low-back pain. Following are the causes of this syndrome except?

- A. Compression of the cauda equina by massive disk herniation or tumor or free fat graft following surgery or trauma or spinal epidural hematoma
- B. Infection which may cause compression by epidural abscess or vascular compromise resulting from local septic thrombophlebitis
- C. Neuropathy caused by inflammation or ischemia
- D. Rheumatoid arthritis
- E. Ankylosing spondylitis

▸▸ Question 6

What is the desirable time of surgery after development of cauda equina syndrome?

- A. Within 48 hours
- B. Within 24 hours
- C. Within 12 hours
- D. Within 6 hours
- E. None of the above

▸▸ Question 7

Which of the following is an indication of surgery in a patient with herniated lumbar disk?

- A. Failure of nonsurgical management which is done for almost 5 to 8 weeks
- B. Patients with cauda equina syndrome
- C. Patients with progressive motor deficit
- D. Intolerable pain despite the use of adequate narcotic pain medication
- E. All of the above

▸▸ **Question 8**

Surgical options for lumbar radiculopathy include transcanal approaches like standard open lumbar laminectomy and diskectomy, microdiskectomy, or sequestrectomy. Which of the following indications are utilized by proponents for intradiskal procedures like automated percutaneous lumbar diskectomy (nucleoplasty), laser disk decompression, percutaneous endoscopic lumbar diskectomy, and intradiskal endothermal therapy?

- A. Contained disk herniation
- B. Best for L4–L5 herniated disk
- C. Not recommended in severe neurologic deficit
- D. All of the above

▸▸ **Question 9**

Common complications after operation for herniated lumbar disk include superficial wound infection, deep wound infection, increased motor deficit, unintended incidental durotomy, recurrent herniated lumbar disk, and postoperative urinary retention. What are the rates of superficial infection, deep infection, and incidental durotomy, respectively?

- A. 0.9 to 5%, less than 1%, and 0.3 to 13%
- B. 1%, 5%, and 13%
- C. 0.1%, 0.5%, and 0.3%
- D. None of the above

▸▸ **Question 10**

What is the possible sequalae of dural opening?

- A. CSF leak (contained or pseudomeningocele or external, CSF fistula)
- B. Herniations of nerve roots through the opening
- C. Associated nerve root contusion, laceration, or injury to the cauda equina
- D. CSF leak may collapse thecal sac and cause bleeding from epidural blood vessels
- E. All of the above

▸▸ **Question 11**

Most herniated lumbar disks occur posteriorly and slightly off to one side within which of the following?

- A. Central canal zone
- B. Foraminal zone
- C. Extraforaminal zone
- D. Far lateral zone
- E. Intravertebrally

▸▸ **Question 12**

A herniated disk at the level of L4–L5 mostly involves root of which of the following?

- A. L3
- B. L4
- C. L5
- D. S1
- E. Filum terminale

▸▸ **Question 13**

A foraminal herniated disk at the level of L4–L5 mostly involves root of which of the following?

- A. L3
- B. L4
- C. L5
- D. S1
- E. Filum terminale

▸▸ **Question 14**

Which of the following is the most specific nerve root tension sign?

- A. Lasegue's test
- B. Cross SLR
- C. Reverse SLR
- D. Hoover test
- E. FABER/Patrick test

▸▸ **Question 15**

Which of the following is a hip motion test for sacroiliitis?

- A. Lasegue's test
- B. Cross SLR
- C. Reverse SLR
- D. Hoover test
- E. FABER/Patrick test

▸▸ **Question 16**

What is the test used to distinguish unilateral functional weakness of iliopsoas from organic weakness using synergistic contraction of the contralateral gluteus medius?

- A. Lasegue's test
- B. Cross SLR
- C. Reverse SLR
- D. Hoover test
- E. FABER/Patrick test

▸▸ **Question 17**

Knee jerk is diminished (Westphal's sign) in herniated lumbar disk of which level?

- A. L2–L3
- B. L3–L4
- C. L4–L5
- D. L5–S1
- E. S1–S2

▸▸ **Question 18**

What is the most consistent finding in cauda equine syndrome?

- A. Urinary retention
- B. Saddle anesthesia
- C. Motor weakness in one limb
- D. Paraplegia
- E. Sciatica

▸▸ **Question 19**

Which of the following is not an intradiskal procedure for lumbar radiculopathy?

- A. Chemonucleolysis
- B. Automated percutaneous lumbar diskectomy
- C. Percutaneous endoscopic intradiskal diskectomy
- D. Sequesterectomy
- E. Laser disk decompression

▸▸ **Question 20**

A diabetic patient with lumbar radiculopathy was operated on and postoperatively he was blind. What is the most common cause?

- A. Anterior ischemic optic neuropathy
- B. Posterior ischemic optic neuropathy
- C. Retinal artery occlusion
- D. Cortical blindness
- E. Diabetic retinopathy

▸▸ **Question 21**

Extreme lateral herniated lumbar disk occurs most commonly at which level?

- A. L1–L2
- B. L2–L3
- C. L3–L4
- D. L4–L5
- E. L5–S1

▸▸ **Question 22**

Which of the following is a less well-documented sequelae of dural opening?

- A. CSF fistula
- B. Herniation of nerve roots through opening
- C. Associated nerve root contusion, laceration, or injury to the cauda equina
- D. CSF leak collapses the thecal sac and may increase blood loss from epidural bleeding
- E. Arachnoiditis

Answers

▸▸ **Answer 1**

Correct answer is B. Traversing nerve root[1]

▸▸ **Answer 2**

Correct answer is E. Bladder symptoms are never present with a herniated lumbar disk[2]

▸▸ **Answer 3**

Correct answer is E. All of the above[3]

▸▸ **Answer 4**

Correct answer is E. All of the above[4]

▸▸ **Answer 5**

Correct answer is D. Rheumatoid arthritis[5]

▸▸ **Answer 6**

Correct answer is B. Within 24 hours[5]

▸▸ **Answer 7**

Correct answer is E. All of the above[6]

▸▸ **Answer 8**

Correct answer is D. All of the above[7]

▸▸ **Answer 9**

Correct answer is A. 0.9 to 5%, less than 1%, and 0.3 to 13%[8]

▸▸ **Answer 10**

Correct answer is E. All of the above[9]

▸▸ **Answer 11**

Correct answer is A. Central canal zone[1]

▸▸ **Answer 12**

Correct answer is C. L5[4]

▸▸ **Answer 13**

Correct answer is B. L4[10]

▸▸ **Answer 14**

Correct answer is B. Cross SLR[3]

▸▸ **Answer 15**

Correct answer is E. FABER/Patrick test[3]

▸▸ **Answer 16**

Correct answer is D. Hoover test[4]

▸▸ **Answer 17**

Correct answer is B. L3–L4[4]

▸▸ **Answer 18**

Correct answer is A. Urinary retention[11]

▸▸ **Answer 19**

Correct answer is D. Sequesterectomy[7]

▸▸ **Answer 20**

Correct answer is A. Anterior ischemic optic neuropathy[12]

▸▸ **Answer 21**

Correct answer is D. L4–L5[10]

▸▸ **Answer 22**

Correct answer is E. Arachnoiditis[9]

References

[1] Greenberg M, ed. Greenberg's Handbook of Neurosurgery. 10th ed. New York: Thieme; 2023:1250
[2] Greenberg M, ed. Greenberg's Handbook of Neurosurgery. 10th ed. New York: Thieme; 2023:1251
[3] Greenberg M, ed. Greenberg's Handbook of Neurosurgery. 10th ed. New York: Thieme; 2023:1252
[4] Greenberg M, ed. Greenberg's Handbook of Neurosurgery. 10th ed. New York: Thieme; 2023:1253
[5] Greenberg M, ed. Greenberg's Handbook of Neurosurgery. 10th ed. New York: Thieme; 2023:1255
[6] Greenberg M, ed. Greenberg's Handbook of Neurosurgery. 10th ed. New York: Thieme; 2023:1256
[7] Greenberg M, ed. Greenberg's Handbook of Neurosurgery. 10th ed. New York: Thieme; 2023:1257
[8] Greenberg M, ed. Greenberg's Handbook of Neurosurgery. 10th ed. New York: Thieme; 2023:1258
[9] Greenberg M, ed. Greenberg's Handbook of Neurosurgery. 10th ed. New York: Thieme; 2023:1260
[10] Greenberg M, ed. Greenberg's Handbook of Neurosurgery. 10th ed. New York: Thieme; 2023:1264
[11] Greenberg M, ed. Greenberg's Handbook of Neurosurgery. 10th ed. New York: Thieme; 2023:1254
[12] Greenberg M, ed. Greenberg's Handbook of Neurosurgery. 10th ed. New York: Thieme; 2023:1261

76 Thoracic Disk Herniation

Questions

▸▸ Question 1

Thoracic disk herniation constitutes only 0.25% of herniated disks and usually occurs at or below T8. These disks are frequently calcified. Pain and sensory disturbance are in a bandlike distribution radiating anteriorly and inferiorly along the involved root's dermatome. What is the indication of surgery in these cases?

- A. Refractory pain
- B. Progressive myelopathy
- C. Both A and B
- D. Radiculopathy
- E. None of the above

▸▸ Question 2

CT should be obtained in cases of thoracic herniated disk along with noncontrast MRI of thoracic spine as most of the disks in this region are calcified. Which of the following are the options for open surgical approaches for these disks?

- A. Posterior midline laminectomy
- B. Posterolateral like lateral gutter (laminectomy plus removal of pedicle), transpedicular, costotransversectomy, and transfacet pedicle sparing
- C. Anterolateral (transthoracic) usually through the pleural space
- D. Lateral extracavitary (retrocoelomic) which is posterior to the pleural space
- E. All of the above

▸▸ Question 3

Which of the following is a correct match of appropriate surgical approach for the given pathology?

- A. Laminectomy for posteriorly located tumor
- B. Posterolateral (transpedicular) for radicular pain with lateral disk herniation or for biopsy of tumor
- C. Lateral (costotransversectomy) for midline disk, good ipsilateral access but poor access to opposite side
- D. Transthoracic for midline lesions especially for reaching both sides of the cord
- E. All of the above

▸▸ Question 4

To access T4–T5 disk space, which rib needs to be removed?

- A. T4
- B. T5
- C. Both A and B
- D. T5 and T6
- E. T4 and T3

▸▸ Question 5

Indications of transthoracic approach for thoracic disk disease include central fragment or calcified disk, and burst fracture of thoracic spine. Following are the advantages of transthoracic approach except?

- A. It provides excellent anterior approach
- B. It causes little compromise of stability
- C. It deals easily with pathology lying posterior to the cord
- D. There is low risk of mechanical cord injury with this approach
- E. All of the above

▸▸ Question 6

Which of the following statements regarding neuromonitoring during thoracic spine disease surgery is correct?

- A. It consists of MEP and SSEP
- B. It is not required for surgery at this level
- C. Injury to cord at this level cannot be prevented
- D. None of the above

▸▸ Question 7

There is risk of injury to radicular artery which may compromise the spinal cord blood supply. How much posterior rib along with transverse process needs to be removed?

- A. 3 to 4 cm
- B. 4 to 5 cm
- C. 5 to 3 cm
- D. More than 5 cm
- E. Less than 6 cm

▸▸ Question 8

What skin incision can be used for costotransversectomy procedure?

- A. Curved paramedian skin incision
- B. Midline incision
- C. Both A and B
- D. T-shaped incision
- E. None of the above

▸▸ Question 9

What is the most common symptom after thoracic disk herniation?

- A. Pain
- B. Sensory changes
- C. Motor changes
- D. All occur at some time

▸▸ Question 10

What is the percentage of occurrence pain in case of thoracic disk disease?
- A. 60%
- B. 23%
- C. 18%
- D. 8%

▸▸ Question 11

About 75% of thoracic disk herniations are below which level?
- A. T6
- B. T7
- C. T8
- D. T10
- E. T12

▸▸ Question 12

For thoracic spine surgery, which of the following is not a posterolateral approach?
- A. Transthoracic
- B. Lateral gutter
- C. Transpedicular
- D. Costotransversectomy
- E. Transfacet pedicle sparing

▸▸ Question 13

For a central disk herniation, especially when calcified, which approach has the lowest incidence of cord injury with the best operative results?
- A. Transfacet pedicle sparing
- B. Transthoracic
- C. Lateral extracavitary approach
- D. Costotransversectomy
- E. Transpedicular approach

▸▸ Question 14

Which of the following is the best approach for radicular pain with lateral disk herniation and biopsy of tumor?
- A. Transfacet pedicle sparing
- B. Transthoracic
- C. Lateral extracavitary approach
- D. Costotransversectomy
- E. Transpedicular approach

▸▸ Question 15

During costotransversectomy, to access the vertebral body of T6, which rib needs to be removed?
- A. 5th
- B. 7th
- C. 5th and 6th
- D. 6th and 7th
- E. 5th, 6th, and 7th

▸▸ Question 16

What is the best approach for midline thoracic spine lesions, especially for reaching both sides of the cord?
- A. Laminectomy
- B. Posterolateral transpedicular
- C. Transpedicular facet sparing
- D. Costotransversectomy
- E. Transthoracic

Answers

▸▸ Answer 1

Correct answer is C. Both A and B[1]

▸▸ Answer 2

Correct answer is E. All of the above[2]

▸▸ Answer 3

Correct answer is E. All of the above[2]

▸▸ Answer 4

Correct answer is B. T5[3]

▸▸ Answer 5

Correct answer is C. It deals easily with pathology lying posterior to the cord[4]

▸▸ Answer 6

Correct answer is A. It consists of MEP and SSEP[2]

▸▸ Answer 7

Correct answer is B. 4 to 5 cm[2]

▸▸ Answer 8

Correct answer is C. Both A and B[3]

▸▸ Answer 9

Correct answer is D. All occur at some time[1]

▸▸ Answer 10

Correct answer is A. 60%[2]

▸▸ **Answer 11**

Correct answer is C. T8[1]

▸▸ **Answer 12**

Correct answer is A. Transthoracic[5]

▸▸ **Answer 13**

Correct answer is B. Transthoracic[2]

▸▸ **Answer 14**

Correct answer is E. Transpedicular approach[2]

▸▸ **Answer 15**

Correct answer is D. 6th and 7th[3]

▸▸ **Answer 16**

Correct answer is E. Transthoracic[2]

References

[1] Greenberg M, ed. Greenberg's Handbook of Neurosurgery. 10th ed. New York: Thieme; 2023:1271
[2] Greenberg M, ed. Greenberg's Handbook of Neurosurgery. 10th ed. New York: Thieme; 2023:1273
[3] Greenberg M, ed. Greenberg's Handbook of Neurosurgery. 10th ed. New York: Thieme; 2023:1274
[4] Greenberg M, ed. Greenberg's Handbook of Neurosurgery. 10th ed. New York: Thieme; 2023:1275
[5] Greenberg M, ed. Greenberg's Handbook of Neurosurgery. 10th ed. New York: Thieme; 2023:1272

77 Cervical Disk Herniation

Questions

►► **Question 1**

Which of the following statements are correct regarding cervical disk syndromes?

- A. C4–C5 herniated cervical disk is only 2%; it causes C5 nerve root compression, diminished deltoid and pectoralis reflexes, motor weakness in deltoid, and paresthesia or hypoesthesia in shoulder
- B. C5–C6 cervical disk herniation is 19%; it causes C6 nerve root compression, diminished biceps and brachioradialis reflex, forearm flexion weakness and paresthesia, and hypesthesia in upper arm, thumb, and radial forearm
- C. C6–C7 cervical disk herniation is 69%; it causes 7 nerve root compression, diminished triceps reflex, motor weakness of forearm extension (wrist drop), and paresthesia hypesthesia in fingers 2 and 3 with all finger tips
- D. C7–T1 cervical disk herniation is 10%; it causes C8 nerve root compression, diminished finger jerk, motor weakness in hand intrinsics, and paresthesia hypesthesia in fingers 4 and 5
- E. All of the above

►► **Question 2**

Evaluation for radiculopathy includes LMN findings which are weakness in one myotome group with atrophy and fasciculations present, sensory loss in dermatome similar to that of myotomal weakness, and eliciting muscle stretch reflexes and positive mechanical signs with reproduction of radicular symptoms with mechanical loading of the head. Evidence of cervical cord involvement (myelopathy) is UMN findings in the lower extremity and presence of pathologic reflexes like Hoffmann's reflex, Babinski sign, and ankle clonus. Following signs are useful in evaluating cervical radiculopathy except?

- A. Painful limitation of neck movement in almost all herniated cervical disk patients. Neck extension usually aggravates pain when cervical disk disease is present. Some patients find relief in evaluating the arm and cupping the back or the top of the head with the hand (abduction relief sign)
- B. Lhermitte's sign (electric shock like sensation radiating down the spine)
- C. Spurling's sign
- D. Axial manual traction of a supine patient with 10 to 15 kg resulting in reduction or disappearance of radicular symptoms is a positive finding
- E. Positive shoulder abduction test in which lifting of hand above head causes reduction or disappearance of radicular signs
- F. Positive Hoffmann's sign

►► **Question 3**

Over 90% of patients with acute cervical radiculopathy due to cervical disk herniation can improve without surgery and regression of an extruded cervical disk has been demonstrated radiographically. Conservative management of cervical disk includes the following except?

- A. Physical therapy which may include intermittent cervical traction (gradually escalating up to 10–15 pounds for 10–15 minutes for two to three times daily)
- B. Use of NSAIDs
- C. Use of short-course tapering steroids
- D. Trigger points injections and facet blocks have no role
- E. Epidural steroid injection (not used as often as in lumbar spine)

►► **Question 4**

Routine anterior approach for cervical spine surgery is usually able to access levels C3 and C7. While in patients with short thick neck, access may be even more limited. Which of the following are advantages of anterior approach over posterior approach?

- A. Safe removal of anterior osteophytes
- B. Fusion of disk space affords immobility, while there is 10% risk of immobility with extensive approach
- C. The only viable means of directly dealing with centrally herniated disk
- D. All of the above

►► **Question 5**

For ACDF, a horizontal skin incision in mediolateral direction is made. C5–C6 disk is at the level of which of the following?

- A. Hyoid bone
- B. Thyroid cartilage
- C. Cricoid cartilage
- D. Cricothyroid membrane
- E. None of the above

►► **Question 6**

Choices of graft for anterior cervical fusion includes autologous graft (from iliac crest), nonautologous bone (cadaveric), bone substitutes (hydroxylapatite), or synthetic (PEEK, titanium) filled with osteogenic material. All of the following are benefits of anterior cervical plating except?

- A. It reduces pseudoarthrosis rate and graft problem
- B. It helps to maintain lordosis
- C. It is recommended for improvement of clinical outcome
- D. It is recommended to improve arm pain

►► **Question 7**

Postoperative check following ACDF includes which of the following?

- A. Checking for evidence of airway obstruction (check for hematoma, respiratory distress, extreme difficulty in swallowing, tracheal deviation)

- B. Weakness of nerve root of the level operated
- C. Long tract signs (Babinski) which may indicate cord compression by spinal epidural hematoma
- D. Hoarseness of voice which may show RLN injury
- E. All of the above

▸▸ Question 8

ACDF complications include the following except?

- A. Exposure injuries (perforation of viscus like pharynx or esophagus or trachea, vocal cord paresis with incidence of 4% permanent and 11% temporary, vertebral artery injury with 0.3% incidence, carotid injury, CSF fistula, Horner syndrome, thoracic duct injury, thrombosis of internal jugular vein)
- B. Spinal cord or nerve root injury
- C. Bone fusion problems like failure of fusion (pseudoarthrosis), anterior kyphotic angulation, graft extrusion
- D. Wound infection, postoperative pneumothorax or hemothorax
- E. All of the above

▸▸ Question 9

Indications for posterior keyhole laminotomy include which of the following?

- A. Monoradiculopathy with posterolateral soft disk sequestration
- B. Radiculopathy in patients who are professional singers or speakers
- C. For lower or upper cervical nerve root compression where anterior approach is more difficult
- D. In patients with herniated disk where it is desired to avoid fusion
- E. All of the above

▸▸ Question 10

Posterior cervical decompression is usually reserved for which of the following cases?

- A. Multiple cervical disks or osteophytes (ACD is usually used to treat only two or three levels without myelopathy)
- B. Where cervical stenosis is more diffuse and more significant as compared to anterior pathology
- C. In professional speakers or singers
- D. All of the above

▸▸ Question 11

A patient presented with weakness of forearm flexion, paresthesias in upper arm and thumb, and diminished biceps reflex. What is the level of herniated cervical disk?

- A. C2–C3
- B. C3–C4
- C. C4–C5
- D. C5–C6
- E. C6–C7

▸▸ Question 12

Which physical examination test for cervical disk herniation is analogous to straight leg raising test for lumbar disk herniation?

- A. Spurling test
- B. Axial manual spinal traction
- C. Shoulder abduction test
- D. FABER test
- E. Patrick test

▸▸ Question 13

What is the accuracy of CT myelogram for cervical disk disease?

- A. 70%
- B. 75%
- C. 80%
- D. 90%
- E. 98%

▸▸ Question 14

Which of the following is the most frequent radiculopathy mimicking carpal tunnel syndrome?

- A. C2
- B. C4
- C. C5
- D. C6
- E. C7

▸▸ Question 15

How many patients with acute cervical radiculopathy due to cervical disk herniation can improve without surgery?

- A. 70%
- B. 80%
- C. 85%
- D. 90%
- E. 98%

▸▸ Question 16

A patient underwent ACDF and developed Horner syndrome. Sympathetic plexus lies within which of the following?

- A. Cricothyroid
- B. Longus coli
- C. Sternocleidomastoid
- D. Omohyoid
- E. Belly of digastric

▸▸ Question 17

The addition of an anterior plate to an ACDF is recommended for what purpose?

- A. Reduce the pseudarthrosis rate
- B. Reduce graft problems
- C. To maintain lordosis
- D. Improve clinical outcome
- E. To improve arm pain

▸▸ Question 18

A patient developed difficulty in swallowing after ACDF. Laryngoscopy for postoperative dysphagia in this case is indicated if symptoms persist for how long?

- A. 24 hours
- B. 3 days
- C. 5 days
- D. > 2 weeks
- E. > 1 month

▸▸ Question 19

What is the most common muscle flap for repair of esophageal perforation?

- A. Sternocleidomastoid
- B. Radial forearm
- C. Pectoralis
- D. Infrahyoid
- E. Omohyoid

Answers

▸▸ Answer 1

Correct answer is E. All of the above[1]

▸▸ Answer 2

Correct answer is F. Positive hoffmann's sign[2]

▸▸ Answer 3

Correct answer is D. Trigger points injections and facet blocks have no role[3]

▸▸ Answer 4

Correct answer is D. All of the above[4]

▸▸ Answer 5

Correct answer is C. Cricoid cartilage[4]

▸▸ Answer 6

Correct answer is C. It is recommended for improvement of clinical outcome[5]

▸▸ Answer 7

Correct answer is E. All of the above[5]

▸▸ Answer 8

Correct answer is E. All of the above[6]

▸▸ Answer 9

Correct answer is E. All of the above[7]

▸▸ Answer 10

Correct answer is D. All of the above[8]

▸▸ Answer 11

Correct answer is D. C5–C6[1]

▸▸ Answer 12

Correct answer is A. Spurling test[2]

▸▸ Answer 13

Correct answer is E. 98%[2]

▸▸ Answer 14

Correct answer is D. C6[2]

▸▸ Answer 15

Correct answer is D. 90%[3]

▸▸ Answer 16

Correct answer is B. Longus coli[4]

▸▸ Answer 17

Correct answer is D. Improve clinical outcome[5]

▸▸ Answer 18

Correct answer is D. > 2 weeks[9]

▸▸ Answer 19

Correct answer is A. Sternocleidomastoid[10]

References

[1] Greenberg M, ed. Greenberg's Handbook of Neurosurgery. 10th ed. New York: Thieme; 2023:1280
[2] Greenberg M, ed. Greenberg's Handbook of Neurosurgery. 10th ed. New York: Thieme; 2023:1282
[3] Greenberg M, ed. Greenberg's Handbook of Neurosurgery. 10th ed. New York: Thieme; 2023:1283
[4] Greenberg M, ed. Greenberg's Handbook of Neurosurgery. 10th ed. New York: Thieme; 2023:1284

[5] Greenberg M, ed. Greenberg's Handbook of Neurosurgery. 10th ed. New York: Thieme; 2023:1285
[6] Greenberg M, ed. Greenberg's Handbook of Neurosurgery. 10th ed. New York: Thieme; 2023:1286
[7] Greenberg M, ed. Greenberg's Handbook of Neurosurgery. 10th ed. New York: Thieme; 2023:1292
[8] Greenberg M, ed. Greenberg's Handbook of Neurosurgery. 10th ed. New York: Thieme; 2023:1291
[9] Greenberg M, ed. Greenberg's Handbook of Neurosurgery. 10th ed. New York: Thieme; 2023:1287
[10] Greenberg M, ed. Greenberg's Handbook of Neurosurgery. 10th ed. New York: Thieme; 2023:1288

78 Cervical Degenerative Disk Disease and Cervical Myelopathy

Questions

▸▸ Question 1

Cervical spinal spondylosis usually implies a more widespread age-related degenerative condition of the cervical spine including various combinations of which of the following?

- A. Congenital cervical spinal stenosis (the shallow cervical canal) and degeneration of the intervertebral disk producing a focal stenosis due to a cervical bar which can be due to an osteophytic spur or protrusion of intervertebral disk material
- B. Hypertrophy of lamina, dura, articular facets, and ligaments (ligamentum flavum, PLL, OPLL, ossification of ligamentum flavum) plus subluxation due to disk and facet joint degeneration
- C. Altered mobility and telescoping of the spine due to loss of height of VBs and disks, which is also called as shingling of laminae
- D. Alteration of normal lordosis curvature including excessive lordosis or kyphosis
- E. All of the above

▸▸ Question 2

In case of myelopathy, the histological findings are degeneration of the central gray matter at the level of compression, degeneration of the posterior column above the lesion, and demyelination of the lateral columns especially corticospinal tracts (anterior spinal tracts are relatively spared). Following are included in the pathogenesis of cervical myelopathy except?

- A. Direct cord compression between osteophytic bars and hypertrophy or infolding of the ligamentum flavum especially if superimposed on congenital narrowing or cervical subluxations
- B. Ischemia due to compression of the vascular structures
- C. Repeated local cord trauma by normal movements in the presence of protruded disks and/or osteophytic bars
- D. Compression due to hypertrophy of the anterior longitudinal ligament

▸▸ Question 3

Cervical spondylosis is the most common cause of myelopathy in patients more than 55 years of age, and cervical spondylotic myelopathy (CSM) is rare in patients less than 40 years of age. CSM develops in almost all patients with more than or equal to 30% narrowing of cross-sectional area of the cervical spinal canal. Clinical problems that can occur with cervical spondylosis include myeloradiculopathy which includes radiculopathy and myelopathy and the second one is pain and paresthesias in the head, neck, and shoulders with little or no suggestion of radiculopathy nor abnormal physical findings. Which of the following statements regarding individual symptoms of CSM is correct?

- A. The earliest motor findings are typically weakness in the triceps and hand intrinsics with wasting of the hand muscles and slow stiff opening and closing of the fist. Clumsiness with fine motor skills (writing, buttoning buttons) is common. There is often proximal weakness of lower extremities (mild to moderate iliopsoas weakness in 54%) and spasticity of the lower extremities
- B. Sensory disturbance may be minimal and when it occurs it is like glove distribution sensory loss in the hands. A sensory level may occur a number of levels below the area of cord compression. Lower extremity often exhibits loss of vibratory sense (in 82% cases) and occasionally has reduced pin prick sensations (9%)
- C. In 72 to 87% of cases, reflexes are hyperactive at a varying distance below the level of stenosis and clonus, Babinski, or Hoffmann's sign may be present. Dynamic Hoffmann's sign may be more sensitive while inverted radial reflex is said to be pathognomonic of CSM
- D. Urinary urgency and frequency are common in CSM, while urinary incontinence is rare. Anal sphincter disturbances are uncommon
- E. All of the above

▸▸ Question 4

Which of the following are included in the cervical spondylotic myelopathic syndromes?

- A. Transverse lesion syndrome: Most frequent syndrome, possibly an end stage of the disease process
- B. Motor system syndrome: Mixture of lower motor neuron findings in the upper extremity and upper motor neuron finding in the lower extremities which can mimic ALS
- C. Central cord syndrome: Motor and sensory involvement producing greater deficit in the upper extremities than the lower extremities results in the so-called numb-clumsy hand syndrome. Lhermitte's sign may be more common in this group
- D. Brown-Sequard syndrome: Upper motor neuron weakness ipsilateral to the side of greater narrowing while contralateral impairment of pain, temperature, and joint position sense
- E. Brachialgia and cord syndrome: Primarily radiculopathy with lesser association with long tract involvement
- F. All of the above

▸▸ Question 5

According to the modified Japanese Orthopedic Association Scale, severe spondylotic myelopathy implies Benzel mJOA grade of how much?

- A. More than or equal to 15
- B. 12 to 14
- C. Less than or equal to 11
- D. More than 9
- E. None of the above

▸▸ **Question 6**

Amyotrophic lateral sclerosis (ALS) is anterior horn motor neuron disease which can mimic motor system syndrome of cervical spondylotic myelopathy (CSM). Triad of ALS are atrophic weakness of hands and forearms, mild lower extremity spasticity, and diffuse hyperreflexia. Which of the following features can help differentiate ALS from CSM?

- A. In ALS sensory symptoms are conspicuously absent while in CSM hand numbness may occur
- B. Bulbar symptoms like dysarthria and hyperactive jaw jerk may occur in ALS but are absent in CSM
- C. ALS causes extensive weakness/muscle atrophy of hands usually with fasciculations
- D. ALS will cause LMN findings in the tongue like visible fasciculations and positive sharp waves on EMG or in the lower extremity like atrophy and fasciculations
- E. CSM or herniated cervical disk usually includes neck and shoulder pain, limitation of neck movements, sensory changes, and LMN findings restricted to one or two spinal cord segments
- F. All of the above

▸▸ **Question 7**

Cervical canal stenosis is spina canal narrowing sufficient to produce spinal cord compression and thereby spinal cord symptoms. Cervical spondylotic myelopathy (CSM) is rare in patients with canal diameter more than 16 mm, and its risk is increased in patients with less than 14-mm diameter. Values less than or equal to 10 mm are likely to be associated with myelopathy while in average patients with CSM, canal diameter is around 11.8 mm. Which of the following findings are found in CSM patients with poor outcome?

- A. Multilevel hyperintensity within the spinal cord parenchyma in T2WI
- B. Single-level T2WI hyperintensity with corresponding T1WI hypointensity
- C. Spinal cord atrophy (transverse area less than 45 mm^2)
- D. Banana-shaped cord in axial images
- E. Snake eyes within the spinal cord on axial T2WI may be related to cystic necrosis of cord and is correlated with poor outcome
- F. All of the above

▸▸ **Question 8**

Nonoperative management of cervical spondylotic myelopathy includes which of the following?

- A. Prolonged immobilization with rigid cervical bracing
- B. Modified activities to eliminate high-risk activities
- C. Bed rest
- D. Anti-inflammatory medications
- E. All of the above

▸▸ **Question 9**

Patients with mJOA score of more than 12 may derive significant improvement from surgery and deterioration from this point may be ominous. For degenerative cervical radiculopathy, patients do better with anterior decompression with/without fusion and cause rapid relief of pain in arm and neck and of sensory loss within 3 to 4 months while relief of symptoms like weakness of wrist extension, elbow extension, shoulder abduction, and internal rotation may take up to how long?

- A. 9 months
- B. 6 months
- C. 3 months
- D. More than or equal to 12 months
- E. More than 18 months

▸▸ **Question 10**

Situations where posterior approach would generally be the initial choice include which of the following?

- A. Congenital cervical stenosis
- B. Disease over more than or equal to three levels
- C. Cases of OPLL
- D. Primary posterior pathology like infolding of ligamentum flavum
- E. All of the above

▸▸ **Question 11**

Hard calcified disks are commonly found in thoracic spine. Which of the following is sometimes called a hard disk in cervical spine?

- A. Shallow canal
- B. Osteophyte
- C. Lamina
- D. Hypertrophied ligamentum flavum
- E. Facet joint capsule

▸▸ **Question 12**

The bow stringing of cervical spinal cord refers to which of the following?

- A. Kyphosis
- B. Lordosis
- C. Ossified posterior longitudinal ligament
- D. Hypertrophied ligamentum flavum
- E. Multilevel disk protrusion

▸▸ **Question 13**

What is the earliest motor finding in cervical spondylotic myelopathy (CSM)?

- A. Weakness of triceps and hand intrinsics
- B. Proximal weakness of lower extremities
- C. Spasticity of lower limb
- D. Weakness of biceps
- E. Weak extension of elbow

▸▸ **Question 14**

During degenerative cervical spine disease, which of the following is usually spared?
- A. Gray matter
- B. Posterior columns
- C. Lateral columns
- D. Corticospinal tracts
- E. Anterior spinal tracts

▸▸ **Question 15**

What is the pathognomonic test for cervical spondylosis myelopathy?
- A. Lhermitte's sign
- B. Hoffmann's sign
- C. Dynamic Hoffmann sign
- D. Inverted radial reflex
- E. Babinski's reflex

▸▸ **Question 16**

Amyotrophic lateral sclerosis may be difficult to differentiate from cervical spondylosis myelopathy and patients with the former are wrongly operated on for the suspicion of the latter. What is a typical feature of ALS that can differentiate it from cervical spondylotic myelopathy (CSM)?
- A. Absence of sensory findings
- B. Absence of bulbar symptoms
- C. Absence of tongue fasciculations
- D. Absence of widespread motor weakness with fasciculations
- E. MR

▸▸ **Question 17**

What is the ratio of the AP diameter of the spinal canal at the mid vertebral body level to the vertebral body at the same location?
- A. Pavlov's
- B. Lhermitte's
- C. Steele's
- D. Babinski's
- E. Spence's

▸▸ **Question 18**

What is the cervical spine canal diameter above which a patient rarely develops myelopathy?
- A. 4 mm
- B. 8 mm
- C. 10 mm
- D. 12 mm
- E. 16 mm

▸▸ **Question 19**

The transverse area of the spinal cord is reduced at the level of maximum compression in cervical spondylosis myelopathy and on axial images what does the cord look like?
- A. Double lumen
- B. Tram track
- C. Owl's eye
- D. Bamboo
- E. Banana

▸▸ **Question 20**

For cervical spondylotic myelopathy (CSM), a posterior approach is favored if the disease spans over how many levels?
- A. > 1 level
- B. > 2 levels
- C. > 3 levels
- D. > 4 levels
- E. > 5 levels

▸▸ **Question 21**

For posterior approach decompression of cervical spine, a standard laminectomy refers to laminectomy at what level?
- A. C1
- B. C2
- C. C3–C6
- D. C2–C7
- E. C1–T1

▸▸ **Question 22**

A motor decline of deltoid muscle strength by ≥ 1 grade within 6 weeks of cervical spine surgery is which postoperative palsy?
- A. C3 palsy
- B. C4 palsy
- C. C5 palsy
- D. C6 palsy
- E. C7 palsy

Answers

▸▸ **Answer 1**

Correct answer is E. All of the above[1]

▸▸ **Answer 2**

Correct answer is D. Compression due to hypertrophy of the anterior longitudinal ligament[1]

▸▸ Answer 3

Correct answer is E. All of the above[2]

▸▸ Answer 4

Correct answer is F. All of the above[3]

▸▸ Answer 5

Correct answer is C. Less than or equal to 11[4]

▸▸ Answer 6

Correct answer is F. All of the above[5]

▸▸ Answer 7

Correct answer is F. All of the above[6]

▸▸ Answer 8

Correct answer is E. All of the above[7]

▸▸ Answer 9

Correct answer is D. More than or equal to 12 months[7]

▸▸ Answer 10

Correct answer is E. All of the above[8]

▸▸ Answer 11

Correct answer is B. Osteophyte[1]

▸▸ Answer 12

Correct answer is A. Kyphosis[1]

▸▸ Answer 13

Correct answer is A. Weakness of triceps and hand intrinsics[9]

▸▸ Answer 14

Correct answer is E. Anterior spinal tracts[1]

▸▸ Answer 15

Correct answer is D. Inverted radial reflex[2]

▸▸ Answer 16

Correct answer is A. Absence of sensory findings[5]

▸▸ Answer 17

Correct answer is A. Pavlov's[6]

▸▸ Answer 18

Correct answer is E. 16 mm[5]

▸▸ Answer 19

Correct answer is E. Banana[6]

▸▸ Answer 20

Correct answer is C. > 3 levels[8]

▸▸ Answer 21

Correct answer is C. C3–C6[8]

▸▸ Answer 22

Correct answer is C. C5 palsy[10]

References

[1] Greenberg M, ed. Greenberg's Handbook of Neurosurgery. 10th ed. New York: Thieme; 2023:1296
[2] Greenberg M, ed. Greenberg's Handbook of Neurosurgery. 10th ed. New York: Thieme; 2023:1298
[3] Greenberg M, ed. Greenberg's Handbook of Neurosurgery. 10th ed. New York: Thieme; 2023:1299
[4] Greenberg M, ed. Greenberg's Handbook of Neurosurgery. 10th ed. New York: Thieme; 2023:1300
[5] Greenberg M, ed. Greenberg's Handbook of Neurosurgery. 10th ed. New York: Thieme; 2023:1301
[6] Greenberg M, ed. Greenberg's Handbook of Neurosurgery. 10th ed. New York: Thieme; 2023:1302
[7] Greenberg M, ed. Greenberg's Handbook of Neurosurgery. 10th ed. New York: Thieme; 2023:1303
[8] Greenberg M, ed. Greenberg's Handbook of Neurosurgery. 10th ed. New York: Thieme; 2023:1304
[9] Greenberg M, ed. Greenberg's Handbook of Neurosurgery. 10th ed. New York: Thieme; 2023:1297
[10] Greenberg M, ed. Greenberg's Handbook of Neurosurgery. 10th ed. New York: Thieme; 2023:1306

79 Spine Measurements

Questions

▸▸ Question 1

Scoliosis is defined as lateral curvature of the spine in the coronal (frontal) plane with Cobb angle more than what?

- A. 8 degrees
- B. 10 degree
- C. 12 degrees
- D. 14 degrees
- E. 16 degrees

▸▸ Question 2

Cobb angle can be measured between two lines, first drawn tangential to the superior endplate of superior vertebra and the second is drawn tangential to the inferior endplate of inferior vertebra. How can this angle be obtained?

- A. Sagittal X-ray
- B. Coronal X-ray
- C. Sagittal CT scan
- D. Coronal MRI films
- E. None of the above

▸▸ Question 3

The absolute value of lumbar spinal lordosis should be about 30 degrees greater than the absolute value of the thoracic kyphosis (e.g., a patient with thoracic kyphosis of 20 degrees should have a lumbar lordosis of approximately −50 degrees). What should be range of lumbar lordosis in normal individuals?

- A. 10 to 30 degrees
- B. 10 to 40 degrees
- C. 20 to 40 degrees
- D. 20 to 50 degrees
- E. 20 to 60 degrees

▸▸ Question 4

Sagittal vertical axis is a horizontal distance from the posterior edge of the S1 endplate to a plumb line dropped from the mid C7 vertebral body. What is its normal value?

- A. < 3 cm
- B. < 7 cm
- C. < 5 cm
- D. < 9 cm
- E. < 1 cm

▸▸ Question 5

Pelvic tilt is the angle between the vertical reference line and a line drawn from the midpoint of the femoral head to the midpoint of the S1 endplate. What should be the normal value of this angle?

- A. 5 to 15 degrees
- B. 10 to 20 degrees
- C. 10 to 25 degrees
- D. 15 to 30 degrees
- E. 20 to 30 degrees

▸▸ Question 6

Pelvic incidence is the angle between a point perpendicular to the S1 endplate and a line drawn from the midpoint of the femoral head to the midpoint of the S1 endplate. What is its normal value approximately?

- A. 35 degrees
- B. 45 degrees
- C. 50 degrees
- D. 55 degrees
- E. 60 degrees

▸▸ Question 7

Sacral slope is the angle between the horizontal reference line and the S1 endplate and it normal value is 36 to 42 degrees. Which of the following statements is correct?

- A. SS = PI − PT
- B. SS = PT − PI
- C. SS = PI + PT
- D. SS = PT multiplied by PI
- E. None of the above

▸▸ Question 8

Lumbar lordosis is the angle between the top of S1 and the top of L1 vertebra. What is its normal value?

- A. 10 to 30 degrees
- B. 20 to 40 degrees
- C. 20 to 50 degrees
- D. 10 to 40 degrees

▸▸ Question 9

Thoracic kyphosis is the angle between top of T4 and the bottom of the T12 vertebrae. What is its normal value?

- A. 41 ± 12 degrees
- B. 39 ± 12 degrees
- C. 37 ± 12 degrees
- D. 43 ± 12 degrees

▸▸ Question 10

The spine is generally kyphotic between T1 and T12 while between L1 and L5 it is what?

- A. Scoliotic
- B. Lordotic
- C. Kyphotic
- D. Hyperacusis
- E. None of the above

▸▸ Question 11

Scoliosis is defined as lateral curvature of the spine in the coronal plane with what Cobb angle?
- A. > 10 degrees
- B. > 15 degrees
- C. > 20 degrees
- D. > 25 degrees
- E. > 30 degrees

▸▸ Question 12

The vertebra whose center is most laterally displaced from the central line is called what?
- A. Center
- B. Apex
- C. Master
- D. Dextro
- E. Levo

▸▸ Question 13

As compared to thoracic spine, the lumbar spine should have lordosis more than what?
- A. 5 degrees
- B. 10 degrees
- C. 15 degrees
- D. 20 degree
- E. 30 degrees

▸▸ Question 14

Pelvic tilt is the angle between the vertical reference line (VRL) and a line drawn from the midpoint of the femoral head to the midpoint of the S1 endplate. Normally, it should be less than what?
- A. 20 degrees
- B. 30 degrees
- C. 40 degrees
- D. 90 degrees
- E. 180 degrees

▸▸ Question 15

Patients with higher sacral slope have a higher chance of developing which of the following?
- A. Spinal stenosis
- B. Spondylolisthesis
- C. Scoliosis
- D. Kyphosis
- E. Lordosis

▸▸ Question 16

Lumbar lordosis (LL) is the angle between the top of S1 and the top of L1. For pelvic harmony, LL should be within how many degrees of pelvic incidence (PI)?
- A. 9
- B. 11
- C. 13
- D. 15
- E. 20

▸▸ Question 17

According to Roussouly classification of lumbar lordosis if the SS = 35–45 degrees, apex of LL is at the center of L4 VB. What is the implication of this type?
- A. LL is distributed over only approximately 3 lumbar levels
- B. Entire spine is hypolordotic and hypokyphotic
- C. Well-balanced spine
- D. LL is distributed over > 5 levels
- E. PI is usually high

Answers

▸▸ Answer 1

Correct answer is B. 10 degree[1]

▸▸ Answer 2

Correct answer is B. Coronal X-ray[1]

▸▸ Answer 3

Correct answer is B. 10 to 40 degrees[2]

▸▸ Answer 4

Correct answer is C. < 5 cm[3]

▸▸ Answer 5

Correct answer is C. 10 to 25 degrees[3]

▸▸ Answer 6

Correct answer is C. 50 degrees[3]

▸▸ Answer 7

Correct answer is A. SS = PI – PT[3]

▸▸ Answer 8

Correct answer is B. 20 to 40 degrees[3]

▸▸ **Answer 9**

Correct answer is A. 41 ± 12 degrees[3]

▸▸ **Answer 10**

Correct answer is B. Lordotic[3]

▸▸ **Answer 11**

Correct answer is A. > 10 degrees[1]

▸▸ **Answer 12**

Correct answer is B. Apex[1]

▸▸ **Answer 13**

Correct answer is E. 30 degrees[2]

▸▸ **Answer 14**

Correct answer is A. 20 degrees[3]

▸▸ **Answer 15**

Correct answer is B. Spondylolisthesis[3]

▸▸ **Answer 16**

Correct answer is A. 9[3]

▸▸ **Answer 17**

Correct answer is C. Well-balanced spine[4]

References

[1] Greenberg M, ed. Greenberg's Handbook of Neurosurgery. 10th ed. New York: Thieme; 2023:1312
[2] Greenberg M, ed. Greenberg's Handbook of Neurosurgery. 10th ed. New York: Thieme; 2023:1313
[3] Greenberg M, ed. Greenberg's Handbook of Neurosurgery. 10th ed. New York: Thieme; 2023:1314
[4] Greenberg M, ed. Greenberg's Handbook of Neurosurgery. 10th ed. New York: Thieme; 2023:1317

80 Idiopathic Scoliosis

Questions

▸▸ Question 1

Scoliosis is defined as lateral curvature of the spine in the coronal plane (frontal plane) with Cobb angle greater than 10 degrees. Which of the following is the type of idiopathic scoliosis which occurs at the age of 10 to 17 years and with overwhelming female predominance?

- A. Congenital scoliosis
- B. Infantile scoliosis
- C. Juvenile scoliosis
- D. Adolescent idiopathic scoliosis
- E. None of the above

▸▸ Question 2

Patients with idiopathic scoliosis are more commonly females and mostly have dextroscoliosis (convex to right side). Imaging for these patients consist of lateral and neutral PA coronal X-rays and left-bending plus right-bending coronal X-rays are done only if surgery is planned. Which of the following statements is incorrect regarding treatment of these patients?

- A. Treatment is based on skeletal maturity and magnitude of scoliosis
- B. Growing patients with curves less than 25 degrees or skeletally mature patients with curves less than 45 to 50 degrees are managed with observation only
- C. Bracing prevents progression but does not correct scoliosis and bracing makes no sense in skeletally mature patients
- D. Use of bracing in patients with curves 25 to 40 degrees who are still growing or in skeletally immature patients with curves more than 45 degrees is done to tide them over until they can have surgery
- E. For growing patients with early scoliosis, there is no need of fixation or vertebral body tethering

▸▸ Question 3

"Reduced growth in areas of compressed cartilage (physes) in the curve concavity may result in progression of scoliosis through development of vertebral body wedging from asymmetric growth"; this principle for adult idiopathic scoliosis is known as what?

- A. Heuber principle
- B. Hueter-Volkmann principle
- C. Heishemer-Volkmann principle
- D. Spence principle
- E. None of the above

▸▸ Question 4

Which of the following physical findings can be found in scoliotic patients?

- A. Shoulder asymmetry, pelvic tilt, age length discrepancy, breast asymmetry, and trunk shift (shift of thorax to one side as compared to the pelvis)
- B. Adams forward bend test which is done by putting the feet of the patient together and forward bending with the knees straight and arms dangling which will result in a rib hump on the convex side of thoracic scoliotic curve
- C. Neurologic examination to look for abdominal cutaneous reflex, deep tendon reflexes, strength, and sensations
- D. Evidence of underlying conditions like arachnodactyly, skin pigment changes, tufts of hair, or dimpling over the spine
- E. All of the above

▸▸ Question 5

Riser staging for assessing skeletal maturity in adolescent patient to guide decisions for bracing and timing of surgery includes following except?

- A. Stage 0 is no ossification center in the iliac crest apophysis
- B. Stages 1, 2, and 3 consist of apophysis of iliac crest up to less than 25%, 25 to 50%, and 50 to 75%, respectively
- C. Stage 4 consists of more than 75% of apophysis of the iliac crest, while stage 5 consists of complete ossification and fusion of the iliac crest apophysis
- D. Grades 0 and 1 are growing rapidly, and scoliosis curve acceleration begins in stage 0
- E. Grades 4 and 5 are growing rapidly

▸▸ Question 6

Which of the following are strong indications of MRI in scoliotic patients?

- A. Early-onset scoliosis in age less than 10 years
- B. Adolescent idiopathic scoliosis in males
- C. Atypical curves like thoracic levoscoliosis, kyphosis
- D. Hyperkyphosis
- E. Neurologic deficit
- F. All of the above

▸▸ Question 7

Major curve in a scoliotic patient is the largest curve and there can be only one major curve which is almost always present at MT (main thoracic from T6 to T11, T12 disk) or TL/L (thoracolumbar/lumbar). There are other two minor curves besides the major curve, which can be structural or nonstructural. Which of the following is a structural criterion of minor curve?

- A. Side-bending residual Cobb angle more than or equal to 25 degrees
- B. A and/or T2–T5 kyphosis more than or equal to plus 20 degrees
- C. A and/or T10–L2 kyphosis more than or equal to plus 20 degrees
- D. All of the above

▸▸ **Question 8**

Lenke classification is the de facto standard for classifying AIS. Following are true regarding this classification except?
- A. Type one is main thoracic
- B. Type two is double thoracic
- C. Type three is double major
- D. Type four is triple major
- E. Type five is thoracolumbar/lumbar
- F. Type six is thoracolumbar/lumbar minor thoracic

▸▸ **Question 9**

Two basic types of braces are TLSO with a goal to wear for 18 to 23 h/d and night time TLSO with a goal to wear for 10 hours per night. Which of the following are contraindications of bracings?
- A. In skeletally mature patients
- B. Thoracic lordosis
- C. Insensate patients or insufficient neuromuscular function
- D. ± significant obesity
- E. Sanders scale 2 to 5 with curves more than or equal to 30 degrees
- F. All of the above

▸▸ **Question 10**

Which of the following are the surgical fusion goals for a scoliotic patient?
- A. Correct scoliosis as much as possible
- B. Restore thoracic kyphosis
- C. Fuse all structural curves
- D. All of the above

▸▸ **Question 11**

Which of the following is usually correct for adolescent idiopathic scoliosis (AIS)?
- A. Presents at 4 to 9 years of age
- B. Overwhelming male dominance
- C. Almost all with dextroscoliosis
- D. Majority are lumbar
- E. Potentially curable with Mehta serial casting

▸▸ **Question 12**

Risser system grades ossification and fusion of the iliac crest apophyses. Ossification of 25 to 50% of the iliac crest apophysis is graded as what stage?
- A. 1
- B. 2
- C. 3
- D. 4
- E. 5

▸▸ **Question 13**

In treatment of AIS, observation is appropriate for which curves?
- A. < 25 degrees
- B. > 25 degrees
- C. < 20 degrees
- D. > 20 degrees
- E. < 30 degrees

▸▸ **Question 14**

Bracing is indicated in AIS for which patients?
- A. Skeletally mature
- B. Insensate patients
- C. Sander stage 1
- D. Sanders stage 3
- E. Thoracic lordosis

▸▸ **Question 15**

How is AdIS different from AIS?
- A. AIS presents with back and LE pain
- B. Coronal and sagittal malalignments are more common in AdIS
- C. Curves are more flexible in AdIS
- D. Sacrum needs to be included in surgical fusion in AIS
- E. In AIS, a degenerative lumbosacral fractional curve is often present as a result of degeneration

Answers

▸▸ **Answer 1**

Correct answer is D. Adolescent idiopathic scoliosis[1]

▸▸ **Answer 2**

Correct answer is E. For growing patients with early scoliosis, there is no need of fixation or vertebral body tethering[1]

▸▸ **Answer 3**

Correct answer is B. Hueter-Volkmann principle[2]

▸▸ **Answer 4**

Correct answer is E. All of the above[3]

▸▸ **Answer 5**

Correct answer is E. Grades 4 and 5 are growing rapidly[3]

▸▸ **Answer 6**

Correct answer is F. All of the above[3]

▸▸ Answer 7

Correct answer is D. All of the above[4]

▸▸ Answer 8

Correct answer is F. Type six is thoracolumbar/lumbar minor thoracic[4]

▸▸ Answer 9

Correct answer is F. All of the above[5]

▸▸ Answer 10

Correct answer is D. All of the above[6]

▸▸ Answer 11

Correct answer is C. Almost all with dextroscoliosis[1]

▸▸ Answer 12

Correct answer is B. 2[3]

▸▸ Answer 13

Correct answer is A. < 25 degrees[7]

▸▸ Answer 14

Correct answer is C. Sander stage 1[5]

▸▸ Answer 15

Correct answer is B. Coronal and sagittal malalignments are more common in AdIS[6]

References

[1] Greenberg M, ed. Greenberg's Handbook of Neurosurgery. 10th ed. New York: Thieme; 2023:1319
[2] Greenberg M, ed. Greenberg's Handbook of Neurosurgery. 10th ed. New York: Thieme; 2023:1320
[3] Greenberg M, ed. Greenberg's Handbook of Neurosurgery. 10th ed. New York: Thieme; 2023:1321
[4] Greenberg M, ed. Greenberg's Handbook of Neurosurgery. 10th ed. New York: Thieme; 2023:1322
[5] Greenberg M, ed. Greenberg's Handbook of Neurosurgery. 10th ed. New York: Thieme; 2023:1324
[6] Greenberg M, ed. Greenberg's Handbook of Neurosurgery. 10th ed. New York: Thieme; 2023:1325
[7] Greenberg M, ed. Greenberg's Handbook of Neurosurgery. 10th ed. New York: Thieme; 2023:1323

81 Lumbar and Thoracic Degenerative Disk Disease

Questions

▸▸ Question 1

Degenerative disk disease in lumbar spine consists of age and wear related decrease in proteoglycan content of the disk, disk desiccation, tear in the annulus fibrosus, disk fibrosis, disk resorption, loss of disk space height, and osteophytes formation. What is the most powerful determinant in developing degenerative disk disease?

- A. Genetic influence and possibly other unidentified factors
- B. Cumulative effects of micro- and macro-traumas
- C. Osteoporosis
- D. Cigarette smoking
- E. Stresses on the spine like excess body weight and loss of muscle tone (primarily abdominal and paraspinal muscles)

▸▸ Question 2

Lumbar spinal stenosis is most common at L4–L5 and then at L3–L4 level. Symptomatic stenosis typically produces neurogenic claudication which classically is gradually progressive back and/or leg pain exacerbated by standing or walking that is relieved by sitting, lying down, or flexing at the waist. It is differentiated with vascular claudication which is usually relieved at rest regardless of position. Which of the following are contributing factors for symptomatic lumbar spinal stenosis?

- A. Congenital narrow spinal canal (short pedicle syndrome)
- B. Hypertrophy of facets and ligamentum flavum abnormalities like hypertrophy, ossification, and infolding (buckling) caused by loss of disk space height
- C. Disk bulging, herniation, collapse, and osteophyte formation
- D. Malalignment of vertebral bodies like spondylolisthesis including anterolisthesis, retrolisthesis, and olisthesis
- E. All of the above

▸▸ Question 3

Lateral recess is the gutter alongside the pedicle, and narrowing of this space causes compression on nerve root en passant (e.g., in case of L4–L5 lateral recess narrowing, L5 nerve root will be involved) while foraminal stenosis (which can be caused by lateral disk herniation, facet hypertrophy, spondylolisthesis, or disk space collapse) causes compression on the exiting nerve root as in above case L4 nerve root. Foraminal stenosis also causes loss of inverted teardrop appearance of the foramen on T1WI or T2WI sagittal MRI images. Which of the following is correct regarding boundaries of lateral recess?

- A. It is bordered anteriorly by the vertebral body
- B. It is bordered laterally by the pedicle
- C. It is bordered posteriorly by the superior articular facet of the inferior vertebral body
- D. All of the above

▸▸ Question 4

Neurogenic claudication (NC) is thought to arise from ischemia of the lumbosacral nerve root, as a result from increased metabolic demand from exercise together with vascular compromise of the nerve root due to pressure from the surrounding structures. Following are the differences between neurogenic claudication and vascular claudication (VC) except?

- A. Distribution of pain in case of NC is dermatomal, while in case of VC, it is sclerotomal (in the distribution of muscle group)
- B. Sensory loss is in the distribution of dermatome in case of NC, while it is stocking distribution in case of VC
- C. NC pain is relieved with rest slowly often in 30 minutes, while VC pain is relieved almost immediately after taking rest
- D. Claudication distance in case of NC is variable from day to day, while it is constant in case of VC
- E. Relief of pain in case of NC is not positional, while in case of VC, it is positional

▸▸ Question 5

Normal AP diameter of lumbar spinal canal on lateral plain film (from spinolaminar line to posterior vertebral body) is 22 to 25 mm, while 15 mm is the lower limit of normal and less than 11 mm is severe lumbar stenosis. Normal ligamentum flavum thickness on CT is less than or equal to 4 to 5 mm. Which of the following statements is correct regarding dimensions of lateral recess on CT?

- A. Lateral recess height of 3 to 4 mm is border line (symptomatic if other lesions like disk bulge is also present)
- B. Less than 3 mm is suggestive of lateral recess syndrome
- C. Less than 2 mm is diagnostic of lateral recess syndrome
- D. All of the above

▸▸ Question 6

In which of the Modic's classification of vertebral endplate changes on MRI, there is high signal drop out (becomes low intensity) on STIR images?

- A. Modic type one (T1WI low intensity signal and T2WI high intensity signal)
- B. Modic type two (both T1WI and T2WI are high intensity signal)
- C. Modic type three (both T1WI and T2WI are low intensity signal)
- D. Modic type four
- E. None of the above

▸▸ Question 7

Unenhanced lumbar MRI is the diagnostic test of choice to see central canal stenosis, lateral recess stenosis, foraminal stenosis, as well as juxtafacet cyst and increased fluid in the facet joint. Narrowed canal may assume a deltoid (also known as tricuspoid) shape with reduction of complete loss of CSF signal on T2WI. What other tests can be used as an adjunct to radiographic evaluation?

- A. Ankle brachial index and bicycle test to rule out vascular claudication
- B. EMG with NCV to exclude peripheral neuropathy when index of suspicion is high
- C. Bone density evaluation to see osteopenia or osteoporosis
- D. Facet blocks
- E. All of the above

▸▸ Question 8

Spondylolisthesis is the displacement (subluxation) of one vertebral body on another in any direction. Most commonly the superior vertebral body is anterior to the posterior one. It is most common at L5 on S1, the next most common is at L4–L5. On axial MRI, it may look like a herniated disk which has been termed as a pseudodisk. Which of the following are the types of spondylolisthesis?

- A. Type 1 is dysplastic which is also called as congenital
- B. Type 2 is isthmic which is further subdivided as lytic, elongated, and acute fracture of pars
- C. Type 3 is degenerative
- D. Type 4 is traumatic
- E. Type 5 is pathologic
- F. All of the above

▸▸ Question 9

Surgical intervention in case of spondylolisthesis is done when symptoms become severe in spite of conservative management. The goals of surgery are pain relief, halting progression of symptoms, and possibly reversal of some existing neurologic deficit. Surgical options include posterior decompression with or without fusion which may include posterior lumbar interbody fusion or transforaminal lumbar interbody fusion. Which of the following are the situations where a fusion should be considered in addition to direct or indirect decompression of the nerves?

- A. Spondylolisthesis (especially grade more than 1)
- B. Symptomatic sagittal imbalance or degenerative scoliosis
- C. Dynamic instability on flexion/extension lateral lumbar spine X-rays
- D. Expectation that decompression will destabilize the spine
- E. Multiple recurrent herniated disk
- F. All of the above

▸▸ Question 10

Gill procedures include which of the following?

- A. Radical decompression of nerve root including removal of the loose posterior elements and total facetectomy
- B. Posterolateral or interbody fusion
- C. Fusion rate may be enhanced with the use of internal fixation, for example, transpedicular screw rod fixation
- D. All of the above

▸▸ Question 11

What is the most powerful determinant in developing degenerative spine disease (DSD)?

- A. Genetic influence
- B. Cumulative effects of micro-trauma and macro-trauma to the spine
- C. Osteoporosis
- D. Cigarette smoking
- E. Excess body weight

▸▸ Question 12

Lumbar spinal stenosis is caused by hypertrophy of facets and ligamentum flavum and may be exacerbated by spondylolisthesis. It occurs most commonly at which level?

- A. L1–L2
- B. L2–L3
- C. L3–L4
- D. L4–L5
- E. L5–S1

▸▸ Question 13

What is the prototypical symptom of lumbar spinal stenosis (LSS)?

- A. Neurogenic claudication
- B. LE spasticity
- C. Sphincter disturbance
- D. Low back ache
- E. Weakness of LE

▸▸ Question 14

What is the clinical feature distinguishing neurogenic claudication from vascular claudication?

- A. Pain in the distribution of muscle group with common vascular supply (sclerotomal)
- B. Relief with rest is slow (often > 30 mins), variable, usually positional (stooped posture or sitting often required)
- C. Claudicating distance is constant every day
- D. Sensory loss in stocking distribution
- E. Reliably reproduced with fixed amount of exercise

▸▸ Question 15

What is the normal AP diameter of lumbar spinal canal on lateral plain film?

- A. 11 to 15 mm
- B. 15 to 18 mm
- C. 18 to 22 mm
- D. 22 to 25 mm
- E. 25 to 28 mm

▸▸ Question 16

Anterior subluxation of one vertebral body (VB) on another is spondylolisthesis. It occurs most commonly at which level?

- A. L1–L2
- B. L2–L3
- C. L3–L4
- D. L4–L5
- E. L5–S1

▸▸ **Question 17**

Commonly a true disk herniation occurs with relation to spondylolisthesis at which level?
- A. At the same level
- B. One level below
- C. One level above
- D. Two levels above
- E. Two levels below

▸▸ **Question 18**

According to the Meyerding grade, spondyloptosis is listhesis of what percent?
- A. > 25%
- B. 25 to 50%
- C. 50 to 75%
- D. 75 to 100%
- E. > 100%

▸▸ **Question 19**

On spine CT, what is the lateral recess height diagnostic of lateral recess syndrome?
- A. 7 mm
- B. 5 mm
- C. 4 mm
- D. 3 mm
- E. 1 mm

▸▸ **Question 20**

In isthmic spondylolisthesis, lesions without sclerosis that show increased uptake on bone scan and MRI high signal changes on STIR may be treated with which of the following?
- A. Boston brace
- B. Steroid
- C. Injection therapy
- D. Crutches
- E. Orthopedic mattress

▸▸ **Question 21**

Which of the following is primarily an extension limiting procedure for lumbar spine that can be used as a stand-alone procedure?
- A. Laminectomy
- B. Anterior lumbar interbody fusion
- C. Transforaminal lumbar interbody fusion
- D. Oblique lumbar interbody fusion
- E. Interspinous spacer

Answers

▸▸ Answer 1

Correct answer is A. Genetic influence and possibly other unidentified factors[1]

▸▸ Answer 2

Correct answer is E. All of the above[2]

▸▸ Answer 3

Correct answer is D. All of the above[2]

▸▸ Answer 4

Correct answer is E. Relief of pain in case of NC is not positional, while in case of VC, it is positional[3]

▸▸ Answer 5

Correct answer is D. All of the above[4]

▸▸ Answer 6

Correct answer is B. Modic type two (both T1WI and T2WI are high intensity signal)[5]

▸▸ Answer 7

Correct answer is E. All of the above[5]

▸▸ Answer 8

Correct answer is F. All of the above[6]

▸▸ Answer 9

Correct answer is F. All of the above[7]

▸▸ Answer 10

Correct answer is D. All of the above[8]

▸▸ Answer 11

Correct answer is A. Genetic influence[1]

▸▸ Answer 12

Correct answer is D. L4–L5[9]

▸▸ Answer 13

Correct answer is A. Neurogenic claudication[9]

▸▸ **Answer 14**

Correct answer is B. Relief with rest is slow (often > 30 mins), variable, usually positional (stooped posture or sitting often required)[3]

▸▸ **Answer 15**

Correct answer is D. 22 to 25 mm[10]

▸▸ **Answer 16**

Correct answer is E. L5–S1[11]

▸▸ **Answer 17**

Correct answer is C. One level above[11]

▸▸ **Answer 18**

Correct answer is E. > 100%[6]

▸▸ **Answer 19**

Correct answer is E. 1 mm[4]

▸▸ **Answer 20**

Correct answer is A. Boston brace[8]

▸▸ **Answer 21**

Correct answer is E. Interspinous spacer[12]

References

[1] Greenberg M, ed. Greenberg's Handbook of Neurosurgery. 10th ed. New York: Thieme; 2023:1327

[2] Greenberg M, ed. Greenberg's Handbook of Neurosurgery. 10th ed. New York: Thieme; 2023:1329

[3] Greenberg M, ed. Greenberg's Handbook of Neurosurgery. 10th ed. New York: Thieme; 2023:1332

[4] Greenberg M, ed. Greenberg's Handbook of Neurosurgery. 10th ed. New York: Thieme; 2023:1334

[5] Greenberg M, ed. Greenberg's Handbook of Neurosurgery. 10th ed. New York: Thieme; 2023:1336

[6] Greenberg M, ed. Greenberg's Handbook of Neurosurgery. 10th ed. New York: Thieme; 2023:1340

[7] Greenberg M, ed. Greenberg's Handbook of Neurosurgery. 10th ed. New York: Thieme; 2023:1343

[8] Greenberg M, ed. Greenberg's Handbook of Neurosurgery. 10th ed. New York: Thieme; 2023:1347

[9] Greenberg M, ed. Greenberg's Handbook of Neurosurgery. 10th ed. New York: Thieme; 2023:1328

[10] Greenberg M, ed. Greenberg's Handbook of Neurosurgery. 10th ed. New York: Thieme; 2023:1333

[11] Greenberg M, ed. Greenberg's Handbook of Neurosurgery. 10th ed. New York: Thieme; 2023:1337

[12] Greenberg M, ed. Greenberg's Handbook of Neurosurgery. 10th ed. New York: Thieme; 2023:1346

82 Adult Spinal Deformity and Degenerative Scoliosis

Questions

►► Question 1

A patient presents with backache radiating to lower limbs which increases during walking. This patient has obvious spinal deformity with scoliosis, forward flexion at the wrist, and walking with knees bent. This patient is more than 60 years of age. Standing coronal view X-ray was done which showed Cobb angle of more than 10 degrees. What is the most probable diagnosis in this case?

- A. Adult degenerative spine disease
- B. Adolescent idiopathic scoliosis
- C. Adult idiopathic scoliosis
- D. Adult spinal deformity
- E. None of the above

►► Question 2

SRS-Schwab classification of adult degenerative spinal deformity has which of the following parameters?

- A. Coronal curve types
- B. Sagittal modifiers
- C. Global alignment
- D. Pelvic tilt
- E. All of the above

►► Question 3

Treatment options for adult degenerative scoliosis are based on clinical symptoms and include the following except?

- A. Observation only
- B. Focal decompression
- C. Surgical correction of deformity and stability using traditional open surgery (decompression by laminectomy, PLIF, TLIF, pedicle screw/rod fixation), minimal invasive spine surgery, and combined (both open and MIS)
- D. Anterior corpectomy and cage fixation
- E. None of the above

►► Question 4

Summary for spinopelvic alignment objectives include the following except?

- A. LL = PI ± 9 degrees
- B. PT less than 20 degrees
- C. PSVL and SSV should be less than 30 degrees
- D. SVA less than 5 cm

►► Question 5

Which of the following is Schwab grade 3 of surgical spine osteotomies?

- A. Resection of the inferior facet and joint capsule
- B. Resection of the superior and inferior facets, ligamentum flavum, and possible lamina and spinous process
- C. Partial wedge resection of the vertebral body and the posterior elements with the pedicles
- D. Partial wedge resection of the vertebral body and the posterior elements with the pedicles plus inclusion of at least a portion of the endplate and one adjacent disk
- E. Complete removal of the vertebra and both adjacent disks

►► Question 6

How much lumbar lordosis can be obtained by Schwab grade 1 osteotomy plus ACR?

- A. 1 degree
- B. 6 degrees
- C. 5 to 10 degrees
- D. 16 degrees
- E. 30 to 40 degrees

►► Question 7

Morbid obesity (BMI more than 40) doubles the risk of complications of all types including cardiac, renal, pulmonary, and wound complications with spine surgery, and mortality is increased by how much?

- A. Doubled
- B. Tripled
- C. Four times increased
- D. Five times increased
- E. None of the above

►► Question 8

Pedicle subtraction can increase LL by 30 to 40 degrees. What is the Schwab grade?

- A. Grade 1
- B. Grade 2
- C. Grade 3
- D. Grade 4
- E. Grade 5

►► Question 9

Coronal balance is measured on AP standing scoliosis X-ray. A plumb line is drawn straight down from the center of the C7 vertebral body. There is coronal imbalance if this falls from midline of the sacrum by more than what?

- A. 2 cm
- B. 3 cm
- C. 4 cm
- D. 5 cm
- E. 6 cm

►► **Question 10**

CT scan in case of adult degenerative scoliotic patient can provide which of the following information?

- A. Any fusions (spontaneous or surgical)
- B. Vacuum disk (which imply hypermobility)
- C. Calcifications (in herniated disks, ligamentum flavum)
- D. For obtaining measurements for surgical instrumentation
- E. All of the above

►► **Question 11**

Before surgery for adult spinal deformity (ASD), surgeons use teriparatide for how long to rapidly increase the strength of osteoporotic bone?

- A. 2 weeks
- B. 4 weeks
- C. 6 weeks
- D. 3 months
- E. 6 months

►► **Question 12**

Standing scoliosis X-ray must image from C7 down to what level?

- A. T7
- B. Midthoracic level
- C. Thoracolumbar junction
- D. L1
- E. Femoral heads

►► **Question 13**

The degree of curve rigidity after scoliosis surgery can be determined with which of the following?

- A. Dynamic standing scoliosis X-ray
- B. Flexion–extension X-rays
- C. CT scan
- D. CT myelogram
- E. MRI with contrast

►► **Question 14**

Pre- and postoperative standing scoliosis X-rays help to confirm that alignment objectives are achieved. Following views are required for adolescent idiopathic scoliosis (AIS) except?

- A. Standing coronal
- B. Lateral
- C. Left bending
- D. Right bending
- E. Sagittal

►► **Question 15**

According to Schwab's classification of surgical osteotomies, a complete removal of the vertebra and both adjacent disks and rib resections extended over multiple vertebral levels is what grade?

- A. Zero
- B. II
- C. III
- D. V
- E. VI

►► **Question 16**

Anterior lumbar interbody fusion (ALIF) is best for lumbar level where the great vessels tend not to interfere with the access, and where every degree of correction produces a more significant amount of improvement in vertical alignment. Which level is this?

- A. L1–L2
- B. L2–L3
- C. L3–L4
- D. L4–L5
- E. L5–S1

►► **Question 17**

Standing scoliosis X-rays provide information about scoliosis and which of the following?

- A. Sagittal balance
- B. Cobb's angle
- C. Anterolisthesis
- D. Retrolisthesis
- F. Dynamic stability

Answers

►► **Answer 1**

Correct answer is A. Adult degenerative spine disease[1]

►► **Answer 2**

Correct answer is E. All of the above[2]

►► **Answer 3**

Correct answer is D. Anterior corpectomy and cage fixation[2]

►► **Answer 4**

Correct answer is C. PSVL and SSV should be less than 30 degrees[2]

►► **Answer 5**

Correct answer is C. Partial wedge resection of the vertebral body and the posterior elements with the pedicles[3]

►► **Answer 6**

Correct answer is D. 16 degrees[4]

▸▸ **Answer 7**

Correct answer is B. Tripled[5]

▸▸ **Answer 8**

Correct answer is C. Grade 3[4]

▸▸ **Answer 9**

Correct answer is C. 4 cm[6]

▸▸ **Answer 10**

Correct answer is E. All of the above[1]

▸▸ **Answer 11**

Correct answer is D. 3 months[1]

▸▸ **Answer 12**

Correct answer is E. Femoral heads[1]

▸▸ **Answer 13**

Correct answer is A. Dynamic standing scoliosis X-ray[6]

▸▸ **Answer 14**

Correct answer is E. Sagittal[6]

▸▸ **Answer 15**

Correct answer is E. VI[7]

▸▸ **Answer 16**

Correct answer is E. L5–S1[4]

▸▸ **Answer 17**

Correct answer is A. Sagittal balance[1]

References

[1] Greenberg M, ed. Greenberg's Handbook of Neurosurgery. 10th ed. New York: Thieme; 2023:1353
[2] Greenberg M, ed. Greenberg's Handbook of Neurosurgery. 10th ed. New York: Thieme; 2023:1354
[3] Greenberg M, ed. Greenberg's Handbook of Neurosurgery. 10th ed. New York: Thieme; 2023:1356
[4] Greenberg M, ed. Greenberg's Handbook of Neurosurgery. 10th ed. New York: Thieme; 2023:1358
[5] Greenberg M, ed. Greenberg's Handbook of Neurosurgery. 10th ed. New York: Thieme; 2023:1360
[6] Greenberg M, ed. Greenberg's Handbook of Neurosurgery. 10th ed. New York: Thieme; 2023:1355
[7] Greenberg M, ed. Greenberg's Handbook of Neurosurgery. 10th ed. New York: Thieme; 2023:1357

83 Special Conditions Affecting Spine

Questions

▸▸ **Question 1**

A patient presents with pain in the back, joint pain, and multiple nerve root compressive symptoms (due to expansion of woven bone, osteoid tissue). Lab work shows elevated alkaline phosphatase and urinary hydroxyproline. CT of spine shows hypertrophic changes at the facet joints and X-rays show cortical thickening, sclerotic changes, and osteolytic areas. Which of the following is correct regarding Paget's disease?

- A. It is a disorder of osteoclasts causing increased rate of bone resorption
- B. Reactive osteoblastic activity with overproduction of new, weaker, woven bone
- C. Initial hot phase
- D. Cold phase in the last
- E. All of the above

▸▸ **Question 2**

A patient presents to neurosurgical OPD with complaints of nonradiating low back pain, morning back stiffness, hip pain with swelling, which is exacerbated by inactivity and improved with exercise. X-ray of this patient shows bridging of syndesmophytes between vertebral bodies creating the so-called bamboo spine appearance and sacroiliitis as well. RA factor in serum of this patient is negative. This patient is diagnosed using Modified New York criteria. What is the diagnosis in this case?

- A. Rheumatoid arthritis
- B. Reiter's syndrome
- C. Forestier's disease
- D. Ankylosing spondylitis
- E. Metastatic prostate cancer

▸▸ **Question 3**

The most common surgical intervention in ankylosing spondylitis is orthopedic total hip arthroplasty, while the most frequent fracture site in ankylosing spondylitis is which of the following?

- A. Lumbar spine
- B. Thoracolumbar spine
- C. Cervical spine
- D. Thoracic spine
- E. Lumbar sacral junction

▸▸ **Question 4**

A 55-year-old male patient presents to OPD with signs of myelopathy and positive Hoffmann's sign. His MRI shows a hypointense signal from C3 to C6 level on T2WI which is obliterating CSF signal with cord compression anteriorly. His CT of cervical spine shows calcified anterior longitudinal ligament behind c4, c5, and c6 vertebral bodies. What is the most common location of OPLL in spine (which is 70 to 75%)?

- A. Cervical
- B. Thoracic
- C. Lumbar
- D. Both cervical and thoracic
- E. None of the above

▸▸ **Question 5**

Which of the following is included in the pathological classification of ossified posterior longitudinal ligament?

- A. Segmental (39%), confined to the space behind the vertebral bodies
- B. Continuous (17%), extending from vertebral body to vertebral body spanning the disk space
- C. Mixed (25%), combined elements of both A and B
- D. Other variants (5%), a rare type of OPLL that is contiguous with the end plates and is confined to the disk space
- E. All of the above

▸▸ **Question 6**

Which of the following statements is correct regarding Nurick grade of disability from cervical spondylosis?

- A. Grade 0: signs or symptoms of root involvement without myelopathy
- B. Grade 1: myelopathy but no difficulty in walking
- C. Grade 2: slight difficulty in walking, able to work
- D. Grade 3: difficulty in walking but not needing assistance, unable to work full time
- E. Grade 4: able to walk only with assistance or walker
- F. Grade 5: chair bound or bed ridden
- G. All of the above

▸▸ **Question 7**

A patient presents to neurosurgical OPD with complaints of backache and anterior wedging of at least 5 degrees of more than or equal to three adjacent thoracic vertebral bodies. Associated findings in Scheuermann's kyphosis include the following except?

- A. End plate irregularities
- B. Posterior narrowing of disk space
- C. Schmorl's nodes
- D. Scoliosis
- E. Spondylolysis in 50%

▸▸ **Question 8**

Rheumatoid arthritis (RA) most commonly involves cervical spine (in 44–88% cases of RA) which can be atlantoaxial subluxation, basilar impression, or subaxial subluxation. Which of the following is included in the Ranawat classification of myelopathy in RA?

- A. Class 1: no neural deficit
- B. Class 2: subjective weakness + hyperreflexia + dysesthesia
- C. Class 3: objective weakness plus long tract signs
- D. Class 3A, ambulatory, and class 3 B, quadriparetic and nonambulatory
- E. All of the above

▸▸ Question 9

Spinal cord infarction can be due to atherosclerosis of radicular arteries in elderly patients, clamping of aorta during surgery, trauma, hypotension, aortic dissection, or embolization of spinal arteries. Acute anterior spinal cord syndrome, which results in motor paralysis below the level of injury, loss of pain and temperature with preserved vibratory and position sense, and loss of sphincter control, is because of involvement of which artery?

- A. Anterior spinal artery
- B. Posterior spinal artery
- C. Radicular arteries
- D. Abdominal aorta
- E. None of the above

▸▸ Question 10

Noncontrast CT scan is probably the most sensitive test for detecting pneumorrhachis as well as air in other body compartments. What are the surgical indications of pneumorrhachis (air in the spinal canal)?

- A. Intracranial hypo-/hypertension refractory to medical management
- B. Significant or persistent CSF leak
- C. Evidence of unidirectional ball valve (tension pneumorrhachis) near at-risk nervous tissue
- D. Herniation or serious injury of adjacent structures (for example, lungs) into the spinal cord
- E. All of the above

▸▸ Question 11

Paget's disease may be asymptomatic or present with pain, radiculopathy, and compression of cranial nerves as they pass through skull foramina. Which of the following is the most commonly affected cranial nerve?

- A. III
- B. VI
- C. VII
- D. VIII
- E. X

▸▸ Question 12

Paget's disease depicts ivory bone. The treatment of the disease includes calcitonin derivatives that mainly act by which of the following mechanisms?

- A. Osteoclast activity reduction
- B. Osteoclast activity stimulation
- C. Osteoblast activity reduction
- D. Osteoblast activity stimulation
- E. Inhibition of intestinal calcium absorption

▸▸ Question 13

Ankylosing spondylitis gives rise to bamboo spine, Andersen lesions, and kyphosis. By definition, which joint is always affected?

- A. Scapulohumeral joint
- B. Sacroiliac joint
- C. Ankle joint
- D. Small joints at wrist
- E. Costovertebral

▸▸ Question 14

Which of the following is a test for monitoring ongoing physical therapy and is done by measuring distraction between skin marks on the back before and after forward flexion to detect reduced mobility of the spine due to fusion?

- A. Schober test
- B. Patrick test
- C. Lhermitte sign
- D. Hoover test
- E. Ankylosing test

▸▸ Question 15

What is the most common level affected by ossified posterior longitudinal ligament?

- A. Cervical
- B. Midthoracic
- C. Thoracolumbar
- D. Lumbar
- E. Lumbosacral

▸▸ Question 16

There are four patterns of ossified posterior longitudinal ligament. When it extends from vertebral body to vertebral body, spanning disk space, it is which pattern?

- A. Segmental
- B. Skipping
- C. Continuous
- D. Punctate
- E. Mixed

▸▸ Question 17

Which is the best test for demonstrating and accurately diagnosing ossified posterior longitudinal ligament?

- A. X-ray

- B. CT with coronal reconstruction
- C. CT myelogram
- D. MRI with contrast
- E. Bone scan

▸▸ **Question 18**

According to Nurick grade of disability from cervical spondylosis, being able to walk only with assistance or walker is which grade?

- A. I
- B. II
- C. III
- D. IV
- E. V

▸▸ **Question 19**

Diffuse idiopathic skeletal hyperostosis (DISH) is characterized in spine by flowing formation of which of the following?

- A. Anterior longitudinal ligament
- B. Posterior longitudinal ligament
- C. Disk desiccation
- D. Osteophytes
- E. Schmorl's nodes

▸▸ **Question 20**

In Scheuermann's kyphosis, when the apex is above T8, the patient can be treated with which of the following?

- A. SOMI brace
- B. Miami J
- C. Philadelphia collar
- D. Milwaukee brace
- E. Abdominal binder

▸▸ **Question 21**

Some surgeons do not operate if the maximal dens–C1 distance is how much?

- A. < 2 cm
- B. < 4 cm
- C. < 6 mm
- D. < 8 mm
- E. < 10 mm

▸▸ **Question 22**

The direct effects of rheumatoid arthritis (RA) on the subaxial spine involves which of the following?

- A. Facet joints posteriorly
- B. Disk space anteriorly
- C. Ligamentous hypertrophy
- D. End plate erosion
- E. Pars defect

▸▸ **Question 23**

What is the incidence of atlantoaxial subluxation (AAS) in Down syndrome (DS)?

- A. 10%
- B. 20%
- C. 30%
- D. 40%
- E. 50%

▸▸ **Question 24**

In Down syndrome, what is the recommended management for asymptomatic atlantoaxial subluxation (AAS) seen on lateral C-spine X-ray with ADI ≤ 4.5 mm and PADI ≥ 14 mm?

- A. No need for further testing
- B. Cervical MRI
- C. Surgical fusion
- D. Prohibit high-risk activity
- E. CT of C spine

▸▸ **Question 25**

With spontaneous SEH, recovery of neurologic deficit without surgery is rare. Improvement is seen when decompression is done within how long?

- A. 6 hours
- B. 12 hours
- C. 24 hours
- D. 48 hours
- E. 72 hours

▸▸ **Question 26**

What is the Ranawat class of a patient with subjective weakness + hyperreflexia + dysesthesia?

- A. I
- B. II
- C. III
- D. IV
- E. V

▸▸ **Question 27**

Anterior atlantodental interval (ADI) gives information about the stability of the C1–C2 joint. The normal ADI in adults is less than what?

- A. 11 mm
- B. 10 mm
- C. 7 mm
- D. 5 mm
- E. 3 mm

▸▸ Question 28

Patients with paralysis from atlantoaxial subluxation in rheumatoid arthritis do not recover with surgery if the preoperative posterior atlantodental interval (PADI) is less than what?

- A. 25 mm
- B. 25 mm
- C. 15 mm
- D. 14 mm
- E. 10 mm

▸▸ Question 29

For transoral odontoidectomy without splitting the mandible, the patient must be able to open the mouth by more than how much?

- A. 5 mm
- B. 10 mm
- C. 15 mm
- D. 20 mm
- E. 25 mm

▸▸ Question 30

Cervicomedullary angle is the angle between a line drawn through the long axis of the medulla on a sagittal MRI and a line drawn through the cervical spinal cord. It correlates with signs of cervicomedullary compression, myelopathy, or C2 radiculopathy when it is less than how much degrees?

- A. 360
- B. 275
- C. 185
- D. 155
- E. 135

Answers

▸▸ Answer 1

Correct answer is E. All of the above[1]

▸▸ Answer 2

Correct answer is D. Ankylosing spondylitis[2]

▸▸ Answer 3

Correct answer is C. Cervical spine[3]

▸▸ Answer 4

Correct answer is A. Cervical[4]

▸▸ Answer 5

Correct answer is E. All of the above[4]

▸▸ Answer 6

Correct answer is G. All of the above[5]

▸▸ Answer 7

Correct answer is B. Posterior narrowing of disk space[6]

▸▸ Answer 8

Correct answer is E. All of the above[7]

▸▸ Answer 9

Correct answer is A. Anterior spinal artery[8]

▸▸ Answer 10

Correct answer is E. All of the above[9]

▸▸ Answer 11

Correct answer is D. VIII[1]

▸▸ Answer 12

Correct answer is A. Osteoclast activity reduction[10]

▸▸ Answer 13

Correct answer is B. Sacroiliac joint[11]

▸▸ Answer 14

Correct answer is A. Schober test[2]

▸▸ Answer 15

Correct answer is A. Cervical[4]

▸▸ Answer 16

Correct answer is C. Continuous[4]

▸▸ Answer 17

Correct answer is C. CT myelogram[12]

▸▸ Answer 18

Correct answer is D. IV[5]

▸▸ Answer 19

Correct answer is D. Osteophytes[13]

▸▸ Answer 20

Correct answer is D. Milwaukee brace[6]

▸▸ Answer 21

Correct answer is C. < 6 mm[14]

▸▸ Answer 22

Correct answer is A. Facet joints posteriorly[7]

▸▸ Answer 23

Correct answer is B. 20%[15]

▸▸ Answer 24

Correct answer is A. No need for further testing[15]

▸▸ Answer 25

Correct answer is E. 72 hours[16]

▸▸ Answer 26

Correct answer is B. II[7]

▸▸ Answer 27

Correct answer is E. 3 mm[14]

▸▸ Answer 28

Correct answer is E. 10 mm[14]

▸▸ Answer 29

Correct answer is E. 25 mm[17]

▸▸ Answer 30

Correct answer is E. 135[18]

References

[1] Greenberg M, ed. Greenberg's Handbook of Neurosurgery. 10th ed. New York: Thieme; 2023:1362
[2] Greenberg M, ed. Greenberg's Handbook of Neurosurgery. 10th ed. New York: Thieme; 2023:1367
[3] Greenberg M, ed. Greenberg's Handbook of Neurosurgery. 10th ed. New York: Thieme; 2023:1368
[4] Greenberg M, ed. Greenberg's Handbook of Neurosurgery. 10th ed. New York: Thieme; 2023:1370
[5] Greenberg M, ed. Greenberg's Handbook of Neurosurgery. 10th ed. New York: Thieme; 2023:1372
[6] Greenberg M, ed. Greenberg's Handbook of Neurosurgery. 10th ed. New York: Thieme; 2023:1375
[7] Greenberg M, ed. Greenberg's Handbook of Neurosurgery. 10th ed. New York: Thieme; 2023:1376
[8] Greenberg M, ed. Greenberg's Handbook of Neurosurgery. 10th ed. New York: Thieme; 2023:1386
[9] Greenberg M, ed. Greenberg's Handbook of Neurosurgery. 10th ed. New York: Thieme; 2023:1388
[10] Greenberg M, ed. Greenberg's Handbook of Neurosurgery. 10th ed. New York: Thieme; 2023:1364
[11] Greenberg M, ed. Greenberg's Handbook of Neurosurgery. 10th ed. New York: Thieme; 2023:1365
[12] Greenberg M, ed. Greenberg's Handbook of Neurosurgery. 10th ed. New York: Thieme; 2023:1371
[13] Greenberg M, ed. Greenberg's Handbook of Neurosurgery. 10th ed. New York: Thieme; 2023:1373
[14] Greenberg M, ed. Greenberg's Handbook of Neurosurgery. 10th ed. New York: Thieme; 2023:1378
[15] Greenberg M, ed. Greenberg's Handbook of Neurosurgery. 10th ed. New York: Thieme; 2023:1381
[16] Greenberg M, ed. Greenberg's Handbook of Neurosurgery. 10th ed. New York: Thieme; 2023:1384
[17] Greenberg M, ed. Greenberg's Handbook of Neurosurgery. 10th ed. New York: Thieme; 2023:1379
[18] Greenberg M, ed. Greenberg's Handbook of Neurosurgery. 10th ed. New York: Thieme; 2023:1380

84 Special Conditions Affecting the Spinal Cord

Questions

▸▸ Question 1

Which of the following is included in the "American/English/French Connection" classification systems of spinal AVMs?

- A. Type 1: Dural AVM (AV fistula) is the most common type of SVM (80%) in adults. This is fed by a radicular artery which forms an AV shunt at the dural root sleeve and drains into an engorged vein. It is further divided into type 1A (single arterial feeder) and type 1B with two or more arterial feeders
- B. Type 2: Also known as spinal glomus AVM it is intramedullary and constitutes 15 to 20% of all AVMs. It is fed by medullary arteries and has worse prognosis than dural AVM
- C. Type 3: Also known as juvenile spinal AVM it occupies the entire cross section of the cord and invades the vertebral body which may cause scoliosis
- D. Type 4: It is intradural perimedullary AVM which is further divided into three types
- E. All of the above

▸▸ Question 2

Which of the following is incorrect regarding Merland's subclassification of type 4 (perimedullary) AV fistulas?

- A. Subtype 1 with single arterial feeder, single AVF, and slow ascending perimedullary venous system
- B. Subtype 2 with multiple arterial supply, multiple AVF, and slow ascending perimedullary venous system
- C. Subtype 3 with multiple arterial feeders, single giant AVF, and giant venous ectasia with rapid venous drainage
- D. Subtype 4 with multiple arterial feeders, multiple AVF, and multiple fast draining veins
- E. All of the above

▸▸ Question 3

Which of the following statements is correct regarding treatment of dural AVF?

- A. Type 1 is mostly treated with surgery
- B. Type 2B is preferably treated with surgery while type 2A is more comfortably treated by neuroradiologic procedures like embolization
- C. Type 3 is treated conservatively
- D. Type 4: Subtype 1 on filum terminale can be treated surgically but on conus medullaris it is difficult to treat surgically. While embolization is difficult for subtype 4. Subtype 3 is treated with embolization
- E. All of the above

▸▸ Question 4

Following are correct regarding spinal meningeal cyst types and their treatment except?

- A. Type 1 is extradural meningeal cysts without spinal nerve root fibers which can be extradural meningeal/arachnoid cysts (type 1A) or sacral meningocele (type 1B) and it is treated by closing the ostium between the cyst and subarachnoid space
- B. Type 2 is extradural meningeal cysts with spinal nerve root fibers (Tarlov perineural cyst, spinal nerve root diverticulum) which is treated by partially resecting cyst wall and oversewing the cyst wall or excising the cyst and involved nerve root
- C. Type 3 is spinal intradural meningeal cyst (intradural arachnoid cyst) which is excised completely unless dense fibrous adhesion prevents this in which case the cyst is marsupialized
- D. Type 4 is both intradural and extradural, which is managed conservatively
- E. None of the above

▸▸ Question 5

A 40-year-old male patient presents with thoracic pain followed by lower extremity symptoms and then myelopathy. This patient also has upper extremity numbness and paresthesias. MRI of thoracic spine of this patient shows indentation or displacement of the spinal cord which is "scalpel sign." This patient has syringomyelia as well. What is the most likely diagnosis in this case?

- A. Spinal arachnoid cyst
- B. Spinal arachnoid web
- C. Spinal meningeal cyst
- D. Syringomyelia
- E. Myelomalacia

▸▸ Question 6

A patient presents with progressive neurologic deterioration over months to years with upper limbs being affected more than the lower limbs. Syringomyelia is also known as syrinx which is cystic cavitation of the spinal cord. What is the most common cause of syrinx formation?

- A. Chari type 1 malformation
- B. Post inflammatory including TB or fungal meningitides or postoperative meningitis
- C. Postoperative syringomyelia
- D. Basilar impression with constriction at the foramen magnum
- E. Spinal tumors

▸▸ Question 7

Major theories of formation of cyst include the following except?

- A. Hydrodynamic (water hammer) theory of Gardner: systolic pulsations are transmitted with each heartbeat from the intracranial cavity to the central canal

- B. William's (craniospinal dissociation) theory: maneuvers that raise CSF pressure (Valsalva, coughing) cause hydrodissection through the spinal cord tissue
- C. Heishima maneuver theory which states that obstruction in the path of CSF causes back pressure which results in formation of syrinx
- D. Heiss-Oldfield theory: occlusion at the foramen magnum causes CSF pulsations during cardiac systole to be transmitted through the Virchow-Robin spaces, which increases the extracellular fluid, which coalesces to form a syrinx

▸▸ Question 8

A patient presents with suspended (cape) dissociated sensory loss (loss of pain and temperature sensation with preserved touch and joint position sense). This patient also has pain in the cervical and occipital region and lower motor weakness of the hand and arm. This patient has low attenuation area within the cord seen on either plain CT or myelogram, and MRI shows hyperintense area within the cord. What is the most likely diagnosis in this patient?

- A. Tumor cyst
- B. Syringomyelia
- C. Central spinal canal
- D. Ventriculus terminalis
- E. None of the above

▸▸ Question 9

The central canal is present within the spinal cord at birth and normally gradually involutes with age. Persistence of the cyst is the normal variant. Which of the following are the differences between syringomyelia and central spinal canal?

- A. Central spinal canal is fusiform or linear on sagittal MRI
- B. Central spinal canal is less than or equal to 4 mm in maximal width while it is wider in case of syringomyelia
- C. Central spinal canal is singular or may be several discontinuous regions in the rostral caudal direction
- D. Central canal is perfectly round in cross section and centrally located on axial MRI
- E. There should be no contrast enhancement in case of central spinal canal if contrast is given
- F. All of the above

▸▸ Question 10

Treatment of syrinx consist of treating the underlying pathology to re-establish subarachnoid CSF flow which includes posterior decompression in case of posterior anomalies like Chiari malformation or decompression if feasible if a site of compression or blockage or tethering is identified. Syrinx shunts indications include syrinx diameter more than 3 to 4 mm with no identifiable cause or blockage that cannot be circumvented due to thick adhesions. What is the syrinx catheter option?

- A. K tube
- B. T tube
- C. M tube
- D. B tube
- E. Both A and B

▸▸ Question 11

In the "American/English/French Connection" classification for spinal vascular malformations, an AVM fed by the radicular artery, which forms an AV shunt at the dural root sleeve, and drains into an engorged spinal vein on the posterior cord is what?

- A. Dural AVM
- B. Intradural AVM
- C. Juvenile spinal AVM
- D. Spinal glomus
- E. Intramedullary

▸▸ Question 12

An intradural perimedullary AVM where there is a direct fistula between anterior spinal artery or artery of Adamkiewicz and draining veins is which subtype of intradural AVMs?

- A. I
- B. II
- C. III
- D. IV
- E. V

▸▸ Question 13

Spetzler classification of spinal AVMs has also added which lesions not included in the "American/English/French Connection" and Hôpital Bicêtre classifications?

- A. Neoplastic lesions
- B. Dorsal malformations
- C. Intramedullary lesions
- D. Extramedullary lesions
- E. Intradural fistulas

▸▸ Question 14

An acute or subacute neurologic deterioration in a patient with a spinal venous malformation (SVM) without evidence of hemorrhage is what?

- A. Coup de poignard of Michon
- B. Foix-Alajouanine syndrome
- C. Artery of Bernasconi & Cassinari
- D. Subacute subarachnoid sclerosis

▸▸ Question 15

Spinal intradural meningeal cysts are what type?

- A. I
- B. IIA
- C. IIB
- D. IIC
- E. III

▸▸ **Question 16**

The juxtafacet cyst (JFC) is most commonly present in which of the following?

- A. Cervical
- B. Cervicothoracic junction
- C. Thoracic
- D. Lumbar
- E. Sacral

▸▸ **Question 17**

What is the most common cause of secondary syringomyelia?

- A. Chiari I malformation
- B. Chiari II malformation
- C. Dandy Walker syndrome
- D. Down syndrome
- E. Rheumatoid arthritis

▸▸ **Question 18**

What is the treatment of choice for syringomyelia associated with Chiari malformation?

- A. Syringostomy
- B. Subarachnoid–subarachnoid shunt
- C. Lumboperitoneal shunt
- D. Posterior decompression
- E. Cordectomy

▸▸ **Question 19**

What is the preferred treatment for syringomyelia secondary to tuberculous meningitis?

- A. Syringostomy
- B. Subarachnoid–subarachnoid shunt
- C. Lumboperitoneal shunt
- D. Posterior decompression
- E. Cordectomy

▸▸ **Question 20**

Hirayama disease is a motor neuron disease predominantly affecting which spinal segments?

- A. c3–c5
- B. c5–c8
- C. c8–t1
- D. t1–t4
- E. t4–t6

Answers

▸▸ Answer 1

Correct answer is E. All of the above[1]

▸▸ Answer 2

Correct answer is E. All of the above[1]

▸▸ Answer 3

Correct answer is D. Type 4: Subtype 1 on filum terminale can be treated surgically but on conus medullaris it is difficult to treat surgically. While embolization is difficult for subtype 4. Subtype 3 is treated with embolization[2]

▸▸ Answer 4

Correct answer is D. Type 4 is both intradural and extradural, which is managed conservatively[3]

▸▸ Answer 5

Correct answer is B. Spinal arachnoid web[4]

▸▸ Answer 6

Correct answer is A. Chari type 1 malformation[5]

▸▸ Answer 7

Correct answer is C. Heishima maneuver theory which states that obstruction in the path of CSF causes back pressure which results in formation of syrinx[5]

▸▸ Answer 8

Correct answer is B. Syringomyelia[6]

▸▸ Answer 9

Correct answer is F. All of the above[7]

▸▸ Answer 10

Correct answer is E. Both A and B[8]

▸▸ Answer 11

Correct answer is A. Dural AVM[9]

▸▸ Answer 12

Correct answer is D. IV[9]

▸▸ Answer 13

Correct answer is A. Neoplastic lesions[10]

▸▸ Answer 14

Correct answer is B. Foix-Alajouanine syndrome[11]

▸▸ Answer 15

Correct answer is E. III[12]

▸▸ Answer 16

Correct answer is D. Lumbar[12]

▸▸ Answer 17

Correct answer is A. Chiari I malformation[13]

▸▸ Answer 18

Correct answer is D. Posterior decompression[14]

▸▸ Answer 19

Correct answer is B. Subarachnoid–subarachnoid shunt[14]

▸▸ Answer 20

Correct answer is C. c8–t1[15]

References

[1] Greenberg M, ed. Greenberg's Handbook of Neurosurgery. 10th ed. New York: Thieme; 2023:1397
[2] Greenberg M, ed. Greenberg's Handbook of Neurosurgery. 10th ed. New York: Thieme; 2023:1399
[3] Greenberg M, ed. Greenberg's Handbook of Neurosurgery. 10th ed. New York: Thieme; 2023:1401
[4] Greenberg M, ed. Greenberg's Handbook of Neurosurgery. 10th ed. New York: Thieme; 2023:1402
[5] Greenberg M, ed. Greenberg's Handbook of Neurosurgery. 10th ed. New York: Thieme; 2023:1406
[6] Greenberg M, ed. Greenberg's Handbook of Neurosurgery. 10th ed. New York: Thieme; 2023:1407
[7] Greenberg M, ed. Greenberg's Handbook of Neurosurgery. 10th ed. New York: Thieme; 2023:1408
[8] Greenberg M, ed. Greenberg's Handbook of Neurosurgery. 10th ed. New York: Thieme; 2023:1410
[9] Greenberg M, ed. Greenberg's Handbook of Neurosurgery. 10th ed. New York: Thieme; 2023:1395
[10] Greenberg M, ed. Greenberg's Handbook of Neurosurgery. 10th ed. New York: Thieme; 2023:1396
[11] Greenberg M, ed. Greenberg's Handbook of Neurosurgery. 10th ed. New York: Thieme; 2023:1398
[12] Greenberg M, ed. Greenberg's Handbook of Neurosurgery. 10th ed. New York: Thieme; 2023:1400
[13] Greenberg M, ed. Greenberg's Handbook of Neurosurgery. 10th ed. New York: Thieme; 2023:1405
[14] Greenberg M, ed. Greenberg's Handbook of Neurosurgery. 10th ed. New York: Thieme; 2023:1411
[15] Greenberg M, ed. Greenberg's Handbook of Neurosurgery. 10th ed. New York: Thieme; 2023:1403

Part XVII

Subarachnoid Hemorrhage and Aneurysms

XVII

85 Aneurysm—Introduction, Grading, and Special Conditions

Questions

▸▸ Question 1

Trauma is the most common cause of subarachnoid hemorrhage. Which of the following statements are correct regarding aneurysmal subarachnoid hemorrhage?

- A. 10 to 15% of patients die before reaching medical care
- B. Mortality is 10% within first few days of aneurysmal subarachnoid hemorrhage
- C. 30-day mortality rate was 46% in one series and in others over half the patients died within 2 weeks of their subarachnoid hemorrhage
- D. Among patients surviving the initial hemorrhage treated without surgery, rebleeding is the major cause of morbidity and mortality, the risk of which is 15 to 20% within 2 weeks. The goal of early surgery is to reduce this risk
- E. About 30% of survivors have moderate to severe disability, with rates of persistent dependence estimated between 8 and 20% in population-based studies
- F. All of the above

▸▸ Question 2

Etiologies of subarachnoid hemorrhage include trauma and spontaneous subarachnoid hemorrhage (which includes ruptured intracranial aneurysms which includes 75 to 80% of spontaneous subarachnoid hemorrhage, cerebral AVM, certain vasculitides, rarely due to tumor or cerebral artery dissection). Which of the following are the risk factors of aneurysmal subarachnoid hemorrhage?

- A. Behavioral including hypertension, cigarette smoking, alcohol abuse, sympathomimetic drugs such as cocaine or amphetamines
- B. Gender and race
- C. History of cerebral aneurysm (unruptured aneurysm, bottleneck shape of aneurysm, and increased ratio of size of aneurysm to parent vessel)
- D. Family history of aneurysms
- E. Genetic syndromes like autosomal dominant polycystic kidney disease or type 4 Ehlers Danlos syndrome
- F. All of the above

▸▸ Question 3

A patient presents with sudden onset of severe headache usually with vomiting, syncope, neck pain, and photophobia. All of the following are causes of coma in a patient with aneurysmal subarachnoid hemorrhage except?

- A. Low ICP
- B. Damage to brain tissue due to intraparenchymal hemorrhage
- C. Hydrocephalus
- D. Diffuse ischemia
- E. Seizure

▸▸ Question 4

What is the gold standard test for evaluation of cerebral aneurysms?

- A. CT angiography of brain
- B. MRA
- C. Catheter angiogram
- D. LP
- E. Plain CT of brain

▸▸ Question 5

Plain CT of brain can predict aneurysm location based on the pattern of blood in 78% of cases while other findings that can be seen on plain CT of brain include ventricular size, hematoma, and amount of blood in cisterns and fissures. What is the size of aneurysms that can be detected on CT angiography with 98% sensitivity and 100% specificity?

- A. More than 1 mm
- B. More than 2 mm
- C. More than 3 mm
- D. More than 4 mm
- E. More than 5 mm

▸▸ Question 6

Lowering the CSF pressure with an LP may possibly precipitate rebleeding by increasing the transmural pressure (the pressure across the aneurysmal wall) which is prevented using less than or equal to 20-gauge spinal needle and removing only a small amount of CSF. Which of the following are the findings that can be obtained using an LP?

- A. Opening pressure usually elevated with subarachnoid hemorrhage
- B. Nonclotting bloody fluid that does not clear with sequential collection tubes and xanthocromia which is yellow coloration of CSF supernatant due to the lysis of RBCs
- C. RBC count is usually more than 1,00,000/mm cube in subarachnoid hemorrhage
- D. Elevated protein due to blood breakdown products
- E. All of the above

▸▸ Question 7

The size of aneurysm dome, neck size of aneurysm, and dome to neck ratio can be obtained using a catheter angiogram. Narrow necks less than 5 mm are ideal for coiling. What is the dome to neck ratio that is associated with higher rate of successful coil occlusion?

- A. More than 1
- B. More than 1.5
- C. More than 2
- D. More than 2.5
- E. More than 3

▸▸ Question 8

Grades 1 and 2 of Hunt and Hess classification are operated upon as soon as the aneurysm is diagnosed while grades more than or equal to 3 are managed until the condition improves to grade 1 or 2. Exception to this include life-threatening hematoma or multiple bleeds which are operated upon regardless of any grade. Which of the following statements is correct regarding Hunt and Hess classification of SAH?

- A. Grade 1 is asymptomatic or mild headache and slight nuchal rigidity
- B. Grade 2 is cranial nerve 3 or 6 palsy with moderate-to-severe headache and nuchal rigidity
- C. Grade 3 is mild focal deficit, lethargy, or confusion
- D. Grade 4 is stupor, moderate-to-severe hemiparesis, and early decerebrate rigidity
- E. Grade 5 is deep coma, decerebrate rigidity, and moribund appearance
- F. All of the above

▸▸ Question 9

Which of the following statements is incorrect regarding WFNS SAH grading?

- A. Grade 0 is intact patient
- B. Grade 1 is GCS score 15 without any major focal deficit
- C. Grade 2 is GCS score 13–14 without any major focal deficit
- D. Grade 3 is GCS score 13–14 with major focal deficit
- E. Grade 4 is GCS score 7–12 with or without major focal deficit
- F. Grade 5 is GCS score 3–6 without major focal deficit

▸▸ Question 10

Acute hydrocephalus (HCP) after SAH can result from blood interfering with CSF flow through the sylvian aqueduct, 4th ventricle, or subarachnoid spaces and/or reabsorption at the arachnoid granulations. What is the best management option for acute hydrocephalus after SAH with poor Hunt and Hess grade?

- A. Urgent ventriculostomy
- B. Keeping the ICP in the range of 15 to 25 mmHg in case of EVD to avoid rapid pressure reduction to decrease the risk of IVC-induced aneurysmal bleeding
- C. Draining CSF slowly after performing an EVD to avoid rapid changes in transmural pressure
- D. Ventriculostomy can cause improvement in 80% of patients with acute hydrocephalus after SAH who are having poor Hunt and Hess grading (grade 4 or 5)
- E. All of the above

▸▸ Question 11

A 70-year-old male presented in the emergency with sudden-onset severe headache followed by loss of consciousness. CT of brain revealed subarachnoid hemorrhage (SAH). What is the most common cause of SAH?

- A. Trauma
- B. Hypertension
- C. Vascular malformations
- D. Telangiectasia
- E. Aneurysm

▸▸ Question 12

A 34-week pregnant woman was brought to the emergency with history of sudden severe headache and altered sensorium. What is the risk of aneurysmal SAH in pregnancy?

- A. 2-fold
- B. 4-fold
- C. 5-fold
- D. 10-fold
- E. No risk

▸▸ Question 13

A 45-year-old female presented in the emergency with sudden loss of consciousness. She has a family history of aneurysms. CT of brain showed SAH. Fundoscopy revealed ocular hemorrhages within vitreous humor. What is this condition is called?

- A. Bouchard syndrome
- B. Turcot syndrome
- C. Terson syndrome
- D. Amyloid angiopathy
- E. Gardener syndrome

▸▸ Question 14

A middle-aged female was referred for definitive treatment for aneurysmal SAH. What is the gold standard test for evaluation of cerebral aneurysms?

- A. CT with contrast
- B. Magnetic resonance arteriogram
- C. Lumbar puncture and CSF examination for xanthochromia
- D. Catheter angiogram
- E. Magnetic resonance venogram

▸▸ Question 15

A middle-aged man presented with sudden-onset headache, altered level of consciousness, and right hemiparesis. On examination, the patient was stuporous with signs of early decerebrate rigidity. What is the Hunt and Hess grade in this case?

- A. 0
- B. 1
- C. 2
- D. 3
- E. 4

▸▸ Question 16

A middle-aged female presented with sudden-onset headache followed by loss of consciousness. On examination, GCS was E1V1M2 with right, dilated, nonreactive pupil and left hemiplegia. What is the WFNS grade for this case?
- A. 1
- B. 2
- C. 3
- D. 4
- E. 5

▸▸ Question 17

Which of the following is safe in management of SAH during pregnancy?
- A. Nimodipine
- B. Mannitol
- C. Iodinated contrast for angiography
- D. Nitroprusside
- E. Phenytoin

▸▸ Question 18

When a ventriculostomy is used, it is recommended to keep ICP in what range?
- A. 7 to 9 mmHg
- B. 9 to 12 mmHg
- C. 12 to 15 mmHg
- D. 15 to 25 mmHg
- E. 25 to 28 mmHg

Answers

▸▸ Answer 1

Correct answer is F. All of the above[1]

▸▸ Answer 2

Correct answer is F. All of the above[2]

▸▸ Answer 3

Correct answer is A. Low ICP[3]

▸▸ Answer 4

Correct answer is C. Catheter angiogram[4]

▸▸ Answer 5

Correct answer is C. More than 3 mm[5]

▸▸ Answer 6

Correct answer is E. All of the above[6]

▸▸ Answer 7

Correct answer is C. More than 2[7]

▸▸ Answer 8

Correct answer is F. All of the above[7]

▸▸ Answer 9

Correct answer is F. Grade 5 is GCS score 3–6 without major focal deficit[8]

▸▸ Answer 10

Correct answer is E. All of the above[9]

▸▸ Answer 11

Correct answer is A. Trauma[10]

▸▸ Answer 12

Correct answer is E. No risk[8]

▸▸ Answer 13

Correct answer is C. Terson syndrome[3]

▸▸ Answer 14

Correct answer is D. Catheter angiogram[11]

▸▸ Answer 15

Correct answer is E. 4[7]

▸▸ Answer 16

Correct answer is E. 5[8]

▸▸ Answer 17

Correct answer is C. Iodinated contrast for angiography[8]

▸▸ Answer 18

Correct answer is D. 15 to 25 mmHg[9]

References

[1] Greenberg M, ed. Greenberg's Handbook of Neurosurgery. 10th ed. New York: Thieme; 2023:1417
[2] Greenberg M, ed. Greenberg's Handbook of Neurosurgery. 10th ed. New York: Thieme; 2023:1418

[3] Greenberg M, ed. Greenberg's Handbook of Neurosurgery. 10th ed. New York: Thieme; 2023:1419
[4] Greenberg M, ed. Greenberg's Handbook of Neurosurgery. 10th ed. New York: Thieme; 2023:1420
[5] Greenberg M, ed. Greenberg's Handbook of Neurosurgery. 10th ed. New York: Thieme; 2023:1421
[6] Greenberg M, ed. Greenberg's Handbook of Neurosurgery. 10th ed. New York: Thieme; 2023:1422
[7] Greenberg M, ed. Greenberg's Handbook of Neurosurgery. 10th ed. New York: Thieme; 2023:1424
[8] Greenberg M, ed. Greenberg's Handbook of Neurosurgery. 10th ed. New York: Thieme; 2023:1425
[9] Greenberg M, ed. Greenberg's Handbook of Neurosurgery. 10th ed. New York: Thieme; 2023:1427
[10] Greenberg M, ed. Greenberg's Handbook of Neurosurgery. 10th ed. New York: Thieme; 2023:1412
[11] Greenberg M, ed. Greenberg's Handbook of Neurosurgery. 10th ed. New York: Thieme; 2023:1423

86 Critical Care of Aneurysm Patients

Questions

▸▸ Question 1

Initial management concerns after aneurysmal SAH (aSAH) include rebleeding, hydrocephalus, delayed cerebral ischemia, hyponatremia with hypovolemia, DVT and pulmonary embolism seizures, and reduced cerebral oxygen delivery. What are the initial management steps that are needed to reduce these risks after aSAH?

- A. Administration of oral nimodipine
- B. Maintaining euvolemia and normal circulating blood volume
- C. Control of blood pressure by keeping the systolic blood pressure below 160 mmHg
- D. Optimizing cerebral blood flow and keeping normal ICP
- E. All of the above

▸▸ Question 2

Methods that may be used to augment cerebral oxygen delivery includes all of the following except?

- A. Optimizing cerebral blood flow by avoiding induced hypertension, avoiding hypotension, and maintaining euvolemia and normal ICP
- B. Elevating oxygen saturation with the goal of 100% saturation in all patients at risk of delayed cerebral ischemia
- C. Maintaining optimal hemoglobin with the goal of 8 to 10 Hgb
- D. Intra-arterial verapamil by endovascular interventionist to improve blood rheology and keep cerebral vascular resistance low
- E. Causing prophylactic hypervolemia

▸▸ Question 3

Arrythmias may occur after aneurysmal subarachnoid hemorrhage. What is the most important monitoring for this risk factor?

- A. Arterial line
- B. Airway monitoring and management with intubation
- C. Maintaining euvolemia
- D. Cardiac monitoring
- E. Intraventricular catheter

▸▸ Question 4

What are the admitting orders for a patient with aneurysmal SAH (aSAH)?

- A. Admit in ICU with VS and neuro check every 1 hour
- B. Elevating head of bed to 30 degrees with low level of external stimulation, restricted visitation, and no loud noises
- C. Nursing care including strict I's and O's monitoring, daily weights, TED stocking with pneumatic compression boots and indwelling Foley catheter if lethargic
- D. Early aggressive fluid therapy to head off cerebral salt wasting which include NS + 20 mEq KCL/L at 2 mL/kg/h (140–150 mL/h)
- E. Medication, oxygenation, and temperature regulation
- F. All of the above

▸▸ Question 5

Which of the following statements is correct regarding medication of a patient admitted in hospital after aneurysmal subarachnoid hemorrhage?

- A. Prophylactic antiseizure medications are given
- B. Analgesics are given along with dexamethasone which may help with headache and neck pain
- C. There is no role of calcium channel blockers in these patients
- D. Stool softener and antiemetics are given
- E. H2 blockers and proton pump inhibitors are given as well

▸▸ Question 6

Risk factors for hyponatremia after SAH include diabetes, CHF, cirrhosis, adrenal insufficiency, or the use of any of the drugs like NSAIDs, acetaminophen, narcotics, and thiazide diuretics. Hyponatremic patients with SAH have incidence of delayed cerebral infarction how much times as compared to normonatremic patients?

- A. Two times
- B. Three times
- C. Four times
- D. Five times
- E. Six times

▸▸ Question 7

Literature review shows that 4 to 26% of SAH patients had onset seizures, 1 to 28% had early seizures (within 2 weeks), and 1 to 35% had late seizures (after 2 weeks). Following are the risk factors for post-SAH seizure except?

- A. Increasing age (more than 65 years)
- B. MCA aneurysm or associated intracerebral or subdural hematoma
- C. Good neurologic grade
- D. Volume of subarachnoid hematoma or rebleeding
- E. Cerebral infarction or vasospasm or hyponatremia

▸▸ Question 8

About 15 to 20% of rebleed in SAH patients occur within 14 days, 50% will rebleed within 6 months; thereafter the risk is 3%/year with a mortality rate of 2%/year. The maximal frequency of rebleed is on which day after SAH (1/3 of these rebleed occur within 3 hours in that day or 1/2 within 6 hours)?

- A. 1st day
- B. 2nd day

- C. 3rd day
- D. 4th day
- E. 5th day

▸▸ Question 9

Which of the following statements is correct regarding correlation of delayed ischemic neurologic deficit (DIND) development with Hunt and Hess grade?

- A. In grade 1, there is 22% chances of DIND
- B. In grade 2, there is 33% chances of DIND
- C. In grade 3, there is 52% chances of DIND
- D. In grade 4, there is 53% chances of DIND
- E. In grade 5, there is 74% chances of DIND
- F. All of the above

▸▸ Question 10

Which of the following statements is incorrect regarding modified grading system of Fisher (correlation between the amount of blood on CT and the risk of vasospasm)?

- A. Grade 0 is no SAH or IVH
- B. Grade 1 is focal or diffuse thin SAH, no IVH with 24% symptomatic vasospasm
- C. Grade 2 is focal or diffuse thin SAH with IVH and has 33% symptomatic vasospasm
- D. Grade 3 is focal or diffuse thick SAH, with no IVH and has 33% chance of vasospasm
- E. Grade 4 is focal or diffuse thick SAH with no IVH and has 40% chance of vasospasm

▸▸ Question 11

Which of the following is not a risk factor for re-bleeding?

- A. Male gender
- B. High-grade SAH
- C. Large aneurysm
- D. SBP > 175 mmHg
- E. Lumbar spinal drainage

▸▸ Question 12

Which method should not be used to augment cerebral oxygen delivery (DO_2)?

- A. Optimizing CBF
- B. Maintaining euvolemia
- C. Nimodipine
- D. Elevate O_2 saturation
- E. Induced hypertension

▸▸ Question 13

A patient with aneurysmal SAH was referred for ICU care. How frequently should the neurological check be performed as a part of initial critical care?

- A. 1 hourly
- B. 2 hourly
- C. 4 hourly
- D. 6 hourly
- E. Twice daily

▸▸ Question 14

A patient with SAH is brought to your ICU. The family is worried about the risk of other such event. After initial hemorrhage, during which time period there is maximal risk of rebleed?

- A. Within 3 hours
- B. Within 6 hours
- C. Within 8 hours
- D. Within 12 hours
- E. Within 24 hours

▸▸ Question 15

ECG of a patient with SAH show inverted T waves, prolonged QT interval, ST elevation, and U waves. The BP of the patient is 100/90. The initial management for neurogenic stress cardiomyopathy in this case includes which of the following?

- A. Dopamine
- B. Dobutamine
- C. Norpine
- D. Milrinone
- E. Potassium

▸▸ Question 16

The management of neurogenic pulmonary edema includes furosemide supplementation along with which of the following?

- A. Alpha blockers
- B. Beta blockers
- C. Ganglion blockers
- D. Dobutamine
- E. Atracurim

▸▸ Question 17

A patient was referred for management of aneurysmal SAH. GCS was 13/15. After a few days the patient deteriorated to GCS 9/15 with left hemiparesis. The clinical vasospasm almost never occurs before which day?

- A. Day 3 post SAH
- B. Day 4 post SAH
- C. Day 5 post SAH
- D. Day 7 post SAH
- E. Day 10 post SAH

▸▸ Question 18

The family of a patient with SAH, admitted in a different hospital, brings the case summary and radiology of the patient to you to discuss referral to your setup and discuss the prognosis. You review the case summary and brain CT of the patient. What is the percentage of symptomatic vasospasm with Fisher grade 2?

- A. 12%
- B. 24%
- C. 33%
- D. 40%
- E. 44%

►► **Question 19**

A patient with SAH is admitted in your ICU. He deteriorated on the 7th postictal day. You order a fresh CT of brain and a transcranial Doppler ultrasound. For severe vasospasm, what is the Lindegaard ratio?

- A. 2
- B. 3 to 5
- C. 4
- D. < 6
- E. > 6

►► **Question 20**

An alert patient was admitted in ICU with aneurysmal SAH. On the 7th day, he developed abulia, drowsiness, confusion, and whispering. The deterioration was attributed to clinical vasospasm. The cluster of these findings is associated with which artery?

- A. Anterior cerebral artery
- B. Middle cerebral artery
- C. Posterior cerebral artery
- D. Posterior inferior cerebellar artery
- E. Anterior inferior cerebellar artery

►► **Question 21**

A patient after clipping of aneurysm is shifted under your care in ICU. How frequently would you get the renal profile as long as the patient is in ICU?

- A. Once daily
- B. Twice daily
- C. On alternate days
- D. Every 3rd day
- E. Only at time of admission to ICU

►► **Question 22**

During round, the consultant ordered to provide triple H therapy/hyperdynamic augmentation to a patient with aneurysmal SAH. What is the initial dose of dopamine to augment blood pressure?

- A. Start at 2.5 µg/kg/min and titrate to 15/20 µg/kg/min
- B. Start at 1 µg/kg/min and titrate to 10 µg/kg/min
- C. Start at 0.5 µg/kg/min and titrate to 10 µg/kg/min
- D. Start at 0.25 µg/kg/min and titrate to 5 µg/kg/min
- E. IV bolus of 10 µg/kg and then maintain at 10 µg/kg/min

Answers

►► **Answer 1**

Correct answer is E. All of the above[1]

►► **Answer 2**

Correct answer is E. Causing prophylactic hypervolemia[1]

►► **Answer 3**

Correct answer is D. Cardiac monitoring[1]

►► **Answer 4**

Correct answer is D. Early aggressive fluid therapy to head off cerebral salt wasting which include NS + 20 mEq KCL/L at 2 mL/kg/h (140–150 mL/h)[2]

►► **Answer 5**

Correct answer is C. There is no role of calcium channel blockers in these patients[3]

►► **Answer 6**

Correct answer is B. Three times[4]

►► **Answer 7**

Correct answer is C. Good neurologic grade[5]

►► **Answer 8**

Correct answer is A. 1st day[3]

►► **Answer 9**

Correct answer is F. All of the above[6]

►► **Answer 10**

Correct answer is E. Grade 4 is focal or diffuse thick SAH with no IVH and has 40% chance of vasospasm[6]

►► **Answer 11**

Correct answer is A. Male gender[7]

►► **Answer 12**

Correct answer is E. Induced hypertension[1]

►► **Answer 13**

Correct answer is A. 1 hourly[8]

►► **Answer 14**

Correct answer is E. Within 24 hours[3]

▸▸ **Answer 15**

Correct answer is D. Milrinone[9]

▸▸ **Answer 16**

Correct answer is D. Dobutamine[9]

▸▸ **Answer 17**

Correct answer is A. Day 3 post SAH[9]

▸▸ **Answer 18**

Correct answer is C. 33%[6]

▸▸ **Answer 19**

Correct answer is E. > 6[2]

▸▸ **Answer 20**

Correct answer is A. Anterior cerebral artery[10]

▸▸ **Answer 21**

Correct answer is B. Twice daily[4]

▸▸ **Answer 22**

Correct answer is A. Start at 2.5 µg/kg/min and titrate to 15/20 µg/kg/min[11]

References

[1] Greenberg M, ed. Greenberg's Handbook of Neurosurgery. 10th ed. New York: Thieme; 2023:1433
[2] Greenberg M, ed. Greenberg's Handbook of Neurosurgery. 10th ed. New York: Thieme; 2023:1444
[3] Greenberg M, ed. Greenberg's Handbook of Neurosurgery. 10th ed. New York: Thieme; 2023:1437
[4] Greenberg M, ed. Greenberg's Handbook of Neurosurgery. 10th ed. New York: Thieme; 2023:1435
[5] Greenberg M, ed. Greenberg's Handbook of Neurosurgery. 10th ed. New York: Thieme; 2023:1436
[6] Greenberg M, ed. Greenberg's Handbook of Neurosurgery. 10th ed. New York: Thieme; 2023:1441
[7] Greenberg M, ed. Greenberg's Handbook of Neurosurgery. 10th ed. New York: Thieme; 2023:1432
[8] Greenberg M, ed. Greenberg's Handbook of Neurosurgery. 10th ed. New York: Thieme; 2023:1434
[9] Greenberg M, ed. Greenberg's Handbook of Neurosurgery. 10th ed. New York: Thieme; 2023:1439
[10] Greenberg M, ed. Greenberg's Handbook of Neurosurgery. 10th ed. New York: Thieme; 2023:1440
[11] Greenberg M, ed. Greenberg's Handbook of Neurosurgery. 10th ed. New York: Thieme; 2023:1447

87 SAH from Cerebral Aneurysm Rupture

Questions

▸▸ Question 1

Aneurysms tend to arise in areas where there is a curve in the parent artery, in the angle between it and a significant branching artery, and point in the direction where the parent artery would have continued had the curve not been present. Also, there is less elastic fiber in the tunica media and adventitia of cerebral blood vessels, the media has less muscle, the adventitia is thinner, and the internal elastic lamina is more prominent. Following are the possible etiologies of aneurysms formation except?

- A. Congenital predisposition
- B. Atherosclerotic changes or hypertension
- C. Embolic
- D. Infectious which are also called as mycotic aneurysms
- E. Trauma is never a cause of aneurysm development

▸▸ Question 2

Saccular aneurysms most commonly occur in the carotid system which accounts for about 85 to 90% of aneurysms, while posterior circulation accounts for 5 to 15% of aneurysms. What is the single most common location of aneurysm (which constitutes 30% of aneurysms)?

- A. AComA
- B. pComA
- C. Middle cerebral artery
- D. Basilar artery
- E. Vertebral artery

▸▸ Question 3

Intraventricular hemorrhage occurs in 13 to 28% of cases of ruptured aneurysms in clinical series. Which of the following statements is incorrect regarding intraventricular hemorrhage and aneurysm location?

- A. Distal PICA aneurysm may rupture directly into the 4th ventricle through the foramen of Luschka
- B. AComA cause IVH by rupturing through the lamina terminalis into the anterior 3rd ventricle or lateral ventricles
- C. Distal basilar artery may rupture through the floor of the 3rd ventricle
- D. Middle cerebral artery aneurysm may rupture through the temporal horn of ventricle
- E. Carotid terminus artery aneurysm may rupture through the floor of the 3rd ventricle

▸▸ Question 4

Oculomotor 3rd nerve palsy occurs mostly in which aneurysm which can result in extraocular muscle palsy, ptosis, and dilated unreactive pupil?

- A. Basilar apex aneurysm
- B. PComA aneurysms
- C. PICA aneurysms
- D. AICA aneurysms
- E. None of the above

▸▸ Question 5

Which of the following are the endovascular techniques to treat aneurysm?

- A. Thrombosing the aneurysm using coiling with Guglielmi electrolytically detachable coils
- B. Thrombosing the aneurysm using Onyx 500 for wide neck or giant ICA aneurysms
- C. Using flow diversion with covered stents
- D. Trapping which can be done by distal and proximal arterial interruption using endovascular techniques
- E. All of the above

▸▸ Question 6

What is the surgical gold standard for aneurysm treatment?

- A. Coiling through endovascular technique
- B. Clipping the aneurysm
- C. Wrapping or coating the aneurysm using muscle or cotton or muslin
- D. Coating the aneurysm using Teflon or fibrin glue
- E. None of the above

▸▸ Question 7

Microsurgical clipping is favorable in patients with intraparenchymal hematomas, favorable dome–neck ratio, younger age, and middle cerebral artery aneurysm. Endovascular coiling may receive increased consideration in which of the following cases?

- A. Elderly patients with age more than 70 years
- B. Those with poor grade WFNS classification
- C. Those with aneurysms of basilar apex
- D. In patients with ruptured aneurysms judged to be technically amenable to both endovascular coiling and neurosurgical clipping, endovascular coiling should be considered
- E. All of the above

▸▸ Question 8

Early surgery after rupture of aneurysm is advocated because it eliminates the risk of rebleeding (which occurs mostly in period immediately post SAH), it facilitates treatment of vasospasm, and it allows lavage to remove potentially vasospasmogenic agent from contact with vessels, including use of thrombolytic agents. Which of the following are the arguments against early surgery in favor of late surgery?

- A. Inflammation and brain edema are most severe immediately post SAH which can damage brain tissue during manipulation

- B. Large clot with mass effect associated with SAH
- C. The presence of solid clot that has not had time to lyse impedes surgery
- D. The risk of intraoperative rupture is higher with early surgery
- E. Incidence of vasospasm possibly increase after early surgery from mechanotrauma to vessels

▸▸ Question 9

Which of the following are the techniques that can be adopted using surgical exposure for aneurysm surgery?

- A. Brain relaxation using hyperventilation, CSF drainage (done only after opening the dura), and diuretics
- B. Cerebral protection by increasing the ischemic tolerance of the CNS using calcium channel blockers, free radical scavengers, and mannitol
- C. Reducing cerebral rate of oxygen consumption by using barbiturates, isoflurane, and prophylactic hypothermia
- D. Using adjunctive cerebral protection techniques using systemic hypotension or focal hypotension by using temporary clips
- E. All of the above

▸▸ Question 10

Which of the following statements is correct regarding the use of temporary clips using aneurysm surgery?

- A. If a long segment of the ICA is being trapped, administer 5,000 unit IV heparin to prevent thrombosis and subsequent emboli
- B. If temporary clip is applied for less than 5 minutes, then there is no need of further intervention
- C. If temporary clip is applied for 10 to 15 minutes, then administration of IV brain protection anesthesia has been shown to significantly decrease infarction rate with intermittent reperfusion
- D. More than 20 minutes of temporary clip is not tolerated
- E. All of the above

▸▸ Question 11

Which is the single most common location of cerebral aneurysms?

- A. Acomm
- B. ACA
- C. MCA
- D. Pcomm
- E. VA-PICA junction

▸▸ Question 12

What is the incidence of spontaneous thrombosis of an aneurysm?

- A. 3 to 6%
- B. 6 to 9%
- C. 9 to 13%
- D. 15 to 18%
- E. 19 to 21%

▸▸ Question 13

A 50-year-old hypertensive patient was referred from DHQ for further management of SAH. Plain CT of brain shows blood predominantly in prepontine and peduncular cisterns and the third ventricle. This suggests aneurysm location as which of the following?

- A. Anterior communicating artery
- B. Anterior cerebral artery
- C. Posterior communicating artery
- D. Middle cerebral srtery
- E. Basilar apex

▸▸ Question 14

A middle-aged smoker presented with sudden-onset severe headache followed by seizures and loss of consciousness. Which of the following aneurysm by location is most commonly associated with seizures?

- A. Anterior communicating artery
- B. Posterior communicating artery
- C. Posterior inferior cerebellar artery
- D. Middle cerebral artery
- E. Anterior cerebral artery

▸▸ Question 15

Facial pain syndromes in the ophthalmic or maxillary nerve distribution that may mimic trigeminal neuralgia can occur with aneurysm in which of the following?

- A. Intracavernous ICA
- B. ACA
- C. AComm
- D. Anterior choroidal artery
- E. pcomm

▸▸ Question 16

Third cranial nerve palsy may be due to aneurysm as well as diabetes. What is an important clinical sign to help differentiate between the two causes?

- A. Pupil dilated in aneurysm
- B. Pupil dilated in diabetes
- C. No effect on pupillary reaction
- D. Ophthalmoplegia
- E. Monocular neuritis

▸▸ Question 17

What is the screening protocol for a patient suffering from adult polycystic kidney disease (APKD) with prior aneurysm?

- A. Plain CT of brain every 2 years
- B. CTA annually
- C. CTA every 2 to 3 years
- D. MRA every 2 to 3 years
- E. MRV every 2 to 3 years

▸▸ Question 18

Treatment options for aneurysms may include all of the following except?

- A. Coiling
- B. Clipping
- C. Wrapping
- D. Antifibrinolytic therapy (e.g., ε-aminocaproic acid [EACA])
- E. Proximal ligation

▸▸ Question 19

A patient with subarachnoid hemorrhage was referred for expert management. After initial resuscitation and basic work-up, angiography studies were performed. Which of the following factors favor endovascular coiling over surgical clipping?

- A. Size < 15 mm
- B. Neck diameter < 5 mm
- C. Dome:neck ratio > 2
- D. A, B, and C
- E. Dome:neck ratio < 1.5

▸▸ Question 20

Regarding basilar apex aneurysm, what is the generally accepted best management option?

- A. Clipping
- B. Coiling
- C. Wrap
- D. Beta blockers
- E. Venodilaters

▸▸ Question 21

Factors that favor choosing early surgery include which of the following?

- A. Good medical condition of the patient
- B. Bad neurologic condition of the patient (H&H grade ≥ 3)
- C. Large amounts of subarachnoid blood
- D. Large clot with mass effect associated with SAH
- E. Early rebleeding, especially multiple rebleeds

▸▸ Question 22

A patient underwent clipping for left ACA aneurysm. Which of the followings is true regarding aneurysmal rest?

- A. Follow-up with serial angiography
- B. Can never expand
- C. If it expands, no need to re-explore
- D. No chance of re-bleed
- E. 10% incidence of re-bleed

▸▸ Question 23

All of the following can be utilized for cerebral protection during aneurysm surgery except?

- A. Barbiturates
- B. Hypothermia to 34°C
- C. Intravenous mannitol
- D. Temporary clipping for 30 minutes
- E. Systemic hypotension

▸▸ Question 24

What is the maximum duration to safely apply a temporary clip?

- A. < 20 minutes
- B. 20 to 25 minutes
- C. 20 to 30 minutes
- D. 25 to 30 minutes
- E. 30 minutes

▸▸ Question 25

Out of the three general stages of aneurysm surgery, intraoperative rupture is most likely to occur during which stage?

- A. Stage I
- B. Stage Ia
- C. Stage II
- D. Stage III
- E. Stage IV

▸▸ Question 26

A patient came into the OPD on the 17th postoperative day of clipping of right MCA aneurysm. What advice will you give regarding the next follow-up visit if the patient remains stable?

- A. CTA at 1 month
- B. CTA at 6 months
- C. CTA at 12 months
- D. CTA at 5 years
- E. CTA at 10 years

Answers

▸▸ Answer 1

Correct answer is E. Trauma is never a cause of aneurysm development[1]

▸▸ Answer 2

Correct answer is A. AComA[1]

▸▸ Answer 3

Correct answer is D. Middle cerebral artery aneurysm may rupture through the temporal horn of ventricle[2]

▸▸ Answer 4

Correct answer is B. PComA aneurysms[3]

▸▸ Answer 5

Correct answer is E. All of the above[4]

▸▸ Answer 6

Correct answer is B. Clipping the aneurysm[5]

▸▸ Answer 7

Correct answer is E. All of the above[6]

▸▸ Answer 8

Correct answer is B. Large clot with mass effect associated with SAH[7]

▸▸ Answer 9

Correct answer is E. All of the above[8]

▸▸ Answer 10

Correct answer is E. All of the above[9]

▸▸ Answer 11

Correct answer is A. Acomm[1]

▸▸ Answer 12

Correct answer is C. 9 to 13%[5]

▸▸ Answer 13

Correct answer is E. Basilar apex[2]

▸▸ Answer 14

Correct answer is D. Middle cerebral artery[2]

▸▸ Answer 15

Correct answer is A. Intracavernous ICA[3]

▸▸ Answer 16

Correct answer is A. Pupil dilated in aneurysm[3]

▸▸ Answer 17

Correct answer is D. MRA every 2 to 3 years[4]

▸▸ Answer 18

Correct answer is D. Antifibrinolytic therapy (e.g., ε-aminocaproic acid [EACA])[4]

▸▸ Answer 19

Correct answer is D. A, B, and C[10]

▸▸ Answer 20

Correct answer is B. Coiling[6]

▸▸ Answer 21

Correct answer is B. Bad neurologic condition of the patient (H&H grade ≥ 3)[7]

▸▸ Answer 22

Correct answer is A. Follow-up with serial angiography[11]

▸▸ Answer 23

Correct answer is D. Temporary clipping for 30 minutes[12]

▸▸ Answer 24

Correct answer is A. < 20 minutes[9]

▸▸ Answer 25

Correct answer is C. Stage II[13]

▸▸ Answer 26

Correct answer is C. CTA at 12 months[14]

References

[1] Greenberg M, ed. Greenberg's Handbook of Neurosurgery. 10th ed. New York: Thieme; 2023:1453
[2] Greenberg M, ed. Greenberg's Handbook of Neurosurgery. 10th ed. New York: Thieme; 2023:1454
[3] Greenberg M, ed. Greenberg's Handbook of Neurosurgery. 10th ed. New York: Thieme; 2023:1455
[4] Greenberg M, ed. Greenberg's Handbook of Neurosurgery. 10th ed. New York: Thieme; 2023:1456
[5] Greenberg M, ed. Greenberg's Handbook of Neurosurgery. 10th ed. New York: Thieme; 2023:1457
[6] Greenberg M, ed. Greenberg's Handbook of Neurosurgery. 10th ed. New York: Thieme; 2023:1460
[7] Greenberg M, ed. Greenberg's Handbook of Neurosurgery. 10th ed. New York: Thieme; 2023:1462
[8] Greenberg M, ed. Greenberg's Handbook of Neurosurgery. 10th ed. New York: Thieme; 2023:1466
[9] Greenberg M, ed. Greenberg's Handbook of Neurosurgery. 10th ed. New York: Thieme; 2023:1465

[10] Greenberg M, ed. Greenberg's Handbook of Neurosurgery. 10th ed. New York: Thieme; 2023:1459
[11] Greenberg M, ed. Greenberg's Handbook of Neurosurgery. 10th ed. New York: Thieme; 2023:1463
[12] Greenberg M, ed. Greenberg's Handbook of Neurosurgery. 10th ed. New York: Thieme; 2023:1464
[13] Greenberg M, ed. Greenberg's Handbook of Neurosurgery. 10th ed. New York: Thieme; 2023:1467
[14] Greenberg M, ed. Greenberg's Handbook of Neurosurgery. 10th ed. New York: Thieme; 2023:1468

88 Aneurysm Type by Location

Questions

▸▸ Question 1

Following statements are correct regarding rupture of anterior communicating artery aneurysm except?

- A. It is associated with intracerebral hematoma in 63% of cases
- B. Intraventricular hematoma is seen in 79% of cases with blood entering the ventricles from the intracerebral hematoma in about one-third of these cases
- C. Acute hydrocephalus is present in 25% of cases
- D. Frontal lobe infarction never occurs after SAH from ruptured AComA
- E. These aneurysms result in blood in the interhemispheric fissure

▸▸ Question 2

Surgical approaches for AComA include pterional approach, subfrontal approach, anterior interhemispheric approach, and transcallosal approach. A right pterional craniotomy is used in all the surgical procedures for AComA except in the following case?

- A. Large AcomA aneurysm pointing to right, in this case left craniotomy, exposes neck before dome
- B. Dominant left A1 feeder to aneurysm (with no filling from right A1), left craniotomy provides proximal control in this case
- C. Additional left-sided aneurysm
- D. Left-sided hematoma causing mass effect
- E. All of the above

▸▸ Question 3

Gyrus rectus resection can be done for exposure of arteries and along with it frontal temporal orbital zygoma removal, splitting of sylvian fissure, and ventricular drainage can also be done. Which of the following are critical branches to preserve during AComA aneurysm surgery?

- A. Recurrent artery of Heubner
- B. Small anterior communicating artery perforators
- C. Frontal polar branches
- D. Anterior temporal branches
- E. Both A and B

▸▸ Question 4

Anterior of the distal anterior cerebral artery (DACA) is usually located at the origin of the frontopolar artery, or at the bifurcation of the pericallosal and callosomarginal arteries at the genu of corpus callosum. Which of the following are usually aneurysms located more distally?

- A. Post-traumatic
- B. Infectious
- C. Mycotic
- D. Tumor embolus
- E. All of the above

▸▸ Question 5

Aneurysms up to 1 cm from ACoA artery may be approached through a standard pterional craniotomy with partial gyrus rectus resection while aneurysms more than 1 cm distal to the anterior communicating artery are approached through which of the following?

- A. Subtemporal craniotomy
- B. Frontal craniotomy using bicoronal skin incision
- C. Orbitotemporal zygomatic approach
- D. Quadrangular flap over Keen's point
- E. None of the above

▸▸ Question 6

Basilar artery aneurysm constitutes only 5% of aneurysms and dome of these aneurysms usually points superiorly. Critical angiographic features to assess for basilar artery aneurysms include which of the following?

- A. Orientation of the aneurysm which is important because posteriorly pointing aneurysm obscure perforators which may be adherent to the aneurysm, making surgery more difficult
- B. Patency of PCAs and SCAs
- C. Patency and size of PComAs to determine if the P1's can be sacrificed because diameter of more than 1 mm is needed to support the collateral flow
- D. Height of the aneurysm relative to the posterior clinoid process which will affect the selection of the surgical approach
- E. All of the above

▸▸ Question 7

Basilar tip aneurysm can be approached through subtemporal or pterional approach. Which of the following statements are correct for comparing subtemporal and pterional approaches?

- A. Subtemporal approach provides less distance to the basilar tip as compared to pterional approach
- B. Subtemporal approach is better than pterional approach for aneurysms projecting posteriorly or posteroinferiorly
- C. Pterional approach needs little or no retraction of temporal lobe as compared to subtemporal approach in which temporal lobe needs to be retracted
- D. There is better visualization of both P1 segments and thalamoperforators using pterional approach as compared to subtemporal approach
- E. All of the above

▸▸ **Question 8**

The carotid artery exits the cavernous sinus and enters the subarachnoid space at the dural constrictions known as the carotid ring (also known as clinoidal ring). The supraclinoid portion of the carotid artery is divided into the following segments except?

- A. Ophthalmic segment which gives rise to ophthalmic artery
- B. Ophthalmic segment which gives superior hypophyseal artery
- C. Communicating segment from the posterior communicating artery origin to the origin of the anterior choroidal artery
- D. Chiasmal segment which gives a branch to optic chiasma
- E. Choroidal segment from the origin of anterior choroidal artery to the terminal bifurcation of the internal carotid artery

▸▸ **Question 9**

What is the correct statement regarding ophthalmic artery aneurysm?

- A. 45% present as subarachnoid hemorrhage
- B. 45% present as visual field defect
- C. Visual field defect can be ipsilateral monocular superior nasal quadrantanopsia or monocular inferior nasal quadrantanopsia or complete loss of vision in one eye with a superior temporal quadrant defect in the contralateral eye
- D. All of the above

▸▸ **Question 10**

What percentage of cerebral aneurysms consist of PICA aneurysms?

- A. 2%
- B. 3%
- C. 4%
- D. 5%
- E. 6%

▸▸ **Question 11**

A patient was found unconscious by his family and was brought to emergency department. After initial resuscitation basic workup and CT of brain were advised. CT scan shows SAH with interhemispheric subdural hematoma. Which is the most likely vessel involved?

- A. Distal anterior cerebral artery
- B. Posterior communicating artery
- C. Posterior inferior cerebellar artery
- D. Anterior inferior cerebellar artery
- E. Vertebral artery

▸▸ **Question 12**

A 46-year-old male presented to ER with severe headache, photophobia, and vomiting. CT of brain shows interhemispheric SAH with IVH. What is the chance for acute hydrocephalus in this patient?

- A. 79%
- B. 63%
- C. 25%
- D. 50%
- E. 100%

▸▸ **Question 13**

CT angiogram of a patient with interhemispheric SAH with IVH shows large anterior communicating artery aneurysm greater than 2.5 cm, pointing superiorly along with ICH. What is the preferred surgical approach in this case?

- A. Interhemispheric approach
- B. Pterional craniotomy
- C. Subfrontal
- D. Transcolossal
- E. Subtemporal

▸▸ **Question 14**

If clipping is planned, right pterional approach is usually preferred. Left pterional approach is preferred in the following except?

- A. Aneurysm pointing to left
- B. Dominant left anterior feeder
- C. Left-sided ICH
- D. Left-sided another aneurysm
- E. Left occipital horn IVH

▸▸ **Question 15**

Regarding distal anterior cerebral artery (DACA) aneurysm, which of the following statements is false?

- A. Usually located at the origin of fronto-polar artery
- B. Can be post-traumatic, infective, or due to tumor emboli
- C. Aneurysms of up to 1 cm from the ACoA may be approached through pterional craniotomy
- D. Incidence of rupture is very less
- E. Both B and C options

▸▸ **Question 16**

A 55-year-old male presented to ER with the worst headache of his life while he was on his way to his office. On examination, he was alert, awake, and oriented with left dilated on reactive pupil with restricted upward, inward, and outward gaze. CT shows aneurysm which impinges on the third cranial nerve. Which of the following is a false statement?

- A. Posterior communicating artery aneurysm occurs commonly with junction to carotid artery
- B. In the presence of fetal circulation, we can sacrifice Pcomm artery without deleterious effects
- C. Pcomm aneurysm points lateral, posterior, and inferior

- D. Surgical clipping may be more advantageous than endovascular coiling to treat oculomotor nerve palsies
- E. None of the above

▸▸ Question 17

MCA aneurysm was incidentally found on CT of brain of a 35-year-old patient. Clipping of aneurysm was planned. Which is the best statement?

- A. Superior temporal gyrus approach has a minimum brain traction and a better proximal control with decreased risk of seizures
- B. Transsylvian approach is not preferred
- C. Temporary clipping is unavoidable in case of rupture
- D. Distal MCA and recurrent perforators from the origin of the major MCA branches are critical branches to be preserved during clipping
- F. None of the above

▸▸ Question 18

Visual field defects in ophthalmic artery aneurysm is about 45% of cases. The most common patterns of field defects may include all except?

- A. Contralateral monocular superior nasal quadrantonopsia
- B. Ipsilateral monocular inferior nasal quadrantonopsia
- C. Ipsilateral blindness with contralateral junctional scotoma
- D. Ipsilateral monocular superior nasal quadrantonopsia

▸▸ Question 19

What is the most common location of posterior circulation aneurysm?

- A. Vertebral artery aneurysm
- B. Posterior inferior cerebellar artery
- C. Vertebrobasilar junction
- D. Basilar tip
- E. Posterior communicating artery aneurysm

▸▸ Question 20

In posterior circulation aneurysm, vertebral artery aneurysms are more commonly associated with which of the following?

- A. Nontraumatic is more common
- B. Dissecting aneurysm is more common
- C. May not arise with VA-PICA junction
- D. Coiling is preferred option
- E. None of the above

▸▸ Question 21

In basilar bifurcation aneurysm, height of aneurysm relative to posterior clinoid affects the selection of approach. Which is the best statement?

- A. In aneurysm greater than 5 mm, inferior approach through supraclinoid approach
- B. 5-mm aneurysm with clinoidal approach
- C. In > 5 mm aneurysm, superior approach through infraclinoidal approach
- D. Transcolossal approach for all sizes
- E. All of the above statements are correct

Answers

▸▸ Answer 1

Correct answer is D. Frontal lobe infarction never occurs after SAH from ruptured AComA[1]

▸▸ Answer 2

Correct answer is E. All of the above[2]

▸▸ Answer 3

Correct answer is E. Both A and B[3]

▸▸ Answer 4

Correct answer is E. All of the above[4]

▸▸ Answer 5

Correct answer is B. Frontal craniotomy using bicoronal skin incision[5]

▸▸ Answer 6

Correct answer is E. All of the above[6]

▸▸ Answer 7

Correct answer is E. All of the above[7]

▸▸ Answer 8

Correct answer is D. Chiasmal segment which gives a branch to optic chiasma[8]

▸▸ Answer 9

Correct answer is D. All of the above[9]

▸▸ Answer 10

Correct answer is B. 3%[10]

▸▸ Answer 11

Correct answer is A. Distal anterior cerebral artery[4]

▸▸ Answer 12

Correct answer is C. 25%[1]

▸▸ **Answer 13**

Correct answer is C. Subfrontal[2]

▸▸ **Answer 14**

Correct answer is A. Aneurysm pointing to left[2]

▸▸ **Answer 15**

Correct answer is D. Incidence of rupture is very less[4]

▸▸ **Answer 16**

Correct answer is B. In the presence of fetal circulation, we can sacrifice Pcomm artery without deleterious effects[11]

▸▸ **Answer 17**

Correct answer is D. Distal MCA and recurrent perforators from the origin of the major MCA branches are critical branches to be preserved during clipping[12]

▸▸ **Answer 18**

Correct answer is A. Contralateral monocular superior nasal quadrantonopsia[9]

▸▸ **Answer 19**

Correct answer is D. Basilar tip[13]

▸▸ **Answer 20**

Correct answer is D. Coiling is preferred option[10]

▸▸ **Answer 21**

Correct answer is B. 5-mm aneurysm with clinoidal approach[7]

References

[1] Greenberg M, ed. Greenberg's Handbook of Neurosurgery. 10th ed. New York: Thieme; 2023:1473
[2] Greenberg M, ed. Greenberg's Handbook of Neurosurgery. 10th ed. New York: Thieme; 2023:1474
[3] Greenberg M, ed. Greenberg's Handbook of Neurosurgery. 10th ed. New York: Thieme; 2023:1774
[4] Greenberg M, ed. Greenberg's Handbook of Neurosurgery. 10th ed. New York: Thieme; 2023:1475
[5] Greenberg M, ed. Greenberg's Handbook of Neurosurgery. 10th ed. New York: Thieme; 2023:1775
[6] Greenberg M, ed. Greenberg's Handbook of Neurosurgery. 10th ed. New York: Thieme; 2023:1482
[7] Greenberg M, ed. Greenberg's Handbook of Neurosurgery. 10th ed. New York: Thieme; 2023:1483
[8] Greenberg M, ed. Greenberg's Handbook of Neurosurgery. 10th ed. New York: Thieme; 2023:478
[9] Greenberg M, ed. Greenberg's Handbook of Neurosurgery. 10th ed. New York: Thieme; 2023:1478
[10] Greenberg M, ed. Greenberg's Handbook of Neurosurgery. 10th ed. New York: Thieme; 2023:1480
[11] Greenberg M, ed. Greenberg's Handbook of Neurosurgery. 10th ed. New York: Thieme; 2023:1476
[12] Greenberg M, ed. Greenberg's Handbook of Neurosurgery. 10th ed. New York: Thieme; 2023:1477
[13] Greenberg M, ed. Greenberg's Handbook of Neurosurgery. 10th ed. New York: Thieme; 2023:1479

89 Special Aneurysms and Nonaneurysmal SAH

Questions

▸▸ **Question 1**

Which of the following are the factors that have been identified as risk for rupture of unruptured aneurysms?

- A. History of previous aneurysmal subarachnoid hemorrhage from a separate aneurysm and multiple aneurysms
- B. Medical conditions like smoking, hypertension, geographic location (North America/Europe < Japan < Finland)
- C. Annual risk of rupture of aneurysms less than 10 mm is estimated to be 0.05%/year by ISUIA study
- D. Larger aneurysms (10–25 mm) are estimated to have 3 to 18%/year risk of rupture
- E. Giant aneurysms have a risk of rupture of around 8 to 50%/year
- F. All of the above statements are correct

▸▸ **Question 2**

Following are the components of PHASES aneurysm rupture risk score except?

- A. Population
- B. Hypertension
- C. Smoking
- D. Age
- E. Size
- F. Earlier rupture from another aneurysm
- G. Site of aneurysm

▸▸ **Question 3**

Following are recommended management strategies for patients with unruptured aneurysms except?

- A. Large and symptomatic aneurysms (especially in younger patients) should be dealt with intervention
- B. Patients with age below 60 years and size of aneurysm less than 7 mm should undergo conservative management if it is anterior circulation aneurysm with no risk factors while if the same size aneurysm in the same patient is found in posterior circulation/PComA with symptoms present and strong family history then intervention should be done for this patient
- C. In a patient less than 60 years of age and aneurysm size more than 7 mm, intervention should be done (surgery or endovascular based on size and location)
- D. Patients more than 60 years of age with aneurysm size less than 7 mm with no family history and no risk factors should be dealt conservatively with medicines
- E. Patients more than 60 years old with aneurysm more 7 to 12 mm in size should be dealt with conservative management if in the anterior circulation or intervention should be done if aneurysm with same size is found in posterior circulation
- F. In patients with aneurysm size more than 12 mm, intervention should never be done regardless of the age or location of aneurysm

▸▸ **Question 4**

Traumatic aneurysms may present with delayed intracranial hemorrhage, recurrent epistaxis, progressive cranial nerve palsy, enlarging skull fracture, or severe headache. What is the common location of traumatic aneurysms that arise due to closed head injury?

- A. A1 portion of anterior cerebral artery
- B. Anterior communicating artery
- C. Distal anterior cerebral artery
- D. Middle cerebral artery
- E. Basilar artery

▸▸ **Question 5**

Mycotic aneurysms are infectious aneurysms that arise due to bacterial infection. These constitute 4% of intracranial aneurysms and have most common location at distal branches of middle cerebral artery. What is the most common pathogen implicated in the pathogenesis of mycotic aneurysms?

- A. *Streptococcus*
- B. *Staphylococcus*
- C. Miscellaneous
- D. *Brucella* species
- E. All of the above

▸▸ **Question 6**

Giant aneurysms are large aneurysms with size of more than 2.5 cm. These are of two types; the first one is saccular aneurysm while the other is fusiform aneurysm. Which of the following are included in the treatment options for these aneurysms?

- A. Direct surgical clipping
- B. Vascular bypass of aneurysm with subsequent clipping
- C. Trapping of aneurysm
- D. Proximal arterial ligation (Hunterian ligation)
- E. Endovascular treatment
- F. All of the above

▸▸ **Question 7**

Aneurysm that fails to be demonstrated on initial angiogram have the following causes except?

- A. Incomplete angiography
- B. Obliteration of aneurysm by the hemorrhage
- C. Thrombosis of aneurysm after SAH
- D. Good filling of aneurysm due to vasodilatation
- E. Aneurysms too small to be visualized

▸▸ **Question 8**

Which of the following are the CT or MRI criteria for diagnosis of pretruncal nonaneurysmal subarachnoid hemorrhage?

- A. Epicenter of bleeding located immediately anterior to and in contact with the brainstem
- B. Blood limited to the prepontine, interpeduncular cisterns, supracellar, interpeduncular, suprasellar, crural, ambient, and/or quadrigeminal cistern
- C. No extension of blood into the sylvian fissure or interhemispheric fissure
- D. Intraventricular blood limited to the filling of the 4th ventricle
- E. All of the above are correct

▸▸ **Question 9**

When should repeat angiography be done in case of subarachnoid hemorrhage of unknown etiology in which there is no aneurysm found on first angiography?

- A. On the 7th day
- B. After 3 days of first angiography
- C. After 10 to 14 days of first angiography
- D. After 18 days
- E. Repeat angiography is never done in such case

▸▸ **Question 10**

When a patient presents with subarachnoid hemorrhage, then following may be the clues to find out which aneurysm has bled except?

- A. Epicenter (area of greatest concentration) of blood on CT or MRI
- B. Area of focal vasospasm has no role in determining the site of bleed
- C. Irregularities in the shape of aneurysm (so-called Murphy's teat)
- D. If no clue is being found, then the largest aneurysm is suspected to have bled
- E. None of the above

Answers

▸▸ **Answer 1**

Correct answer is F. All of the above statements are correct[1]

▸▸ **Answer 2**

Correct answer is C. Smoking[1]

▸▸ **Answer 3**

Correct answer is F. In patients with aneurysm size more than 12 mm, intervention should never be done regardless of the age or location of aneurysm[2]

▸▸ **Answer 4**

Correct answer is C. Distal anterior cerebral artery[3]

▸▸ **Answer 5**

Correct answer is Answer: A. *Streptococcus*[4]

▸▸ **Answer 6**

Correct answer is F. All of the above[5]

▸▸ **Answer 7**

Correct answer is D. Good filling of aneurysm due to vasodilatation[6]

▸▸ **Answer 8**

Correct answer is E. All of the above are correct[7]

▸▸ **Answer 9**

Correct answer is C. After 10 to 14 days of first angiography[6]

▸▸ **Answer 10**

Correct answer is B. Area of focal vasospasm has no role in determining the site of bleed[8]

References

[1] Greenberg M, ed. Greenberg's Handbook of Neurosurgery. 10th ed. New York: Thieme; 2023:1487
[2] Greenberg M, ed. Greenberg's Handbook of Neurosurgery. 10th ed. New York: Thieme; 2023:1489
[3] Greenberg M, ed. Greenberg's Handbook of Neurosurgery. 10th ed. New York: Thieme; 2023:1491
[4] Greenberg M, ed. Greenberg's Handbook of Neurosurgery. 10th ed. New York: Thieme; 2023:1493
[5] Greenberg M, ed. Greenberg's Handbook of Neurosurgery. 10th ed. New York: Thieme; 2023:1494
[6] Greenberg M, ed. Greenberg's Handbook of Neurosurgery. 10th ed. New York: Thieme; 2023:1495
[7] Greenberg M, ed. Greenberg's Handbook of Neurosurgery. 10th ed. New York: Thieme; 2023:1497
[8] Greenberg M, ed. Greenberg's Handbook of Neurosurgery. 10th ed. New York: Thieme; 2023:1490

Part XVIII

Vascular Malformations

XVIII

90 Vascular Malformations

Questions

▸▸ Question 1

Arteriovenous malformations (AVMs) are dilated arteries and veins with dysplastic vessels in which arterial blood flows directly into veins without any capillary bed and no intervening neural parenchyma. Which of the following statements are correct regarding AVM?

- A. Risk of first-time hemorrhage is 1%/year
- B. Risk of recurrent ICH is 5%/year
- C. 5-year risk of first seizure is 8% for unruptured AVM
- D. 5-year risk of epilepsy after a first seizure is 58%
- E. All of the above

▸▸ Question 2

What is the most common presentation of AVM which is about 58%?

- A. Hemorrhage
- B. Seizures
- C. Mass effect
- D. Ischemia
- E. Increased ICP

▸▸ Question 3

About 7% of patients with AVM have aneurysms. These aneurysms are classified into five types. Following statements regarding classification of these aneurysms are true except?

- A. Type 1 aneurysm is proximal on ipsilateral major artery feeding AVM
- B. Type 1A is aneurysm on proximal major artery related but contralateral to AVM
- C. Type 2 is aneurysm on distal superficial feeding artery
- D. Type 4 is aneurysm on artery related to AVM
- E. Type 3 is aneurysm on proximal or distal deep feeding artery

▸▸ Question 4

Characteristics of AVM on MRI include flow void on T1WI or T2WI within the AVM, feeding arteries, draining veins, and increased intensity on partial flip angle. What are the characteristics of AVM on angiography?

- A. Tangle of vessels
- B. Large feeding artery
- C. Large draining veins
- D. Draining veins are visualized in the same image as arteries
- E. All of the above

▸▸ Question 5

Following statements are correct regarding Spetzler Martin AVM grading system except?

- A. Size of AVM less than 3 cm, 3 to 6 cm, and more than 6 cm are given 1, 2, and 3 scores, respectively
- B. Score 1 is given if AVM is on eloquent brain area and score 0 is given if it is on noneloquent area
- C. If pattern of venous drainage is deep then score is 1 and if it is superficial then score is 0
- D. Class A (S-M grades 1 and 2) is treated without surgery
- E. Class C (S-M grades 4 and 5) is treated without surgery

▸▸ Question 6

Which of the following statements is correct regarding pros and cons of surgery and radiation treatment for AVM?

- A. Surgery eliminates the risk of bleeding almost immediately while therapeutic response of stereotactic radiosurgery takes about 1 to 3 years during which time period risk of bleeding is about the same as natural history
- B. Surgery is an invasive procedure with high cost while stereotactic radiosurgery is a noninvasive procedure which is done on outpatient basis
- C. Seizure control improves in both surgery and radiotherapy but in the latter group it is subjected to reduction or obliteration of nidus
- D. Radiosurgery is limited to lesions less than or equal to 3 cm in size with obliteration rate of 70 to 80% and delayed side effects including radiation necrosis, brain edema, and cyst formation
- E. All of the above

▸▸ Question 7

Following are the basic tenets of AVM surgery except?

- A. Exposure should be wide
- B. Feeding arteries are isolated and occluded before draining veins
- C. Excision of whole nidus is necessary to protect against rebleeding
- D. En passant vessels and adjacent arteries are identified and preserved
- E. Dissection is done directly on nidus of AVM while working in sulci and gyri whenever possible without damaging brain parenchyma
- F. In lesions that are low flow on angiography, preoperative embolization is considered

▸▸ Question 8

For resected AVMs, follow-up is done with intraoperative or early postoperative angiogram to confirm complete removal of nidus, and residual nidus if present should be re-resected. If nidus is completely removed, then repeat catheter angiogram should be done at 1 and 5 years. Following radiosurgery, MRI/MRA should be done at 6 months interval and if SRS-induced obliteration is demonstrated, then catheter angiogram should be done to confirm. What are the causes of delayed postoperative deterioration in case of AVM?

- A. Normal perfusion pressure breakthrough phenomenon, which is characterized by postoperative swelling or hemorrhage and it is thought to be due to loss of autoregulation
- B. Occlusive hyperemia: in the immediate postoperative period it is due to obstruction of normal venous outflow from the adjacent normal brain, while in a delayed presentation, it is due to delayed thrombosis of draining veins or dural sinus
- C. Rebleeding from a retained nidus of AVM
- D. Seizures
- E. All of the above

▸▸ Question 9

Dural arteriovenous fistula is a vascular abnormality in which an arteriovenous shunt is contained within the leaflets of the dura mater, exclusively supplied by branches of the internal/external carotid or vertebral arteries. It presents with pulsatile tinnitus, occipital bruit, headache, and visual impairment with papilledema. Which of the following statements is incorrect regarding Cognard angiographic classification of dural AVMs?

- A. Type 1 is normal anterograde flow into the dural venous sinus and it is benign
- B. Type 2a is drainage into a sinus with retrograde flow within the sinus, 2b is drainage into a sinus with retrograde flow into cortical veins, and type 2a + b is drainage into a sinus with retrograde flow within the sinus and cortical veins
- C. Type 3 is direct drainage into a cortical vein without venous ectasia
- D. Type 4 is direct drainage into a cortical vein with venous ectasia
- E. Type 5 is direct drainage into spinal perimedullary veins in exclusion of all of the above

▸▸ Question 10

Carotid cavernous fistula (CCF) is presented with orbital/retro-orbital pain, chemosis, pulsatile proptosis, ocular or cranial bruit, deterioration of visual acuity, diplopia, or pupillary dilatation. Which of the following is the type of CCF which is direct high flow shunts between the internal carotid artery and cavernous sinus?

- A. Type A
- B. Type B
- C. Type C
- D. Type D
- E. All of the above

Answers

▸▸ Answer 1

Correct answer is E. All of the above[1]

▸▸ Answer 2

Correct answer is A. Hemorrhage[2]

▸▸ Answer 3

Correct answer is D. Type 4 is aneurysm on artery related to AVM[3]

▸▸ Answer 4

Correct answer is E. All of the above[4]

▸▸ Answer 5

Correct answer is D. Class A (S-M grades 1 and 2) is treated without surgery[5]

▸▸ Answer 6

Correct answer is E. All of the above[6]

▸▸ Answer 7

Correct answer is F. In lesions that are low flow on angiography, preoperative embolization is considered[7]

▸▸ Answer 8

Correct answer is E. All of the above[8]

▸▸ Answer 9

Correct answer is E. Type 5 is direct drainage into spinal perimedullary veins in exclusion of all of the above[9]

▸▸ Answer 10

Correct answer is A. Type A[10]

References

[1] Greenberg M, ed. Greenberg's Handbook of Neurosurgery. 10th ed. New York: Thieme; 2023:1504

[2] Greenberg M, ed. Greenberg's Handbook of Neurosurgery. 10th ed. New York: Thieme; 2023:1505

[3] Greenberg M, ed. Greenberg's Handbook of Neurosurgery. 10th ed. New York: Thieme; 2023:1507

[4] Greenberg M, ed. Greenberg's Handbook of Neurosurgery. 10th ed. New York: Thieme; 2023:1508

[5] Greenberg M, ed. Greenberg's Handbook of Neurosurgery. 10th ed. New York: Thieme; 2023:1509

[6] Greenberg M, ed. Greenberg's Handbook of Neurosurgery. 10th ed. New York: Thieme; 2023:1510

[7] Greenberg M, ed. Greenberg's Handbook of Neurosurgery. 10th ed. New York: Thieme; 2023:1511

[8] Greenberg M, ed. Greenberg's Handbook of Neurosurgery. 10th ed. New York: Thieme; 2023:1512

[9] Greenberg M, ed. Greenberg's Handbook of Neurosurgery. 10th ed. New York: Thieme; 2023:1516

[10] Greenberg M, ed. Greenberg's Handbook of Neurosurgery. 10th ed. New York: Thieme; 2023:1519

91 Angiographically Occult Vascular Malformations

Questions

▸▸ Question 1

Angiographically occult (cryptic) vascular malformations refer to cerebrovascular malformations that are not demonstrable on technically satisfactory catheter angiography. Which of the following are the etiologies of such condition?

- A. Lesions that have hemorrhaged in which bleeding may obliterate the lesion or the clot may temporarily compress the lesion
- B. Sluggish flow of blood within abnormal vessels
- C. Small size of the abnormal vessels
- D. May require very late angiographic films (i.e., delayed films) to visualize due to late filling
- E. All of the above

▸▸ Question 2

Angiographically occult vascular malformation most commonly present with which of the following?

- A. Seizures or headache
- B. Progressive neurologic symptoms
- C. One-sided body weakness
- D. Memory deficit
- E. Urinary incontinence

▸▸ Question 3

Osler Weber Rendu syndrome, also known as hereditary hemorrhagic telangiectasia or capillary telangiectasia, is slightly enlarged capillaries with low flow. It is usually incidentally found at necropsy and has very low risk of hemorrhage (except possibly in brainstem) with intervening neural tissue. Associated cerebrovascular malformations with it include the following except?

- A. AVMs
- B. Vein of Galen malformation
- C. Venous angiomas
- D. Aneurysms
- E. Telangiectasia

▸▸ Question 4

Osler Weber Rendu syndrome may show a well-demarcated homogenous or mottled high density with some form of contrast enhancement on CT of brain. On T2WI, there is found reticulated core of increased and decreased intensity, and a prominent surrounding rim of reduced intensity may be present. What is the most suitable treatment option for this disease?

- A. Surgery is indicated for evacuation of hematoma or for recurrent hemorrhages
- B. Stereotactic radiosurgery is the most suitable option
- C. Embolization is superior to all other modalities
- D. Treatment is only with medication
- E. There is no known treatment for this disease

▸▸ Question 5

Cavernous malformation is an angiographically occult lesion with low flow vessels and no intervening neural parenchyma or arteries. What is the study of choice for this lesion (on which it appears as popcorn pattern)?

- A. CT angiography of brain
- B. MRI, especially gradient echo or SWI
- C. Catheter angiogram
- D. CT with IV contrast
- E. PET scan

▸▸ Question 6

Cavernoma or cavernous hemangioma or angioma or hemangioma is a well-circumscribed, benign vascular hamartoma consisting of irregular thick and thin-walled sinusoidal vascular channels located within the brain but lacking intervening neural parenchyma, large feeding arteries, or large draining veins. Structural characteristics of this lesion include which of the following?

- A. Comprised of dilated endothelial lined capillary vessels (caverns) with defective tight junctions
- B. No identifiable arterial feeders on angiography
- C. Often associated with a developmental venous anomaly (DVA)
- D. No functional brain tissue with the encapsulated core
- E. All of the above

▸▸ Question 7

Cavernous malformation constitutes 5 to 13% of CNS vascular malformations. What is the most common location of these lesions?

- A. Brainstem
- B. Supratentorial
- C. Basal ganglia
- D. Spinal cord
- E. Cerebellum

▸▸ Question 8

Which of the following is incorrect regarding Zabramski classification of cavernous malformations?

- A. Type 1 is subacute hemorrhage with a rim of hemosiderin-laden macrophages and gliotic brain

- B. Type 2 is loculated areas of hemorrhage and thrombus of varying age with a rim of gliotic, hemosiderin-stained brain, with large lesions that may have areas of calcifications
- C. Type 3 is chronic resolved hemorrhage with hemosiderin staining within and around the cavernous malformation
- D. Some lesions in type 4 category were found to be telangiectasia
- E. Type 5 presents with intralesional hemorrhage

▸▸ Question 9

Which of the following statements is incorrect regarding surgical management of cavernous malformations (CMs)?

- A. Surgery is not recommended for asymptomatic CMs, especially those that are deep or in eloquent areas or brainstem, or with multiple CMs
- B. Consider surgery for solitary asymptomatic CMs if easily accessible and not in eloquent brain, to prevent future hemorrhage, because of psychological burden, expensive time-consuming follow-ups, to facilitate lifestyle or career decision, or in patients who might need to be on anticoagulants
- C. Early CM resection is considered (≤ 6 weeks from hemorrhage) in patients with seizures, especially when medically refractory, if the CM is the likely cause of the seizure
- D. Consider surgery in symptomatic easily accessible CMs (surgical morbidity and mortality is equivalent to living with the CM for 1–2 years after a first bleed)
- E. Consider surgery after a symptomatic second bleed in a brainstem cavernous malformation
- F. Consider radiosurgery in solitary CMs with previous symptomatic hemorrhage if the CM is located in eloquent areas that have an unacceptably high risk with surgery
- G. All of the above are correct

▸▸ Question 10

Stereotactic localization or intraoperative ultrasound is particularly helpful in localizing the cavernous malformation. What is the goal of surgery in case of cavernous malformation?

- A. Only decompression
- B. Decompression with removal of hematoma
- C. Complete resection of the lesion
- D. Removing only symptomatic portion of the lesion
- E. None of the above

▸▸ Question 11

The reason for a vascular lesion being angiographically cryptic does not include which of the following?

- A. Lesions that have hemorrhaged
- B. The bleeding may obliterate the lesion
- C. The clot may temporarily compress the lesion
- D. Fast flow
- E. May require delayed film to visualize due to late filling

▸▸ Question 12

Multiple lesions in hereditary hemorrhagic telangiectasia are not associated with which of the following?

- A. Osler Weber Rendu syndrome
- B. Louis-Barr
- C. Myburn Mason
- D. Sturge Weber
- E. Multiple endocrine neoplasia type I

▸▸ Question 13

In hereditary hemorrhagic telangiectasia (HHT), surgery is indicated mainly for which of the following?

- A. Unruptured lesion
- B. Diagnosis
- C. Thalamic location
- D. 1st hemorrhage
- E. Well-controlled seizures

▸▸ Question 14

A patient is admitted with seizures and ICH. What is the typical MRI radiologic sign for cavernoma?

- A. Popcorn
- B. Spokes of wheel
- C. Sunburst
- D. Sunset
- E. Caput medusae

▸▸ Question 15

Which of the following is a risk factor for formation of cavernous malformation?

- A. Trauma
- B. Radiotherapy
- C. Diabetes
- D. Smoking
- E. Ehlers Danlos disease

▸▸ Question 16

When is a hemorrhage considered to have occurred in cavernous malformation?

- A. Only lesion growth without signal change
- B. Presence of hemosiderin without signs of a recent hemorrhage
- C. The appearance of blood-degradation products without lesion growth
- D. Edema with blood degradation products
- E. Blood products without clinical symptoms

▸▸ Question 17

According to Zabramski classification of cavernous malformations loculated areas of hemorrhage and thrombus of varying age with a rim of gliotic, hemosiderin-stained brain with calcifications had an annual hemorrhage rate of how much?

- A. 8.9%
- B. 12.3%

- C. 17.6%
- D. 20.1%
- E. 23.7%

▸▸ Question 18

Early cavernous malformation (CM) resection (≤6 weeks from hemorrhage) should be considered in patients with which of the following?

- A. Seizures, especially when medically refractory, if the CM is the likely cause of the seizure
- B. Asymptomatic CMs
- C. Deep CM
- D. Brainstem CM
- E. Multiple CMs

Answers

▸▸ Answer 1

Correct answer is E. All of the above[1]

▸▸ Answer 2

Correct answer is A. Seizures or headache[1]

▸▸ Answer 3

Correct answer is B. Vein of Galen malformation[1]

▸▸ Answer 4

Correct answer is A. Surgery is indicated for evacuation of hematoma or for recurrent hemorrhages[2]

▸▸ Answer 5

Correct answer is B. MRI, especially gradient echo or SWI[2]

▸▸ Answer 6

Correct answer is E. All of the above[3]

▸▸ Answer 7

Correct answer is B. Supratentorial[3]

▸▸ Answer 8

Correct answer is E. Type 5 presents with intralesional hemorrhage[4]

▸▸ Answer 9

Correct answer is G. All of the above are correct[5]

▸▸ Answer 10

Correct answer is C. Complete resection of the lesion[6]

▸▸ Answer 11

Correct answer is D. Fast flow[1]

▸▸ Answer 12

Correct answer is E. Multiple endocrine neoplasia type I[1]

▸▸ Answer 13

Correct answer is B. Diagnosis[2]

▸▸ Answer 14

Correct answer is A. Popcorn[7]

▸▸ Answer 15

Correct answer is B. Radiotherapy[3]

▸▸ Answer 16

Correct answer is D. Edema with blood degradation products[8]

▸▸ Answer 17

Correct answer is D. 20.1%[4]

▸▸ Answer 18

Correct answer is A. Seizures, especially when medically refractory, if the CM is the likely cause of the seizure[5]

References

[1] Greenberg M, ed. Greenberg's Handbook of Neurosurgery. 10th ed. New York: Thieme; 2023:1524
[2] Greenberg M, ed. Greenberg's Handbook of Neurosurgery. 10th ed. New York: Thieme; 2023:1525
[3] Greenberg M, ed. Greenberg's Handbook of Neurosurgery. 10th ed. New York: Thieme; 2023:1526
[4] Greenberg M, ed. Greenberg's Handbook of Neurosurgery. 10th ed. New York: Thieme; 2023:1528
[5] Greenberg M, ed. Greenberg's Handbook of Neurosurgery. 10th ed. New York: Thieme; 2023:1530
[6] Greenberg M, ed. Greenberg's Handbook of Neurosurgery. 10th ed. New York: Thieme; 2023:1532
[7] Greenberg M, ed. Greenberg's Handbook of Neurosurgery. 10th ed. New York: Thieme; 2023:1529
[8] Greenberg M, ed. Greenberg's Handbook of Neurosurgery. 10th ed. New York: Thieme; 2023:1527

Part XIX

Stroke and Occlusive Cerebrovascular Disease

XIX

92 Stroke—General Information and Physiology

Questions

▸▸ Question 1

Following statements are correct except?

- A. Transient ischemic attack (TIA) is transient neuronal dysfunction secondary to focal ischemia of brain, spinal cord, or retina without (permanent) acute infarction (10–15% of patients with TIA have stroke within 3 months)
- B. Stroke is permanent (irreversible) death of neurons caused by hyperperfusion of a region of the brain or brainstem
- C. Watershed infarct is ischemic infarction in a territory located at the periphery of two bordering arterial distributions due to a disturbance in flow in one or both of the arteries
- D. Normal cerebral blood flow is 45 to 60 mL/100-g tissue/min
- E. Normal cerebral metabolic rate of oxygen consumption averages about 3.0 to 3.8 mL/100-g tissue/min

▸▸ Question 2

The effects of ICA stenosis/occlusion may be ameliorated by collateral blood flow. Potential alternate routes for blood to reach brain tissue include the following except?

- A. Flow through circle of Willis from contralateral ICA through anterior communicating artery and from forward flow through the ipsilateral posterior communicating artery
- B. Retrograde flow through ophthalmic artery parasitizing blood from both ECAs via facial artery, maxillary artery, transverse facial artery, and superficial temporal artery
- C. Proximal maxillary artery
- D. Cortical–cortical anastomoses
- E. Dural–dural anastomosis

▸▸ Question 3

A patient presents with expressive aphasia + mild hemiparesis (upper extremity more than lower extremity, proximal muscle weaker than distal) in neurosurgical emergency. What is the most likely blood vessel involved in this case?

- A. Anterior choroidal artery
- B. Recurrent medial striate artery (of Heubner)
- C. Posterior cerebral artery
- D. Anterior cerebral artery
- E. Anterior inferior cerebral artery

▸▸ Question 4

A patient presents with vertigo, nausea and vomiting, diplopia, oscillopsia, hiccups with ipsilateral facial pain, paresthesias, impaired sensation, ataxia of limbs, Horner syndrome dysphagia, and hoarseness of voice. This patient is diagnosed with lateral medullary syndrome (also known as Wallenberg's syndrome). What is the most likely artery occluded in this syndrome?

- A. AICA
- B. Posterior cerebral artery
- C. Anterior cerebral artery
- D. Posterior inferior cerebral artery
- E. Anterior choroidal artery

▸▸ Question 5

Small infarcts in deep noncortical cerebrum or brainstem result from occlusion of penetrating branches of cerebral arteries. Size of infarcts ranges from 3 to 20 mm. Which of the following is the typical location for lacunar infarcts?

- A. Putamen and caudate
- B. Thalamus
- C. Pons and internal capsule
- D. Convolutional white matter
- E. All of the above

▸▸ Question 6

Trauma is the most common cause of stroke in young adults making 22% of total stroke causes in young adults. What is the second most common cause of stroke in young adults (comprising about 20% of stroke cases)?

- A. Atherosclerosis
- B. Embolisms with source from cardiac origin or fat embolism syndrome or paradoxical embolism
- C. Vasculopathy or coagulopathy
- D. Peripartum
- E. Both A and B

▸▸ Question 7

Carotid artery lesions are considered symptomatic if there are one or more lateralizing ischemic episodes appropriate to the distribution of the lesion. What is the acceptable initial screening test for carotid artery stenosis?

- A. Catheter angiogram
- B. Doppler
- C. CTA
- D. MRA
- E. All of the above except A

▸▸ Question 8

What are the medical management options for carotid artery stenosis?

- A. Antiplatelet therapy including aspirin, P2Y12 receptor blockers, combination of dipyridamole and ASA
- B. Antihypertensive therapy
- C. Good control of diabetes

- D. Antilipid therapy
- E. Patients with asymptomatic atrial fibrillation should be treated with anticoagulation
- F. Intervention to help patients to quit smoking
- G. All of the above

▸▸ Question 9

Which of the following statements is incorrect regarding practice guidelines of asymptomatic carotid stenosis?

- A. Carotid endarterectomy is reasonable in asymptomatic patients with more than 70% stenosis if risk of perioperative stroke, MI, and death is low
- B. Prophylactic carotid artery stenting may be considered in highly selected patients with asymptomatic ICA stenosis (more than 60% by angiography, more than 70% by validated Doppler ultrasound)
- C. In patients with age more than 80 years, the effectiveness of revascularization over medical therapy alone is not well recognized
- D. It is reasonable to choose carotid artery stenting over carotid endarterectomy when revascularization is not indicated in patients with anatomy favorable for surgery
- E. None of the above

▸▸ Question 10

What is the gold standard test for carotid artery stenosis?

- A. Catheter angiogram
- B. Doppler ultrasound
- C. CT angiography brain
- D. Magnetic resonance imaging
- E. All of the above

▸▸ Question 11

What is the cerebral blood flow (mL/100-g tissue/min) for normal brain at rest?

- A. 15 to 30
- B. 30 to 45
- C. 45 to 60
- D. 55 to 80
- E. > 70

▸▸ Question 12

What is the typical EEG change for ischemic brain?

- A. Flat line
- B. Tall alpha waves
- C. Increased amplitude
- D. Frequency > 50 Hz
- E. Bizarre pattern

▸▸ Question 13

Marie-Fox syndrome/lateral pontine syndrome is associated with the occlusion of which of the following?

- A. Posterior inferior cerebellar artery
- B. Anterior inferior cerebellar artery
- C. Anterior choroidal artery
- D. Superior cerebellar artery
- E. Inferior petrosal vein

▸▸ Question 14

Lacunar infarct most commonly involves which of the following locations?

- A. Putamen
- B. Thalamus
- C. Pons
- D. Internal capsule
- E. Convulational white matter

▸▸ Question 15

Pure motor hemiparesis sparing face indicates a lacune in which of the following?

- A. Medullary pyramid
- B. Posteroventral thalamus
- C. Lower basis pontis
- D. Posterior limb of internal capsule
- E. Mesencephalothalamus

▸▸ Question 16

What is the most common cause of ischemic stroke?

- A. Trauma
- B. Embolism with a recognized source
- C. Atherosclerosis
- D. Fat embolism
- E. Hypercoagulable states

▸▸ Question 17

What is the most frequently associated risk factor for ischemic stroke?

- A. Diabetes mellitus
- B. Hypertension
- C. Smoking
- D. Chronic alcoholism
- E. Obesity

▸▸ Question 18

What is the gold standard test for internal carotid artery stenosis?

- A. CT angiography
- B. Catheter angiogram
- C. 2D TOF MRI
- D. B mode duplex ultrasound
- E. MRA

▸▸ Question 19

What is the loading dose of clopidogrel for internal carotid artery stenosis?

- A. 75 mg
- B. 150 mg
- C. 225 mg
- D. 500 mg
- E. 1500 mg

▸▸ Question 20

According to ECST measurements for internal carotid artery stenosis, what is the degree of stenosis for which surgery does not have any clear benefit for symptomatic patients?

- A. 65
- B. 70
- C. 75
- D. 91
- E. 95

Answers

▸▸ Answer 1

Correct answer is B. Stroke is permanent (irreversible) death of neurons caused by hyperperfusion of a region of the brain or brainstem[1]

▸▸ Answer 2

Correct answer is E. Dural–dural anastomosis[2]

▸▸ Answer 3

Correct answer is B. Recurrent medial striate artery (of Heubner)[3]

▸▸ Answer 4

Correct answer is D. Posterior inferior cerebral artery[3]

▸▸ Answer 5

Correct answer is E. All of the above[4]

▸▸ Answer 6

Correct answer is E. Both A and B[5]

▸▸ Answer 7

Correct answer is E. All of the above except A[6]

▸▸ Answer 8

Correct answer is G. All of the above[6]

▸▸ Answer 9

Correct answer is D. It is reasonable to choose carotid artery stenting over carotid endarterectomy when revascularization is not indicated in patients with anatomy favorable for surgery[7]

▸▸ Answer 10

Correct answer is A. Catheter angiogram[8]

▸▸ Answer 11

Correct answer is C. 45 to 60[9]

▸▸ Answer 12

Correct answer is A. Flat line[9]

▸▸ Answer 13

Correct answer is B. Anterior inferior cerebellar artery[3]

▸▸ Answer 14

Correct answer is A. Putamen[4]

▸▸ Answer 15

Correct answer is A. Medullary pyramid[10]

▸▸ Answer 16

Correct answer is A. Trauma[10]

▸▸ Answer 17

Correct answer is A. Diabetes mellitus[11]

▸▸ Answer 18

Correct answer is B. Catheter angiogram[11]

▸▸ Answer 19

Correct answer is C. 225 mg[7]

▸▸ Answer 20

Correct answer is A. 65[12]

References

[1] Greenberg M, ed. Greenberg's Handbook of Neurosurgery. 10th ed. New York: Thieme; 2023:1537
[2] Greenberg M, ed. Greenberg's Handbook of Neurosurgery. 10th ed. New York: Thieme; 2023:1538

[3] Greenberg M, ed. Greenberg's Handbook of Neurosurgery. 10th ed. New York: Thieme; 2023:1539
[4] Greenberg M, ed. Greenberg's Handbook of Neurosurgery. 10th ed. New York: Thieme; 2023:1540
[5] Greenberg M, ed. Greenberg's Handbook of Neurosurgery. 10th ed. New York: Thieme; 2023:1542
[6] Greenberg M, ed. Greenberg's Handbook of Neurosurgery. 10th ed. New York: Thieme; 2023:1547
[7] Greenberg M, ed. Greenberg's Handbook of Neurosurgery. 10th ed. New York: Thieme; 2023:1548
[8] Greenberg M, ed. Greenberg's Handbook of Neurosurgery. 10th ed. New York: Thieme; 2023:1546
[9] Greenberg M, ed. Greenberg's Handbook of Neurosurgery. 10th ed. New York: Thieme; 2023:1536
[10] Greenberg M, ed. Greenberg's Handbook of Neurosurgery. 10th ed. New York: Thieme; 2023:1541
[11] Greenberg M, ed. Greenberg's Handbook of Neurosurgery. 10th ed. New York: Thieme; 2023:1543
[12] Greenberg M, ed. Greenberg's Handbook of Neurosurgery. 10th ed. New York: Thieme; 2023:1545

93 Evaluation and Treatment for Acute Ischemic Stroke

Questions

▸▸ Question 1

In case of acute stroke, treatment benefits are time dependent. Initial evaluation steps include history/physical examination, noncontrast brain CT, blood glucose level, and CTA in some cases. What is the optimal time of administration of tissue plasminogen activator alteplase in a patient with acute ischemic stroke?

- A. Within 3.5 hours
- B. Within 4 hours
- C. Within 4.5 hours
- D. Within 5 hours
- E. Within 6 hours

▸▸ Question 2

Following are included in the NIH stroke scale except?

- A. Level of consciousness, level of consciousness questions, and level of consciousness commands
- B. Best gaze and visual
- C. Facial palsy, motor arm, motor leg, limb ataxia, and sensory
- D. Ophthalmoplegia and dysphagia
- E. Best language and dysarthria
- F. Extinction and inattention and distal motor function

▸▸ Question 3

Which of the following statements is incorrect regarding treatment of hypertension in a patient with acute ischemic stroke?

- A. If diastolic blood pressure is more than 140 mmHg, then 20 to 30% reduction is desirable with cardene infusion or IV labetalol is the agent of choice
- B. Systolic blood pressure more than 230 or diastolic blood pressure 120 to 140 for 20 minutes is treated with 10 mg slow IV infusion over 2 minutes of labetalol. The dosage of labetalol is doubled every 10 minutes (20, 40, 80, then 160 mg IV slow until controlled or total of 300 mg is given)
- C. Maintenance is effective dose of labetalol every 6 to 8 hours for SBP more than 180 or DBP more than 110
- D. SBP 180 to 230 or DBP more than 105 to 120 is treated with oral labetalol
- E. If labetalol is contraindicated, nicardipine is never used

▸▸ Question 4

What are the indications of emergency surgery in case of acute stroke?

- A. Herniation from subdural hematoma
- B. Suboccipital craniectomy for progressive neurologic deterioration due to brainstem compression from cerebellar hemorrhage or infarction
- C. Decompressive craniectomy for malignant MCA territory stroke
- D. Carotid endarterectomy for high-grade carotid stenosis ipsilateral to fluctuating neuro deficit
- E. All of the above

▸▸ Question 5

Which of the following are the early signs of infarction within 6 hours (hyperacute) of onset of ischemic stroke?

- A. Hyperdense artery sign
- B. Focal low attenuation within the gray matter and loss of the gray–white interface
- C. Attenuation of the lentiform nucleus or mass effect with effacement of cerebral sulci or with midline shift
- D. Lost of the insular ribbon sign which is hypodensity involving the insular cortex, susceptible to ischemia due to poor collaterals
- E. Infarction with IV contrast which occurs in only 33% of cases
- F. All of the above

▸▸ Question 6

Most strokes can be identified as low density after 24 hours. When does stroke approaches that of CSF density?

- A. At 1 to 2 weeks
- B. At 3 weeks
- C. At 6 weeks
- D. At 3 months
- E. None of the above

▸▸ Question 7

Preoperative management of carotid endarterectomy includes acetylsalicylic acid 325 mg TID for at least 2 days or preferably for 5 days. Postoperative management after the procedure includes ICU monitoring with BP at 110 to 115 mmHg and avoidance of antiplatelet therapy for 24 to 48 hours postoperatively. Which of the following are the postoperative complications that can occur after the procedure?

- A. Disruption of arteriotomy closure
- B. Stroke
- C. Postoperative TIAs and seizures
- D. Cerebral hypoperfusion syndrome
- E. Cranial nerve injury

▸▸ Question 8

Indications of carotid endarterectomy includes stroke in evolution, crescendo TIAs, or following intra-arterial thrombolysis. Emergent carotid endarterectomy (CEA) is indicated for residual critical carotid stenosis. Which of the following are the possible techniques for management of thrombus?

- A. Spontaneous extrusion is attempted using back pressure
- B. If A fails then removal using smoothened suction catheter is attempted
- C. If B fails then balloon embolectomy catheter is used by passing it as far as base of the skull
- D. Intraoperative angiogram is obtained unless thrombus emerges and backflow is excellent
- E. Plicate ICA (avoid creating a blind pouch at origin) if there is good backflow or if satisfactory angiography cannot be obtained
- F. All of the above

▸▸ Question 9

What is the most sensitive test to detect ischemic stroke within 24 hours of occurrence?

- A. MRI with contrast
- B. CT with contrast
- C. DWI MRI
- D. CT angiography of brain
- E. CT perfusion

▸▸ Question 10

Contraindications for administration of tissue plasminogen activator includes intracerebral hemorrhage, patients with history of more than 10 cerebral microbleeds, clinical presentation of SAH, active internal bleeding, known intracranial aneurysm, or SVM, known bleeding diathesis, serious head trauma, and systolic blood pressure more than 185 mmHg or diastolic blood pressure more than 110 mmHg. Which of the following are included in the eligibility criteria in the administration of tissue plasminogen activator?

- A. Age above 18 years
- B. Time since last seen normal less than or equal to 4.5 hours prior to administration
- C. AIS in adults with known sickle disease
- D. tPA is reasonable in otherwise eligible patients with history of less than or equal to 10 cerebral microbleeds on MRI
- E. All of the above

Answers

▸▸ Answer 1

Correct answer is C. Within 4.5 hours[1]

▸▸ Answer 2

Correct answer is D. Ophthalmoplegia and dysphagia[2]

▸▸ Answer 3

Correct answer is E. If labetalol is contraindicated, nicardipine is never used[3]

▸▸ Answer 4

Correct answer is E. All of the above[4]

▸▸ Answer 5

Correct answer is F. All of the above[4]

▸▸ Answer 6

Correct answer is B. At 3 weeks[4]

▸▸ Answer 7

Correct answer is D. Cerebral hypoperfusion syndrome[5]

▸▸ Answer 8

Correct answer is F. All of the above[6]

▸▸ Answer 9

Correct answer is C. DWI MRI[7]

▸▸ Answer 10

Correct answer is E. All of the above[8]

References

[1] Greenberg M, ed. Greenberg's Handbook of Neurosurgery. 10th ed. New York: Thieme; 2023:1553
[2] Greenberg M, ed. Greenberg's Handbook of Neurosurgery. 10th ed. New York: Thieme; 2023:1556
[3] Greenberg M, ed. Greenberg's Handbook of Neurosurgery. 10th ed. New York: Thieme; 2023:1558
[4] Greenberg M, ed. Greenberg's Handbook of Neurosurgery. 10th ed. New York: Thieme; 2023:1559
[5] Greenberg M, ed. Greenberg's Handbook of Neurosurgery. 10th ed. New York: Thieme; 2023:1568
[6] Greenberg M, ed. Greenberg's Handbook of Neurosurgery. 10th ed. New York: Thieme; 2023:1571
[7] Greenberg M, ed. Greenberg's Handbook of Neurosurgery. 10th ed. New York: Thieme; 2023:1560
[8] Greenberg M, ed. Greenberg's Handbook of Neurosurgery. 10th ed. New York: Thieme; 2023:1563

94 Cerebral Arterial Dissections and Moyamoya Disease

Questions

▸▸ Question 1

Following statements are correct except?

- A. Cerebral arterial dissection can be spontaneous, post-traumatic, or iatrogenic
- B. Dissection means extravasation of blood between the intima and media, creating luminal narrowing or occlusion
- C. Dissecting aneurysm is dissection of blood between the media and adventitia or at the media causing aneurysmal dilatation which may rupture into the subarachnoid space
- D. Pseudoaneurysm is rupture of artery with subsequent encapsulation of the extravascular hematoma, and may or may not produce luminal narrowing
- E. Cerebral arterial dissection may present with TIA or Horner syndrome but never present with pain

▸▸ Question 2

The lesion common to all dissections is hemorrhage outside of the vascular lumen due to pathological transintimal extravasation of blood from the true lumen into the vessel wall. What is the most common site of spontaneous intracranial dissection?

- A. Basilar artery
- B. Vertebral artery
- C. Internal carotid artery
- D. Middle cerebral artery
- E. Anterior cerebral artery

▸▸ Question 3

Cerebral arterial dissection may cause symptoms by embolization secondary to platelet aggregation, dislodged thrombus causing reduced distal flow, or subarachnoid hemorrhage. The most common presentation in patients with age less than 30 years is due to dissection of which artery?

- A. Vertebral artery
- B. Basilar artery
- C. Internal carotid artery
- D. Posterior cerebral artery
- E. Anterior cerebral artery

▸▸ Question 4

What is the definitive diagnostic study for cerebral arterial dissection?

- A. CT of brain with IV contrast
- B. CT angiogram of brain
- C. Catheter angiography of brain
- D. MRI of brain with IV contrast
- E. Plain CT of brain

▸▸ Question 5

What is the most common clinical feature of spontaneous internal carotid artery dissection?

- A. Focal cerebral ischemia
- B. Headache
- C. Oculosympathetic palsy
- D. Bruit
- E. Amaurosis fugax

▸▸ Question 6

Traumatic dissections of vertebral artery tend to occur where it crosses bony prominences, for example, at the c1–c2 junction or where it enters the foramen transversarium usually at c6. Whereas spontaneous VA dissections are associated with fibromuscular dysplasia, migraine, and oral contraceptive pills. What is the prominent early finding in spontaneous extradural dissection of VA?

- A. TIAs or stroke
- B. Cerebellar infarction
- C. Neck pain over posterior cervical region or over occiput
- D. Lateral medullary syndrome
- E. Dysphagia

▸▸ Question 7

Moyamoya disease looks like "puff of cigarette smoke" due to secondary formation of an anastomotic collateral capillary network at the base of the brain. Progressive spontaneous occlusion of which arteries lead to this disease?

- A. Vertebral arteries
- B. Basilar arteries
- C. Both internal carotid arteries
- D. Posterior inferior cerebral arteries
- E. None of the above

▸▸ Question 8

Intracranial aneurysms are frequently associated with moyamoya disease. It may be as a result of increased flow through dilated collaterals or it may be that patients with moyamoya may also have a congenital defect in the arterial wall that predisposes them to aneurysms. What are the types of aneurysms that are associated with moyamoya disease?

- A. Aneurysms at the circle of Willis
- B. Aneurysms in the peripheral portion of cerebral arteries, for example, posterior/anterior choroidal or Heubner's artery
- C. Within moyamoya vessels
- D. All of the above

▸▸ Question 9

What is the most common presentation of moyamoya disease?

- A. Ischemic infarcts/TIAs
- B. Hemorrhage
- C. Aneurysms
- D. Ischemic infarcts/TIAs in children and hemorrhage in adults
- E. None of the above

▸▸ Question 10

Medical treatment for moyamoya disease includes antiplatelet drugs, anticoagulation, or vasodilators while surgical option includes revascularization. Cerebral angiography is necessary to delineate the degree of stenosis as well as to evaluate potential extracranial donor vessels for revascularization. Which of the following is the angiographic finding in the moyamoya disease (Suzuki stages)?

- A. Stage 1 is stenosis of suprasellar ICA, usually bilateral
- B. Stage 2 is development of moyamoya vessels at the base of brain. ACA, MCA, and PCA are dilated
- C. Stage 3 is increasing ICA stenosis and prominence of moyamoya vessels (most cases diagnosed at this stage). Maximal basal moyamoya
- D. Stage 4 is entire circle of Willis and PCAs occluded, extracranial collaterals start to appear, and moyamoya vessels begin to diminish
- E. Stage 5 is further progression of stage 4 with intensification of ECA collaterals and reduction of moyamoya-associated vessels
- F. Stage 6 is occlusion of ICA and major cerebral arteries and complete absence of moyamoya vessels
- G. All of the above

▸▸ Question 11

Which of the following is the most common vessel involved in cerebral arterial dissection?

- A. Basilar artery
- B. Vertebral artery
- C. Internal carotid artery
- D. External carotid artery
- E. Common carotid artery

▸▸ Question 12

The angiographic radiologic signs for cerebral arterial dissection include all of the following except?

- A. String and pearl
- B. Wavy ripple
- C. Sunburst
- D. String of beads
- E. Double lumen

▸▸ Question 13

Which of the following is the most common site of pain in spontaneous ICA dissections?

- A. Orbital or periorbital
- B. Auricular or mastoid
- C. Frontal
- D. Temporal
- E. Over carotid artery

▸▸ Question 14

For vertebral artery dissection, oral anticoagulation should be continued for how long?

- A. 24 hours
- B. 21 days
- C. 1 month
- D. 6 months
- E. 1 year

▸▸ Question 15

Which of the following is the most common initial symptom of spontaneous internal carotid artery dissection?

- A. Unilateral headache
- B. Seizures
- C. Altered level of conscious
- D. Facial palsy
- E. Proptosis

▸▸ Question 16

In a patient with dissection involving dominant vertebral artery, who does not tolerate occlusion what is the best alternative?

- A. Clipping proximal to PICA origin
- B. Trapping the aneurysm between clips
- C. Clipping VA distal to PICA take off
- D. Huntarian ligation
- E. Side-to-side PICA–PICA anastomosis

▸▸ Question 17

Which of the following is a likely etiology of primary moyamoya disease?

- A. Graves' disease
- B. Elevated basic fibroblast growth factor
- C. History of cerebral inflammatory disease
- D. Previous head trauma
- E. Radiation therapy for skull base glioma in children

▸▸ **Question 18**

What is the radiologic sign on CT angiogram for moyamoya disease?
- A. Tangled ball
- B. Puff of smoke
- C. Chimney
- D. Coconut
- E. Sunburst

▸▸ **Question 19**

CT angiogram shows bilateral stenosis of suprasellar ICA. What is the angiographic stage of moyamoya disease in this case?
- A. 1
- B. 2
- C. 3
- D. 4
- E. 5

▸▸ **Question 20**

Which of the angiographic stages of moyamoya disease should be considered for revascularization?
- A. 1–2
- B. 2–4
- C. 5
- D. 4–6
- E. All of the stages

▸▸ **Question 21**

How long after an acute ischemic attack should revascularization procedure be attempted for moyamoya disease?
- A. > 2 weeks after the most recent attack
- B. > 4 weeks
- C. > 6 weeks
- D. > 2 months
- E. > 6 months

▸▸ **Question 22**

Which of the following procedures has the highest potential to revascularize ischemic tissue in moyamoya disease?
- A. Encephalomyosynangiosis
- B. Encephaloduroateriosynangiosis
- C. Omental transposition
- D. Frontal burr holes
- E. Ribbon EDAS

Answers

▸▸ **Answer 1**

Correct answer is E. Cerebral arterial dissection may present with TIA or Horner syndrome but never present with pain[1]

▸▸ **Answer 2**

Correct answer is B. Vertebral artery[2]

▸▸ **Answer 3**

Correct answer is C. Internal carotid artery[2]

▸▸ **Answer 4**

Correct answer is C. Catheter angiography of brain[3]

▸▸ **Answer 5**

Correct answer is A. Focal cerebral ischemia[4]

▸▸ **Answer 6**

Correct answer is C. Neck pain over posterior cervical region or over occiput[5]

▸▸ **Answer 7**

Correct answer is C. Both internal carotid arteries[6]

▸▸ **Answer 8**

Correct answer is D. All of the above[7]

▸▸ **Answer 9**

Correct answer is D. Ischemic infarcts/TIAs in children and hemorrhage in adults[7]

▸▸ **Answer 10**

Correct answer is G. All of the above[8]

▸▸ **Answer 11**

Correct answer is B. Vertebral artery[2]

▸▸ **Answer 12**

Correct answer is C. Sunburst[3]

▸▸ **Answer 13**

Correct answer is A. Orbital or periorbital[3]

▸▸ **Answer 14**

Correct answer is D. 6 months[5]

▸▸ **Answer 15**

Correct answer is A. Unilateral headache[3]

▸▸ **Answer 16**

Correct answer is E. Side-to-side PICA–PICA anastomosis[5]

▸▸ Answer 17

Correct answer is B. Elevated basic fibroblast growth factor[6]

▸▸ Answer 18

Correct answer is B. Puff of smoke[8]

▸▸ Answer 19

Correct answer is A. 1[8]

▸▸ Answer 20

Correct answer is B. 2–4[9]

▸▸ Answer 21

Correct answer is D. > 2 months[9]

▸▸ Answer 22

Correct answer is C. Omental transposition[9]

References

[1] Greenberg M, ed. Greenberg's Handbook of Neurosurgery. 10th ed. New York: Thieme; 2023:1576
[2] Greenberg M, ed. Greenberg's Handbook of Neurosurgery. 10th ed. New York: Thieme; 2023:1577
[3] Greenberg M, ed. Greenberg's Handbook of Neurosurgery. 10th ed. New York: Thieme; 2023:1578
[4] Greenberg M, ed. Greenberg's Handbook of Neurosurgery. 10th ed. New York: Thieme; 2023:1579
[5] Greenberg M, ed. Greenberg's Handbook of Neurosurgery. 10th ed. New York: Thieme; 2023:1580
[6] Greenberg M, ed. Greenberg's Handbook of Neurosurgery. 10th ed. New York: Thieme; 2023:1581
[7] Greenberg M, ed. Greenberg's Handbook of Neurosurgery. 10th ed. New York: Thieme; 2023:1582
[8] Greenberg M, ed. Greenberg's Handbook of Neurosurgery. 10th ed. New York: Thieme; 2023:1583
[9] Greenberg M, ed. Greenberg's Handbook of Neurosurgery. 10th ed. New York: Thieme; 2023:1584

95 Other Vascular Occlusive Conditions

Questions

▸▸ Question 1

What are the patterns of stroke with total internal carotid artery occlusion?

- A. Whole hemispheric stroke
- B. Watershed infarct
- C. Carotid stump syndrome in which there are continued cerebral or retinal symptoms due to inadequacy of collaterals or due to emboli formed in the turbulent flow
- D. Whole brain ischemic symptoms
- E. All of them except D

▸▸ Question 2

Intra-arterial thrombolysis within 6 hours of onset of symptoms may increase recanalization rate and clinical improvement without significant increase in hemorrhagic transformation as compared to intravenous thrombolytic therapy. Surgical options for these cases include carotid endarterectomy. Which patient is the candidate for surgical intervention in case of total internal carotid artery occlusion?

- A. Patients with acute neuro deficit associated with total occlusion presenting after about 2 hours
- B. Patients with extremely poor neuro deficit
- C. Patients with acute neuro deficit associated with total occlusion of internal carotid artery within 2 hours of symptoms onset
- D. Patients without persistent neuro deficit with total ICA occlusion
- E. Both C and D

▸▸ Question 3

A patient presents with symptoms of dizziness, vertigo, nausea, vomiting, loss of balance, and headache. This patient also has signs of truncal and appendicular ataxia, nystagmus, and dysarthria. This patient's scan showed compression and obliteration of basal cisterns and 4th ventricle, hydrocephalus, and tight posterior fossa. In 1 hour, this patient develops deep coma and is found to have cerebellar infarct. What is the management option at this stage of the patient?

- A. Conservative and counselling of the attendants
- B. Surgical decompression with brain frontal lobectomy
- C. Suboccipital craniectomy
- D. Suboccipital craniectomy with enlargement of foramen magnum
- E. Only supportive therapy with ventilatory support

▸▸ Question 4

A patient presents with severe drowsiness, dense hemiplegia, early parenchymal hypodensity involving more than 50% of the MCA distribution on brain CT, midline shift of more than 8 to 10 mm, and hyperdense artery sign in MCA. What are the options of management in case of malignant middle cerebral artery infarction (which carries mortality of up to 80%)?

- A. Conventional measures to control ICP
- B. A + Hemicraniectomy
- C. Agents to lyse clot
- D. Hyperventilation, mannitol, or barbiturate coma
- E. Both C and D

▸▸ Question 5

Guidelines for hemicraniectomy in a patient with malignant MCA infarct include age less than 70 years, more strongly considered in nondominant hemisphere, and CT or clinical evidence of acute complete ICA or MCA infarcts with direct signs of impending or complete severe hemispheric brain swelling. When should hemicraniectomy be performed to decrease the mortality and increase functional outcome?

- A. Within 24 hours
- B. Within 48 hours
- C. Within 6 hours
- D. Within 12 hours
- E. Within 72 hours

▸▸ Question 6

Causes of cardiogenic brain embolism include acute myocardial infarction, atrial fibrillation, prosthetic heart valves, paradoxical embolism, or endocarditis. Which of the following are the components of CHADS2 scoring system for risk of stroke with atrial fibrillation?

- A. CHF
- B. HTN
- C. Smoking
- D. Age more than 75 years
- E. Diabetes mellitus

▸▸ Question 7

Following are the management steps for cardiogenic brain ischemic stroke except?

- A. CT should be obtained within 48 hours
- B. Anticoagulation should be used for large infarcts
- C. Heparin and warfarin are started simultaneously
- D. An INR of 2 to 3 appears satisfactory
- E. ASA is only about half as effective as warfarin but may be sufficient for those without associated risk factors

▸▸ Question 8

Criteria for clinical diagnosis of vertebral basilar insufficiency include any two of the following: motor or sensory symptoms or both occurring bilaterally in the same event, diplopia which is due to upper brainstem involvement, dysarthria which is due to lower brainstem involvement, or homonymous hemianopia which is due to ischemia of occipital cortex. What are the surgical treatment options for this condition?

- A. Vertebral endarterectomy
- B. Transposition of VA to ICA
- C. Bypass grafting
- D. C1 and C2 posterior arthrodesis in case of os odontoideum
- E. All of the above

▸▸ Question 9

The most frequently involved sinus in cerebral venous thrombosis is superior sagittal sinus or left transverse sinus. Following are the signs on noncontrast that can help diagnose case of cerebral venous thrombosis except?

- A. Hyperdense sign or cortical vein of high density or clots in cortical veins
- B. Hemorrhage
- C. Small ventricles
- D. Venous infarct and white matter edema never occur with it
- E. Triangular shaped high density within the sinus posteriorly near the torcular herophili on axial CT images

▸▸ Question 10

For EC/ICA bypass graft, the type of graft depends on preoperative determination of amount of flow augmentation necessary, the size of recipient graft, and availability of donor vessel. What type of graft is used for high flow vessel with 70 to 140 mL/min flow rate?

- A. Superficial temporal artery
- B. Saphenous vein graft
- C. Radial artery graft
- D. Occipital artery
- E. All of the above

▸▸ Question 11

What is the overall rate of subsequent ischemic stroke ipsilateral to the occluded carotid artery?

- A. 2.9% per year
- B. 3.9% per year
- C. 4.9% per year
- D. 5.9% per year
- E. 6.9% per year

▸▸ Question 12

The emergency operations for acute neurological deficit associated with total occlusion of ICA should not be performed after how long?

- A. 2 hours
- B. 3 hours
- C. 4 hours
- D. 6 hours
- E. 12 hours

▸▸ Question 13

In case of cerebellar infarction, surgical decompression should not be attempted in presence of which of the following symptoms?

- A. Abducens (VI) nerve palsy, loss of ipsilateral gaze (compression of VI nucleus and lateral gaze center)
- B. Peripheral facial nerve paresis (compression of facial colliculus), confusion, and somnolence (may be partly due to developing hydrocephalus)
- C. Babinski sign, hemiparesis, lethargy
- D. Small but reactive pupils coma posturing → flaccidity, ataxic respirations
- E. Dysphagia, dysarthria, Horner syndrome, ipsilateral facial numbness, crossed sensory loss

▸▸ Question 14

For malignant MCA infarct, mortality is reduced if hemicraniectomy is performed within what time?

- A. 48 hours
- B. 96 hours
- C. 3 days
- D. 5 days
- E. 7 days

▸▸ Question 15

Paradoxical cardiogenic embolism can occur with which of the following?

- A. Left ventricular hypertrophy
- B. Patent foramen ovale
- C. Subacute bacterial endocarditis
- D. Moyamoya disease
- E. Prosthetic heart valves

▸▸ Question 16

Which of the following is not a component of CHAD2 scoring system?

- A. Congestive cardiac failure
- B. Hypertension
- C. Age
- D. Diabetes
- E. Hypercholesterolemia

▸▸ Question 17

Criteria for clinical diagnosis of vertebrobasilar insufficiency include all of the following except?

- A. Diplopia
- B. Dysarthria

- C. Homonymous hemianopsia
- D. Repetitive speech
- E. Motor symptoms

▸▸ Question 18

Which of the following investigations is diagnostic but potentially dangerous in bow hunter stroke?
- A. CTA
- B. CTV
- C. MRV
- D. Dynamic cerebral angiography
- E. Digital subtraction angiography

▸▸ Question 19

Which of the following is the most commonly involved sinus in cerebral venous thrombosis?
- A. Straight sinus
- B. Superior sagittal sinus
- C. Inferior sagittal sinus
- D. Occipital sinus
- E. Cavernous sinus

▸▸ Question 20

In dural sinus thrombosis, postcontrast CT shows which radiologic sign near torcular herophili?
- A. Sunburst
- B. Popcorn
- C. String
- D. Delta
- E. C shaped

▸▸ Question 21

The type of graft used for EC/IC bypass depends on preoperative determination of amount of flow augmentation necessary, the size of the recipient graft, and the availability of donor vessel. What is the rate of flow through the radial artery graft?
- A. 15 to 25 mL/min
- B. 25 to 40 mL/min
- C. 40 to 70 mL/min
- D. 60 to 120 mL/min
- E. 70 to 140 mL/min

Answers

▸▸ Answer 1

Correct answer is E. All of them except D[1]

▸▸ Answer 2

Correct answer is E. Both C and D[2]

▸▸ Answer 3

Correct answer is D. Suboccipital craniectomy with enlargement of foramen magnum[3]

▸▸ Answer 4

Correct answer is B. A + Hemicraniectomy[3]

▸▸ Answer 5

Correct answer is B. Within 48 hours[3]

▸▸ Answer 6

Correct answer is C. Smoking[4]

▸▸ Answer 7

Correct answer is B. Anticoagulation should be used for large infarcts[5]

▸▸ Answer 8

Correct answer is E. All of the above[6]

▸▸ Answer 9

Correct answer is D. Venous infarct and white matter edema never occur with it[7]

▸▸ Answer 10

Correct answer is B. Saphenous vein graft[8]

▸▸ Answer 11

Correct answer is D. 5.9% per year[1]

▸▸ Answer 12

Correct answer is A. 2 hours[1]

▸▸ Answer 13

Correct answer is E. Dysphagia, dysarthria, Horner syndrome, ipsilateral facial numbness, crossed sensory loss[3]

▸▸ Answer 14

Correct answer is A. 48 hours[3]

▸▸ Answer 15

Correct answer is B. Patent foramen ovale[4]

▸▸ Answer 16

Correct answer is E. Hypercholesterolemia[4]

►► **Answer 17**

Correct answer is D. Repetitive speech[5]

►► **Answer 18**

Correct answer is D. Dynamic cerebral angiography[9]

►► **Answer 19**

Correct answer is B. Superior sagittal sinus[10]

►► **Answer 20**

Correct answer is D. Delta[11]

►► **Answer 21**

Correct answer is C. 40 to 70 mL/min[8]

References

[1] Greenberg M, ed. Greenberg's Handbook of Neurosurgery. 10th ed. New York: Thieme; 2023:1587

[2] Greenberg M, ed. Greenberg's Handbook of Neurosurgery. 10th ed. New York: Thieme; 2023:1588

[3] Greenberg M, ed. Greenberg's Handbook of Neurosurgery. 10th ed. New York: Thieme; 2023:1589

[4] Greenberg M, ed. Greenberg's Handbook of Neurosurgery. 10th ed. New York: Thieme; 2023:1590

[5] Greenberg M, ed. Greenberg's Handbook of Neurosurgery. 10th ed. New York: Thieme; 2023:1591

[6] Greenberg M, ed. Greenberg's Handbook of Neurosurgery. 10th ed. New York: Thieme; 2023:1592

[7] Greenberg M, ed. Greenberg's Handbook of Neurosurgery. 10th ed. New York: Thieme; 2023:1596

[8] Greenberg M, ed. Greenberg's Handbook of Neurosurgery. 10th ed. New York: Thieme; 2023:1602

[9] Greenberg M, ed. Greenberg's Handbook of Neurosurgery. 10th ed. New York: Thieme; 2023:1593

[10] Greenberg M, ed. Greenberg's Handbook of Neurosurgery. 10th ed. New York: Thieme; 2023:1595

[11] Greenberg M, ed. Greenberg's Handbook of Neurosurgery. 10th ed. New York: Thieme; 2023:1597

96 Intracerebral Hemorrhage in Older Adults

Questions

▸▸ Question 1

Which of the following are the risk factors of spontaneous intracerebral hemorrhage in adults?

- A. Age: the incidence increases after 55 years of age and doubles with each decade of age until the age of more than 80 years when incidence is 25 times that during previous decade
- B. Gender: more common men
- C. Previous stroke
- D. Alcohol consumption
- E. Cigarette smoking and street drugs
- F. Liver dysfunction
- G. All of the above

▸▸ Question 2

Common arterial feeders of ICH include lenticulostriates, thalamoperforators, and paramedian branches of basilar artery. What is the most common site of spontaneous ICH which constitutes about 50%?

- A. Striate boyd (basal ganglia) in which putamen is the most common
- B. Thalamus
- C. Pons
- D. Cerebellum
- E. Cerebral white matter

▸▸ Question 3

Lobar hemorrhages are more common in people with high alcohol consumption, and it can involve frontal, parietal, occipital, or temporal lobe. Following are the etiologies of lobar hemorrhage except?

- A. Extension of deep hemorrhage
- B. Amyloid angiopathy
- C. Hemorrhagic tumor
- D. Hemorrhagic transformation of ischemia can never cause it
- E. AVM
- F. Aneurysm

▸▸ Question 4

What is the factor that constitutes up to two-thirds of the cerebellar hemorrhages?

- A. Hypertension
- B. AVM
- C. Aneurysm
- D. Smoking
- E. Diabetes mellitus

▸▸ Question 5

Cerebral amyloid angiopathy (CAA) is pathologic deposition of beta amyloid protein within the media of small meningeal and cortical vessels without evidence of systemic amyloidosis. Definite diagnosis of CAA can be made only on full postmortem. Which of the following is probably CAA with supporting pathological evidence for CAA?

- A. Lobar, cortical, or corticosubcortical hemorrhage
- B. Some degree of vascular amyloid deposition in biopsy specimen
- C. Absence of another diagnostic lesion
- D. All of the above

▸▸ Question 6

Malignant tumors most commonly involving ICH include the following except?

- A. Glioblastoma
- B. Lymphoma
- C. Medulloblastomas and gliomas
- D. Renal cell carcinoma and bronchogenic carcinoma
- E. Metastatic tumors like melanoma or choriocarcinoma

▸▸ Question 7

Delayed deterioration after the initial hemorrhage is usually due to any combination of the following?

- A. Rebleeding
- B. Edema
- C. Hydrocephalus
- D. Seizures
- E. Increased ICP
- F. All of the above

▸▸ Question 8

Following statements are correct regarding variation of brain MRI signal characteristics of intraparenchymal blood over time except?

- A. Hyperacute blood is within first 6 hours; it consists of oxy-Hgb and appears isointense on T1 and hyperintense on T2 MRI
- B. Acute is from 6 to 72 hours, which consists of deoxy-Hgb which appears isointense on T1 and hypointense on T2
- C. Early subacute which is from 3 to 7 days; it consists of met-Hgb (intracellular) which is hyperintense on T1 and hypointense on T2 MRI
- D. Late subacute is from 7 to 14 days which consist of met-Hgb (extracellular) which is hyperintense on both T1 and T2 images
- E. Chronic which is more than 14 days and consists of hemosiderin. It appears hyperintense on both T1 and T2 MRI images

▸▸ Question 9

ICH scores of 0, 1, 2, 3, 4, 5, and 6 correlate with 30-day mortality of 0, 13, 26, 72, 97, 100, and 100%, respectively. Which of the following are the components of ICH score?

- A. GCS (with score 2 for GCS 3–4, score 1 for GCS 5–12, score 0 for GCS 13–15)
- B. Age (with age above 80 years comprising score 1 while below 80 years it is 0)
- C. Location (1 for infratentorial and 0 for supratentorial)
- D. ICH volume (1 for > 30 mL while 0 for < 30 mL)
- E. Intraventricular blood (1 for presence and 0 for absence)
- F. All of the above

▸▸ Question 10

Indications for ventriculostomy after ICH include which of the following?

- A. Acute hydrocephalus and management of ICP
- B. For evacuation of ICH in brain parenchyma
- C. For low GCS patients
- D. In patients who are not surgical candidates with large ICH
- E. In patients who cannot tolerate surgery

▸▸ Question 11

What is the most common site for spontaneous ICH?

- A. Basal ganglia
- B. Thalamus
- C. Pons
- D. Cerebellum
- E. Brainstem

▸▸ Question 12

What is the source of putaminal hemorrhage in spontaneous ICH?

- A. Lenticulostriate
- B. Thalamoperforators
- C. Basilar artery
- D. Vertebral artery
- E. Extension from cortical ICH

▸▸ Question 13

Hemorrhagic transformation of an ischemic stroke where the hemorrhage is extending beyond the margins of the ischemia is categorized as which type?

- A. Type I
- B. Type II
- C. Type III
- D. Type IV
- E. Complex

▸▸ Question 14

The diagnosis of cerebral amyloid angiopathy is best confirmed with which of the following?

- A. Postmortem histopathology
- B. Catheter angiogram
- C. CTA
- D. MRA
- E. MRV

▸▸ Question 15

Which of the following metastatic tumors is not associated with ICH?

- A. Melanoma
- B. Bronchogenic carcinoma
- C. Renal cell carcinoma
- D. Choricarcinoma
- E. Prostate carcinoma

▸▸ Question 16

A patient presented with hemisensory loss following an ICH. What is the most likely location of the ICH?

- A. Thalamus
- B. Basal ganglia
- C. Brainstem
- D. Cerebellum
- E. Putaminal

▸▸ Question 17

In case of lobar hemorrhage, contralateral hemiparesis along with hemisensory deficit is associated with which of the following?

- A. Cerebellar
- B. Frontal
- C. Temporal
- D. Parietal
- E. Occipital

▸▸ Question 18

After ICH, what is the incidence of rebleed within first 3 hours?

- A. 15%
- B. 33%
- C. 45%
- D. 54%
- E. 100%

▸▸ Question 19

After ICH, the size of clot decreases at what rate per day?

- A. 0.25 mm
- B. 0.75 mm
- C. 1 mm
- D. 1.25 mm
- E. 10 mm

▸▸ **Question 20**

A 95-year-old patient presented with severe headache followed by seizures and loss of consciousness. The GCS was 7/15. Plain CT of brain revealed a 50-mL ICH in the left parietal region with intraventricular extension. What is the ICH score in this case?

- A. 2
- B. 3
- C. 4
- D. 5
- E. 6

▸▸ **Question 21**

In an ICH that is hyperintense on T1 and hypointense on T2 MRI, what is the phase of the ICH?

- A. Hyperacute
- B. Acute
- C. Early subacute
- D. Late subacute
- E. Chronic

▸▸ **Question 22**

How long should oral anticoagulant (OAC) use be avoided after OAC-associated ICH inpatients without mechanical heart valves to decrease the risk of recurrent ICH?

- A. For at least 1 week
- B. For at least 2 weeks
- C. For at least 3 weeks
- D. For at least 4 weeks
- E. For at least 5 weeks

Answers

▸▸ **Answer 1**

Correct answer is G. All of the above[1]

▸▸ **Answer 2**

Correct answer is A. Striate boyd (basal ganglia) in which putamen is the most common[1]

▸▸ **Answer 3**

Correct answer is D. Hemorrhagic transformation of ischemia can never cause it[2]

▸▸ **Answer 4**

Correct answer is D. Smoking[3]

▸▸ **Answer 5**

Correct answer is D. All of the above[4]

▸▸ **Answer 6**

Correct answer is C. Medulloblastomas and gliomas[4]

▸▸ **Answer 7**

Correct answer is F. All of the above[5]

▸▸ **Answer 8**

Correct answer is E. Chronic which is more than 14 days and consists of hemosiderin. It appears hyperintense on both T1 and T2 MRI images[6]

▸▸ **Answer 9**

Correct answer is F. All of the above[7]

▸▸ **Answer 10**

Correct answer is A. Acute hydrocephalus and management of ICP[8]

▸▸ **Answer 11**

Correct answer is A. Basal ganglia[1]

▸▸ **Answer 12**

Correct answer is A. Lenticulostriate[1]

▸▸ **Answer 13**

Correct answer is B. Type II[9]

▸▸ **Answer 14**

Correct answer is A. Postmortem histopathology[3]

▸▸ **Answer 15**

Correct answer is E. Prostate carcinoma[3]

▸▸ **Answer 16**

Correct answer is A. Thalamus[5]

▸▸ **Answer 17**

Correct answer is D. Parietal[2]

▸▸ **Answer 18**

Correct answer is B. 33%[5]

▸▸ **Answer 19**

Correct answer is B. 0.75 mm[10]

▸▸ **Answer 20**

Correct answer is C. 4[6]

▸▸ **Answer 21**

Correct answer is C. Early subacute[6]

▸▸ **Answer 22**

Correct answer is D. For at least 4 weeks[11]

References

[1] Greenberg M, ed. Greenberg's Handbook of Neurosurgery. 10th ed. New York: Thieme; 2023:1609
[2] Greenberg M, ed. Greenberg's Handbook of Neurosurgery. 10th ed. New York: Thieme; 2023:1610
[3] Greenberg M, ed. Greenberg's Handbook of Neurosurgery. 10th ed. New York: Thieme; 2023:1612
[4] Greenberg M, ed. Greenberg's Handbook of Neurosurgery. 10th ed. New York: Thieme; 2023:1613
[5] Greenberg M, ed. Greenberg's Handbook of Neurosurgery. 10th ed. New York: Thieme; 2023:1615
[6] Greenberg M, ed. Greenberg's Handbook of Neurosurgery. 10th ed. New York: Thieme; 2023:1618
[7] Greenberg M, ed. Greenberg's Handbook of Neurosurgery. 10th ed. New York: Thieme; 2023:1619
[8] Greenberg M, ed. Greenberg's Handbook of Neurosurgery. 10th ed. New York: Thieme; 2023:1623
[9] Greenberg M, ed. Greenberg's Handbook of Neurosurgery. 10th ed. New York: Thieme; 2023: 1610
[10] Greenberg M, ed. Greenberg's Handbook of Neurosurgery. 10th ed. New York: Thieme; 2023:1616
[11] Greenberg M, ed. Greenberg's Handbook of Neurosurgery. 10th ed. New York: Thieme; 2023:1622

97 ICH in Young Adults and Pediatrics

Questions

▸▸Question 1

What is the most common cause of spontaneous ICH in young adults?
- A. Ruptured AVM
- B. Arterial hypertension
- C. Ruptured saccular aneurysm
- D. Sympathomimetic drug abuse
- E. Tumor

▸▸ Question 2

Intracerebral hemorrhage of the newborn occurs primarily in the premature infants. Alternate terms for this include subependymal hemorrhage, germinal matrix hemorrhage, and periventricular intraventricular hemorrhage. Intraventricular hemorrhage arises from extension of subependymal hemorrhage through ependymal lining of ventricles and occurs in how many cases of subependymal hemorrhage?
- A. 50%
- B. 60%
- C. 70%
- D. 80%
- E. 90%

▸▸ Question 3

The metabolically active germinal matrix is susceptible to hypotension and hypoperfusion which can lead to infarction. The germinal matrix is a valuable watershed zone which is supplied by which artery?
- A. Heubner's artery from anterior cerebral artery
- B. Terminal branches of the lateral striate arteries from the middle cerebral artery
- C. Anterior choroidal artery from the internal carotid or middle cerebral artery
- D. All of the above

▸▸ Question 4

What is the pathogenesis of periventricular intraventricular hemorrhage in the preterm infant?
- A. Postnatal hypoxia due to respiratory distress syndrome related to hyaline membrane disease, pneumothorax, or anemia can deprive the metabolically active germinal matrix of oxygen. This ischemia makes them vulnerable to infarction and rupture
- B. Hypercapnia maximally dilates the thin-walled vessels of the germinal matrix. If this is followed by sudden increase in perfusion this can lead to rupture of vessels
- C. Increased venous pressure from any cause like labor or positive pressure ventilation can lead to hemorrhage in germinal matrix
- D. In dehydration followed by rapid resuscitation with hyperosmolar solutions with associated increase in systemic blood pressure, the germinal matrix is at risk of hemorrhage
- E. All of the above

▸▸ Question 5

Which of the following are risk factors for periventricular intraventricular hemorrhage in premature infants?
- A. Those associated primarily with increased CBF or CPP
- B. Younger gestational age and low birth weight
- C. Acute amnionitis and failure to give antenatal steroids
- D. APGARs score less than 4 at 2 minutes and less than 8 at 5 minutes
- E. Use of recreational drugs by the mother or maternal aspirin use
- F. Smoking by the mother
- G. Acidosis and coagulopathies

▸▸ Question 6

Which of the following are the grades of subependymal hemorrhage?
- A. Grade 1 is subependymal hemorrhage
- B. Grade 2 is IVH without ventricular dilatation
- C. Grade 3 is IVH with ventricular dilatation
- D. Grade 4 is IVH with parenchymal hemorrhage
- E. All of the above

▸▸ Question 7

What can be the steps for prevention of periventricular intraventricular hemorrhage?
- A. Good prenatal care and avoiding preterm delivery with antenatal steroids
- B. Indomethacin and antenatal vitamin K given IM more than 4 hours prior to delivery
- C. Sluicing umbilical cord and delaying umbilical cord clamping by 30 to 120 seconds in premature infants increased hematocrit and decreased PIVH in 5 of 7 studies
- D. Using surfactant
- E. All of the above

▸▸ Question 8

Following are the pathophysiologic effects of periventricular intraventricular hemorrhage (PIVH) except?
- A. Destruction of germinal matrix and direct injury to neural tissue from hematoma
- B. Reduction of CBF in the whole brain due to elevated ICP
- C. Decreased CPP leads to periventricular leukomalacia and cerebral infarction
- D. Injury to brain stem
- E. Periventricular hemorrhagic infarction, hydrocephalus, and seizures

▸▸ **Question 9**

What is the indication of surgical intervention in a patient with periventricular intraventricular hemorrhage (PIVH)?
- A. Progressive ventriculomegaly
- B. Periventricular hemorrhage
- C. Progressive ventriculomegaly with the OFC crossing percentile curves and clinical evidence of increased ICP
- D. Progressive ventriculomegaly with OFC crossing percentile curves without clinical evidence of increased ICP
- E. None of the above

▸▸ **Question 10**

What are the indications and requirements of insertion of VP shunt or conversion of sub Q reservoir to VP shunt?
- A. Symptomatic hydrocephalus or progressive ventriculomegaly
- B. Infant is extubated (and thus off ventilator)
- C. Infant weight more than or equal to 2,000 g
- D. CSF protein ideally less than 100 mg/dL
- E. No evidence of NEC
- F. All of the above

▸▸ **Question 11**

What is the most common cause of spontaneous ICH in young adults?
- A. Ruptured AVM
- B. Arterial hypertension
- C. Ruptured saccular aneurysm
- D. Sympathomimetic drug abuse
- E. Tumor

▸▸ **Question 12**

What is the site of hemorrhage at > 29-week gestational age?
- A. Head of caudate nucleus
- B. Lentiform nucleus
- C. Intraventricular
- D. Cerebellar vermis
- E. Lobar

▸▸ **Question 13**

Risk factors for periventricular intraventricular hemorrhage (PIVH) do not include which of the following?
- A. Blood pressure fluctuations
- B. Younger gestational age (GA)
- C. Low birth weight
- D. Acute amnionitis
- E. Antenatal steroids

▸▸ **Question 14**

Regarding ICH in newborns, an intraventricular hemorrhage with ventricular dilation, what is the subependymal hemorrhage grade?
- A. 1
- B. 2
- C. 3
- D. 4
- E. 5

▸▸ **Question 15**

Post periventricular intraventricular hemorrhage (PIVH) hydrocephalus usually occurs for how long after the hemorrhage?
- A. 1 to 3 weeks
- B. 3 days
- C. 5 days
- D. 3 to 5 weeks
- E. 48 hours

▸▸ **Question 16**

To allow ventricles to expand to facilitate catheterization, reservoir should not be tapped before inserting a new ventricular catheter for at least how long?
- A. 12 hours
- B. 24 hours
- C. 36 hours
- D. 48 hours
- E. 72 hours

Answers

▸▸ **Answer 1**

Correct answer is A. Ruptured AVM[1]

▸▸ **Answer 2**

Correct answer is D. 80%[2]

▸▸ **Answer 3**

Correct answer is D. All of the above[2]

▸▸ **Answer 4**

Correct answer is E. All of the above[2]

▸▸ **Answer 5**

Correct answer is F. Smoking by the mother[2]

▸▸ **Answer 6**

Correct answer is E. All of the above[3]

▸▸ **Answer 7**

Correct answer is E. All of the above[3]

▸▸ **Answer 8**

Correct answer is D. Injury to brain stem[4]

▸▸ **Answer 9**

Correct answer is C. Progressive ventriculomegaly with the OFC crossing percentile curves and clinical evidence of increased ICP[5]

▸▸ **Answer 10**

Correct answer is F. All of the above[6]

▸▸ **Answer 11**

Correct answer is A. Ruptured AVM[1]

▸▸ **Answer 12**

Correct answer is A. Head of caudate nucleus[2]

▸▸ **Answer 13**

Correct answer is E. Antenatal steroids[2]

▸▸ **Answer 14**

Correct answer is C. 3[3]

▸▸ **Answer 15**

Correct answer is A. 1 to 3 weeks[7]

▸▸ **Answer 16**

Correct answer is B. 24 hours[6]

References

[1] Greenberg M, ed. Greenberg's Handbook of Neurosurgery. 10th ed. New York: Thieme; 2023:1630
[2] Greenberg M, ed. Greenberg's Handbook of Neurosurgery. 10th ed. New York: Thieme; 2023:1631
[3] Greenberg M, ed. Greenberg's Handbook of Neurosurgery. 10th ed. New York: Thieme; 2023:1632
[4] Greenberg M, ed. Greenberg's Handbook of Neurosurgery. 10th ed. New York: Thieme; 2023:1634
[5] Greenberg M, ed. Greenberg's Handbook of Neurosurgery. 10th ed. New York: Thieme; 2023:1635
[6] Greenberg M, ed. Greenberg's Handbook of Neurosurgery. 10th ed. New York: Thieme; 2023:1636
[7] Greenberg M, ed. Greenberg's Handbook of Neurosurgery. 10th ed. New York: Thieme; 2023:1633

Part XX

Outcome Assessment

XX

98 Outcome Assessment

Questions

▸▸ Question 1

A 60-year-old patient is known case of GBM grade 4. He requires occasional assistance but can take care of most of his needs. What would be his Karnofsky performance score?

- A. 80
- B. 70
- C. 60
- D. 50
- E. 40

▸▸ Question 2

A 40-year-old patient had road traffic accident 2 months ago. He performs daily routine in highly familiar environment in a nonconfused but automatic "robot-like" fashion. His skills deteriorate in unfamiliar environment. He lacks realistic planning for future. What would be his Ranchos Los Amigos cognitive score?

- A. Confused agitated
- B. Confused-appropriate
- C. Automatic-appropriate
- D. Purposeful-appropriate
- E. None

▸▸ Question 3

If a patient is having severe disability (conscious but disabled) and his dependence for daily support may be institutionalized, what would be his Glasgow outcome score?

- A. 0
- B. 1
- C. 2
- D. 3
- E. 4

▸▸ Question 4

A 30-year-old man had trauma 2 weeks ago. He is unable to walk without assistance and unable to attend to his own bodily needs without assistance. What would be his modified Rankin score?

- A. 5
- B. 4
- C. 3
- D. 2
- E. 1

▸▸ Question 5

As for functional independence measure (FIM) for evaluation of disabilities of spinal cord injuries, if a patient requires minimal assistance and can carry out > 75% activities on his or her own what would be the score?

- A. 6
- B. 4
- C. 2
- D. 1
- E. 0

▸▸ Question 6

Karnofsky performance scale (KPS) is often used for grading functional status in patients with cancer. What is the KPS score that often identifies patients with a worse prognosis for any given treatment?

- A. < 80
- B. < 70
- C. < 60
- D. < 50
- E. < 40

▸▸ Question 7

Which of the following is correct regarding Karnofsky performance scale in cancer patients?

- A. Score 80 to 100 are able to carry on normal activity and work with no special care needed
- B. Score 50 to 70 are unable to work. They are able to live at home and care for most personal needs with variable assistance required
- C. Score 0 to 30 are unable to care for themselves. They require equivalent of institutional or hospital care and the disease may be rapidly progressing
- D. All of the above

▸▸ Question 8

Which of the following is incorrect regarding WHO performance score?

- A. Grade 0 is fully active, with no performance restriction as a result of the disease
- B. Grade 1 is restriction in physically strenuous activity. The patient is ambulatory and able to do light work
- C. Grade 2 is unable to perform any activities and nonambulatory
- D. Grade 3 is only able to perform limited self-care
- E. Grade 4 is completely disabled and not able to perform self-care
- F. Grade 5 is dead

▸▸ Question 9

Ranchos Los Amingos scale is often used in rating disability following what?

- A. Spine injury
- B. Cancer patient
- C. Head injury
- D. Quadriplegia
- E. None of the above

▸▸ Question 10

Which of the following is correct regarding Ranchos Los Amigos cognitive scale?

- A. Level 1 is no response to pain, touch, sigh, or sound
- B. Level 2 is generalized reflex response to pain
- C. Level 3 is localized response
- D. Level 4 is confused agitated
- E. Level 5 is confused and nonagitated
- F. Level 6 is confused appropriate
- G. Level 7 is automatic appropriate
- H. Level 8 is purposeful appropriate
- I. All of the above

▸▸ Question 11

Which of the following is correct regarding Glasgow outcome scale extended and original?

- A. Score 1 is dead
- B. Score 2 is vegetative
- C. Scores 3 and 4 are severely disabled
- D. Scores 5 and 6 are moderately disabled
- E. Scores 7 and 8 are good recovery
- F. All of the above

▸▸ Question 12

Which of the following is incorrect regarding modified Rankin scale?

- A. Grade 0 is no symptoms at all
- B. Grade 1 is no significant disability despite symptoms
- C. Grade 2 is slight disability with unable to carry out all activities
- D. Grade 3 is moderate disability requiring some help
- E. Grade 4 is moderately severe disability and unable to walk without assistance
- F. Grade 5 is severe disability, bedridden, and incontinent
- G. None of the above

▸▸ Question 13

Of all the factors in Barthel index, what is the most difficult one?

- A. Personal hygiene
- B. Self bathing
- C. Feeding
- D. Toilet
- E. Stair climbing

▸▸ Question 14

Following are included in functional independence measure for spinal cord injury except?

- A. Self-care
- B. Sphincter control
- C. Power
- D. Mobility
- E. Locomotion

▸▸ Question 15

What does functional independence score of 7 mean?

- A. Modified independence
- B. Complete independence
- C. Minimal assistance
- D. Moderate assistance
- E. Maximal assistance

Answers

▸▸ Answer 1

Correct answer is C. 60[1]

▸▸ Answer 2

Correct answer is C. Automatic-appropriate[2]

▸▸ Answer 3

Correct answer is D. 3[2]

▸▸ Answer 4

Correct answer is B. 4[3]

▸▸ Answer 5

Correct answer is B. 4[4]

▸▸ Answer 6

Correct answer is B. < 70[1]

▸▸ Answer 7

Correct answer is D. All of the above[1]

▸▸ Answer 8

Correct answer is C. Grade 2 is unable to perform any activities and nonambulatory[2]

▸▸ Answer 9

Correct answer is C. Head injury[2]

▸▸ **Answer 10**

Correct answer is I. All of the above[3]

▸▸ **Answer 11**

Correct answer is F. All of the above[3]

▸▸ **Answer 12**

Correct answer is G. None of the above[3]

▸▸ **Answer 13**

Correct answer is B. Self bathing[4]

▸▸ **Answer 14**

Correct answer is C. Power[4]

▸▸ **Answer 15**

Correct answer is B. Complete independence[4]

References

[1] Greenberg M, ed. Greenberg's Handbook of Neurosurgery. 10th ed. New York: Thieme; 2023:1640
[2] Greenberg M, ed. Greenberg's Handbook of Neurosurgery. 10th ed. New York: Thieme; 2023:1641
[3] Greenberg M, ed. Greenberg's Handbook of Neurosurgery. 10th ed. New York: Thieme; 2023:1642
[4] Greenberg M, ed. Greenberg's Handbook of Neurosurgery. 10th ed. New York: Thieme; 2023:1643

Part XXI

Differential Diagnosis

XXI

99 Differential Diagnosis by Location or Radiographic Finding—Intracranial

Questions

▸▸ Question 1

The differential diagnosis of a solitary intraparenchymal lesion in an adult p-fossa is what until proven otherwise?
- A. Abscess
- B. Metastasis
- C. Hemangioma
- D. Hemorrhage
- E. Medulloblastoma

▸▸ Question 2

PHACES syndrome: acronym for a group of findings including which of the following?
- A. Posterior fossa malformations
- B. Truncal hemangioma
- C. Arterial anomalies of the head and neck
- D. Coarctation of the aorta and cardiac defects
- E. Eye anomalies and sternal cleft

▸▸ Question 3

Differentiating feature of medulloblastoma and ependymoma are all of the following except?
- A. Ependymoma which tends to grow into the 4th ventricle from the floor
- B. Ependymoma may grow through the foramen of Luschka and/or Magendie
- C. Ependymomas tend to be inhomogeneous on T1WI MRI
- D. The exophytic component of ependymomas tends to be high signal on T2WI MRI
- E. Calcifications are more common in medulloblastoma

▸▸ Question 4

Tumor passing from the posterior fossa to the middle fossa though the incisura is highly suggestive of which of the following?
- A. Vestibular schwannoma
- B. Epidermoid cyst
- C. Cysticercosis
- D. Arachnoid cyst
- E. Lipoma

▸▸ Question 5

All of the following are long tract signs found in foramen magnum lesion except?
- A. Brisk muscle stretch reflexes
- B. Loss of abdominal cutaneous reflexes
- C. Neurogenic bladder
- D. Contralateral Horner syndrome
- E. Nystagmus: classically downbeat

▸▸ Question 6

Which of following is not included in D/Dx of corpus callosum lesion?
- A. Lymphoma
- B. MS plaque
- C. Lipoma
- D. Diffuse axonal injury from trauma
- E. None of the above

▸▸ Question 7

Following conditions can lead to pituitary pseudotumor formation except?
- A. Primary hyperthyroidism
- B. Primary hypogonadism
- C. Pregnancy
- D. Ectopic GHRH secretion
- E. Intracranial hypotension

▸▸ Question 8

Differentiating features of juxta sellar meningioma from macroadenoma are all except?
- A. Homogenous contrast enhancement
- B. Dural tail
- C. Suprasellar epicenter
- D. Pushing the carotids laterally
- E. None of the above

▸▸ Question 9

All of the following are included in metastatic workup of intracranial lesions except?
- A. CT of chest
- B. CT of abdomen
- C. Bone scan
- D. PSA
- E. Mammogram

▸▸ Question 10

What is the most common malignancy of the skull?
- A. Osteogenic sarcoma
- B. Chondrogenic sarcoma
- C. Hemangiosarcoma
- D. Fibrosarcoma
- E. None of the above

▸▸ Question 11

Classic X-ray finding of "starburst" appearance is seen in which of the following?
- A. Hemangioblastoma
- B. Metastasis
- C. Multiple myeloma
- D. Lymphoma
- E. Brown tumor of hyperparathyroidism

▸▸ Question 12

Meningiomas of CPA present with which of the following?
- A. Early facial nerve involvement
- B. Early hearing loss
- C. Less trigeminal neuralgia like pain than VS
- D. Tinnitus
- E. Rarely calcified

▸▸ Question 13

Which of the following features favor nasal glioma in contrast to encephalocele?
- A. Pulsatile
- B. Positive Furstenberg sign
- C. Absence of stalk
- D. Probe can be passed laterally
- E. Presence of hypertelorism

▸▸ Question 14

Which of the following are the non-neoplastic thalamic lesions in pediatric and adult patients?
- A. Cavernous angioma
- B. Granuloma
- C. Heterotopias
- D. AVM
- E. Hamartoma

▸▸ Question 15

A patient presents with 2 months history of short-term memory deficit, seizures, and psychiatric symptoms of anxiety, depression, and behavioral changes. His MRI shows bilateral abnormalities highly restricted to medial temporal lobes on T2 FLAIR and CSF shows pleocytosis: WBCs > 5/mm^3. On EEG, epileptic or slow-wave activity involving the temporal lobes is seen. What is the most likely diagnosis?
- A. Mesial temporal sclerosis
- B. Herpes encephalitis
- C. Autoimmune limbic encephalitis
- D. Temporal hamartoma
- E. PCA ischemic infarct

▸▸ Question 16

By the rule of thumb "the differential diagnosis of a solitary intraparenchymal lesion in an adult posterior fossa is metastasis, metastasis, metastasis until proven otherwise." Other differential diagnoses in P-fossa of adults include hemangioblastoma, cerebellar astrocytoma, brainstem glioma, choroid plexus tumor, cerebellar liponeurocytoma, abscess, cavernous hemangioma, or hemorrhage. Differential in pediatric posterior fossa includes medulloblastoma (27%), cerebellar astrocytoma (27%), brain stem gliomas (28%), ependymoma, choroid plexus papilloma, and metastasis. How can medulloblastoma be differentiated from ependymoma?
- A. Medulloblastoma arise from the roof of the 4th ventricle and most are solid while ependymoma arise from the floor of the 4th ventricle
- B. The 4th ventricle drapes around the medulloblastoma forming "banana sign" while ependymoma tends to grow through the foramen of Luschka or/and Magendie
- C. Ependymoma tends to homogenous on T1WI while medulloblastoma tends to be heterogenous
- D. The exophytic component of ependymomas tends to be high signal on T2WI MRI while medulloblastoma is only mildly hyperintense
- E. Calcifications are more common in ependymomas while in MB these are less than 10%
- F. All of the above

▸▸ Question 17

What is the most common cerebellopontine (CP) angle lesion among the following CP angle lesions listed below?
- A. Vestibular schwannoma
- B. Meningioma
- C. Epidermoid
- D. Arachnoid cyst
- E. Trigeminal neuroma or facial nerve neuroma

▸▸ Question 18

How can vestibular schwannoma be differentiated from meningioma in CP angle region?
- A. VS presents with progressive unilateral hearing loss usually with tinnitus, and facial nerve signs and symptoms occur late. In case of CP angle meningioma, early facial nerve involvement is more common, and hearing loss is usually late
- B. Trigeminal neuralgia like pain is more common with CP angle meningioma as compared to VS
- C. On imaging VS shows heterogenous signal and nonuniform enhancement while VP angle meningioma shows homogenous signal and enhancement
- D. Medium size tumor in case of VS look like ice cream in the cone (trumpet sign) with the tumor forming an acute angle between the tumor and petrous bone and enlargement of IAC is often present while in case of meningioma, IAC is usually not enlarged with the tumor flat against the petrous bone forming an obtuse angle with the bone
- E. Calcifications and bony hypertrophy may occur in case of meningioma while in case of VS these are often absent
- F. All of the above

▸▸ Question 19

A patient presents in neurosurgical OPD with complaints of craniocervical junction pain in the neck and occiput with increase in pain with increased head movement. This patient also has numbness and tingling in fingers with dissociated sensory loss (loss of pain and temperature contralateral to the lesion with preservation of tactile sensation). There is spastic weakness of the extremities which usually starts in the ipsilateral upper limb, then the ipsilateral lower limb, then the contralateral lower limb, and finally contralateral upper limb (rotatory paralysis). Following are the differential diagnosis of foramen magnum lesion except?

- A. Meningioma
- B. Chordoma
- C. Ependymoma
- D. Neurilemmoma
- E. Epidermoid
- F. Chondroma
- G. Chondrosarcoma

▸▸ Question 20

Enhancing ring of tumor may be incomplete and irregular while in case of abscess, the ring is usually complete, often thinner and smoother than the tumor. Abscess is usually brighter than the tumor on DWI MRI. MR spectroscopy is ideal for differentiating the tumor from the abscess with the abscess showing reduced NAA, Cr, and choline while the tumor shows increased choline peak. What are the differential diagnoses in case of ring-enhancing lesions?

- A. Metastasis (including lymphoma)
- B. Abscess
- C. Glioma (astrocytoma usually glioblastoma)
- D. Infarct
- E. Contusion
- F. Demyelination
- G. Radiation
- H. All of the above

▸▸ Question 21

Differential diagnosis of tumors in sellar, suprasellar, or parasellar region includes pituitary tumors (adenohypophyseal tumors and neurohypophyseal tumors), pituitary pseudotumors (thyrotroph hyperplasia, gonadotroph hyperplasia, somatotroph hyperplasia), juxtasellar or suprasellar tumors, or masses (craniopharyngioma, Rathke cleft cyst, meningioma, germ cell tumors, hypothalamic tumors, optic nerve or chiasma tumors). Which of the following are the differentiating points between hypophysitis and adenoma?

- A. Enlargement of hypophyistis is symmetric while in case of adenoma it is asymmetric
- B. Pituitary stalk is thickened and nontapering in case of hypophysitis while it is not thickened, tapering, and deviated in case of adenoma
- C. Sellar floor is spared in hypophysitis while it may be eroded in case of tumor
- D. Enhancement is intense and may be heterogenous in case of adenoma, while it is less intense and usually homogenous in case of hypophysitis
- E. Mean size at the time of presentation of hypophysitis is 3-cm cube in case of hypophysitis, while it is 10-cm cube in case of adenoma

▸▸ Question 22

Differential of orbital tumors in adults include neoplastic lesions (cavernous hemangioma, capillary hemangioma, lymphangioma, melanoma, retinoblastoma, lymphoma), congenital lesion (retinopathy of prematurity, persistent hyperplastic primary vitreous), infectious, inflammatory, and vascular lesions. What is the most common orbital lesion in pediatric patients among the following?

- A. Dermoid cyst
- B. Hemangioma
- C. Rhabdomyosarcoma
- D. Optic nerve glioma
- E. Lymphangioma

▸▸ Question 23

Following statements are correct regarding the type of intraventricular lesion by location except?

- A. Meningioma is the most common tumor in the atrium of lateral ventricle (trigone) in adults more than 30 years of age while in case of children less than 5 years of age, choroid plexus papilloma is the most common lesion at this location
- B. Astrocytoma is the most common lesion in the frontal horn of ventricle and then meningioma
- C. At the foramen of Monro region, SEGAs are most common in people 6 to 30 years of age with pilocytic astrocytoma in the second and CPP in the third number at this location, while in case of adults more than 30 years, metastasis is the most common tumor at this location
- D. The most common lesion at the 3rd ventricle is colloid cyst, then craniopharyngioma, and then astrocytoma
- E. Epidermoid is the most common lesion in the 4th ventricle and then comes medulloblastoma and ependymoma

▸▸ Question 24

What is the most common periventricular solid enhancing lesion?

- A. Ependymoma
- B. Lymphoma
- C. Metastatic carcinoma
- D. Ventriculitis
- E. Medulloblastoma

▸▸ Question 25

How can an encephalocele be differentiated from nasal glioma?

- A. Encephalocele is frequently pulsatile while nasal glioma is nonpulsatile
- B. Encephalocele swells with Valsalva maneuver while nasal glioma does not
- C. Presence of hypertelorism suggests encephalocele while it does not correlate with nasal glioma
- D. Probe can be passed lateral to encephalocele while it cannot be passed lateral to a nasal glioma
- E. Encephalocele is attached to the CNS with a stalk while nasal glioma does not
- F. All of the above

Answers

►► Answer 1

Correct answer is B. Metastasis[1]

►► Answer 2

Correct answer is B. Truncal hemangioma[2]

►► Answer 3

Correct answer is E. Calcifications are more common in medulloblastoma[2]

►► Answer 4

Correct answer is B. Epidermoid cyst[2]

►► Answer 5

Correct answer is D. Contralateral Horner syndrome[3]

►► Answer 6

Correct answer is E. None of the above[4]

►► Answer 7

Correct answer is A. Primary hyperthyroidism[4]

►► Answer 8

Correct answer is D. Pushing the carotids laterally[5]

►► Answer 9

Correct answer is C. Bone scan[6]

►► Answer 10

Correct answer is A. Osteogenic sarcoma[6]

►► Answer 11

Correct answer is A. Hemangioblastoma[7]

►► Answer 12

Correct answer is A. Early facial nerve involvement[8]

►► Answer 13

Correct answer is C. Absence of stalk[5]

►► Answer 14

Correct answer is E. Hamartoma[9]

►► Answer 15

Correct answer is C. Autoimmune limbic encephalitis[10]

►► Answer 16

Correct answer is F. All of the above[1]

►► Answer 17

Correct answer is A. Vestibular schwannoma[2]

►► Answer 18

Correct answer is F. All of the above[8]

►► Answer 19

Correct answer is C. Ependymoma[3]

►► Answer 20

Correct answer is H. All of the above[11]

►► Answer 21

Correct answer is D. Enhancement is intense and may be heterogenous in case of adenoma, while it is less intense and usually homogenous in case of hypophysitis[12]

►► Answer 22

Correct answer is A. Dermoid cyst[13]

►► Answer 23

Correct answer is E. Epidermoid is the most common lesion in the 4th ventricle and then comes medulloblastoma and ependymoma[14]

►► Answer 24

Correct answer is B. Lymphoma[15]

►► Answer 25

Correct answer is F. All of the above[16]

References

[1] Greenberg M, ed. Greenberg's Handbook of Neurosurgery. 10th ed. New York: Thieme; 2023:1646
[2] Greenberg M, ed. Greenberg's Handbook of Neurosurgery. 10th ed. New York: Thieme; 2023:1647
[3] Greenberg M, ed. Greenberg's Handbook of Neurosurgery. 10th ed. New York: Thieme; 2023:1649
[4] Greenberg M, ed. Greenberg's Handbook of Neurosurgery. 10th ed. New York: Thieme; 2023:1653
[5] Greenberg M, ed. Greenberg's Handbook of Neurosurgery. 10th ed. New York: Thieme; 2023:1654
[6] Greenberg M, ed. Greenberg's Handbook of Neurosurgery. 10th ed. New York: Thieme; 2023:1661
[7] Greenberg M, ed. Greenberg's Handbook of Neurosurgery. 10th ed. New York: Thieme; 2023:1662
[8] Greenberg M, ed. Greenberg's Handbook of Neurosurgery. 10th ed. New York: Thieme; 2023:1648
[9] Greenberg M, ed. Greenberg's Handbook of Neurosurgery. 10th ed. New York: Thieme; 2023:1673
[10] Greenberg M, ed. Greenberg's Handbook of Neurosurgery. 10th ed. New York: Thieme; 2023:1672
[11] Greenberg M, ed. Greenberg's Handbook of Neurosurgery. 10th ed. New York: Thieme; 2023:1652
[12] Greenberg M, ed. Greenberg's Handbook of Neurosurgery. 10th ed. New York: Thieme; 2023:1655
[13] Greenberg M, ed. Greenberg's Handbook of Neurosurgery. 10th ed. New York: Thieme; 2023:1658
[14] Greenberg M, ed. Greenberg's Handbook of Neurosurgery. 10th ed. New York: Thieme; 2023:1669
[15] Greenberg M, ed. Greenberg's Handbook of Neurosurgery. 10th ed. New York: Thieme; 2023:1670
[16] Greenberg M, ed. Greenberg's Handbook of Neurosurgery. 10th ed. New York: Thieme; 2023:1674

100 Differential Diagnosis by Location or Radiographic Finding—Spine

Questions

▸▸ Question 1

Atlantoaxial subluxation in rheumatoid arthritis is due to which of the following?
- A. Erosion of insertion points of the TAL
- B. Congenital laxity of the TAL
- C. Disruption (tear) of the TAL
- D. Avulsion of the insertion points of the TAL
- E. Incompetence of the odontoid process

▸▸ Question 2

Fractures due to metastatic involvement show which of the following?
- A. Hyperintense on T1WI and hyperintense on T2WI
- B. Hypointense on T1WI and hyperintense on T2WI
- C. Isointense on T1WI and hypointense on T2WI
- D. Hypointense on T1WI and hypointense on T2WI
- E. Hyperintense on T1WI and hypointense on T2WI

▸▸ Question 3

Criteria for vertebra plana include all of the following except?
- A. Increased density of vertebra
- B. Spares neural arches
- C. Normal disk and intervertebral disk space
- D. Intervertebral vacuum cleft sign
- E. Kyphosis

▸▸ Question 4

Destruction of the disk space which often involves at least two adjacent vertebral levels is highly suggestive of which of the following?
- A. Tumor
- B. Potts disease
- C. Pyogenic infection
- D. Metastasis
- E. None of the above

▸▸ Question 5

What is the most common sacral neoplasm?
- A. Chordoma
- B. Osteoma
- C. Metastasis
- D. Giant cell tumor
- E. Teratoma

▸▸ Question 6

In which type of sacral agenesis, there is partial bilaterally symmetric defects in the sacrum, iliac bones articulate with S1, and distal segments of the sacrum and coccyx fail to develop?
- A. Type 1
- B. Type 2
- C. Type 3
- D. Type 4
- E. Type 5

▸▸ Question 7

Nodular enhancing lesions in spine occur in all of the following except?
- A. Neurofibromatosis
- B. Drop metastasis
- C. Meningioma
- D. Schwannoma
- E. Neurofibroma

▸▸ Question 8

Which of the following is the cause of atlantoaxial subluxation?
- A. Incompetence of transverse atlantal ligament (TAL) which can be due to rheumatoid arthritis (causes erosion of insertion point of TAL), traumatic, congenital laxity of TAL (in Down syndrome), retropharyngeal infection, or chronic steroid use
- B. Incompetence of odontoid process which can be due to odontoid fractures, os odontoideum, erosion of odontoid due to rheumatoid arthritis, neoplastic erosion of odontoid (metastasis), local infection, or congenital absence
- C. Congenital absence of tectorial membrane
- D. Basilar invagination
- E. Both A and B

▸▸ Question 9

Which of the following are the etiologies of pathologic fracture of spine?
- A. Osteoporosis
- B. Neoplasm (metastasis, lymphoma, hemangioma)
- C. Infection
- D. Avascular necrosis of vertebral bodies (with excessive use of steroids)
- E. All of the above

▸▸ Question 10

All of the following are destructive lesions of spine except?
- A. Neoplastic (metastatic or primary bone tumors like chordoma, osteoid osteoma, hemangioma)
- B. Paget's disease
- C. Infection like vertebral osteomyelitis
- D. Ankylosing spondylitis

- E. Chronic renal failure causing spondyloarthropathy resembling infection

►► Question 11

Following are the causes of vertebral hyperostosis except?

- A. Paget's disease
- B. Osteoblastic metastasis (prostate in men and breast in women)
- C. Marfan's syndrome or Ehlers Danlos syndrome
- D. Osteoid osteoma or osteoblastoma
- E. Bone island (also known as enostosis)

►► Question 12

Which of the following is the most common sacral neoplasm?

- A. Metastasis
- B. Giant cell tumor
- C. Chordoma
- D. Teratoma
- E. None of the above

►► Question 13

Sacral agenesis is associated with increased incidence of spinal abnormalities like syrinx, tethered cord, lipoma, and lipomyelomeningocele. Which of the following are the types of sacral agenesis?

- A. Type 1: partial unilateral agenesis
- B. Type 2: partial bilaterally symmetric defects in the sacrum
- C. Type 3: total sacral agenesis plus iliac bone fuses with the lowest segment of the lumbar spine present
- D. Type 4: total sacral agenesis plus iliac bones fuse posteriorly in the midline
- E. All of the above

►► Question 14

Following are the causes of enhancing nerve roots except?

- A. Tumor (meningeal carcinomatosis and lymphoma)
- B. Infection (CMV)
- C. Inflammatory (Guillain–Barre, arachnoiditis)
- D. Neurofibromatosis

►► Question 15

Which of the following are the differential of nodular enhancing lesions in the spinal canal?

- A. Neurofibromatosis
- B. Drop metastasis
- C. Neurofibroma
- D. Schwannoma
- E. All of the above

►► Question 16

Which of the following are the differentials of intraspinal cysts?

- A. Spinal meningeal cysts
- B. Cystic neurofibroma
- C. Ependymoma
- D. Syringomyelia
- E. Dilated central canal
- F. All of the above

►► Question 17

Which of the following are the differentials of diffuse enhancement of nerve roots/cauda equina?

- A. Guillain Barre
- B. Meningitis
- C. CMV
- D. Lymphoma
- E. Sarcoid
- F. All of the above

Answers

►► Answer 1

Correct answer is A. Erosion of insertion points of the TAL[1]

►► Answer 2

Correct answer is B. Hypointense on T1WI and hyperintense on T2WI[2]

►► Answer 3

Correct answer is E. Kyphosis[3]

►► Answer 4

Correct answer is C. Pyogenic infection[4]

►► Answer 5

Correct answer is C. Metastasis[4]

►► Answer 6

Correct answer is B. Type 2[5]

►► Answer 7

Correct answer is C. Meningioma[5]

►► Answer 8

Correct answer is E. Both A and B[6]

▸▸ **Answer 9**

Correct answer is E. All of the above[7]

▸▸ **Answer 10**

Correct answer is B. Paget's disease[3]

▸▸ **Answer 11**

Correct answer is C. Marfan's syndrome or Ehlers Danlos syndrome[4]

▸▸ **Answer 12**

Correct answer is A. Metastasis[5]

▸▸ **Answer 13**

Correct answer is E. All of the above[5]

▸▸ **Answer 14**

Correct answer is D. Neurofibromatosis[8]

▸▸ **Answer 15**

Correct answer is E. All of the above[5]

▸▸ **Answer 16**

Correct answer is F. All of the above[5]

▸▸ **Answer 17**

Correct answer is F. All of the above[5]

References

[1] Greenberg M, ed. Greenberg's Handbook of Neurosurgery. 10th ed. New York: Thieme; 2023:1667
[2] Greenberg M, ed. Greenberg's Handbook of Neurosurgery. 10th ed. New York: Thieme; 2023:1667,1668
[3] Greenberg M, ed. Greenberg's Handbook of Neurosurgery. 10th ed. New York: Thieme; 2023:1679
[4] Greenberg M, ed. Greenberg's Handbook of Neurosurgery. 10th ed. New York: Thieme; 2023:1680
[5] Greenberg M, ed. Greenberg's Handbook of Neurosurgery. 10th ed. New York: Thieme; 2023:1681
[6] Greenberg M, ed. Greenberg's Handbook of Neurosurgery. 10th ed. New York: Thieme; 2023:1677
[7] Greenberg M, ed. Greenberg's Handbook of Neurosurgery. 10th ed. New York: Thieme; 2023:1678
[8] Greenberg M, ed. Greenberg's Handbook of Neurosurgery. 10th ed. New York: Thieme; 2023:1682

101 Differential Diagnosis (DDx) by Signs and Symptoms—Primarily Intracranial

Questions

▸▸ **Question 1**

What is the most common cause of syncope?
- A. Reflex-mediated such as vasovagal or Valsalva/stress-induced
- B. Cardiac valvular etiology or arrhythmia
- C. Orthostatic due to autonomic dysregulation, dehydration, or polypharmacy
- D. Cerebrovascular due to stroke
- E. Seizure

▸▸ **Question 2**

Most of transient ischemic attack (TIA) resolve within how long?
- A. < 5 minutes
- B. < 10 minutes
- C. < 20 minutes
- D. < 30 minutes
- E. < 40 minutes

▸▸ **Question 3**

Wide base gait is defined as gait with feet spread of how much?
- A. > 1 to 2 inch apart
- B. > 2 to 4 inch apart
- C. > 4 to 6 inch apart
- D. > 6 to 8 inch apart
- E. > 8 to 10 inch apart

▸▸ **Question 4**

A patient presented with abdominal cramps, dry mouth, and diarrhea followed by symmetrical cranial nerve palsies, diplopia, ptosis, loss of accommodation, and pupillary light reflex and descending weakness. Sensory disturbances are absent. Sensorium is clear. What is the most likely diagnosis?
- A. Graves' disease
- B. Myasthenia gravis
- C. Giant cell arteritis
- D. Botulism
- E. Pseudotumor cerebri

▸▸ **Question 5**

All of the following are causes of facial diplegia except?
- A. Mobius syndrome
- B. Guillain Barre syndrome
- C. Lyme disease
- D. Lhermitte Duclos syndrome
- E. Sarcoidosis

▸▸ **Question 6**

A 30-year-old patient presented with binocular vision loss after head trauma. All of the following are causes of binocular vision loss except?
- A. Amaurosis fugax
- B. Bilateral PCA flow impairment
- C. Bilateral occipital lobe injury
- D. Raised ICP
- E. Epileptic blindness

▸▸ **Question 7**

Exophthalmos is defined as anterior displacement of globe by how much?
- A. > 14 mm
- B. > 16 mm
- C. > 18 mm
- D. > 20 mm
- E. > 22 mm

▸▸ **Question 8**

What is the most common cause of unilateral proptosis?
- A. Orbital tumor
- B. Infection (cellulitis)
- C. Hemorrhage
- D. Thyroid disease
- E. Cavernous sinus occlusion

▸▸ **Question 9**

Which of the following investigations is not helpful for diagnosis (nonsensitive, nonspecific) of pulsatile tinnitus?
- A. MRI
- B. MRV
- C. Carotid USG
- D. Angiogram
- E. None of the above

▸▸ **Question 10**

How frequently is treatment required for arachnoid cyst?
- A. 10%
- B. 20%
- C. 30%
- D. 40%
- E. 50%

▸▸ Question 11

Syncope is defined as one or more episodes of brief loss of consciousness with prompt recovery. Which of the following are the etiologies of syncope?

- A. Cerebrovascular (subarachnoid hemorrhage, intracerebral hemorrhage, brainstem infarction, pituitary apoplexy, vertebrobasilar insufficiency, rarely with migraine)
- B. Cardiovascular (carotid sinus syncope, vasopressor syncope, cardiac standstill, orthostatic hypotension)
- C. Infections (meningitis, encephalitis)
- D. Metabolic hypoglycemia
- E. All of the above

▸▸ Question 12

Following are the causes of transient neurologic deficit except?

- A. Transient ischemic attack
- B. Migraine
- C. Spinocerebellar degeneration
- D. Seizures
- E. TIA like syndrome (tumor TIA)

▸▸ Question 13

Wide based gait is a gait with feet spread more than 2 to 4 inches apart. Which of the following are included in the differentials of this symptom?

- A. Idiopathic normal pressure hydrocephalus
- B. Cerebellar ataxia
- C. Sensorimotor peripheral neuropathy
- D. Vestibular ataxia
- E. Myelopathy
- F. All of the above

▸▸ Question 14

Following are the causes of diplopia except?

- A. Cranial nerve palsy of any one or a combination of cranial nerves 3, 4, and 6
- B. Intraorbital mass compressing extraocular muscles
- C. Grave's disease
- D. Myasthenia gravis
- E. Friderichsen syndrome
- F. Giant cell arteritis

▸▸ Question 15

Following are included in the most probable cause of gradual onset of anosmia except?

- A. Allergic rhinitis and sinus disease
- B. Intracranial neoplasms
- C. Head trauma
- D. Nasal polyps
- E. Intracranial neoplasms like olfactory groove meningioma

▸▸ Question 16

Marble bone disease is a group of genetic disorders of defective osteoclastic resorption of bone resulting in increased bone density, which may be transmitted either as autosomal dominant or recessive. What is the other name of this disease?

- A. Paget's disease
- B. Marfan syndrome
- C. Osteopetrosis
- D. Osteoporosis
- E. None of the above

▸▸ Question 17

All of the following are included in the differentials of binocular blindness except?

- A. Bilateral posterior cerebral artery flow impairment
- B. Amaurosis fugax due to giant cell arteritis or TIAs
- C. Bilateral vitreous hemorrhage
- D. Trauma with bilateral occipital lobe injury
- E. Posterior ischemic optic neuropathy usually in the setting of shock

▸▸ Question 18

Exophthalmos is abnormal protrusion of eyeball. It can be pulsatile or nonpulsatile. All of the following are included in nonpulsatile exophthalmos except?

- A. Intraorbital tumors like optic glioma, optic sheath neuroma, lymphoma or Graves disease or enlargement of periorbital fat
- B. Carotid cavernous fistula or transmitted intracranial pulsations due to defect in orbital roof or vascular tumors
- C. Inflammatory or hemorrhage or third nerve palsy
- D. Cavernous sinus occlusion
- E. Pseudo exophthalmos

▸▸ Question 19

Ptosis is drooping of upper eyelid. Ptosis can be pupil sparing or not pupil sparing. Etiologies of pupil sparing ptosis includes the following except?

- A. Congenital
- B. Traumatic injury to eyelid or traumatic roof fracture
- C. Neurogenic involving third nerve palsy due to compression from tumors or pituitary apoplexy
- D. Myogenic ptosis due to botulism toxin or myasthenia gravis
- E. None of the above

▸▸ Question 20

Following are the causes of macrocephaly with ventricular enlargement except?

- A. Hydranencephaly
- B. Constitutional ventriculomegaly

- C. External hydrocephalus
- D. Hydrocephalus ex vacuo
- E. Obstructive hydrocephalus

Answers

▸▸ **Answer 1**

Correct answer is A. Reflex-mediated such as vasovagal or Valsalva/stress-induced[1]

▸▸ **Answer 2**

Correct answer is C. < 20 minutes[2]

▸▸ **Answer 3**

Correct answer is B. > 2 to 4 inch apart[3]

▸▸ **Answer 4**

Correct answer is D. Botulism[4]

▸▸ **Answer 5**

Correct answer is D. Lhermitte Duclos syndrome[5]

▸▸ **Answer 6**

Correct answer is A. Amaurosis fugax[5]

▸▸ **Answer 7**

Correct answer is C. > 18 mm[6]

▸▸ **Answer 8**

Correct answer is D. Thyroid disease[6]

▸▸ **Answer 9**

Correct answer is C. Carotid USG[7]

▸▸ **Answer 10**

Correct answer is C. 30%[8]

▸▸ **Answer 11**

Correct answer is E. All of the above[2]

▸▸ **Answer 12**

Correct answer is C. Spinocerebellar degeneration[3]

▸▸ **Answer 13**

Correct answer is F. All of the above[3]

▸▸ **Answer 14**

Correct answer is E. Friderichsen syndrome[4]

▸▸ **Answer 15**

Correct answer is C. Head trauma[4]

▸▸ **Answer 16**

Correct answer is C. Osteopetrosis[5]

▸▸ **Answer 17**

Correct answer is B. Amaurosis fugax due to giant cell arteritis or TIAs[6]

▸▸ **Answer 18**

Correct answer is B. Carotid cavernous fistula or transmitted intracranial pulsations due to defect in orbital roof or vascular tumors[9]

▸▸ **Answer 19**

Correct answer is C. Neurogenic involving third nerve palsy due to compression from tumors or pituitary apoplexy[9]

▸▸ **Answer 20**

Correct answer is C. External hydrocephalus[8]

References

[1] Greenberg M, ed. Greenberg's Handbook of Neurosurgery. 10th ed. New York: Thieme; 2023:1684
[2] Greenberg M, ed. Greenberg's Handbook of Neurosurgery. 10th ed. New York: Thieme; 2023:1685
[3] Greenberg M, ed. Greenberg's Handbook of Neurosurgery. 10th ed. New York: Thieme; 2023:1686
[4] Greenberg M, ed. Greenberg's Handbook of Neurosurgery. 10th ed. New York: Thieme; 2023:1687
[5] Greenberg M, ed. Greenberg's Handbook of Neurosurgery. 10th ed. New York: Thieme; 2023:1689
[6] Greenberg M, ed. Greenberg's Handbook of Neurosurgery. 10th ed. New York: Thieme; 2023:1690
[7] Greenberg M, ed. Greenberg's Handbook of Neurosurgery. 10th ed. New York: Thieme; 2023:1693
[8] Greenberg M, ed. Greenberg's Handbook of Neurosurgery. 10th ed. New York: Thieme; 2023:1692
[9] Greenberg M, ed. Greenberg's Handbook of Neurosurgery. 10th ed. New York: Thieme; 2023:1691

102 Differential Diagnosis (DDx) by Signs and Symptoms—Primarily Spine and Other

Questions

▸▸ Question 1

Which one of the following does not present as a spinal epidural mass?

- A. Bone fracture
- B. Extramedullary hematopoiesis
- C. Vertebral Paget disease
- D. Bony compression secondary to incompetence of odontoid process or transverse atlantal ligament
- E. Cervical or thoracic spinal stenosis

▸▸ Question 2

A 17-year-old male patient presents with insidious asymmetrical painless wasting of the distal UE muscles. What is the most likely diagnosis?

- A. Epidural lipomatosis
- B. Vertebral Paget disease
- C. OPLL
- D. Hirayama disease
- E. Idiopathic spinal cord herniation

▸▸ Question 3

All are signs of ALS except?

- A. It is an upper and lower motor neuron disease
- B. Slight spasticity of LEs
- C. Atrophic weakness of the hands and forearms
- D. Fasciculations in the UE
- E. Loss of sphincter control

▸▸ Question 4

What is the most common cause of sciatica?

- A. Diskitis
- B. Spinal stenosis
- C. Lumber disk herniation
- D. Tumor
- E. None of the above

▸▸ Question 5

A patient presents with pain in the sciatic distribution and weakness of external rotation and abduction of the hip. On clinical examination, Freiberg test and Pace test are positive. What is the most likely diagnosis?

- A. Piriformis syndrome
- B. Femoral neuropathy
- C. Diabetic neuropathy
- D. Sacral tumor
- E. Herniated lumbar intervertebral disk

▸▸ Question 6

What is the most common etiology of pure motor hemiplegia?

- A. Ischemic lacunar infarct
- B. Tumor of motor strip
- C. Brainstem ischemic infarct
- D. Foramen magnum lesions
- E. Acute subdural hematoma

▸▸ Question 7

Which of the following conditions presents with descending paralysis with ophthalmoplegia?

- A. Guillain-Barre syndrome
- B. Tick borne paralysis
- C. Myasthenia gravis
- D. Spinal infections
- E. Ascending hematomyelia

▸▸ Question 8

In sacral plexus lesions, which of the following muscles will be spared on EMG?

- A. Gluteus maximus
- B. Gluteus medius
- C. Gluteus minimus
- D. Piriformis
- E. Both A and B

▸▸ Question 9

Which of the following feature suggests L4 radiculopathy?

- A. Iliopsoas weakness
- B. Quadriceps weakness
- C. Preservation of power in thigh adductors
- D. Sensory loss in anterior thigh
- E. Intact sensations from knee to medial malleolus

▸▸ Question 10

In patients with foot drop, which of the following muscles must be spared to differentiate common peroneal nerve palsy from L4–L5 radiculopathy?

- A. Anterior tibialis
- B. Posterior tibialis
- C. Extensor digitorum longus
- D. Extensor hallucis longus
- E. None of the above

▸▸ Question 11

Which of the following is not an etiology of Lhermitte's sign?

- A. Multiple sclerosis
- B. Cervical spondylosis
- C. Subacute combined degeneration
- D. Central cord syndrome
- E. Anterior cord syndrome

▸▸ Question 12

All of the following are the congenital causes of myelopathy except?

- A. Arnold Chiari malformation
- B. Tethered cord or syringomyelia
- C. Cervical or thoracic spine stenosis
- D. Neurenteric cyst or hereditary spastic paraplegia
- E. Cord compression that occurs with some mucopolysaccharidoses

▸▸ Question 13

Which of the following are the possible causes of myelopathy?

- A. Congenital
- B. Acquired
- C. Neoplastic (primary spine tumors, carcinomatous meningitis, or epidural metastasis)
- D. Vascular (spinal cord infarction, vascular malformation)
- E. All of the above

▸▸ Question 14

Causes of sciatica include congenital (meningeal cyst, conjoined nerve root), acquired (spinal stenosis, juxtafacet cyst, nerve root sheath cyst), infections, neoplastic, inflammatory, and vascular. What is the most common cause of sciatica?

- A. Radiculopathy due to herniated lumbar disk
- B. Bone or soft tissue tumors along the course of sciatic nerve
- C. Diskitis
- D. Spinal stenosis, spondylosis/spondylolysis/spondylolisthesis
- E. Nerve root sheath cyst

▸▸ Question 15

Which of the following are the points to differentiate femoral neuropathy from L4 radiculopathy?

- A. Distribution of sensory loss in femoral neuropathy is anterior thigh, while in case of L4 radiculopathy, it is dermatome from knee to medial malleolus sparing anterior thigh
- B. Iliopsoas is weak in case of femoral neuropathy while it is normal in case of L4 radiculopathy
- C. Thigh adductors are normal in case of femoral neuropathy while it may be weak in case of L4 radiculopathy
- D. Quadriceps are weak in case of both femoral neuropathy and in L4 radiculopathy
- E. All of the above

▸▸ Question 16

Following are the possible causes of acute paraplegia or quadriplegia except?

- A. In infancy spinal muscular atrophy, spinal cord injury, congenital myopathies, infantile botulism
- B. Traumatic spinal cord injury
- C. Congenital (achondroplasia, syringomyelia)
- D. Spinocerebellar degeneration
- E. Metabolic (thallium poisoning, central pontine myelinolysis)
- F. Infections
- G. Peripheral neuromuscular disorders (GBS, myopathies)

▸▸ Question 17

Following are the causes of hemiplegia or hemiparesis due to insult within the brain except?

- A. Lesions of the contralateral internal capsule
- B. Lesions of the brain stem
- C. Lesions of the cervicomedullary junction
- D. Unilateral spinal cord lesion
- E. Brain tumor or traumatic epidural or subdural hematoma

▸▸ Question 18

Which of the following are the differentials of ascending paralysis?

- A. GBS
- B. Tick-borne paralysis
- C. Spinal infection
- D. Patients with a prior spinal cord injury which can be due to ascending hematomyelia or post-traumatic syringomyelia
- E. All of the above

▸▸ Question 19

Chronic low-back pain is pain in back after 3 months. What are the causes of chronic low-back pain?

- A. Degenerative conditions like spinal stenosis, degenerative spondylolisthesis
- B. Spondyloarthropathies like ankylosing spondylitis
- C. Osteitis condensans ilii which is increased density in the ilium which is usually found in pregnant women
- D. Psychological overlay
- E. All of the above

▸▸ **Question 20**

Foot drop is because of weakness of anterior tibialis muscle which is innervated by deep peroneal nerve. What is the most common cause of foot drop?

- A. L4/L5 radiculopathy
- B. Common peroneal nerve palsy
- C. Parasagittal lesion in the brain
- D. Lumbosacral plexus neuropathy
- E. Muscular dystrophy

▸▸ **Question 21**

Lhermitte's sign is electric shock like sensation radiating down the spine usually provoked by neck flexion. Which of the following are the etiologies in which this sign can be positive?

- A. Multiple sclerosis
- B. Cervical spondylosis
- C. Cervical cord tumor
- D. Cervical disk herniation
- E. Chiari type 1 malformation
- F. All of the above

Answers

▸▸ **Answer 1**

Correct answer is E. Cervical or thoracic spinal stenosis[1]

▸▸ **Answer 2**

Correct answer is D. Hirayama disease[2]

▸▸ **Answer 3**

Correct answer is E. Loss of sphincter control[3]

▸▸ **Answer 4**

Correct answer is C. Lumber disk herniation[3]

▸▸ **Answer 5**

Correct answer is A. Piriformis syndrome[4]

▸▸ **Answer 6**

Correct answer is A. Ischemic lacunar infarct[5]

▸▸ **Answer 7**

Correct answer is D. Spinal infections[5]

▸▸ **Answer 8**

Correct answer is E. Both A and B[6]

▸▸ **Answer 9**

Correct answer is B. Quadriceps weakness[7]

▸▸ **Answer 10**

Correct answer is B. Posterior tibialis[7]

▸▸ **Answer 11**

Correct answer is E. Anterior cord syndrome[8]

▸▸ **Answer 12**

Correct answer is C. Cervical or thoracic spine stenosis[9]

▸▸ **Answer 13**

Correct answer is E. All of the above[3]

▸▸ **Answer 14**

Correct answer is A. Radiculopathy due to herniated lumbar disk[4]

▸▸ **Answer 15**

Correct answer is E. All of the above[10]

▸▸ **Answer 16**

Correct answer is D. Spinocerebellar degeneration[11]

▸▸ **Answer 17**

Correct answer is D. Unilateral spinal cord lesion[5]

▸▸ **Answer 18**

Correct answer is E. All of the above[5]

▸▸ **Answer 19**

Correct answer is E. All of the above[12]

▸▸ **Answer 20**

Correct answer is A. L4/L5 radiculopathy[7]

▸▸ **Answer 21**

Correct answer is F. All of the above[8]

References

[1] Greenberg M, ed. Greenberg's Handbook of Neurosurgery. 10th ed. New York: Thieme; 2023:1696

[2] Greenberg M, ed. Greenberg's Handbook of Neurosurgery. 10th ed. New York: Thieme; 2023:1697
[3] Greenberg M, ed. Greenberg's Handbook of Neurosurgery. 10th ed. New York: Thieme; 2023:1700
[4] Greenberg M, ed. Greenberg's Handbook of Neurosurgery. 10th ed. New York: Thieme; 2023:1701
[5] Greenberg M, ed. Greenberg's Handbook of Neurosurgery. 10th ed. New York: Thieme; 2023:1704
[6] Greenberg M, ed. Greenberg's Handbook of Neurosurgery. 10th ed. New York: Thieme; 2023:1707
[7] Greenberg M, ed. Greenberg's Handbook of Neurosurgery. 10th ed. New York: Thieme; 2023:1708
[8] Greenberg M, ed. Greenberg's Handbook of Neurosurgery. 10th ed. New York: Thieme; 2023:1712
[9] Greenberg M, ed. Greenberg's Handbook of Neurosurgery. 10th ed. New York: Thieme; 2023:1696
[10] Greenberg M, ed. Greenberg's Handbook of Neurosurgery. 10th ed. New York: Thieme; 2023:1702
[11] Greenberg M, ed. Greenberg's Handbook of Neurosurgery. 10th ed. New York: Thieme; 2023:1703
[12] Greenberg M, ed. Greenberg's Handbook of Neurosurgery. 10th ed. New York: Thieme; 2023:1706

Part XXII

Procedures, Interventions, Operations

XXII

103 Intraoperative Dyes, OR Equipment, Surgical Hemostasis, and Bone Extenders

Questions

▸▸ Question 1

Owing to risk of developing paraparesis, quadriplegia, multiple cranial nerves, dementia, and hydrocephalus, which of the following dyes must not be used as stain in neurosurgical procedures?

- A. Indigo carmine
- B. Methylene blue
- C. Flourescien
- D. Indocyanine green
- E. Gentian violet

▸▸ Question 2

For children below 3 years of age, the knob of Mayfield head holder clamp housing the tension spring and gauge is tightened up to how much?

- A. 20 to 30 lbs
- B. 30 to 40 lbs
- C. 40 to 50 lbs
- D. 50 to 60 lbs
- E. Not applicable

▸▸ Question 3

Microfibrillar collagen promotes adhesion and aggregation of platelets and leads to chemical hemostasis. It is rendered ineffective if platelets count is how much?

- A. < 50,000/mL
- B. < 40,000/mL
- C. < 30,000/mL
- D. < 20,000/mL
- E. < 10,000/mL

▸▸ Question 4

Which of the following is an important imaging view of MRI to identify L5–S1 disk space for preoperative localization of level by identifying sacral ala?

- A. Sagittal view
- B. Coronal view
- C. Axial view
- D. Both A and B
- E. Both A and C

▸▸ Question 5

If best osteoconductive and osteogenic properties are required, which bone graft is preferable?

- A. Cancellous bone graft
- B. Cortical bone graft
- C. Vascularized autograft
- D. Bone marrow aspirate
- E. Devascularized bone graft

▸▸ Question 6

Bone growth stimulators are indicated to be used in all of following conditions except?

- A. Diabetes
- B. Inflammatory arthritis
- C. Systemic vascular disease
- D. Malignancy
- E. Cigarette smokers

▸▸ Question 7

Which of the following dural substitutes is absorbable, retains suture, and can be used with dural sealant?

- A. Tutopatch®
- B. Neuro-Patch®
- C. DuraGen®
- D. Durepair®
- E. DuraMatrix®

▸▸ Question 8

What is the lateral limit of safe region for posterior iliac crest bone graft in order to protect superior cluneal nerves crossing iliac crest?

- A. 3 cm
- B. 5 cm
- C. 6 cm
- D. 8 cm
- E. 9 cm

▸▸ Question 9

Indigo carmine is a blue dye that can be used intrathecally to locate CSF leaks. Fluorescein is another dye which can be used intrathecally or IV. Fluorescein is used in diluted form because it can cause which of the following side effects?

- A. Brain stem herniations
- B. Increased ICP
- C. Seizures
- D. Blindness
- E. Memory impairment

▸▸ **Question 10**

A patient is given IT dye after which he/she develops quadriplegia, multiple cranial nerve palsy, dementia, and hydrocephalus. Which dye is given to this patient?

- A. Indigo carmine
- B. Methylene blue
- C. Fluorescein
- D. Indigo cyanine
- E. Ultravist

▸▸ **Question 11**

For spine cases, the ideal location of observer's eye piece is directly opposite the surgeon. For intracranial work, the observer's eye piece is placed to the right of the operators except in which of the following cases where it is placed to the left?

- A. Transsphenoidal surgery
- B. Right posterior fossa craniotomy in lateral oblique position
- C. For supine position surgery with head tilt toward one side
- D. For craniotomy of posterior fossa in prone position
- E. Both A and B

▸▸ **Question 12**

Pin-based head fixation include the Mayfield head holder or head frame. Following are the indications for pin stabilization except?

- A. Craniotomy for most intracranial vascular operations
- B. Craniotomy for most tumor operations especially if there is need of retractor system that attaches to the Mayfield head holder
- C. When intraoperative image guidance system is used
- D. For craniotomy in patients less than 3 years of age
- E. In cervical spine often used for posterior cervical operations

▸▸ **Question 13**

Which of the following are the complications of pin head fixation?

- A. Malposition of pins through unintended anatomic structure like pinna, orbit, superficial artery, or poor fixation by not properly placing pins close to the equator
- B. Skin penetration by pins which can cause injury to intracranial structures
- C. Skin necrosis or skull fracture
- D. Slippage of any of the joints or connections to the OR table or clamp breakage or bleeding from pin site
- E. All of the above

▸▸ **Question 14**

All of the following are included in the mechanical means of hemostasis except?

- A. Bone wax use
- B. Ligature
- C. Use of monopolar or bipolar cautery
- D. Use of silver clips (hemoclips)
- E. None of the above

▸▸ **Question 15**

All of the following are means of chemical hemostasis except?

- A. Gelatin sponge
- B. Oxidized cellulose
- C. Bone wax
- D. Microfibrillar collagen
- E. Thrombin

▸▸ **Question 16**

All of the following are included in the allograft for use as dural substitutes except?

- A. Reconstituted material like processed gelatin
- B. Processed intact natural materials like ovine or bovine
- C. Fascia lata or galea or pericranium
- D. Synthetic materials like polyesterurethane
- E. Biosynthetic materials like cellulose

▸▸ **Question 17**

Which of the following are the components of bone graft that are important for fusion?

- A. Osteoinduction which is recruitment of mesenchymal cells and the stimulation of these cells to develop into osteoblast or osteoclasts
- B. Osteogenesis which is formation of new bone by host or graft mesenchymal stem cells
- C. Osteoconduction which is the structure of the graft that acts as a scaffold upon which new bone and blood vessels form
- D. Mechanical stability which is the structural anatomical biomechanical support
- E. All of the above

▸▸ **Question 18**

Which of the following bone graft material has the best osteogenic property?

- A. Cancellous graft
- B. Cortical autograft
- C. Bone marrow aspirate
- D. Vascularized autograft
- E. Demineralized bone matrix

Answers

▸▸ **Answer 1**

Correct answer is B. Methylene blue[1]

▸▸ Answer 2

Correct answer is E. Not applicable[2]

▸▸ Answer 3

Correct answer is E. < 10,000/mL[3]

▸▸ Answer 4

Correct answer is C. Axial view[4]

▸▸ Answer 5

Correct answer is A. Cancellous bone graft[5]

▸▸ Answer 6

Correct answer is D. Malignancy[6]

▸▸ Answer 7

Correct answer is A. Tutopatch®[3]

▸▸ Answer 8

Correct answer is D. 8 cm[6]

▸▸ Answer 9

Correct answer is C. Seizures[1]

▸▸ Answer 10

Correct answer is B. Methylene blue[1]

▸▸ Answer 11

Correct answer is E. Both A and B[1]

▸▸ Answer 12

Correct answer is D. For craniotomy in patients less than 3 years of age[2]

▸▸ Answer 13

Correct answer is E. All of the above[7]

▸▸ Answer 14

Correct answer is C. Use of monopolar or bipolar cautery[3]

▸▸ Answer 15

Correct answer is C. Bone wax[3]

▸▸ Answer 16

Correct answer is C. Fascia lata or galea or pericranium[3]

▸▸ Answer 17

Correct answer is E. All of the above[5]

▸▸ Answer 18

Correct answer is A. Cancellous graft[5]

References

[1] Greenberg M, ed. Greenberg's Handbook of Neurosurgery. 10th ed. New York: Thieme; 2023:1716
[2] Greenberg M, ed. Greenberg's Handbook of Neurosurgery. 10th ed. New York: Thieme; 2023:1717
[3] Greenberg M, ed. Greenberg's Handbook of Neurosurgery. 10th ed. New York: Thieme; 2023:1719
[4] Greenberg M, ed. Greenberg's Handbook of Neurosurgery. 10th ed. New York: Thieme; 2023:1721
[5] Greenberg M, ed. Greenberg's Handbook of Neurosurgery. 10th ed. New York: Thieme; 2023:1722
[6] Greenberg M, ed. Greenberg's Handbook of Neurosurgery. 10th ed. New York: Thieme; 2023:1725
[7] Greenberg M, ed. Greenberg's Handbook of Neurosurgery. 10th ed. New York: Thieme; 2023:1718

104 Craniotomies—General Information and Cortical Mapping

Questions

▸▸ **Question 1**

Intraoperative brain swelling etiologies include all of the following except?

- A. Extraparenchymal bleeding: from a vessel or intraoperative aneurysm rupture
- B. Intracerebral hemorrhage
- C. Venous outflow obstruction
- D. Vasodilatation induced by hypocarbia
- E. Severe diffuse cerebral edema

▸▸ **Question 2**

What is the last life-saving measure for uncontrollable intraoperative brain swelling?

- A. Reverse Trendelenburg position
- B. Removal of swollen brain
- C. Decompressive craniectomy
- D. Apply pressure on the brain
- E. Place the head in neutral position

▸▸ **Question 3**

Cranioplasty following posterior fossa surgery for vestibular schwannoma reduced the incidence of postoperative headache to how much?

- A. 4%
- B. 17%
- C. 50%
- D. 70%
- E. 100%

▸▸ **Question 4**

What is the incidence of postoperative headache after posterior fossa surgery?

- A. 100%
- B. 80%
- C. 95%
- D. 97%
- E. 90%

▸▸ **Question 5**

A patient who underwent tumor resection and awake craniotomy develops lethargy, confusion, severe headache, nausea, vomiting, and seizures. For awake craniotomy, skull block is being done for which local anesthetic agents injection must be applied at how many regions?

- A. 1 region
- B. 2 regions
- C. 3 regions
- D. 4 regions
- E. 5 regions

▸▸ **Question 6**

Definitive treatment of syndrome of trephination is indicated if headache does not settle within how long?

- A. 2 months
- B. 3 months
- C. 4 months
- D. 5 months
- E. 6 months

▸▸ **Question 7**

During awake craniotomies, what is the maximum current that can be used to stimulate any area of cortex?

- A. 2 mA
- B. 4 mA
- C. 6 mA
- D. 8 mA
- E. 10 mA

▸▸ **Question 8**

Which of the following nerves must not be anesthetized during awake craniotomies?

- A. Supraorbital nerve
- B. Facial nerve
- C. Postauricular nerve
- D. Lesser occipital nerve
- E. Third occipital nerve

▸▸ **Question 9**

During awake craniotomy, total speech arrest occurs by stimulating which area of nondominant hemisphere?

- A. Pars opercularis
- B. Frontal operculum
- C. Posterior middle temporal gyrus
- D. Anterior supramarginal gyrus
- E. None of the above

▸▸ **Question 10**

Which of the following is a contraindication of awake craniotomy?

- A. Thalamic tumor
- B. Epileptic foci in eloquent brain area
- C. Removal of brainstem tumors

- D. Tumor near motor strip
- E. Significant speech/motor deficits

▸▸ Question 11

The FDA released a number of recommendations for use of drill to reduce injury during craniotomy which are the following?

- A. Selection of appropriate perforator based on the skull thickness (pediatric vs. adults)
- B. Keeping the perforator perpendicular to the skull throughout the drilling process
- C. Do on rock, rotate, or change the angel of the device during drilling
- D. Avoid using excessive pressure on the drill
- E. Use caution when drilling through areas of irregular bone contour, curvature, or variations in thickness or drilling where bone might be diseased or incompetent
- F. All of the above

▸▸ Question 12

All of the following are etiologies of intraoperative brain swelling except?

- A. Extraparenchymal bleeding from a vessel or intraoperative aneurysm rupture
- B. Intracerebral hemorrhage
- C. Venous outflow obstruction
- D. Vasoconstriction induced by hypercapnia
- E. Severe diffuse cerebral edema following stroke or traumatic brain injury

▸▸ Question 13

Management of intraoperative brain swelling include finding out the cause and treating that cause. Other measures that should be taken for decreasing brain swelling include which of the following?

- A. Elevation of head of bed
- B. Making sure the jugular veins are not kinked
- C. Ruling out hypercarbia, making sure that endotracheal tube is not kinked, and checking the patient's end tidal pCO_2
- D. Measures to lower ICP are adopted, which includes giving mannitol, draining CSF, tapping and draining ventricle, having the anesthesiologist hyperventilate the patient's pCO_2 to 30 to 35 mmHg
- E. Emergency intubation for patients are undergoing awake craniotomy and intraoperative ultrasound or CT of brain
- F. All of the above

▸▸ Question 14

The overall risk of postoperative hemorrhage is 0.8 to 1.1%. Which hematomas constitute 43 to 60% of these?

- A. Intraparenchymal
- B. Epidural
- C. Subdural
- D. Intrasellar
- E. Mixed

▸▸ Question 15

What are the postoperative medications that are given to a patient after craniotomy for brain tumor?

- A. Dexamethasone and H2 antagonist
- B. Antiepileptic drugs
- C. Cardene drip to keep systolic BP less than 160 mmHg and diastolic BP less than 100 mmHg
- D. Prophylactic antibiotics are continued
- E. Acetaminophen and codeine are also given for pain relief
- F. All of the above

▸▸ Question 16

All of the following are causes of postoperative deterioration of patients after craniotomy except?

- A. Hematoma or cerebral infarction (from compromise of normal arteries or veins)
- B. Postoperative seizures or acute hydrocephalus
- C. Syringomyelia formation
- D. Pneumocephalus or brain edema
- E. Persistent anesthetic effect or vasospasm

▸▸ Question 17

What are the causes of postoperative headache in a patient after craniotomy?

- A. Traction of the dura when the bone is not replaced
- B. Traction on dura due to tight dural closure
- C. Temporalis or nuchal muscle dissection
- D. Nerve entrapment in the closing suture or healing scar
- E. Intradural blood and/or CSF leak
- F. All of the above

▸▸ Question 18

Phase reversal technique can be used to see primary sensory or motor cortex. What is the use of intraoperative cortical mapping in a patient undergoing craniotomy?

- A. Motor strip localization
- B. Sensory cortex localization
- C. Speech centers determination
- D. All of the above

▸▸ Question 19

Indications of awake craniotomy include surgery in eloquent brain area, removal of brain stem tumors, or for some seizure surgery to look for seizure focus. All of the following are contraindications of awake craniotomy except?

- A. Patients who are unable to cooperate

- B. Very young or very elderly patients
- C. Confused patients
- D. Those with significant speech deficit already present
- E. Those with no language barrier

▸▸ Question 20

What is the typical sequence of anesthesia in case of awake craniotomy?
- A. In the preoperative holding area, precedex is started
- B. Induction of anesthesia is given using propofol and skull block is applied
- C. Inhalational anesthesia is started and continued until dura starts to open, at which point inhalational anesthesia is stopped
- D. Remifentanil is given for pain control with neurophysiologic resting performed at this time
- E. Once the intracranial part of the operation is complete, general anesthesia is given again and the operation is completed
- F. All of the following

Answers

▸▸ Answer 1

Correct answer is D. Vasodilatation induced by hypocarbia[1]

▸▸ Answer 2

Correct answer is B. Removal of swollen brain[1]

▸▸ Answer 3

Correct answer is A. 4%[2]

▸▸ Answer 4

Correct answer is B. 80%[2]

▸▸ Answer 5

Correct answer is D. 4 regions[3]

▸▸ Answer 6

Correct answer is B. 3 months[2]

▸▸ Answer 7

Correct answer is E. 10 mA[4]

▸▸ Answer 8

Correct answer is B. Facial nerve[3]

▸▸ Answer 9

Correct answer is A. Pars opercularis[4]

▸▸ Answer 10

Correct answer is E. Significant speech/motor deficits[3]

▸▸ Answer 11

Correct answer is F. All of the above[1]

▸▸ Answer 12

Correct answer is D. Vasoconstriction induced by hypercapnia[1]

▸▸ Answer 13

Correct answer is F. All of the above[1]

▸▸ Answer 14

Correct answer is A. Intraparenchymal[5]

▸▸ Answer 15

Correct answer is F. All of the above[2]

▸▸ Answer 16

Correct answer is C. Syringomyelia formation[2]

▸▸ Answer 17

Correct answer is F. All of the above[2]

▸▸ Answer 18

Correct answer is D. All of the above[6]

▸▸ Answer 19

Correct answer is E. Those with no language barrier[3]

▸▸ Answer 20

Correct answer is F. All of the following[7]

References

[1] Greenberg M, ed. Greenberg's Handbook of Neurosurgery. 10th ed. New York: Thieme; 2023:1728
[2] Greenberg M, ed. Greenberg's Handbook of Neurosurgery. 10th ed. New York: Thieme; 2023:1731
[3] Greenberg M, ed. Greenberg's Handbook of Neurosurgery. 10th ed. New York: Thieme; 2023:1733

[4] Greenberg M, ed. Greenberg's Handbook of Neurosurgery. 10th ed. New York: Thieme; 2023:1735

[5] Greenberg M, ed. Greenberg's Handbook of Neurosurgery. 10th ed. New York: Thieme; 2023:1729

[6] Greenberg M, ed. Greenberg's Handbook of Neurosurgery. 10th ed. New York: Thieme; 2023:1732

[7] Greenberg M, ed. Greenberg's Handbook of Neurosurgery. 10th ed. New York: Thieme; 2023:1734

105 Posterior Fossa Craniotomies

Questions

▸▸ Question 1

Advantages of sitting position for posterior fossa craniotomies include improved drainage of blood and CSF out of the surgical site, enhanced venous drainage which helps reduce venous bleeding, easy ventilation, and patients' head can be kept at exactly midline. Which of the following are included in the disadvantages of sitting position?

- A. Possible air embolism
- B. Fatigue of operator's hand and risk of postoperative hematoma at the surgical site
- C. Possible brachial plexus injury and mid cervical quadriplegia
- D. Extent of postoperative pneumocephalus is more pronounced and venous pooling of blood in the lower extremities
- E. All of the above

▸▸ Question 2

Air embolism is suspected in any operative case in which the surgical site is higher than the heart. Transesophageal echocardiography and precordial Doppler ultrasound are the tests to see air embolism in heart. Following are included in the treatment of air embolism except?

- A. The site of air entry is found and occluded and the patient's head is lowered if at all possible
- B. Jugular venous compression or aspiration of air from right atrium
- C. Nitrous oxide is given if it is not being used
- D. Patient is ventilated with 100% oxygen
- E. Pressors volume expanders are used to maintain blood pressure

▸▸ Question 3

Lateral oblique position is also known as Park Bench position. Axillary roll is used for the down-side arm and upper arm is supported on pillows or towels. Adhesive tape is used to pull down the upper shoulder. Thorax is usually elevated to what degrees in such cases?

- A. 10 to 15 degrees
- B. 20 to 25 degrees
- C. 30 to 35 degrees
- D. 40 to 45 degrees
- E. It is kept flat

▸▸ Question 4

Indications for paramedian suboccipital craniectomy include all of the following except?

- A. Access to CPA lesions like vestibular schwannoma or for microvascular decompression
- B. For lesions in the cerebellar hemisphere
- C. For access to the posterior communicating artery aneurysms
- D. For access to the vertebral artery for aneurysms or for vertebral endarterectomy
- E. For access to the anterolateral brain stem

▸▸ Question 5

Which of the following statements are correct regarding access to CP angle lesions through paramedian incision?

- A. A slightly curved retromastoid incision is made 5 mm medial to the mastoid notch
- B. 5–4-6 incision (5 mm medial to mastoid notch, 6 cm above notch, and 4 cm below notch) is made for approach to the fifth nerve like in microvascular decompression
- C. 5–5-5 incision (5 mm medial to mastoid notch, 5 cm above notch, and 5 cm below notch) is used for microvascular decompression for hemifacial spasm or for small vestibular schwannoma
- D. 5–4-6 incision (5 mm medial to notch, 4 cm above notch, and 6 cm below notch) is used for glossopharyngeal neuralgia
- E. All of the above

▸▸ Question 6

For microvascular decompression, a craniectomy of 2 cm is used in the angle between transverse sinus and sigmoid sinus while for small tumors (< 2.5 cm), a 4-cm craniectomy is used in the same space. What are the boundaries of craniectomy for large tumors?

- A. Transverse sinus superiorly
- B. Foramen magnum inferiorly
- C. Sigmoid sinus laterally
- D. Midline medially
- E. All of the above

▸▸ Question 7

Burr hole for placement of emergency ventriculostomy is done at Frazier point which is 3 to 4 cm from midline and how much distance from the inion?

- A. 6 to 7 cm above the inion
- B. 3 to 4 cm above the inion
- C. 6 to 7 cm above the inion in adults, while 3 to 4 cm above inion in children
- D. 8 cm above inion in adults, while 5 cm above inion in children
- E. None of the above

►► **Question 8**

For midline suboccipital craniectomies, Y-shaped durotomy is often used and craniectomy is done with no intention of replacing the bone. What is the advantage of not replacing the bone at this location?

- A. It is cumbersome to place bone here
- B. It can dip into cerebellum when the patient lies on head
- C. It there is postoperative swelling, the inelastic bone will cause more pressure to be transmitted to the brainstem
- D. There is more chance of postoperative infection if bone is placed
- E. None of the above

►► **Question 9**

The two main approaches for the 4th ventricle are transvermian approach and telovelar approach. Following statements are correct regarding these approaches except?

- A. Transvermian approach gives wider and slightly more rostral exposure than telovelar approach
- B. The risks of caudal vermis syndrome, cerebellar mutism, and injury to caudate nucleus are more in case of transvermian approach
- C. No nerve tissue is harmed in case of telovelar approach
- D. Telovelar approach causes decreased access to the lateral recess of the 4th ventricle
- E. Telovelar approach provides narrower corridor as compared to transvermian approach

►► **Question 10**

The causes of CSF fistula are abnormal CSF hydrodynamics, poor wound closure, or subarachnoid scarring. The treatment of CSF fistula includes elevation of the head of bed, lumbar subarachnoid drainage, reinforcement of skin incisions, or surgical correction. What are the treatment options for suboccipital pseudomeningocele?

- A. Noninvasive measures like expectant management, fluid restriction, head wrapping, keeping head of bed elevated, and acetazolamide use
- B. Percutaneous aspiration
- C. Direct surgical exploration with multilayer closure
- D. Lumbar drainage or ventricular drainage
- E. All of the above

Answers

►► **Answer 1**

Correct answer is E. All of the above[1]

►► **Answer 2**

Correct answer is C. Nitrous oxide is given if it is not being used[2]

►► **Answer 3**

Correct answer is A. 10 to 15 degrees[3]

►► **Answer 4**

Correct answer is C. For access to the posterior communicating artery aneurysms[4]

►► **Answer 5**

Correct answer is E. All of the above[5]

►► **Answer 6**

Correct answer is E. All of the above[6]

►► **Answer 7**

Correct answer is C. 6 to 7 cm above the inion in adults, while 3 to 4 cm above inion in children[7]

►► **Answer 8**

Correct answer is C. It there is postoperative swelling, the inelastic bone will cause more pressure to be transmitted to the brainstem[8]

►► **Answer 9**

Correct answer is D. Telovelar approach causes decreased access to the lateral recess of the 4th ventricle[9]

►► **Answer 10**

Correct answer is E. All of the above[10]

References

[1] Greenberg M, ed. Greenberg's Handbook of Neurosurgery. 10th ed. New York: Thieme; 2023:1737

[2] Greenberg M, ed. Greenberg's Handbook of Neurosurgery. 10th ed. New York: Thieme; 2023:1738

[3] Greenberg M, ed. Greenberg's Handbook of Neurosurgery. 10th ed. New York: Thieme; 2023:1739

[4] Greenberg M, ed. Greenberg's Handbook of Neurosurgery. 10th ed. New York: Thieme; 2023:1740

[5] Greenberg M, ed. Greenberg's Handbook of Neurosurgery. 10th ed. New York: Thieme; 2023: 1740

[6] Greenberg M, ed. Greenberg's Handbook of Neurosurgery. 10th ed. New York: Thieme; 2023:1742

[7] Greenberg M, ed. Greenberg's Handbook of Neurosurgery. 10th ed. New York: Thieme; 2023: 1742

[8] Greenberg M, ed. Greenberg's Handbook of Neurosurgery. 10th ed. New York: Thieme; 2023:1743

[9] Greenberg M, ed. Greenberg's Handbook of Neurosurgery. 10th ed. New York: Thieme; 2023:1744

[10] Greenberg M, ed. Greenberg's Handbook of Neurosurgery. 10th ed. New York: Thieme; 2023:1746

106 Supratentorial Craniotomies

Questions

▸▸ **Question 1**

Which of the following is not an ideal indication of pterional craniotomy?

- A. All aneurysms of anterior circulation
- B. Basilar tip aneurysms
- C. Direct surgical approach to cavernous sinus
- D. Primarily sellar PitNET
- E. Craniopharyngioma

▸▸ **Question 2**

What is the head rotation required in pterional craniotomy for exposure of Acom artery aneurysm?

- A. 30 degrees from vertical
- B. 45 degrees from vertical
- C. 60 degrees from vertical
- D. 75 degrees from vertical
- E. 90 degrees from vertical

▸▸ **Question 3**

What must be linear incision for small craniectomy in temporal region for laterally located vestibular schwannoma?

- A. 0.5 cm anterior to the EAC, extending 7 to 8 cm above the zygomatic arch
- B. 1 cm anterior to the EAC, extending 7 to 8 cm above the zygomatic arch
- C. 0.5 cm anterior to the EAC, extending 3 to 4 cm above the zygomatic arch
- D. 2 cm anterior to the EAC, extending 7 to 8 cm above the zygomatic arch
- E. 1.5 cm anterior to the EAC, extending 7 to 8 cm above the zygomatic arch

▸▸ **Question 4**

Without the use of mapping techniques to localize speech, one can usually safely resect up to how much from the temporal tip in dominant hemisphere?

- A. 3 to 4 cm
- B. 4 to 5 cm
- C. 6 to 7 cm
- D. 7 to 8 cm
- E. 1 to 2 cm

▸▸ **Question 5**

Which of the following points is not considered a danger point during frontal craniotomy?

- A. Motor speech area
- B. Anterior cerebral artery
- C. Sensory speech area
- D. Superior sagittal sinus
- E. Corpus callosum

▸▸ **Question 6**

Sylvian fissure is considered a danger point in temporal craniotomy owing to the presence of which structure?

- A. ACA
- B. MCA
- C. Wernicke's area
- D. Sylvian vein
- E. None of the above

▸▸ **Question 7**

All of the following are indications of pterional craniotomies except?

- A. For aneurysms which include anterior circular aneurysms and basilar tip aneurysms
- B. Direct surgical approach to cavernous sinus
- C. Suprasellar tumors like pituitary adenoma or craniopharyngioma
- D. Third ventricular tumors like colloid cyst
- E. Sphenoid wing meningioma tumors

▸▸ **Question 8**

For pterional approach, skin incision is started 1 cm anterior to the tragus from the zygomatic arch with curving slightly anteriorly and staying behind the hairline to widow's peak. Which of the following statements are correct regarding position of head?

- A. It is kept 30 degrees from vertical for posterior exposure, for example, for ICA, P comm, carotid terminus, or basilar bifurcation aneurysms
- B. 45 degrees from vertical for middle exposure, for example, for ICA–MCA aneurysms
- C. 60 degrees from vertical for anterior circle of Willis exposure, for example, for a-comm aneurysms, suprasellar tumors
- D. All of the above

▸▸ **Question 9**

The sylvian fissure can be exposed by starting at a point where the carotid artery penetrates the fissure and working laterally (which is easier when prolific veins overlie the junction of the frontal and temporal lobes) or by working from lateral aspect of fissure medially. Which artery crosses the sylvian fissure which needs to be spared during opening of fissure?

- A. Middle cerebral artery
- B. Anterior cerebral artery
- C. Internal carotid artery
- D. Artery of sylvian fissure
- E. No artery crosses the sylvian fissure

▸▸ Question 10

Which of the following are the indications of temporal craniotomy?

- A. Temporal lobe biopsy or temporal lobectomy
- B. Temporal lobe hematoma evacuation or tumors of temporal lobe
- C. Small laterally placed vestibular schwannomas or for access to the floor of the middle cranial fossa
- D. Access to the medial temporal lobe
- E. All of the above

▸▸ Question 11

To access the temporal tip, incision is placed midway between the lateral canthus and which of the following?

- A. Mastoid notch
- B. Tragus
- C. External auditory canal
- D. Inion
- E. Mastoid tip

▸▸ Question 12

For dominant temporal lobe lobectomy, safe resection up to 4 to 5 cm from the temporal tip can be used, while on nondominant hemisphere, it is 6 to 7 cm. It is best to amputate the temporal lobe backward from the tip and medially up to incisura to prevent damage to brainstem. What structure of brain is at risk of injury at this region?

- A. Broca's area
- B. Wernicke's area
- C. Motor cortex
- D. Auditory brain cortex
- E. None of the above

▸▸ Question 13

Which of the following are the indications of frontal craniotomy?

- A. Access to the frontal lobe of brain for infiltrating brain tumors
- B. Approach to the 3rd ventricle
- C. Approach to sellar tumors in some situations
- D. Repair of ethmoidal CSF fistula
- E. All of the above

▸▸ Question 14

Danger points in case of frontal craniotomy are the following except?

- A. Anterior cerebral arteries in midline
- B. Injury to Wernicke's area
- C. Injury to superior sagittal sinus with excessive bleeding
- D. Injury to corpus callosum
- E. Injury to Broca's area

▸▸ Question 15

What is the most commonly injured artery during deep dissection of the sylvian fissure?

- A. Middle cerebral artery
- B. Anterior cerebral artery
- C. Internal carotid artery
- D. Anterior choroidal artery
- E. None of the above

▸▸ Question 16

Large bifrontal skin incision from ear to ear is also known what?

- A. Pterional skin incision
- B. Modified Frazier's incision
- C. Souttar skin incision
- D. Frontal temporal zygomatic skin incision
- E. None of the above

Answers

▸▸ Answer 1

Correct answer is D. Primarily sellar PitNET[1]

▸▸ Answer 2

Correct answer is C. 60 degrees from vertical[2]

▸▸ Answer 3

Correct answer is A. 0.5 cm anterior to the EAC, extending 7 to 8 cm above the zygomatic arch[3]

▸▸ Answer 4

Correct answer is B. 4 to 5 cm[4]

▸▸ Answer 5

Correct answer is C. Sensory speech area[5]

▸▸ Answer 6

Correct answer is B. MCA[5]

▸▸ Answer 7

Correct answer is D. Third ventricular tumors like colloid cyst[1]

►► Answer 8

Correct answer is D. All of the above[2]

►► Answer 9

Correct answer is E. No artery crosses the sylvian fissure[6]

►► Answer 10

Correct answer is E. All of the above[7]

►► Answer 11

Correct answer is C. External auditory canal[3]

►► Answer 12

Correct answer is B. Wernicke's area[4]

►► Answer 13

Correct answer is E. All of the above[5]

►► Answer 14

Correct answer is B. Injury to Wernicke's area[5]

►► Answer 15

Correct answer is A. Middle cerebral artery[4]

►► Answer 16

Correct answer is C. Souttar skin incision[5]

References

[1] Greenberg M, ed. Greenberg's Handbook of Neurosurgery. 10th ed. New York: Thieme; 2023:1748
[2] Greenberg M, ed. Greenberg's Handbook of Neurosurgery. 10th ed. New York: Thieme; 2023:1749
[3] Greenberg M, ed. Greenberg's Handbook of Neurosurgery. 10th ed. New York: Thieme; 2023:1752
[4] Greenberg M, ed. Greenberg's Handbook of Neurosurgery. 10th ed. New York: Thieme; 2023:1753
[5] Greenberg M, ed. Greenberg's Handbook of Neurosurgery. 10th ed. New York: Thieme; 2023:1754
[6] Greenberg M, ed. Greenberg's Handbook of Neurosurgery. 10th ed. New York: Thieme; 2023:1750
[7] Greenberg M, ed. Greenberg's Handbook of Neurosurgery. 10th ed. New York: Thieme; 2023:1751

107 Approaches to the Lateral and Third Ventricles, Decompressive Craniectomies, and Cranioplasty

Questions

▸▸ Question 1

Which of following approaches to trigone of lateral ventricles is not used if neurology of the patient is intact?

- A. Lateral temporal parietal
- B. Superior parietal occipital
- C. Tanscallosal
- D. Transtemporal horn
- E. Occipital lobe incision or occipital lobectomy

▸▸ Question 2

Which approach is preferred for tumors in the 3rd ventricle extending into lateral ventricle with gross hydrocephalus?

- A. Transcallosal approach
- B. Transsphenoidal approach
- C. Transcortical approach
- D. Subfrontal approach
- E. Subtemporal approach

▸▸ Question 3

What are the parameters for craniotomy while using transcallosal approach to the 3rd ventricle so as to preserve important structures?

- A. 3 cm anterior and 3 cm posterior to coronal suture
- B. 4 cm anterior and 3 cm posterior to coronal suture
- C. 2 cm anterior and 4 cm posterior to coronal suture
- D. 4 cm anterior and 2 cm posterior to coronal suture
- E. 4 cm anterior and 4 cm posterior to coronal suture

▸▸ Question 4

To prevent complication of disconnection syndrome, callosotomy performed must not exceed how much?

- A. 0.5 cm
- B. 2.5 cm
- C. 3.5 cm
- D. 4.5 cm
- E. 1.5 cm

▸▸ Question 5

Bilateral forniceal lesions can result in loss of short-term memory and ability for new learning, which can be avoided while approaching the 3rd ventricle via all methods except?

- A. Stay as close to midline as possible
- B. If needed open foramen of Monro laterally
- C. Making incision posteriorly sacrificing thalamostriate vein
- D. Incising the anterosuperior margin of the foramen through the column of both fornices
- E. Interforniceal approach

▸▸ Question 6

After decompressive craniectomy, bone flap can be stored externally for future reimplantation by saturating with sterile preservative solution (e.g., RPMI medium). It must be stored at what temperature?

- A. −80°C
- B. −70°C
- C. −60°C
- D. −50°C
- E. −40°C

▸▸ Question 7

In noncontaminated situations, cranioplasty can be done after how long?

- A. 1 to 2 weeks
- B. 3 to 4 weeks
- C. 5 to 10 weeks
- D. 6 to 12 weeks
- E. 6 months

▸▸ Question 8

For transcallosal approach to the lateral or third ventricle, thorax should be elevated up to what degrees?

- A. 10 degrees
- B. 20 degrees
- C. 30 degrees
- D. 40 degrees
- E. 50 degrees

▸▸ Question 9

Which of the following statements are correct regarding approaches to the lateral ventricle?

- A. Approaches to the atrium (trigone) include middle temporal gyrus, lateral temporal parietal approach, superior parietal occipital approach, transcallosal, transtemporal horn, and through occipital lobe incision or occipital lobectomy
- B. Approach to frontal horn is through middle frontal gyrus
- C. Midventricular body approach includes through transcallosal and middle frontal gyrus approach
- D. Temporal horn is approached by dissection through middle temporal gyrus and transtemporal horn
- E. All of the above

▸▸ Question 10

Approaches to the third ventricle include which of the following?

- A. Transcortical approach
- B. Transcallosal approach
- C. Subfrontal approach
- D. Transsphenoidal approach
- E. Subtemporal approach
- F. All of the above

▸▸ Question 11

Transcallosal approach to the lateral or third ventricle is performed through an interhemispheric approach to the corpus callosum via a parietal craniotomy, usually right sided in a left hemisphere dominant patient. Following statements are correct regarding indications of this approach except?

- A. Colloid cysts is excised through this approach
- B. Craniopharyngiomas in the third ventricle can also be approached through this approach
- C. Cysticercosis cyst cannot be removed through this approach
- D. Thalamic gliomas can also be removed using this approach
- E. AVM can also be excised using this approach

▸▸ Question 12

During approach to corpus callosum through interhemispheric approach, the two cingulate gyri can be easily mistaken for the corpus callosum. This error may be compounded by mistaking the callosomarginal arteries for the pericallosal arteries. What are the differentiating points between corpus callosum and cingulate gyrus?

- A. Corpus callosum is a pure white structure
- B. Corpus callosum is usually deeper than one anticipates
- C. Corpus callosum is appreciated beneath the paired pericallosal arteries
- D. Image-guided surgery or measuring the depth of the corpus callosum on the preoperative MRI may help
- E. All of the above are correct

▸▸ Question 13

The callosotomy is usually performed between the two pericallosal arteries. Disconnection syndrome can occur with it which is more common with posterior callosotomy where more information crosses. The risk is reduced by creating the callosotomy of what distance?

- A. < 5.5 cm
- B. < 4.5 cm
- C. < 3.5 cm
- D. < 2.5 cm
- E. < 1.5 cm

▸▸ Question 14

Venous infarction during interhemispheric approach can occur because of which of the following?

- A. Damage to the critical cortical draining veins
- B. Damage or thrombosis of superior sagittal sinus
- C. Damage to thalamostriate veins
- D. Damage to vein of Trolard
- E. Both A and B

▸▸ Question 15

Transcortical approach to the lateral or third ventricle is used for tumors of atrium of lateral ventricle, tumor of the roof of the third ventricle, or third ventricular tumors with significant extension onto lateral ventricle. Which of the following are the approaches included in transcortical approach?

- A. Posterior parietal approach
- B. Middle temporal gyrus
- C. Middle frontal gyrus
- D. All of the above

▸▸ Question 16

Indications for cranioplasty include cosmetic restoration of the external skull appearance, relief of symptoms (pain or tenderness, syndrome of trephined or focal deficit related to the defect), protection from trauma, reduction of irritation of brain, and improving from cognitive deficits. Contraindications of cranioplasty include infection, brain protruding from the confines of skull, or untreated hydrocephalus. What materials can be used for cranioplasty?

- A. The patient's own bone
- B. Polymethylmethacrylate (PMMA)
- C. Titanium
- D. Prefabricated custom bone flaps like PMMA, polyether ether ketone, titanium, or acrylic
- E. Split-thickness calvaria
- F. All of the above

▸▸ Question 17

Which of the following is the complication of cranioplasty that constitutes 8% of total complications?

- A. Infection
- B. Hematoma (epidural or subdural)
- C. Seizures
- D. Brain injury
- E. Hydrocephalus

▸▸ Question 18

For noncontaminated situations like stroke, re-implantation can be considered after about how long?

- A. 2 to 4 weeks
- B. 6 to 12 weeks
- C. 2 to 4 months
- D. 8 to 10 months
- E. None of the above

Answers

▸▸ Answer 1

Correct answer is E. Occipital lobe incision or occipital lobectomy[1]

▸▸ Answer 2

Correct answer is C. Transcortical approach[1]

▸▸ Answer 3

Correct answer is D. 4 cm anterior and 2 cm posterior to coronal suture[2]

▸▸ Answer 4

Correct answer is B. 2.5 cm[3]

▸▸ Answer 5

Correct answer is D. Incising the anterosuperior margin of the foramen through the column of both fornices[3]

▸▸ Answer 6

Correct answer is A. −80° C[4]

▸▸ Answer 7

Correct answer is D. 6 to 12 weeks[4]

▸▸ Answer 8

Correct answer is B. 20 degrees[2]

▸▸ Answer 9

Correct answer is E. All of the above[1]

▸▸ Answer 10

Correct answer is F. All of the above[1]

▸▸ Answer 11

Correct answer is C. Cysticercosis cyst cannot be removed through this approach[2]

▸▸ Answer 12

Correct answer is E. All of the above are correct[3]

▸▸ Answer 13

Correct answer is D. < 2.5 cm[3]

▸▸ Answer 14

Correct answer is E. Both A and B[5]

▸▸ Answer 15

Correct answer is D. All of the above[6]

▸▸ Answer 16

Correct answer is F. All of the above[4]

▸▸ Answer 17

Correct answer is A. Infection[4]

▸▸ Answer 18

Correct answer is B. 6 to 12 weeks[7]

References

[1] Greenberg M, ed. Greenberg's Handbook of Neurosurgery. 10th ed. New York: Thieme; 2023:1757
[2] Greenberg M, ed. Greenberg's Handbook of Neurosurgery. 10th ed. New York: Thieme; 2023:1758
[3] Greenberg M, ed. Greenberg's Handbook of Neurosurgery. 10th ed. New York: Thieme; 2023:1760
[4] Greenberg M, ed. Greenberg's Handbook of Neurosurgery. 10th ed. New York: Thieme; 2023:1764
[5] Greenberg M, ed. Greenberg's Handbook of Neurosurgery. 10th ed. New York: Thieme; 2023:1761
[6] Greenberg M, ed. Greenberg's Handbook of Neurosurgery. 10th ed. New York: Thieme; 2023:1762
[7] Greenberg M, ed. Greenberg's Handbook of Neurosurgery. 10th ed. New York: Thieme; 2023:1766

108 Spine—Cervical

Questions

▸▸ **Question 1**

What is the percentage of patients undergoing transoral removal of the odontoid process who required posterior fusion afterwards due to ligamentous instability?

- A. 20%
- B. 45%
- C. 75%
- D. 80%
- E. 90%

▸▸ **Question 2**

Transoral approach for odontoidectomy is preferred if the patient is able to open mouth up to how much?

- A. 55 mm
- B. 45 mm
- C. 35 mm
- D. 25 mm
- E. 15 mm

▸▸ **Question 3**

What is the range of motion reduced after occipitocervical fusion?

- A. Flexion/extension: reduced by 30%
- B. Lateral rotation: 15 degrees is lost
- C. Lateral bending: 8 degrees is lost
- D. Flexion/extension: reduced by 20%
- E. Both A and C

▸▸ **Question 4**

What screws are used for atlanto-occipital transarticular fusion?

- A. 22 to 24 mm cannulated lag screws
- B. 24 to 28 mm cannulated lag screws
- C. 28 to 32 mm cannulated lag screws
- D. 32 to 34 mm cannulated lag screws
- E. 34 to 36 mm cannulated lag screws

▸▸ **Question 5**

All of the following are considered to be contraindications of anterior odontoid fixation?

- A. All fractures of the C2 vertebral body
- B. Disruption of transverse atlantal ligament (TAL)
- C. Large odontoid fracture gap
- D. Irreducible fracture
- E. Pathological odontoid fracture

▸▸ **Question 6**

While drilling for placement of C2 pedicle screws, if brisk bleeding occurs after withdrawing the drill, what is the next best step?

- A. Abort procedure immediately
- B. Placement of screw at drilled site
- C. Screw placement on both sides
- D. Securing hemostasis by locating the bleed site
- E. None of the above

▸▸ **Question 7**

For LMS placement by Magerl method where is the entry point?

- A. 2 mm medial to midpoint
- B. 3 mm medial to midpoint
- C. 1 mm medial to midpoint
- D. 2 mm superior to midpoint
- E. 2 mm inferior to midpoint

▸▸ **Question 8**

Which of the following are the anterior approaches to the cervical spine?

- A. Anterior odontoid screw
- B. For upper cervical spine (c1–c3) transoral approach including odontoidectomy
- C. For upper cervical spine (c1–c3) extrapharyngeal approach including medial extrapharyngeal approach and lateral extrapharyngeal approach
- D. For c3–c7 cervical spine, standard anterior cervical diskectomy approach is used
- E. All of the above

▸▸ **Question 9**

Indications for anterior transoral odontoidectomy includes anterior extradural compression of the cervicomedullary junction as with pannus from rheumatoid arthritis, irreducible basilar invagination, tumors of c2, or infection. Following are the preoperative requirements for transoral approach except?

- A. Patient's mouth can be opened at least up to 25 mm. If not, then other approaches like translabiomandibular should be considered
- B. For conditions resulting in malalignment or basilar invagination, cervical traction for 1 or more days is sometimes required
- C. Radiographic evaluation cervical MRI with and without contrast to define the soft tissue pathology, and CT of the craniocervical junction with sagittal and coronal reconstruction
- D. Intradural pathology is best dealt with this approach because watertight dural closure is easier and there are very

low chances of postoperative meningitis in case of intradural pathology
- E. CTA should be done to assess position and involvement of the vertebral arteries. Measuring the distance between vertebral arteries provides useful information

▸▸ Question 10

Which of the following statements are correct regarding transoral surgery?
- A. Video laryngoscope and second choice fiberoptic bronchoscopy are now the intubation methods of choice
- B. Three-point fixation with a Mayfield head holder is typically used
- C. A specialized retractor, for example, Crockard transoral retractor or a conventional Dingman retractor, is used
- D. The tubercle of the atlas can be palpated through the posterior pharynx to locate the midline and for craniocaudal orientation with infiltration of mucosa of posterior pharynx with 1% lidocaine with epinephrine
- E. A 3-cm long vertical incision is used with a working window of 20 to 25 mm between the two vertebral arteries
- F. Occipitocervical fusion or posterior c1–c2 arthrodesis is often used in case of basilar invagination or c1–c2 instability alone respectively
- G. All of the above

▸▸ Question 11

Indications of occipitocervical fusion includes traumatic occipitoatlantal dislocation, absence of a complete arch of c1, congenital anomalies of the occipitocervical joints, upward migration of odontoid into the foramen magnum, or marked irreducible shifts of c1 or c2. The occipital screws are cortical screws (narrow pitched) with distal blunt tip (to avoid dural injury) and have dimensions of 4.5-mm diameter or 8- to 12-mm length. Following are the options of occipitocervical fusion except?
- A. Keel plate (placed centrally over the thickest portion of the occipital bone) which is connected via rods to the cervical screws (c2 pedicle screw and c3 lateral mass screws)
- B. Occipital condyle–C1 polyaxial screws
- C. Occipital–c1 (also known as atlantooccipital) transarticular screws
- D. c1–c2 transarticular screws
- E. Looped rod wired to the occiput via wire cables placed through holes drilled in the occiput which reduces the range of motion to only 31% of normal

▸▸ Question 12

The entry point of occipital condyle screws is 4 to 5 mm lateral to foramen magnum and 1 to 2 mm rostral to the atlantooccipital joint. Screws are 3.5-mm diameter polyaxial screws and bicortical purchase is obtained using screws of 20- to 24-mm length. Following are the structures that are needed to be preserved while using these screws except?
- A. Hypoglossal nerve in hypoglossal canal
- B. Carotid arteries
- C. Vertebral arteries
- D. Accessory nerve
- E. Jugular bulb

▸▸ Question 13

Horizontal skin incision is given at c5–c6 level for anterior odontoid screw fixation. Indication for this procedure is a reducible odontoid type 2 fracture or type 3 fracture where fracture line is in the cephalad portion of the body of c2 in an elderly patient. Which of the following are the contraindications of this procedure?
- A. Fracture of c2 vertebral body
- B. Disruption of transverse atlantal ligament
- C. Large odontoid fracture gap
- D. Irreducible fracture
- E. Patients with short thick neck and barrel chest or pathologic odontoid fracture
- F. All of the above

▸▸ Question 14

Indications of atlantoaxial fusion includes instability of c1–c2 joint due to incompetence of transverse atlantal ligament or because of incompetence of odontoid process, hangman's fracture, or vertebrobasilar insufficiency. How much of head rotation is lost after c1–c2 fusion?
- A. 30%
- B. 40%
- C. 50%
- D. 60%
- E. 70%

▸▸ Question 15

Which of the following are the surgical options for c1–c2 fusion?
- A. Rigid instrumentation with c1 lateral mass and c2 pedicle screws
- B. Posterior cervical wiring and fusion
- C. Halifax clamps and fusion
- D. Odontoid compression screws
- E. Combined anterolateral and posterior bone grafting
- F. All of the above

▸▸ Question 16

Options for c2 screws include which of the following?
- A. Pedicle screws
- B. Lateral mass screws
- C. c1–c2 transarticular screws
- D. Translaminar screws
- E. All of the above

▸▸ **Question 17**

Cervical laminoplasty is a procedure which is similar to laminectomy except that the decompressed posterior elements are not removed. Following are the advantages of this procedure except?

- A. Lower incidence of postoperative kyphosis
- B. It might protect against some posterior trauma
- C. There is no impact on postoperative range of motion in extension after this procedure
- D. Provides decompression of cervical cord
- E. None of the above

Answers

▸▸ **Answer 1**

Correct answer is C. 75%

▸▸ **Answer 2**

Correct answer is D. 25 mm[1]

▸▸ **Answer 3**

Correct answer is E. Both A and C[2]

▸▸ **Answer 4**

Correct answer is C. 28 to 32 mm cannulated lag screws[3]

▸▸ **Answer 5**

Correct answer is A. All fractures of the C2 vertebral body[4]

▸▸ **Answer 6**

Correct answer is B. Placement of screw at drilled site[5]

▸▸ **Answer 7**

Correct answer is A. 2 mm medial to midpoint[6]

▸▸ **Answer 8**

Correct answer is E. All of the above[1]

▸▸ **Answer 9**

Correct answer is D. Intradural pathology is best dealt with this approach because watertight dural closure is easier and there are very low chances of postoperative meningitis in case of intradural pathology[7]

▸▸ **Answer 10**

Correct answer is G. All of the above[2]

▸▸ **Answer 11**

Correct answer is D. c1–c2 transarticular screws[3]

▸▸ **Answer 12**

Correct answer is D. Accessory nerve[3]

▸▸ **Answer 13**

Correct answer is F. All of the above[8]

▸▸ **Answer 14**

Correct answer is C. 50%[5]

▸▸ **Answer 15**

Correct answer is F. All of the above[10]

▸▸ **Answer 16**

Correct answer is E. All of the above[11]

▸▸ **Answer 17**

Correct answer is C. There is no impact on postoperative range of motion in extension after this procedure[12]

References

[1] Greenberg M, ed. Greenberg's Handbook of Neurosurgery. 10th ed. New York: Thieme; 2023:1771
[2] Greenberg M, ed. Greenberg's Handbook of Neurosurgery. 10th ed. New York: Thieme; 2023:1773
[3] Greenberg M, ed. Greenberg's Handbook of Neurosurgery. 10th ed. New York: Thieme; 2023:1774
[4] Greenberg M, ed. Greenberg's Handbook of Neurosurgery. 10th ed. New York: Thieme; 2023:1775
[5] Greenberg M, ed. Greenberg's Handbook of Neurosurgery. 10th ed. New York: Thieme; 2023:17780
[6] Greenberg M, ed. Greenberg's Handbook of Neurosurgery. 10th ed. New York: Thieme; 2023:1785
[7] Greenberg M, ed. Greenberg's Handbook of Neurosurgery. 10th ed. New York: Thieme; 2023:1772
[8] Greenberg M, ed. Greenberg's Handbook of Neurosurgery. 10th ed. New York: Thieme; 2023:1776
[9] Greenberg M, ed. Greenberg's Handbook of Neurosurgery. 10th ed. New York: Thieme; 2023:1778
[10] Greenberg M, ed. Greenberg's Handbook of Neurosurgery. 10th ed. New York: Thieme; 2023:1779
[11] Greenberg M, ed. Greenberg's Handbook of Neurosurgery. 10th ed. New York: Thieme; 2023:1783
[12] Greenberg M, ed. Greenberg's Handbook of Neurosurgery. 10th ed. New York: Thieme; 2023:1787

109 Spine—Thoracic and Lumbar

Questions

▸▸ Question 1

For anterior access to midthoracic spine, why left-sided approach may be preferred?

- A. Heart does not impede access
- B. Mediastinum does not block access
- C. Brachiocephalic vein does not interfere with exposure
- D. It is easier to mobilize aorta
- E. It is easier to mobilize vena cava

▸▸ Question 2

Screws for smaller pedicles (usually T1–T4, especially in females) usually require the smallest screw diameter—typically 4.5 mm. What is the typical length?

- A. 5 to 10 mm
- B. 10 to 15 mm
- C. 20 to 25 mm
- D. 30 to 35 mm
- E. 45 to 50 mm

▸▸ Question 3

Which of the following is not an advantage of anatomic ("freehand") thoracic pedicle screw placement technique?

- A. Accuracy as good as or better than other techniques
- B. Avoids the challenges of getting fluoro aligned for each level in a scoliotic spine, especially when a rotational component is present
- C. Releases joints which facilitates reduction of scoliosis
- D. Can be used if anatomy is distorted by previous fusions or congenital anomalies
- E. Not impeded in areas that are difficult to image on fluoroscopy

▸▸ Question 4

In freehand thoracic pedicle screw placement technique, pedicle breach rates are highest between which levels?

- A. T1 and T3
- B. T2 and T4
- C. T4 and T6
- D. T6 and T8
- E. T10 and T12

▸▸ Question 5

For anterior lumbar interbody fusion (ALIF), what is the usual incision?

- A. Costotransversectomy
- B. Anterolateral
- C. Trans-sternal
- D. Grid iron
- E. Pfannenstiel's

▸▸ Question 6

What is the medial angle for lumbar pedicle screw at L1?

- A. 5 degrees medially
- B. 10 degrees medially
- C. 15 degrees medially
- D. 20 degrees medially
- E. 25 degrees medially

▸▸ Question 7

According to Gertzbein classification of pedicle screw medial breach, a breach distance of > 4 mm is what grade?

- A. 0
- B. 1
- C. 2
- D. 3
- E. 4
- F. 5

▸▸ Question 8

What should be the diameter of lumbosacral pedicle screws in adult lumbar spine?

- A. ≥ 2 mm
- B. ≥ 3 mm
- C. ≥ 4 mm
- D. ≥ 5 mm
- E. ≥ 6 mm

▸▸ Question 9

Approach for upper thoracic spine or for cervicothoracic junction is through sternal splitting procedure which can give access up to T3 or from T5 level. For mid or lower thoracic levels, transthoracic or retropleural approach is used. Which of the following is the most appropriate statement about advantages of right-sided thoracotomy over left-sided thoracotomy?

- A. The heart, mediastinum, or brachiocephalic vein do not impede access through right-sided approach
- B. It is easier to make position on the right side as compared to the left side
- C. Aorta is easier to mobilize and retract than vena cava on the right side
- D. There is no impedance of inflow of blood into the heart while using right-sided approach
- E. None of the above

▸▸ Question 10

Which of the following are the options for thoracic screws placement?

- A. By using intraoperative fluoroscopy
- B. Using anatomic (free hand) thoracic pedicle screw placement method based on anatomic landmarks
- C. Performing small laminotomies and assessing position of the pedicle either by visualization or by palpating medial and superior aspects of pedicles using a dissector
- D. By using image guidance that is fitted with instruments with specialized markers that are tracked in real time by cameras that project the drill or screw location on CT or on X-ray
- E. All of the above

▸▸ Question 11

What is the uniform entry point for free hand pedicle screw placement?

- A. 1 mm inferior to the junction of the lateral edge of the superior facet and the transverse process
- B. 3 mm inferior to the junction of the lateral edge of the superior facet and the transverse process
- C. 4 mm inferior to the junction of the lateral edge of the superior facet and the transverse process
- D. 5 mm inferior to the junction of the lateral edge of the superior facet and the transverse process
- E. 7 mm inferior to the junction of the lateral edge of the superior facet and the transverse process

▸▸ Question 12

Which of the following statements is correct regarding entry points and direction of screw placement in pedicles?

- A. Entry point in the T1, T2, T3, and T12 is even with the middle of the transverse process
- B. Entry point in the T7, T8, and T9 is even with the top of the transverse process
- C. For levels T4, T5, and T6, the entry point gradually move slightly superiorly at each level from mid transverse process at T3 to the top of the transverse process at T7
- D. The mediolateral trajectory is slightly lateral (−5 degree) at T12; at T11 it is 0 degree; from here upward it increases medially at 2 degrees per level up to T1 where it is 27 degrees medially
- E. All of the above

▸▸ Question 13

What is the typical thoracic screw length?

- A. 30 to 35 mm
- B. 35 to 40 mm
- C. 40 to 45 mm
- D. 45 to 50 mm
- E. 50 to 55 mm

▸▸ Question 14

Entry point in the lumbar spine for screws is at the base of transverse process at the intersection of the center of the transverse process and the lateral aspect of superior facet. Which of the following statements is correct regarding medial angle of the pedicle screws?

- A. At L1 it is 5 degrees medially
- B. At L2 it is 10 degrees medially
- C. At L3 it is 15 degrees medially
- D. At L4 it is 20 degrees medially
- E. At L5 and S1 it is 25 degrees medially
- F. At S2 it is 40 to 45 degrees laterally
- G. All of the above

▸▸ Question 15

What is the recommended titanium rod diameter for lumbar pedicle screw fixation?

- A. 4.5 mm
- B. 5.5 mm
- C. 6.5 mm
- D. 7.5 mm
- E. 3.5 mm

▸▸ Question 16

What is the use of postoperative X-rays after fixation and fusion?

- A. To see alignment
- B. Position of graft is used
- C. Integrity of hardware
- D. Lucencies around screws which may indicate motion and implies nonunion
- E. All of the above

▸▸ Question 17

What is the postoperative care for PLIF or TLIF or ALIF?

- A. For single-level lumbar LLIF, the patient is mobilized in the immediate postoperative period without a brace
- B. Hip flexion pain on the approach side is anticipated during the immediate postoperative period
- C. Transient hip flexion weakness related to psoas muscle manipulation is usually self-limited and improves by 8 weeks postoperatively
- D. In case of significant leg weakness, a lumbar CT or MRI is indicated to rule out compression by a psoas hematoma
- E. All of the above

▸▸ Question 18

Which of the following is incorrect regarding Gertzbein classification of pedicle screw medial breach?

- A. Grade 0 is no breach

- B. Grade 1 is breach of less than 2 mm
- C. Grade 2 is breach of 2 to 4 mm
- D. Grade 3 is breach of more than 4 mm
- E. Grade 4 is breach of more than 6 mm

Answers

▸▸ Answer 1

Correct answer is D. It is easier to mobilize aorta[1]

▸▸ Answer 2

Correct answer is C. 20 to 25 mm[2]

▸▸ Answer 3

Correct answer is D. Can be used if anatomy is distorted by previous fusions or congenital anomalies[3]

▸▸ Answer 4

Correct answer is C. T4 and T6[3]

▸▸ Answer 5

Correct answer is E. Pfannenstiel's[4]

▸▸ Answer 6

Correct answer is A. 5 degrees medially[5]

▸▸ Answer 7

Correct answer is D. 3[6]

▸▸ Answer 8

Correct answer is D. ≥ 5 mm[7]

▸▸ Answer 9

Correct answer is A. The heart, mediastinum, or brachiocephalic vein do not impede access through right-sided approach[1]

▸▸ Answer 10

Correct answer is E. All of the above[8]

▸▸ Answer 11

Correct answer is B. 3 mm inferior to the junction of the lateral edge of the superior facet and the transverse process[4]

▸▸ Answer 12

Correct answer is E. All of the above[4]

▸▸ Answer 13

Correct answer is B. 35 to 40 mm[4]

▸▸ Answer 14

Correct answer is G. All of the above[5]

▸▸ Answer 15

Correct answer is B. 5.5 mm[6]

▸▸ Answer 16

Correct answer is E. All of the above[9]

▸▸ Answer 17

Correct answer is E. All of the above[10]

▸▸ Answer 18

Correct answer is E. Grade 4 is breach of more than 6 mm[6]

References

[1] Greenberg M, ed. Greenberg's Handbook of Neurosurgery. 10th ed. New York: Thieme; 2023:1790

[2] Greenberg M, ed. Greenberg's Handbook of Neurosurgery. 10th ed. New York: Thieme; 2023:1792

[3] Greenberg M, ed. Greenberg's Handbook of Neurosurgery. 10th ed. New York: Thieme; 2023:1793

[4] Greenberg M, ed. Greenberg's Handbook of Neurosurgery. 10th ed. New York: Thieme; 2023:1795

[5] Greenberg M, ed. Greenberg's Handbook of Neurosurgery. 10th ed. New York: Thieme; 2023:1797

[6] Greenberg M, ed. Greenberg's Handbook of Neurosurgery. 10th ed. New York: Thieme; 2023:1799

[7] Greenberg M, ed. Greenberg's Handbook of Neurosurgery. 10th ed. New York: Thieme; 2023:1796

[8] Greenberg M, ed. Greenberg's Handbook of Neurosurgery. 10th ed. New York: Thieme; 2023:1791

[9] Greenberg M, ed. Greenberg's Handbook of Neurosurgery. 10th ed. New York: Thieme; 2023:1809

[10] Greenberg M, ed. Greenberg's Handbook of Neurosurgery. 10th ed. New York: Thieme; 2023:1804

110 Miscellaneous Surgical Procedures

Questions

▸▸ **Question 1**

What should be the size of spinal needle for percutaneous ventricular tap in adults?
- A. 14 to 16 Ga
- B. 16 to 18 Ga
- C. 18 to 20 Ga
- D. 20 to 22 Ga
- E. 22 to 24 Ga

▸▸ **Question 2**

To drain subdural collections and to obtain fluid for diagnostic tests such as culture, repeat taps may be used, but surgery should be considered after how many taps?
- A. 2 to 3 taps
- B. 3 to 4 taps
- C. 4 to 5 taps
- D. 5 to 6 taps
- E. 6 to 7 taps

▸▸ **Question 3**

Which of following is not considered a contraindication of lumbar puncture?
- A. Risk of tonsillar herniation
- B. Platelet count > $50,000/mm^3$
- C. Suspected aneurysmal SAH
- D. Infection at puncture site
- E. Complete spinal block

▸▸ **Question 4**

For estimating true total CSF protein content with a traumatic tap, what is the correction applied?
- A. Subtract 1 mg/100 mL of protein for every 1,000 RBC/mm^3
- B. Subtract 10 mg/100 mL of protein for every 1,000 RBC/mm^3
- C. Subtract 1 mg/100 mL of protein for every 500 RBC/mm^3
- D. Subtract 1 mg/100 mL of protein for every 700 RBC/mm^3
- E. Subtract 10 mg/100 mL of protein for every 100 RBC/mm^3

▸▸ **Question 5**

What is the mortality risk for delaying treatment of acute bacterial meningitis?
- A. Increase by 10% per hour
- B. Increase by 11% per hour
- C. Increase by 12% per hour
- D. Increase by 13% per hour
- E. Increase by 15% per hour

▸▸ **Question 6**

Which of the following factors are found not to affect the incidence of post LP H/A?
- A. Age of the patient
- B. Pregnancy
- C. Volume of fluid removed during LP
- D. Prior history of headache
- E. Needle size

▸▸ **Question 7**

What should be the trajectory for insertion of ventricular catheter from Kocher's point?
- A. Toward nasion
- B. Toward ipsilateral medial canthus in coronal plane
- C. Toward contralateral medial canthus in coronal plane
- D. Toward ipsilateral medial canthus in AP plane
- E. Toward EAM in coronal plane

▸▸ **Question 8**

What should be the length of ventricular catheter inserted from Frazier burr hole with stylet initially?
- A. 3 cm
- B. 4 cm
- C. 5 cm
- D. 6 cm
- E. 7 cm

▸▸ **Question 9**

Tip of VA catheter in children should be advanced up to which level?
- A. T4
- B. T5
- C. T6
- D. T8
- E. T10

▸▸ **Question 10**

All of following are considered locations for making an opening in the floor of the third ventricle during ETV except?
- A. In the midline
- B. In the region of the tuber cinereum
- C. Anterior to the infundibular recess
- D. Anterior to the mammillary bodies
- E. Anterior to the tip of the basilar artery

▸▸ **Question 11**

During sural nerve biopsy, sural nerve is differentiated by which point from lesser saphenous vein?

- A. Nerve has many branches at right angle
- B. Vein has branches at right angle
- C. Nerve lies superficial and posterior to vein
- D. Vein has branches at acute angle
- E. None of the above

▸▸ Question 12

What is the actual cable tension for titanium alloy cables for spine fusion?
- A. 20 lbs
- B. 30 lbs
- C. 40 lbs
- D. 60 lbs
- E. Depends on quality of bone

▸▸ Question 13

Following are the contraindications of lumbar puncture except?
- A. Risk of tonsillar herniation (known or suspected intracranial mass or noncommunicating hydrocephalus)
- B. Infection in the region desired of lumbar puncture
- C. Coagulopathy
- D. Can be used without any hazard in suspected SAH
- E. Caution in patients with complete spinal block

▸▸ Question 14

The intercristal line passes through (in most adults) which of the following?
- A. At L4 spinous process
- B. Between L4 and L5 spinous processes
- C. Between L3 and L4 spinous processes
- D. At L5 spinous process
- E. Both A and B

▸▸ Question 15

What is the desirable spinal needle size for diagnostic purpose?
- A. 16 G
- B. 18 G
- C. 20 G
- D. 22 G
- E. 24 G

▸▸ Question 16

What is the normal opening pressure in the left lateral decubitus position during performing an LP?
- A. 12.2 ± 3.4 cm H_2O
- B. 14.2 ± 3.4 cm H_2O
- C. 11 cm H_2O
- D. 9 cm H_2O
- E. 17 cm H_2O

▸▸ Question 17

In case of traumatic tap, how can we get WBC count that is other than peripheral blood in a nonanemic patient?
- A. By subtracting 1 WBC for every 500 RBC
- B. By subtracting 1 WBC for every 700 RBC
- C. By subtracting 1 WBC for every 100 RBC
- D. By subtracting 1 WBC for every 1000 RBC
- E. By subtracting 1 WBC for every 1200 RBC

▸▸ Question 18

Which of the following are the differentiating points between traumatic tap and subarachnoid hemorrhage on LP?
- A. RBC count is less than 2,000/mm cube in traumatic tap while in case of SAH it is usually more than 1,00,000 RBC/mm cube
- B. Clearing of RBCs from the first tube to the last tube declines as CSF drains in case of traumatic tap, while in case of SAH, it changes little as CSF drains
- C. Ratio of WBC to RBC is similar to ratio in peripheral blood in case of traumatic tap, while it usually promotes leukocytosis in case of SAH
- D. Supernatant in case of traumatic tap is clear, while it is xanthochromic in case of SAH
- E. All of the above

▸▸ Question 19

Which of the following are the treatment options for headache after LP?
- A. Flat in bed for at least 24 hours
- B. Hydration per oral or IV
- C. Analgesics for headache
- D. Tight abdominal binder
- E. Deoxycortisone acetate 5 mg IM every 88 hours
- F. Caffeine sodium benzoate 500 mg in 2 mL IV every 8 hours up to 3 days max
- G. High-dose steroids
- H. Blood patch if refractory
- I. All of the above

▸▸ Question 20

Which of the following are the indications of lumbar catheter CSF drainage?
- A. To reduce CSF pressure at the site of CSF leak (e.g., dural breach during spine surgery or for spontaneous CSF fistula)
- B. To reduce intracranial pressure in case of communicating hydrocephalus
- C. To reduce CSF pressure to attempt to increase perfusion of the spinal cord, for example, during surgery for aortic abdominal aneurysms
- D. All of the above

▸▸ **Question 21**

Which of the following are the indications of ventricular catheterization?

- A. Intracranial pressure measurement
- B. Temporary CSF diversion in case of hydrocephalus when definite shunting is not immediately indicated or practical
- C. For management of infected shunt occasionally in case of meningitis when repeated LPs or a lumbar drain is not suitable
- D. For intrathecal drug administration
- E. All of the above

▸▸ **Question 22**

What are the VP shunt postoperative orders?

- A. Flat in bed to avoid overshunting and possible postoperative hematoma, with gradual mobilization
- B. If peritoneal end is new or revised, do not feed until bowel sound resumes
- C. Shunt series X-rays for future comparison
- D. All of the above

Answers

▸▸ **Answer 1**

Correct answer is B. 16 to 18 Ga[1]

▸▸ **Answer 2**

Correct answer is D. 5 to 6 taps[1]

▸▸ **Answer 3**

Correct answer is B. Platelet count > 50,000/mm^3[1]

▸▸ **Answer 4**

Correct answer is A. Subtract 1 mg/100 mL of protein for every 1,000 RBC/mm^3[2]

▸▸ **Answer 5**

Correct answer is D. Increase by 13% per hour[3]

▸▸ **Answer 6**

Correct answer is C. Volume of fluid removed during LP[4]

▸▸ **Answer 7**

Correct answer is B. Toward ipsilateral medial canthus in coronal plane[5]

▸▸ **Answer 8**

Correct answer is D. 6 cm[6]

▸▸ **Answer 9**

Correct answer is E. T10[7]

▸▸ **Answer 10**

Correct answer is C. Anterior to the infundibular recess[8]

▸▸ **Answer 11**

Correct answer is B. Vein has branches at right angle[9]

▸▸ **Answer 12**

Correct answer is E. Depends on quality of bone[10]

▸▸ **Answer 13**

Correct answer is D. Can be used without any hazard in suspected SAH[11]

▸▸ **Answer 14**

Correct answer is E. Both A and B[11]

▸▸ **Answer 15**

Correct answer is C. 20 G[11]

▸▸ **Answer 16**

Correct answer is A. 12.2 ± 3.4 cm H_2O[2]

▸▸ **Answer 17**

Correct answer is B. By subtracting 1 WBC for every 700 RBC[12]

▸▸ **Answer 18**

Correct answer is E. All of the above[12]

▸▸ **Answer 19**

Correct answer is I. All of the above[13]

▸▸ **Answer 20**

Correct answer is D. All of the above[14]

▸▸ **Answer 21**

Correct answer is E. All of the above[5]

▸▸ **Answer 22**

Correct answer is D. All of the above[15]

References

[1] Greenberg M, ed. Greenberg's Handbook of Neurosurgery. 10th ed. New York: Thieme; 2023:1811
[2] Greenberg M, ed. Greenberg's Handbook of Neurosurgery. 10th ed. New York: Thieme; 2023:1813
[3] Greenberg M, ed. Greenberg's Handbook of Neurosurgery. 10th ed. New York: Thieme; 2023:1815
[4] Greenberg M, ed. Greenberg's Handbook of Neurosurgery. 10th ed. New York: Thieme; 2023:1816
[5] Greenberg M, ed. Greenberg's Handbook of Neurosurgery. 10th ed. New York: Thieme; 2023:1821
[6] Greenberg M, ed. Greenberg's Handbook of Neurosurgery. 10th ed. New York: Thieme; 2023:1822
[7] Greenberg M, ed. Greenberg's Handbook of Neurosurgery. 10th ed. New York: Thieme; 2023:1828
[8] Greenberg M, ed. Greenberg's Handbook of Neurosurgery. 10th ed. New York: Thieme; 2023:1829
[9] Greenberg M, ed. Greenberg's Handbook of Neurosurgery. 10th ed. New York: Thieme; 2023:1833
[10] Greenberg M, ed. Greenberg's Handbook of Neurosurgery. 10th ed. New York: Thieme; 2023:1835
[11] Greenberg M, ed. Greenberg's Handbook of Neurosurgery. 10th ed. New York: Thieme; 2023:1812
[12] Greenberg M, ed. Greenberg's Handbook of Neurosurgery. 10th ed. New York: Thieme; 2023:1814
[13] Greenberg M, ed. Greenberg's Handbook of Neurosurgery. 10th ed. New York: Thieme; 2023:1817
[14] Greenberg M, ed. Greenberg's Handbook of Neurosurgery. 10th ed. New York: Thieme; 2023:1818
[15] Greenberg M, ed. Greenberg's Handbook of Neurosurgery. 10th ed. New York: Thieme; 2023:1827

111 Functional Neurosurgery and Stereotactic Neurosurgery

Questions

▸▸ Question 1

What is the desirable level of platelets for stereotactic brain biopsy?

- A. ≥ 10,000/mL
- B. ≥ 30,000/mL
- C. ≥ 50,000/mL
- D. ≥ 1,00,000/mL
- E. ≥ 1,50,000/mL

▸▸ Question 2

Which of following is not included in indications of deep brain stimulation?

- A. Movement disorders
- B. Obesity
- C. Hypotension
- D. Epilepsy
- E. Drug addiction

▸▸ Question 3

If tremor is predominant symptom of Parkinson's disease, then what should be the target of stimulation?

- A. Ventralis intermedius nucleus of the thalamus
- B. Pedunculopontine nucleus
- C. Subthalamic nucleus
- D. Anterior limb of internal capsule
- E. Globus pallidus

▸▸ Question 4

Immediately after DBS, anti-Parkinson drugs are continued without any change in dosage for how long?

- A. 1 month
- B. 2 months
- C. 3 months
- D. 4 months
- E. 5 months

▸▸ Question 5

In the treatment of dystonia, pallidal stimulation has best results for which of the following types of dystonia?

- A. Postanoxic dystonia
- B. Postencephalitic dystonia
- C. Primary dystonia
- D. Perinatal dystonia
- E. Poststroke dystonias

▸▸ Question 6

Local injection of botulinum toxin works for which of the following types of torticollis?

- A. Retrocollis
- B. Anterocollis
- C. Lateral collis
- D. Extrapyramidal torticollis
- E. Horizontal type

▸▸ Question 7

A patient had H/O spinal trauma 3 months ago. Now the patient has increased tone in limbs but could move limbs passively with ease. According to Ashworth score of spasticity grading, what would be the grade?

- A. 1
- B. 2
- C. 3
- D. 4
- E. 5

▸▸ Question 8

What are the selection criteria for baclofen pump?

- A. Age < 18 years
- B. Not able to give informed consent
- C. Moderate new-onset spasticity
- D. Spasticity responsive to oral baclofen
- E. No CSF block

▸▸ Question 9

What is the maximum dose of dantrolene recommended for spasticity?

- A. 25 mg/d
- B. 25 mg BID
- C. 50 mg BID
- D. 100 mg TID
- E. 100 mg QID

▸▸ Question 10

Which of the following is not an ideal candidate for dorsal rhizotomy?

- A. Most often used in children > 2 years of age
- B. Some surgeons reserve SDR for patients who have failed IT baclofen
- C. Mild-to-moderate LE weakness with the ability to walk or maintain antigravity posture
- D. Spasticity hampers gait and/or development of motor skills
- E. Arms worse than legs

▸▸ Question 11

What is the only movement disorder which persists in sleep?

- A. Tourette's syndrome
- B. Parkinson's tremors
- C. Palatal myoclonus
- D. Essential tremors
- E. None of the above

▸▸ Question 12

In trigeminal neuralgia, if immediate relief of pain is required, which procedure should not be used due to its latency?

- A. Radiofrequency rhizotomy
- B. Stereotactic radiosurgery
- C. Balloon compression
- D. Glycerol injection
- E. MVD

▸▸ Question 13

Once stimulation is achieved during RFR, how should lesioning be done?

- A. 30 to 40°C × 90 sec
- B. 60 to 70°C × 90 sec
- C. 70 to 80°C × 90 sec
- D. 80 to 90°C × 90 sec
- E. 20 to 30°C × 90 sec

▸▸ Question 14

Functional neurosurgery (FN) involves the use of electrical stimulation, ablative therapy, or therapeutic infusions to mask or relieve symptoms of aberrant neurophysiology. FN may be used in the treatment of which of the following?

- A. Movement disorders
- B. Microvascular compression syndromes
- C. Autonomic dysfunction or psychiatric disease
- D. Pain or epilepsy
- E. All of the above

▸▸ Question 15

Following are the indications of stereotactic surgery except?

- A. Biopsy for deeply located cerebral lesions or brain stem lesions or for multiple lesions
- B. Catheter placement for drainage of deep lesions or for indwelling catheter placement for intratumoral chemotherapy
- C. Electrode placement for epilepsy or for deep brain stimulation
- D. Lesion generation for movement disorder or for treatment of chronic pain
- E. It cannot be used for evacuation of intracerebral hemorrhage
- F. Stereotactic radiosurgery or for localization of lesion for open craniotomy

▸▸ Question 16

What is the most frequent complication of stereotactic radiosurgery?

- A. Seizure
- B. Hemorrhage
- C. Headache
- D. Memory impairment
- E. Hearing impairment

▸▸ Question 17

Deep brain stimulation (DBS) is the use of electrical stimulation through surgically implanted electrodes to produce neuromodulation of electrical signals for the purpose of symptom improvement. The conditions that may be treated using DBS include which of the following?

- A. Movement disorders like parkinsonism or dystonia
- B. Epilepsy
- C. Pain
- D. Potential uses include psychiatric disorders, obesity, or drug addiction
- E. All of the above

▸▸ Question 18

An early treatment for Parkinson's disease was ligation of anterior choroidal artery. Pallidotomy of which area of thalamus is most effective in diminishing tremors?

- A. Anterolateral thalamus
- B. Ventrolateral thalamus
- C. Anterodorsal thalamus
- D. Anteromedial thalamus
- E. Mediolateral thalamus

▸▸ Question 19

Anterodorsal pallidotomy became an accepted procedure in the long-term improvement of rigidity while tremors and bradykinesia did not improve with it. What are the other areas that can be targeted in the treatment of Parkinson's disease?

- A. Globus pallidus pars interna
- B. Ventral intermediate nucleus of thalamus
- C. Ventrolateral thalamus
- D. Ventralis intermediate nucleus of thalamus
- E. All of the above

▸▸ Question 20

Following are the indications for surgical treatment of Parkinson disease except?

- A. Patients refractory to medical treatment
- B. Patients with significant dementia
- C. Primary indication is patients with levodopa-induced dyskinesias
- D. Gait and postural instability
- E. Patients primarily with rigidity and bradykinesia (unilateral or bilateral), on-off fluctuations, or dystonia

►► Question 21

Which of the following are the contraindications of surgical treatment of Parkinson's disease?
- A. Patients with significant dementia
- B. Patients at risk of intracerebral hemorrhage
- C. Patients with ipsilateral hemianopsia
- D. Age more than or equal to 85 years
- E. Patients with secondary parkinsonism
- F. Patients with normal dopamine transport scan which may rule out PD as the cause of tremors
- G. All of the above

►► Question 22

Significant improvement of levodopa-induced dyskinesias occurred in 90% cases after surgical treatment for Parkinson's disease, rigidity improved in 75% cases while tremors improved in 57% of cases. What is the percentage of improvement of bradykinesia after surgical treatment?
- A. 70%
- B. 85%
- C. 95%
- D. 60%
- E. 40%

►► Question 23

Which of the following steps are included in the deep brain stimulation technique?
- A. Medications (antitremors or antiparkinsonism) are withheld the morning of the procedure to bring out symptoms
- B. A stereotactic frame is applied under local anesthetic parallel to orbitomeatal line
- C. Radiologic target localization is done using MRI or CT of brain
- D. Awake or asleep placement of DBS electrodes is done
- E. All of the above

Answers

►► Answer 1

Correct answer is D. ≥ 100,000[1]

►► Answer 2

Correct answer is C. Hypotension[2]

►► Answer 3

Correct answer is A. Ventralis intermedius nucleus of the thalamus[3]

►► Answer 4

Correct answer is B. 2 months[3]

►► Answer 5

Correct answer is C. Primary dystonia[4]

►► Answer 6

Correct answer is A. Retrocollis[5]

►► Answer 7

Correct answer is C. 3[6]

►► Answer 8

Correct answer is E. No CSF block[7]

►► Answer 9

Correct answer is E. 100 mg QID[8]

►► Answer 10

Correct answer is E. Arms worse than legs[9]

►► Answer 11

Correct answer is C. Palatal myoclonus[10]

►► Answer 12

Correct answer is B. Stereotactic radiosurgery[11]

►► Answer 13

Correct answer is B. 60 to 70 °C × 90 sec[12]

►► Answer 14

Correct answer is E. All of the above[13]

►► Answer 15

Correct answer is E. It cannot be used for evacuation of intracerebral hemorrhage[1]

►► Answer 16

Correct answer is B. Hemorrhage[1]

►► Answer 17

Correct answer is E. All of the above[2]

►► Answer 18

Correct answer is B. Ventrolateral thalamus[2]

►► Answer 19

Correct answer is E. All of the above[3]

▸▸ Answer 20

Correct answer is B. Patients with significant dementia[3]

▸▸ Answer 21

Correct answer is G. All of the above[3]

▸▸ Answer 22

Correct answer is B. 85%[3]

▸▸ Answer 23

Correct answer is E. All of the above[4]

References

[1] Greenberg M, ed. Greenberg's Handbook of Neurosurgery. 10th ed. New York: Thieme; 2023:1839
[2] Greenberg M, ed. Greenberg's Handbook of Neurosurgery. 10th ed. New York: Thieme; 2023:1840
[3] Greenberg M, ed. Greenberg's Handbook of Neurosurgery. 10th ed. New York: Thieme; 2023:1841
[4] Greenberg M, ed. Greenberg's Handbook of Neurosurgery. 10th ed. New York: Thieme; 2023:1842
[5] Greenberg M, ed. Greenberg's Handbook of Neurosurgery. 10th ed. New York: Thieme; 2023:1844
[6] Greenberg M, ed. Greenberg's Handbook of Neurosurgery. 10th ed. New York: Thieme; 2023:1845
[7] Greenberg M, ed. Greenberg's Handbook of Neurosurgery. 10th ed. New York: Thieme; 2023:1848
[8] Greenberg M, ed. Greenberg's Handbook of Neurosurgery. 10th ed. New York: Thieme; 2023:1846
[9] Greenberg M, ed. Greenberg's Handbook of Neurosurgery. 10th ed. New York: Thieme; 2023:1851
[10] Greenberg M, ed. Greenberg's Handbook of Neurosurgery. 10th ed. New York: Thieme; 2023:1871
[11] Greenberg M, ed. Greenberg's Handbook of Neurosurgery. 10th ed. New York: Thieme; 2023:1862
[12] Greenberg M, ed. Greenberg's Handbook of Neurosurgery. 10th ed. New York: Thieme; 2023: 1847
[13] Greenberg M, ed. Greenberg's Handbook of Neurosurgery. 10th ed. New York: Thieme; 2023:1838

112 Neurovascular Compression Syndromes

Questions

▸▸ Question 1

Which of the following vessels is the main offender in disabling positional vertigo?

- A. SCA
- B. AICA
- C. PICA
- D. VA
- E. BA

▸▸ Question 2

What is the treatment of status trigeminus?

- A. IV diazepam
- B. IV epival
- C. IV carbamazepine
- D. IV phenobarbital
- E. IV levetiracetam

▸▸ Question 3

In which of the following, trigeminal neuralgia (TGN) is more common?

- A. Right side
- B. Left side
- C. Bilaterally
- D. In v1 distribution
- E. In all three divisions

▸▸ Question 4

Which of the following is best for v3 neuralgia?

- A. Radiofrequency
- B. Balloon compression
- C. Glycerol injection
- D. Motor cortex stimulation
- E. SRS

▸▸ Question 5

What is the dose of SRS used for TGN at the center of lesion?

- A. 30 to 40 Gy
- B. 40 to 50 Gy
- C. 50 to 60 Gy
- D. 60 to 70 Gy
- E. 70 to 80 Gy

▸▸ Question 6

How is percutaneous trigeminal radiofrequency rhizotomy (RFR) lesioning done?

- A. 60 to 70°C × 30 sec
- B. 60 to 70°C × 60 sec
- C. 60 to 70°C × 90 sec
- D. 70 to 90°C × 90 sec
- E. 70 to 90°C × 60 sec

▸▸ Question 7

What is the success rate of microvascular decompression (MVD) for TGN?

- A. 30 to 50%
- B. 50 to 75%
- C. 75 to 80%
- D. 80 to 90%
- E. 90 to 95%

▸▸ Question 8

Which of the following is an effective medical management for hemifacial spasm?

- A. Carbamazepine
- B. Phenytoin
- C. Botulinum toxin
- D. Baclofen
- E. Dantrolene

▸▸ Question 9

Tic convulsif is a combination of which of the following?

- A. GeN + hemifacial spasm
- B. GeN + focal UE fits
- C. Hemifacial spasm + focal UE fits
- D. GeN + status trigeminus
- E. Hemifacial spasm + glossopharyngeal neuralgia

▸▸ Question 10

Post vagal section for glossopharyngeal neuralgia, 24 hours monitoring is required for which of the following?

- A. BP
- B. Syncope
- C. Cardiovascular complications
- D. Respiratory failure
- E. Neck hematoma

▸▸ Question 11

Which of the following are neurovascular compression syndromes?

- A. Trigeminal neuralgia due to 5th cranial nerve involvement
- B. Hemifacial spasm due to 7th cranial nerve involvement
- C. Geniculate neuralgia or disabling positional vertigo due to 7th cranial nerve (nevus intermedius) or 8th cranial nerve involvement respectively

- D. Glossopharyngeal neuralgia due to 9th cranial nerve involvement
- E. All of the above

▸▸ Question 12

TGN is caused by compression on 5th nerve by which artery?

- A. Anterior inferior cerebellar artery
- B. Posterior inferior cerebellar artery
- C. Superior cerebellar artery
- D. Vertebral artery
- E. Posterior inferior cerebellar artery

▸▸ Question 13

What percentage of trigeminal neuralgia patients will ultimately fail medical therapy and require surgery?

- A. 25%
- B. 50%
- C. 75%
- D. 85%
- E. 95%

▸▸ Question 14

Which of the following is included in the medical therapy of TGN?

- A. Carbamazepine (Tegretol) 100 mg PO BID, increased by 200 mg/d up to maximum of 1,200 mg/d divided TID
- B. Oxcarbazepine (Trileptal) 300 mg PO BID, increased by 600 mg/d every week up to maximum of 2,400 mg/d
- C. Baclofen 5 mg PO TID, increase every day by 5 mg/dose up to maximum of 80 mg/d in QID
- D. Gabapentin started with 100 mg PO BID, titrate to 5 to 7 mg/kg/d (3,600 mg/d maximum)
- E. All of the above

▸▸ Question 15

Complications of percutaneous radiofrequency include all of the following except?

- A. Partial masseter weakness
- B. Oculomotor paresis (usually temporary)
- C. Bitemporal hemianopsia
- D. Reduced hearing (secondary to paresis of tensor tympani)
- E. Neuroparalytic keratitis (keratitis due to fifth nerve deficit which impairs sensation)

▸▸ Question 16

Radiofrequency rhizotomy, glycerol injection into Meckel's cave, mechanotrauma by inflation of no. 4 Fogarty catheter balloon, or injection of sterile boiling water is used to selectively destroy A delta and C fibers while preserving A alpha and beta fibers. All of these procedures come under which heading?

- A. Blocking the trigger
- B. Percutaneous trigeminal rhizotomy
- C. Intradural retrogasserian trigeminal nerve section
- D. Stereotactic radiosurgery
- E. Peripheral trigeminal nerve branch procedures to block or ablate the division involved with pain

▸▸ Question 17

For stereotactic radiosurgery, 4 to 5 mm isocenter in the trigeminal nerve root entry zone is used which is identified on MRI. What is the dose of radiation that is used for this procedure?

- A. 50 to 60 Gy
- B. 60 to 70 Gy
- C. 70 to 80 Gy
- D. 80 to 90 Gy
- E. 40 to 50 Gy

▸▸ Question 18

What is the postoperative care after percutaneous trigeminal rhizotomy?

- A. Ice pack to face on the side of procedure for 4 hours
- B. Soft diet
- C. Routine activity when alert
- D. Avoid narcotics
- E. If corneal reflex is impaired, then natural tear drops 2 to 3 drops every 2 hours is used on the affected side
- F. All of the above

▸▸ Question 19

How is dura opened during microvascular decompression for trigeminal neuralgia?

- A. Curvilinear with each end at the sinus and convexity away from the junction
- B. Inverted T shaped
- C. In x shape
- D. In y-shaped pattern
- E. Both A and B

▸▸ Question 20

Hemifacial spasm is typically caused by compression of facial nerve by which of the following?

- A. PICA
- B. SCA
- C. VA
- D. AICA
- E. MCA

Answers

►► Answer 1

Correct answer is B. AICA[1]

►► Answer 2

Correct answer is C. IV carbamazepine[1]

►► Answer 3

Correct answer is A. Right side[2]

►► Answer 4

Correct answer is A. Radiofrequency[3]

►► Answer 5

Correct answer is E. 70 to 80 Gy[4]

►► Answer 6

Correct answer is C. 60 to 70°C × 90 sec[5]

►► Answer 7

Correct answer is C. 75 to 80%[6]

►► Answer 8

Correct answer is C. Botulinum toxin[7]

►► Answer 9

Correct answer is A. GeN + hemifacial spasm[8]

►► Answer 10

Correct answer is C. Cardiovascular complications[9]

►► Answer 11

Correct answer is E. All of the above[1]

►► Answer 12

Correct answer is C. Superior cerebellar artery[1]

►► Answer 13

Correct answer is C. 75%[1]

►► Answer 14

Correct answer is E. All of the above[3]

►► Answer 15

Correct answer is C. Bitemporal hemianopsia[10]

►► Answer 16

Correct answer is B. Percutaneous trigeminal rhizotomy[3]

►► Answer 17

Correct answer is C. 70 to 80 Gy[11]

►► Answer 18

Correct answer is F. All of the above[5]

►► Answer 19

Correct answer is E. Both A and B[12]

►► Answer 20

Correct answer is D. AICA[13]

References

[1] Greenberg M, ed. Greenberg's Handbook of Neurosurgery. 10th ed. New York: Thieme; 2023:1857
[2] Greenberg M, ed. Greenberg's Handbook of Neurosurgery. 10th ed. New York: Thieme; 2023:1859
[3] Greenberg M, ed. Greenberg's Handbook of Neurosurgery. 10th ed. New York: Thieme; 2023:1861
[4] Greenberg M, ed. Greenberg's Handbook of Neurosurgery. 10th ed. New York: Thieme; 2023:1864
[5] Greenberg M, ed. Greenberg's Handbook of Neurosurgery. 10th ed. New York: Thieme; 2023:1866
[6] Greenberg M, ed. Greenberg's Handbook of Neurosurgery. 10th ed. New York: Thieme; 2023:1867
[7] Greenberg M, ed. Greenberg's Handbook of Neurosurgery. 10th ed. New York: Thieme; 2023:1871
[8] Greenberg M, ed. Greenberg's Handbook of Neurosurgery. 10th ed. New York: Thieme; 2023:1873
[9] Greenberg M, ed. Greenberg's Handbook of Neurosurgery. 10th ed. New York: Thieme; 2023:1874
[10] Greenberg M, ed. Greenberg's Handbook of Neurosurgery. 10th ed. New York: Thieme; 2023:1863
[11] Greenberg M, ed. Greenberg's Handbook of Neurosurgery. 10th ed. New York: Thieme; 2023:1865
[12] Greenberg M, ed. Greenberg's Handbook of Neurosurgery. 10th ed. New York: Thieme; 2023:1868
[13] Greenberg M, ed. Greenberg's Handbook of Neurosurgery. 10th ed. New York: Thieme; 2023:1870

113 Pain Procedures

Questions

▸▸ Question 1

For unilateral pain in head, face, neck, and upper extremity, what is the pain procedure to be done?

- A. Cingulotomy
- B. Cordotomy
- C. Commisural myelotomy
- D. Stereotactic mesencephalotomy
- E. Dorsal rhizotomy

▸▸ Question 2

The success of cordotomy is known by which of the following?

- A. Loss of pinprick sensation on the affected site
- B. Weakness of the affected side
- C. Ipsilateral Horner syndrome
- D. Muscle tetany on the affected side
- E. None of the above

▸▸ Question 3

Which of following is considered to be a relative contraindication of spinal cord stimulation?

- A. Failed back syndrome
- B. Regional pain syndrome
- C. Cancer pain
- D. Diabetic neuropathy
- E. Postherpetic neuralgia

▸▸ Question 4

For commissural myelotomy, where is laminectomy done?

- A. Single level above highest dermatome involved in pain
- B. Two levels above highest dermatome involved in pain
- C. Three levels above highest dermatome involved in pain
- D. Two levels below highest dermatome involved in pain
- E. Three levels below highest dermatome involved in pain

▸▸ Question 5

Dorsal root entry lesions are indicated for all except?

- A. Phantom pain
- B. Cancer pain
- C. Spinal cord injuries
- D. Postherpetic neuralgia
- E. Deafferentation pain

▸▸ Question 6

What is the most common complication of cordotomy?

- A. Ataxia
- B. Ipsilateral paresis
- C. Bladder dysfunction
- D. Postcordotomy dysesthesia
- E. Sleep-induced apnea

▸▸ Question 7

Which of the following are the types of pain procedures which are being used currently?

- A. Electrical stimulation (deep brain stimulation or spinal cord stimulation)
- B. Direct drug administration into the CNS (spinal, epidural, intrathecal, or intraventricular)
- C. Intracranial ablative procedures (cingulotomy, medial thalamotomy)
- D. Spinal ablative surgical procedures like cordotomy or cordectomy or commissural myelotomy
- E. Sympathectomy or peripheral nerve procedures like nerve block
- F. All of the above

▸▸ Question 8

Cordotomy is the procedure of choice for unilateral pain below C5 dermatomal level. Which of the following fibers are interrupted in this procedure?

- A. Lateral spinothalamic tract fibers
- B. Anterior spinothalamic tract fibers
- C. Posterior spinothalamic tract fibers
- D. Medial spinothalamic tract fibers
- E. All of the above

▸▸ Question 9

Following are the postcordotomy complications except?

- A. Ataxia
- B. Ipsilateral paresis
- C. Sleep-induced apnea never occurs with it
- D. Bladder dysfunction
- E. Postcordotomy dysfunction

▸▸ Question 10

In experienced hands, 94% of patients will achieve at least significant pain relief at the time of hospital discharge. This level of analgesia falls with time. At 1 year, what percentage of patients will be pain free?

- A. 80%
- B. 70%
- C. 60%
- D. 50%
- E. 40%

▸▸ Question 11

Commissural myelotomy is performed for interruption of pain fibers crossing in the anterior commissure on their way to the lateral spinothalamic tract. It is done for bilateral or midline pain primarily below the thoracic levels. What percentage of patients have complete pain relief after the operation?
- A. 50%
- B. 60%
- C. 70%
- D. 80%
- E. 90%

▸▸ Question 12

Administration of narcotics can be done in epidural space or intrathecally for pain relief. Which of the following are the advantages of CSN administration of narcotics over systemic narcotics?
- A. It causes less sedation or confusion
- B. It causes less interference with GI motility
- C. It causes less nausea and vomiting
- D. All of the above

▸▸ Question 13

Which of the following are the indications of spinal cord stimulation?
- A. Failed back surgery syndrome and complex regional pain syndrome are FDA-approved indications
- B. Diabetic neuropathy or refractory angina pectoris
- C. Postthoracotomy pain
- D. Postherpetic neuralgia or painful limb ischemia
- E. All of the above

▸▸ Question 14

Dorsal root entry zone lesions appear to be most effective in treating all of the following except?
- A. Deafferentation pain resulting from nerve root evulsion
- B. Spinal cord injuries with pain around the lowest spared dermatome
- C. Postherpetic neuralgia
- D. Generally used for cancer pain
- E. Postamputation phantom limb pain

▸▸ Question 15

Which of the following are the potential complications of spinal cord stimulation?
- A. Lead migration or lead breakage
- B. Infection
- C. Hardware malfunction or unwanted stimulation
- D. CSF leak, radicular pain, intermittent interference with cardiac pacemaker
- E. All of the above

▸▸ Question 16

Nociceptive pain syndromes are more likely to be benefitted from stimulation of which of the following?
- A. Periventricular gray matter
- B. Periaqueductal gray matter
- C. Basal ganglia region
- D. Thalamus stimulation
- E. Both A and B

Answers

▸▸ Answer 1

Correct answer is D. Stereotactic mesencephalotomy[1]

▸▸ Answer 2

Correct answer is C. Ipsilateral Horner syndrome[2]

▸▸ Answer 3

Correct answer is C. Cancer pain[3]

▸▸ Answer 4

Correct answer is C. Three levels above highest dermatome involved in pain[4]

▸▸ Answer 5

Correct answer is B. Cancer pain[5]

▸▸ Answer 6

Correct answer is A. Ataxia[6]

▸▸ Answer 7

Correct answer is F. All of the above[7]

▸▸ Answer 8

Correct answer is A. Lateral spinothalamic tract fibers[7]

▸▸ Answer 9

Correct answer is C. Sleep-induced apnea never occurs with it[6]

▸▸ Answer 10

Correct answer is C. 60%[6]

▸▸ Answer 11

Correct answer is B. 60%[6]

▸▸ Answer 12

Correct answer is D. All of the above[8]

▸▸ Answer 13

Correct answer is E. All of the above[9]

▸▸ Answer 14

Correct answer is D. Generally used for cancer pain[5]

▸▸ Answer 15

Correct answer is E. All of the above[10]

▸▸ Answer 16

Correct answer is E. Both A and B[5]

References

[1] Greenberg M, ed. Greenberg's Handbook of Neurosurgery. 10th ed. New York: Thieme; 2023:1877
[2] Greenberg M, ed. Greenberg's Handbook of Neurosurgery. 10th ed. New York: Thieme; 2023:1878–1879
[3] Greenberg M, ed. Greenberg's Handbook of Neurosurgery. 10th ed. New York: Thieme; 2023:1833
[4] Greenberg M, ed. Greenberg's Handbook of Neurosurgery. 10th ed. New York: Thieme; 2023:1880
[5] Greenberg M, ed. Greenberg's Handbook of Neurosurgery. 10th ed. New York: Thieme; 2023:1886
[6] Greenberg M, ed. Greenberg's Handbook of Neurosurgery. 10th ed. New York: Thieme; 2023:1879
[7] Greenberg M, ed. Greenberg's Handbook of Neurosurgery. 10th ed. New York: Thieme; 2023:1878
[8] Greenberg M, ed. Greenberg's Handbook of Neurosurgery. 10th ed. New York: Thieme; 2023:1881
[9] Greenberg M, ed. Greenberg's Handbook of Neurosurgery. 10th ed. New York: Thieme; 2023:1883
[10] Greenberg M, ed. Greenberg's Handbook of Neurosurgery. 10th ed. New York: Thieme; 2023:1884

114 Seizure Surgery

Questions

►► **Question 1**

Region of cortex produces interictal spikes detected on scalp or invasive EEG, magnetoencephalography (MEG), or triggered fMRI. Isolated spikes that generally do not produce clinical symptoms are called?

- A. Epileptogenic zone
- B. Ictal onset zone
- C. Symptomatogenic zone
- D. Irritative zone
- E. Functional deficit zone

►► **Question 2**

What surgical procedure is recommended for drop attacks?

- A. Hemispherectomy
- B. Amygdalohippocampectomy
- C. Callosotomy
- D. Temporal lobectomy
- E. None of the above

►► **Question 3**

Resection of 6 to 7 cm of temporal lobe on nondominant side can lead to which of the following?

- A. Partial contralateral upper quadrant homonymous hemianopsia
- B. Complete contralateral upper quadrantanopsia
- C. Partial contralateral lower quadrant homonymous hemianopsia
- D. Speech deficit
- E. Memory disturbance

►► **Question 4**

After seizure surgery, antiepileptic drugs must be continued for how long?

- A. 2 months
- B. 6 months
- C. 1 to 2 years
- D. 2 to 4 years
- E. No need

►► **Question 5**

Follow-up MRI after seizure surgery is obtained after how long?

- A. 1 month
- B. 3 months
- C. 6 months
- D. 1 year
- E. 2 years

►► **Question 6**

After seizure surgery, if there is worthwhile reduction in seizures, then what would be the class according to the modified Engel classification?

- A. Class I
- B. Class II
- C. Class III
- D. Class IV
- E. None of the above

►► **Question 7**

Which of the following is the largest group of surgical candidates among the types of seizures that are amenable to seizure surgery?

- A. Focal onset seizures of temporal origin
- B. Focal onset seizures of extratemporal origin
- C. Symptomatic generalized seizures
- D. Unilateral, multifocal epilepsy associated with infantile hemiplegia syndrome
- E. All of the above

►► **Question 8**

Noninvasive evaluation techniques for seizures include all of the following except?

- A. Video EEG monitoring
- B. CAT scan
- C. PET scan
- D. Wada test or intracarotid amytal test
- E. SPECT scan and MEG

►► **Question 9**

Which of the following are the surgical techniques of seizure surgery?

- A. Resections (resection of epileptic focus or anterior temporal lobectomy or resection of neocortical areas)
- B. Disconnections (section of corpus callosum, functional hemispherectomy)
- C. Stimulations (vagus stimulation or deep brain stimulation)
- D. All of the above

►► **Question 10**

Following are the indications of corpus callosotomy except?

- A. Frequent episodes of atonic seizures

- B. Possibly for generalized seizure disorder with unilateral hemisphere damage
- C. Patients with speech and dominant handedness in opposite hemisphere
- D. Some patients with generalized seizures without identifiable, resectable focus

▸▸ **Question 11**

Disconnection syndrome can occur with commissural resection which includes left tactile anomia, left-sided dyspraxia, pseudohemianopsia, right-sided anomia for smell, or decreased spontaneity of speech. How much time a patient usually requires to adapt to most daily activities?

- A. 2 to 3 months
- B. 8 to 9 months
- C. 1 to 2 years
- D. 3 to 4 years
- E. 6 to 7 years

▸▸ **Question 12**

Which of the following are the approaches for selective amygdalohippocampectomy?

- A. Transcortical through inferior temporal gyrus
- B. Transsylvian
- C. Subtemporal through temporal fossa approach
- D. All of the above

▸▸ **Question 13**

Risks of seizure surgery include all of the following except?

- A. Removal of essential areas of cortex
- B. Memory impairment
- C. Injury to medullary core underlying cortical resection
- D. Injury to vessels in area of resection
- E. Injury to nearby cranial nerves

▸▸ **Question 14**

Postoperative management for seizure surgery includes all of the following except?

- A. Observation in ICU for 24 hours
- B. Load appropriately with IV phenytoin or Keppra
- C. 10 mg dexamethasone IV before surgery followed by every 8 hours as necessary
- D. Antiseizure medication is not needed beyond 2 to 4 weeks
- E. Neuropsychiatric evaluation should be done after 6 to 12 months

▸▸ **Question 15**

Which of the following are included in the modified Engel and ILAE classification of seizure surgery outcome?

- A. Class 1 is seizure-free or residual auras
- B. Class 2 is rare disabling seizure (less than three complex partial seizures per year)
- C. Class 3 is worthwhile improvement
- D. Class 4 is no worthwhile seizure improvement
- E. All of the above

▸▸ **Question 16**

Following are ablative techniques other than seizure surgery except?

- A. Radiofrequency ablation
- B. MRI-guided laser interstitial thermal therapy
- C. Stereotactic radiosurgery of mesial temporal lobe
- D. Application of local block to prevent occurrence of seizures

Answers

▸▸ **Answer 1**

Correct answer is D. Irritative zone[1]

▸▸ **Answer 2**

Correct answer is C. Callosotomy[2]

▸▸ **Answer 3**

Correct answer is A. Partial contralateral upper quadrant homonymous hemianopsia[3]

▸▸ **Answer 4**

Correct answer is C. 1 to 2 years[4]

▸▸ **Answer 5**

Correct answer is B. 3 months[4]

▸▸ **Answer 6**

Correct answer is C. Class III[5]

▸▸ **Answer 7**

Correct answer is A. Focal onset seizures of temporal origin[1]

▸▸ **Answer 8**

Correct answer is D. Wada test or intracarotid amytal test[6]

▸▸ **Answer 9**

Correct answer is D. All of the above[7]

▸▸ **Answer 10**

Correct answer is C. Patients with speech and dominant handedness in opposite hemisphere[2]

▸▸ **Answer 11**

Correct answer is A. 2 to 3 months[3]

▸▸ **Answer 12**

Correct answer is D. All of the above[3]

▸▸ **Answer 13**

Correct answer is B. Memory impairment[4]

▸▸ **Answer 14**

Correct answer is D. Antiseizure medication is not needed beyond 2 to 4 weeks[4]

▸▸ **Answer 15**

Correct answer is E. All of the above[5]

▸▸ **Answer 16**

Correct answer is D. Application of local block to prevent occurrence of seizures[4]

References

[1] Greenberg M, ed. Greenberg's Handbook of Neurosurgery. 10th ed. New York: Thieme; 2023:1889
[2] Greenberg M, ed. Greenberg's Handbook of Neurosurgery. 10th ed. New York: Thieme; 2023:1892
[3] Greenberg M, ed. Greenberg's Handbook of Neurosurgery. 10th ed. New York: Thieme; 2023:1893
[4] Greenberg M, ed. Greenberg's Handbook of Neurosurgery. 10th ed. New York: Thieme; 2023:1894
[5] Greenberg M, ed. Greenberg's Handbook of Neurosurgery. 10th ed. New York: Thieme; 2023:1895
[6] Greenberg M, ed. Greenberg's Handbook of Neurosurgery. 10th ed. New York: Thieme; 2023:1890
[7] Greenberg M, ed. Greenberg's Handbook of Neurosurgery. 10th ed. New York: Thieme; 2023:1891

115 Radiation Therapy (XRT)

Questions

▸▸ Question 1

CNS tumors that are very radiosensitive includes all of the following except?
- A. Gliosarcoma
- B. Germinoma
- C. Metastatic lung cancer
- D. Lymphoma
- E. Choriocarcinoma

▸▸ Question 2

For most metastatic spine tumors treated with conventional radiation therapy (i.e., not stereotactic radiosurgery), what is the usual fractionation?
- A. 20 Gy administered over 10 fractions
- B. 30 Gy administered over 10 fractions
- C. 60 Gy administered over 10 fractions
- D. 30 Gy administered over 5 fractions
- E. 30 Gy administered over 20 fractions

▸▸ Question 3

For acute spinal cord paralysis from lymphoma, if emergency surgery is not a consideration, what is the emergency radiation that can be given in the 1st fraction?
- A. 2 Gy
- B. 3 Gy
- C. 4 Gy
- D. 6 Gy
- E. 8 Gy

▸▸ Question 4

In chronic, progressive myelopathy, what is the commonly reported radiation myelopathy type?
- A. I
- B. II
- C. III
- D. IV
- E. V

▸▸ Question 5

What is the source of particle generation PET scan?
- A. Cyclotron
- B. Tungsten
- C. Cobalt 60
- D. Cobalt 62
- E. Chromium

▸▸ Question 6

A patient presented with sudden-onset loss of consciousness. According to Virginia Radiosurgery AVM Scale, a 3 cm^3 thalamic AVM presenting with hemorrhage will be awarded how many points?
- A. 1
- B. 2
- C. 3
- D. 4
- E. 5

▸▸ Question 7

An old female patient with breast cancer presents with first-time seizures. What is the recommended dose of SRS for a 25-mm metastatic brain lesion?
- A. 10 Gy
- B. 18 Gy
- C. 24 Gy
- D. 28 Gy
- E. 30 Gy

▸▸ Question 8

A patient presented with unilateral hearing loss, tinnitus, and disequilibrium. What is the recommended single dose SRS for hearing preservation and to minimize new onset or worsening of cranial nerve deficits?
- A. 12 Gy
- B. 16 Gy
- C. 18 Gy
- D. 20 Gy
- E. 25 Gy

▸▸ Question 9

A young female presented with galactorrhea amenorrhea and visual field defects. What is the usual SRS dose for secretory pituitary tumors?
- A. 10 Gy
- B. 12 Gy
- C. 20 Gy
- D. 25 Gy
- E. 30 Gy

▸▸ Question 10

What is the rate of clinical improvement after interstitial brachytherapy?
- A. 100%
- B. 90%

- C. 75%
- D. 50%
- E. Rare chances

▸▸ Question 11

What are the four Rs of radiobiology that are referred by radiation oncologists?

- A. Repair of sublethal damage
- B. Reoxygenation of tumor cells that were hypoxic before radiotherapy
- C. Repopulation of tumor cells
- D. Redistribution of cell within the cell cycle
- E. All of the above

▸▸ Question 12

All of the following are the CNS tumors that are very radiosensitive except?

- A. Lymphoma
- B. Thyroid adenocarcinoma
- C. Germ cell tumors
- D. Metastatic small cell cancer

▸▸ Question 13

Radiation therapy is the main treatment modality for radiosensitive spinal metastasis. Even tumors that are considered radioresistant can respond to radiotherapy. What is the usual fractionated therapy for spinal tumors?

- A. 20 Gy administrated over 10 fractions
- B. 30 Gy administrated over 10 fractions
- C. 40 Gy administrated over 10 fractions
- D. 50 Gy administrated over 10 fractions
- E. 60 Gy administrated over 10 fractions

▸▸ Question 14

Following are the side effects of spinal radiation except?

- A. Radiation myelopathy
- B. Due to overlap, radiation injury to GI tract
- C. Bone marrow hyperactivity
- D. Growth retardation in children
- E. Risk of development of cavernous malformation of spinal cord

▸▸ Question 15

Small artery injury because of radiation therapy causes which phase of radiation injury?

- A. Acute phase
- B. Early delayed which starts from few weeks to 2 to 3 months following completion of radiation therapy
- C. Late delayed phase which remains from 3 months to 12 years
- D. None of the above

▸▸ Question 16

Manifestation of radiation effects includes all of the following except?

- A. Decreased cognition
- B. Radiation necrosis
- C. Injury to optic pathways or injury to hypothalamic pituitary axis
- D. Primary hyperthyroidism
- E. May induce formation of new tumor or malignant transformation or leukoencephalopathy

▸▸ Question 17

Which of the following tests can be done to differentiate radiation necrosis from recurrent tumor?

- A. MRI spectroscopy
- B. DWI
- C. Nuclear brain scan
- D. Computerized radionuclide studies including SPECT or PET
- E. All of the above

▸▸ Question 18

Which of the following are included in the treatment of radiation necrosis which may cause mass effect or otherwise toxicity?

- A. Steroids
- B. Bevacizumab
- C. Reoperation or excision
- D. Hyperbaric oxygen and anticoagulation
- E. All of the above

▸▸ Question 19

Types of radiation myelopathy include which of the following?

- A. Type 1 is mild form with mild sensory symptoms which commonly resolves within several months
- B. Type 2 is injury to anterior horn cells with lower motor neuron signs in arms or legs
- C. Type 3 is described only in experimental animals after doses larger than normal radiation. Complete cord lesion within hours occurs due to injury to blood vessels
- D. Type 4 is chronic progressive myelopathy which is commonly reported
- E. All of the above

▸▸ Question 20

Following are indications of stereotactic radiosurgery except?

- A. Vascular lesions including AVMs or cavernous malformations

- B. Tumors which include lesions less than 3 cm which can be metastasis, vestibular schwannomas, meningiomas, pituitary adenomas, or gliomas
- C. Compressive tumors of the spinal cord, brain stem, or optic structures
- D. Functional disorders like trigeminal neuralgia or intractable chronic pain, movement disorders of psychiatric disease

Answers

▸▸ **Answer 1**

Correct answer is A. Gliosarcoma[1]

▸▸ **Answer 2**

Correct answer is B. 30 Gy administered over 10 fractions[2]

▸▸ **Answer 3**

Correct answer is E. 8 Gy[2]

▸▸ **Answer 4**

Correct answer is D. IV[3]

▸▸ **Answer 5**

Correct answer is A. Cyclotron[4]

▸▸ **Answer 6**

Correct answer is C. 3[5]

▸▸ **Answer 7**

Correct answer is B. 18 Gy[6]

▸▸ **Answer 8**

Correct answer is A. 12 Gy[6]

▸▸ **Answer 9**

Correct answer is D. 25 Gy[7]

▸▸ **Answer 10**

Correct answer is E. Rare chances[8]

▸▸ **Answer 11**

Correct answer is E. All of the above[1]

▸▸ **Answer 12**

Correct answer is B. Thyroid adenocarcinoma[1]

▸▸ **Answer 13**

Correct answer is B. 30 Gy administrated over 10 fractions[2]

▸▸ **Answer 14**

Correct answer is C. Bone marrow hyperactivity[9]

▸▸ **Answer 15**

Correct answer is C. Late delayed phase which remains from 3 months to 12 years[2]

▸▸ **Answer 16**

Correct answer is D. Primary hyperthyroidism[4]

▸▸ **Answer 17**

Correct answer is E. All of the above[4]

▸▸ **Answer 18**

Correct answer is E. All of the above[10]

▸▸ **Answer 19**

Correct answer is E. All of the above[3]

▸▸ **Answer 20**

Correct answer is C. Compressive tumors of the spinal cord, brain stem, or optic structures[11]

References

[1] Greenberg M, ed. Greenberg's Handbook of Neurosurgery. 10th ed. New York: Thieme; 2023:1898
[2] Greenberg M, ed. Greenberg's Handbook of Neurosurgery. 10th ed. New York: Thieme; 2023:1899
[3] Greenberg M, ed. Greenberg's Handbook of Neurosurgery. 10th ed. New York: Thieme; 2023:1902
[4] Greenberg M, ed. Greenberg's Handbook of Neurosurgery. 10th ed. New York: Thieme; 2023:1900
[5] Greenberg M, ed. Greenberg's Handbook of Neurosurgery. 10th ed. New York: Thieme; 2023:1906
[6] Greenberg M, ed. Greenberg's Handbook of Neurosurgery. 10th ed. New York: Thieme; 2023:1908
[7] Greenberg M, ed. Greenberg's Handbook of Neurosurgery. 10th ed. New York: Thieme; 2023:1909
[8] Greenberg M, ed. Greenberg's Handbook of Neurosurgery. 10th ed. New York: Thieme; 2023:1910
[9] Greenberg M, ed. Greenberg's Handbook of Neurosurgery. 10th ed. New York: Thieme; 2023:1989
[10] Greenberg M, ed. Greenberg's Handbook of Neurosurgery. 10th ed. New York: Thieme; 2023:1901
[11] Greenberg M, ed. Greenberg's Handbook of Neurosurgery. 10th ed. New York: Thieme; 2023:1904

116 Endovascular Neurosurgery

Questions

▸▸ Question 1

What is evaluation of flow through the posterior communicating arteries by vertebral injection with simultaneous common carotid artery compression in the neck called?

- A. Allcock test
- B. Wada test
- C. Froin's
- D. Queckensdest's
- E. Widal

▸▸ Question 2

Reversal of aspirin can be achieved with which of the following?

- A. Protamine sulfate
- B. Vitamin K
- C. RBC transfusion
- D. FFPs
- E. Platelets

▸▸ Question 3

According to weight-based protocol, heparin is given as 70 units/kg followed by maintenance intravenous dose of how much (units/kg/h)?

- A. 18
- B. 22
- C. 25
- D. 28
- E. 30

▸▸ Question 4

Lidocaine overdose is reversed with which of the following given intravenously?

- A. Calcium
- B. Potassium
- C. Magnesium
- D. Albumin
- E. Lipid emulsion

▸▸ Question 5

Which aneurysm feature is a not a high risk for rupture?

- A. Irregular shape
- B. Size > 7 mm
- C. Aspect ratio > 2.7
- D. Posterior circulation
- E. 10-mm cavernous segment aneurysm

▸▸ Question 6

For chemical spasmolysis to treat vasospasm, what is the drug of first choice?

- A. Verapamil
- B. Nimodipine
- C. Beta blockers
- D. Steroids
- E. Alpha blockers

▸▸ Question 7

Which of the following is the hallmark for aggressive dural arteriovenous fistula (DAVF)?

- A. Cortical venous reflux
- B. Intracerebral hemorrhage
- C. Focal neurological deficit
- D. Increased intraocular pressure
- E. Audible bruit

▸▸ Question 8

The method of choice for carotid-cavernous fistula (CCF) is transarterial embolization with which of the following?

- A. Coil
- B. Clip
- C. Onyx
- D. NCBA
- E. PVA

▸▸ Question 9

Which of the following is not included in the 5 Ds of vertebrobasilar insufficiency?

- A. Diplopia
- B. Dysarthria
- C. Defective vision
- D. Drop attacks
- E. Diastematomyelia

▸▸ Question 10

Which of the following statements regarding risk of cerebral angiography is incorrect?

- A. Arterial dissection can occur because of it
- B. Perforation of artery or aneurysm can occur during the procedure
- C. Air embolism is the most common complication of cerebral angiography
- D. Cerebral angiography can also cause embolic thrombus
- E. There can also be puncture site complications like hematoma formation or embolism distal to puncture site

▸▸ **Question 11**

Indications and case selection of aspirin include diagnostic cerebral angiography, coil embolization of aneurysms, stent complications, balloon test occlusion, or therapeutic occlusion of large arteries. What is the maximum dose of aspirin that is used in 1 day?

- A. 275 mg
- B. 300 mg
- C. 325 mg
- D. 350 mg
- E. 375 mg

▸▸ **Question 12**

Daily dose of clopidogrel is 75 mg. Following are the indications of clopidogrel use except?

- A. Coil embolization of wide neck cerebral aneurysms where stent will be used
- B. Stent implantation
- C. Therapeutic occlusion of large arteries
- D. Parent artery coil prolapse or herniation
- E. Thrombus or clot on coil phenomena
- F. All of the above

▸▸ **Question 13**

Heparin is used in embolization of brain AVM or dural AVF, cervical or intracranial angioplasty, intra- or extracranial stent implantation, or balloon test occlusion of carotid, vertebral, or other large cerebral arteries. Which of the following is used for reversal of heparin?

- A. FFPs
- B. Warfarin
- C. Protamine sulfate
- D. Steroids
- E. Analgesics

▸▸ **Question 14**

All of the following are included in the exclusion criteria of tissue plasminogen activator except?

- A. History of previous intracranial hemorrhage
- B. Recent intracranial or intraspinal surgery
- C. Diagnosis of ischemic stroke with onset of symptoms in less than or equal to 3 hours
- D. Intracranial neoplasm, AVM, or aneurysm
- E. Active internal bleeding or elevated blood pressure

▸▸ **Question 15**

What is the intravenous dose of tissue plasminogen activator?

- A. 0.7 mg/kg
- B. 0.9 mg/kg
- C. 1.1 mg/kg
- D. 1.3 mg/kg
- E. 1.5 mg/kg

▸▸ **Question 16**

Which of the following is used for reversal of tissue plasminogen?

- A. Cryoprecipitate
- B. Tranexamic acid
- C. Protamine sulfate
- D. FFPs
- E. All of the above

▸▸ **Question 17**

Which of the following are the factors that affect the selection of aneurysm for treatment?

- A. Ruptured or unruptured aneurysms (ruptured aneurysms need to be treated urgently)
- B. Symptoms other than rupture like cranial nerve palsy or loss of vision or ischemia as aneurysms causing these kind of symptoms are at increased risk of rupture
- C. Large aneurysms (size more than 7–10 mm) are more likely to rupture than small aneurysms
- D. An irregular-shaped aneurysm is at increased risk of rupture than a spherical saccular aneurysm
- E. All of the above

▸▸ **Question 18**

Which of the following are the endovascular options for treatment of neurosurgical patients?

- A. Coiling
- B. Coiling with stenting
- C. Balloon-assisted coiling
- D. Dual catheter technique
- E. All of the above

▸▸ **Question 19**

Following are the treatments of aneurysmal rupture during coiling except?

- A. Inflate balloon if balloon-assisted coiling
- B. Immediately lower blood pressure
- C. Immediately anticoagulation is given
- D. An extraventricular drainage
- E. All of the above

Answers

▸▸ **Answer 1**

Correct answer is A. Allcock test[1]

▸▸ Answer 2

Correct answer is E. Platelets[2]

▸▸ Answer 3

Correct answer is A. 18[3]

▸▸ Answer 4

Correct answer is E. Lipid emulsion[4]

▸▸ Answer 5

Correct answer is E. 10-mm cavernous segment aneurysm[5]

▸▸ Answer 6

Correct answer is A. Verapamil[6]

▸▸ Answer 7

Correct answer is A. Cortical venous reflux[7]

▸▸ Answer 8

Correct answer is A. Coil[8]

▸▸ Answer 9

Correct answer is E. Diastematomyelia[9]

▸▸ Answer 10

Correct answer is C. Air embolism is the most common complication of cerebral angiography[5]

▸▸ Answer 11

Correct answer is C. 325 mg[2]

▸▸ Answer 12

Correct answer is F. All of the above[2]

▸▸ Answer 13

Correct answer is C. Protamine sulfate[10]

▸▸ Answer 14

Correct answer is E. Active internal bleeding or elevated blood pressure[11]

▸▸ Answer 15

Correct answer is B. 0.9 mg/kg[12]

▸▸ Answer 16

Correct answer is A. Cryoprecipitate[12]

▸▸ Answer 17

Correct answer is E. All of the above[5]

▸▸ Answer 18

Correct answer is C. Balloon-assisted coiling[13]

▸▸ Answer 19

Correct answer is E. All of the above[14]

References

[1] Greenberg M, ed. Greenberg's Handbook of Neurosurgery. 10th ed. New York: Thieme; 2023:1914
[2] Greenberg M, ed. Greenberg's Handbook of Neurosurgery. 10th ed. New York: Thieme; 2023:1915
[3] Greenberg M, ed. Greenberg's Handbook of Neurosurgery. 10th ed. New York: Thieme; 2023:1916
[4] Greenberg M, ed. Greenberg's Handbook of Neurosurgery. 10th ed. New York: Thieme; 2023:1920
[5] Greenberg M, ed. Greenberg's Handbook of Neurosurgery. 10th ed. New York: Thieme; 2023:1923
[6] Greenberg M, ed. Greenberg's Handbook of Neurosurgery. 10th ed. New York: Thieme; 2023: 1925
[7] Greenberg M, ed. Greenberg's Handbook of Neurosurgery. 10th ed. New York: Thieme; 2023:1928
[8] Greenberg M, ed. Greenberg's Handbook of Neurosurgery. 10th ed. New York: Thieme; 2023:1930
[9] Greenberg M, ed. Greenberg's Handbook of Neurosurgery. 10th ed. New York: Thieme; 2023:1931
[10] Greenberg M, ed. Greenberg's Handbook of Neurosurgery. 10th ed. New York: Thieme; 2023:1917
[11] Greenberg M, ed. Greenberg's Handbook of Neurosurgery. 10th ed. New York: Thieme; 2023:1918
[12] Greenberg M, ed. Greenberg's Handbook of Neurosurgery. 10th ed. New York: Thieme; 2023:1919
[13] Greenberg M, ed. Greenberg's Handbook of Neurosurgery. 10th ed. New York: Thieme; 2023:1924
[14] Greenberg M, ed. Greenberg's Handbook of Neurosurgery. 10th ed. New York: Thieme; 2023:1925

Index

A

B

J

K

L

M

P

Q

R

S

T

U

V

W

X

Y

Z